PULMONARY PHYSIOLOGY IN CLINICAL PRACTICE

The Essentials for Patient Care and Evaluation

PULMONARY PHYSIOLOGY IN CLINICAL PRACTICE

The Essentials for Patient Care and Evaluation

LAWRENCE MARTIN, M.D., FACP, FCCP

Chief, Pulmonary Division
The Mt. Sinai Medical Center
Cleveland, Ohio

Associate Professor of Medicine
Case Western Reserve University School of Medicine

JOEL A. MICHAEL. PH.D.
DEPARTMENT OF PHYSIOLOGY
RUSH MEDICAL COLLEGE
1750 W. HARRISON STREET
CHICAGO, IL 60612

with 222 illustrations

The C. V. Mosby Company

ST. LOUIS • WASHINGTON, D.C. • TORONTO   1987

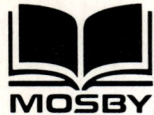

A TRADITION OF PUBLISHING EXCELLENCE

Editor: Dennis Carson
Assistant editor: Elizabeth Raven
Project editor: Patricia Gayle May
Book design: Nancy Steinmeyer
Cover design: Gail Morey Hudson
Production: Marilyn K. Wynd

Copyright © 1987 by The C.V. Mosby Company

All rights reserved. No part of this publication may be reproduced, stored in a retrieval system, or transmitted, in any form or by any means, electronic, mechanical, photocopying, recording, or otherwise, without prior written permission of the publisher.

Printed in the United States of America

The C.V. Mosby Company
11830 Westline Industrial Drive, St. Louis, Missouri 63146

Library of Congress Cataloging in Publication Data

Martin, Lawrence
 Pulmonary physiology in clinical practice.

 Includes bibliographies and index.
 1. Lungs. 2. Respiration. 3. Lungs—Diseases.
I. Title. [DNLM: 1. Lung—physiology. 2. Respiration Disorders—physiopathology. WF 600 M3806p]
QP121.M367 1987   616.2   86-18105
ISBN 0-8016-3192-0

GW/VHP/VHP 9 8 7 6 5 4 3 2 1   01/A/003

To my wife
Ruth
and my children
Joanna, **Rachel**, and **Amy**
and to my parents
Harry and **Sadie**

Preface

A generation ago, care of patients with lung disease required tools no more sophisticated than a stethoscope and chest x-ray. Blood gases, pulmonary function tests, hemodynamic monitoring, and artificial ventilation were available, but not widely utilized or understood by practicing physicians. Today, blood gas and spirometry have achieved equal footing with the ECG, blood count, and serum electrolytes as basic tools in patient care and evaluation. In addition, artificial ventilation and hemodynamic monitoring are now employed in all critical care areas.

Another major change has been the expansion of medical personnel involved in patient care and evaluation. It used to be that only the physician and nurse were involved in direct patient care. Today, respiratory patients are also likely to have contact with respiratory therapists, chest physical therapists, pulmonary technicians, and, at teaching hospitals, medical and nursing students.

It should be evident that the better anyone—nurse or doctor, therapist or student—understands pulmonary physiology, the better care he or she can give patients. Hence the need for this book. Though there are many excellent physiology texts, few explain pulmonary physiology as it relates directly to patient care and patient evaluation. This book is based on extensive experience in teaching pulmonary physiology to medical personnel, at all levels of training. This experience has shown that it is artificial to teach one type of physiology to medical students, and another to nurses, respiratory therapists, or pulmonary technicians. There is a fundamental, basic core of pulmonary physiology, and it is the same regardless of the intended audience. This basic core, as it directly relates to patient care, is the subject of this book.

Pulmonary Physiology in Clinical Practice is not a general review of pulmonary physiology, but rather covers only the essentials for clinical practice; anyone studying to care for respiratory patients should find it useful and rewarding. Several aspects of physiology covered in larger or more basic texts will not be found here. Those wishing a comprehensive or basic science review of pulmonary physiology are referred to one of the several excellent texts listed in Appendix G.

Although many students find respiratory physiology difficult to grasp at first, all agree the effort is ultimately worthwhile. In no other field of medicine is an understanding of physiology so directly relevant to patient care. Management is often closely based on blood gas values, spirometric results, hemodynamic measurements, etc. Adequate care of patients in respiratory failure, especially those receiving artificial ventilation, is simply not possible without knowledge of basic pulmonary physiology.

Included with each chapter are clinical problems to enhance your understanding; detailed answers are provided in Appendix A. It is highly recommended that you work through each problem before reviewing the answer. A summary is provided near the end of each chapter. Finally, at the end of each chapter is a list of ten true-false questions; if you can easily answer them, chances are good you understand the material.

Several additional appendices are provided to complement the chapters and provide additional information. Those readers who have access to IBM-compatible microcomputers may wish to sample computer programs we have written in the area of cardiopulmonary medicine. Information about these freely available programs can be found in Appendix H.

Lawrence Martin, M.D.
Cleveland

Acknowledgments

This book grew out of syllabus material originally written for medical students at Case Western Reserve University. I have since used chapters from the book to teach many other groups, including house staff, respiratory therapists, and nurses. Without students to teach, there would be no book, and to them I am particularly indebted. I would also like to acknowledge those many students—too numerous to list—who brought to my attention typographical or factual errors while the manuscript was in draft form.

I would like to offer a special thank you to the following people:

Jose Katz, M.D., Shaul Margaliot, M.D., and Linda Haacke, R.R.T., M.D., for their meticulous and thorough reviews; Lawrence McCastle, R.R.T., for his review of Chapter 10; Robert Martin, M.D., for his review of Chapter 10; Brian Jeffreys, R.C.P.T., for his invaluable assistance in developing computer software (listed in Appendix H); Barbara Zaremsky, for her cheerful and unstinting secretarial assistance; Nancy Heim, for her wonderful illustrations; Elizabeth Raven of The C.V. Mosby Company, for her guidance and understanding during the book's preparation; Gayle May, of The C.V. Mosby Company, for her detailed editing and cheerful handling of my numerous changes; Alan Salm, M.D., Brian Jeffreys, and Kristina Suchy, for their able photographic assistance; and Stephen Reich, M.D., for the Mencken quote used in Chapter 7. Finally, I want to thank Matthew Levy, M.D., whose recommendation of this book to the publisher started the whole project.

Contents

Introduction
    Historical perspective   1

1   Clinical approach   7
    Schema for diagnosis and management   7
    History   9
    Physical examination   10
    Chest x-ray examination   12
    Spirometry   18
    Arterial blood gas analysis   19
    Sputum examination   20
    Other tests and procedures   20
    Evaluation of dyspnea   21
    Bedside vs. laboratory   25
    Summary   25
    Review questions   26

2   Structure and function   27
    Gas properties   27
    The atmosphere   28
    Gas laws   30
    ATPS, BTPS, and STPD   31
    Gases in solution   32
    Breathing—an overview of gas exchange   33
    Lung disease and the respiratory system   41
    Summary   42
    Review questions   42

3 Lung mechanics   43

Breathing—a mechanical function   43
Pressure, volume, and flow   44
Generation of airway pressures   44
Lung compliance   46
Airway resistance   48
Lung volumes and capacities   49
Functional residual capacity   50
Forced vital capacity   52
Flow-volume curves and loops   57
Determinants of expiratory airflow   60
Small airways disease and dynamic compliance   64
Clinical value of using spirometry   65
Patterns of respiratory disease   66
Interpretation of spirometry   68
Mechanics and gas exchange—correlation?   71
Summary   73
Review questions   73

4 P_{CO_2} and alveolar ventilation   74

Ventilation—minute, alveolar, and dead space   74
P_{CO_2}—its relation to alveolar ventilation and carbon dioxide production   75
P_{CO_2} and the respiratory quotient   77
Hyperventilation and hypoventilation   78
Clinical importance of the P_{CO_2} equation   79
P_{CO_2} in the clinical setting   79
Physiologic basis for hypercapnia   80
V_D/V_T and the Bohr dead space equation   82
Dangers of hypercapnia   83
Pa_{CO_2} and need for ventilatory assistance   84
Noninvasive measurement of P_{CO_2} 85
Pa_{CO_2}—its relationship to oxygenation and acid-base balance   86
Summary   87
Review questions   87

Contents

5 Oxygen transfer — 88

Clinical questions 88
Lung oxygen transfer 88
Oxygen diffusion and diffusing capacity 90
Alveolar oxygen pressure 92
Arterial oxygen pressure 93
Alveolar-arterial oxygen pressure difference 93
Pao_2/Pao_2 and Pao_2/Fio_2 95
Causes of low Pao_2 95
Nonrespiratory causes of low Pao_2 96
Respiratory causes of low Pao_2 98
Ventilation-perfusion imbalance 98
Shunts and venous admixture 103
How V/Q imbalance reduces Pao_2 and increases $Paco_2$ 104
Low mixed venous oxygen—effect on Pao_2 106
V/Q imbalance in patients—variable effect on oxygen and carbon dioxide 107
Summary 110
Review questions 110

6 Is the patient adequately oxygenated? — 112

Clinical assessment 112
Hypoxemia vs. hypoxia 113
The oxygenation cycle 114
Sao_2 and oxygen content 115
Shifts of oxygen dissociation curve and P_{50} 116
Carbon monoxide 118
Carbon monoxide exposure and its effects 120
Methemoglobinemia and sulfhemoglobinemia 121
Causes of reduced Sao_2 122
Oxygen delivery 123
Fick equation 123
Mixed venous oxygen saturation 124
Summary 127
Review questions 127

7 Acid-base balance — 129

Hydrogen ion homeostasis   129
Concept of pH   130
Buffer systems   130
Henderson-Hasselbalch equation   131
Does the patient have an acid-base disorder?   132
Calculated vs. measured HCO_3^- 132
Acid-base nomogram   132
Acidemia and alkalemia   134
Acidosis and alkalosis   134
Anion gap   137
Primary vs. compensatory processes   137
Acid-base map   138
In vivo titration curve for carbon dioxide   139
Base excess   140
Acute vs. chronic respiratory disorders   140
Acute vs. chronic metabolic disorders   141
Mixed acid-base disorders   143
Clinical approach to acid-base diagnosis   144
Summary   144
Review questions   145

8 Pulmonary circulation — 147

Pulmonary vs. systemic circulation   147
Pulmonary hypertension and right heart failure   149
Causes of pulmonary hypertension   150
Assessment of hemodynamic status   152
Swan-Ganz catheterization   153
Insertion of Swan-Ganz catheter—pressure tracings   156
Hemodynamic measurements and calculations   158
Pulmonary artery wedge pressure—measurement   161
Pulmonary artery wedge pressure—what does it represent?   165
Pitfalls and complications in hemodynamic monitoring   170
Hemodynamic monitoring in clinical practice   171
Summary   173
Review questions   174

Contents

9 Oxygen therapy — 175

Oxygen as a drug 175
Terminology in oxygen therapy 179
When to institute oxygen therapy 179
Classification of oxygen therapy 180
Low-supplemental FIO_2 therapy 180
High-supplemental FIO_2 therapy 184
Potential harm from oxygen therapy 184
Positive airway pressure and oxygen therapy 187
Hyperbaric oxygen 187
Monitoring oxygen therapy—clinical signs and PaO_2 188
Blood transfusion—effect on PaO_2 and oxygen content 190
Artificial blood 190
Methods of home oxygen therapy 190
Indications for home oxygen therapy 193
Summary 194
Review questions 195

10 Artificial ventilation — 197

Intubation and artificial ventilation 197
Indications for artificial ventilation 200
Mode of artificial ventilation and FIO_2 201
Normal breathing vs. ventilator breathing 201
Controlled ventilation 202
Assist-control ventilation 202
Intermittent mandatory ventilation 204
Ventilator settings 206
Ventilator compliance 209
High-frequency ventilation 209
Positive end expiratory pressure 211
Continuous positive airway pressure 212
Complications of artificial ventilation 213
Ventilator weaning 215
Summary 217
Review questions 217

11 Respiratory failure — 219

Definition of respiratory failure 219
Physiologic classification of respiratory failure 220
Clinical classification of respiratory failure 220
Acute vs. chronic respiratory failure 221
Pulmonary edema 221
Shunt equation 223
Adult respiratory distress syndrome 225
Physiologic manifestations of ARDS 227
Management of ARDS 228
A case of oxygenation respiratory failure 229
Respiratory failure in chronic obstructive pulmonary disease 233
A case of combined ventilatory and oxygenation failure in COPD 234
Summary 237
Review questions 237

12 Exercise physiology — 239

Exercise physiology 239
What happens during exercise? 239
Metabolism during exercise—aerobic vs. anaerobic 240
$Paco_2$ during exercise 241
The exercise test 242
Physiologic changes during exercise 244
Normal exercise parameters 249
Clinical use of physiologic exercise testing 249
Clinical interpretation of physiologic exercise testing 250
Summary 254
Review questions 254

13 Pleural effusions — 256

Pleural fluid dynamics 261
Transudates vs. exudates 262

Contents   xvii

Diagnostic procedures   264
Determining cause of exudative effusion   266
Selected pleural fluid laboratory tests   268
Mechanism of pleural fluid acidosis   270
Use of laboratory tests in specific exudative effusions   271
Pneumothorax   275
Chest tube drainage   276
Obliteration of the pleural space   279
Pleural effusion, lung mechanics, and gas exchange   280
Summary   281
Review questions   281

14 Sleep disorders   283

The study of sleep disorders   283
Polysomnography   284
Normal sleep   286
Sleep apnea   289
Obstructive sleep apnea   292
Pickwickian syndrome   294
Ondine's curse   295
Treatment of sleep apnea   295
Cheyne-Stokes breathing   298
Summary   299
Review questions   300

15 Newborn and infant   301

Changes at birth   301
Apgar score   304
The pediatric history   305
Vital signs   306
Physical examination   309
Chest x-ray examination   312
Pulmonary function tests   313
Blood gases   314
Ventilation-perfusion imbalance   317
Oxygen therapy   317
Hemodynamic assessment   318
Sudden infant death syndrome   319

Infant respiratory distress syndrome 320
Summary 322
Review questions 323

Appendix

- **A** Answers to clinical problems 325
- **B** Normal values for FVC and FEV_1 357
- **C** Basic equations and formulas 360
- **D** Abbreviations and symbols 362
- **E** Glossary 364
- **F** Common clinical conditions 372
- **G** General references 382
- **H** Microcomputer programs 384

PULMONARY PHYSIOLOGY
IN CLINICAL PRACTICE
The Essentials for Patient Care and Evaluation

introduction
Historical perspective

Look around your hospital. Did it always have a pulmonary function laboratory? An intensive care unit? Facilities for cardiac catheterization? A computerized laboratory? If it is newly built or only a few years old, the answer is probably "yes" to all these questions. But if you work in a hospital built before 1950, the answer to all is "no." Since the end of World War II, there has been a technologic revolution in patient care. In our daily practice we use machines, prescribe drugs, and perform operations inconceivable a few decades ago.

For the most part, diseases that we treat are not new. Certain microorganisms may be newly recognized (e.g., acquired immune deficiency syndrome virus and Legionella bacterium), and some conditions may be more common than in years past (e.g., lung cancer and myocardial infarction), but the basic disease processes are the same. There have always been patients suffering from cardiac and respiratory failure, pneumonia, lung abscess, shock, and asthma. How did physicians cope with these patients 200 years ago? A century ago? Fifty, twenty, even ten years ago? The answers to these general questions provide a historical perspective, which can be defined as the viewing of our current situation in light of medical history.

There is sometimes a tendency to think that the way we care for patients is the only way, the best way, the universal way. Not so, of course. By examining how medical problems were handled in the past, we can better appreciate today's medical environment and perhaps can glimpse what practice might be like years hence. Medical care has changed radically over the generations and will surely continue to change in dramatic ways.

To illustrate how medical practice has changed, the following four cases are presented; each case is from the medical literature and is representative of "state-of-the-art" medical practice for its era.

Case I (Laennec, 1818)

A man, aged 29, caught a severe catarrh from exposure to much cold in the beginning of October, which he neglected. . . . This catarrh, after a few weeks, was followed by spitting of blood for several days and, subsequently, by a continual cough, dyspnoea, and emaciation. In the beginning of February he come into hospital. At this time he was evidently in a confirmed consumption—being affected with great emaciation, frequent cough, yellow opaque sputa, dyspnoea, diarrhea. . . . Things continued much in the same way until the 17th, when the supervention of more febrile symptoms indicated a slight peripneumony. On applying the cylinder, it was found that respiration was not at all audible on the anterior and lateral portions of the left side of the chest; while percussion gave a much distincter sound than on the right side; and succussion of the trunk produced the characteristic noise of fluctuation. From all these circumstances, being convinced of the existence of both air and pus in the cavity of the pleura, and seeing no other means of alleviating the patient, I proposed the operation of empyema. This however was not performed, as he died the same day.

This case is from one of the earliest "classics" of respiratory medicine, published in 1818, Laennec's *Treatise on the Diseases of the Chest*. In 1816 Laennec (1781-1826) invented the stethoscope (the "cylinder" in this case report). From that point onward, for about 100 years, the stethoscope was the premier tool for diagnosing chest diseases premortem. Not until the introduction of chest radiology in the early 1900's was a better tool available.

At his autopsy, this patient was found to have had tuberculous empyema, which Laennec diagnosed after careful dissection. Without antibiotics, it is unlikely that even "operation of empyema" would have helped. Of course, anesthesia was also unavailable to relieve the pain of surgery.

Laennec was a master diagnostician. He "fixed definitely the clinical picture of the disease [tuberculosis] . . . having separated it by means of auscultation and his pathological studies from all similar affections of the lungs" (Walsh, 1907). Unfortunately, like all doctors of his era, Laennec could not offer meaningful treatment for tuberculosis. The next case, from half a century later, shows a different approach to tuberculosis (phthisis pulmonalis).

Case II (Mackey, 1869)

Phthisis pulmonalis. Mrs. W.—age 31, who had lost her father and sisters of consumption, consulted me in Dec. 1867. For the last six months had had cough, for the last three had emaciated, and at this time had the prostration, night sweats, diarrhea, and hectic of the third stage of phthisis; hemoptysis had occurred several times: the expectoration was generally purulent. There were violent pains, especially over left chest, and examination revealed a fine crepitus at apex of left lung. The patient was treated with ordinary medicines, and improved gradually. Opium in the form of an atomized spray was found to be the best medicine for relieving cough, and procuring sleep; tincture of steel and carbolic acid used in the same manner relieved, to a certain extent, the profuse expectoration; and although the case became complicated with a peri-uterine haematocele, in February 1868 she rallied from this also.

It was July 1868 before she could walk as far as my house. Her principal symptoms then were debility, pains in the chest, cough, and copious muco-purulent sputum. At this point she began inhalations of oxygen in the proportion of 6 pints to 60 of air, increasing to 12 pints. She took inhalations at intervals of two days, and then found the above symptoms so relieved as to be able to omit all treatment for a time. She herself attributed great benefit to the gas, and was taking no other special medicine at the time. Since then she has borne fairly well the cares of a large family. She has gained flesh, and though there is still a frequent cough, and sputum, a mucous rale about the left apex (I examined the chest two days ago), the progress of the disease is arrested for a time at least.

Today both Laennec's and Mackey's patients would have a chest x-ray examination, which would no doubt show abnormalities. Sputum examination and culture would confirm the diagnosis, and both patients would receive antituberculous therapy. But it was only in 1882 that Robert Koch discovered the tuberculous bacillus, in 1895 that Roentgen discovered x-rays, and in the 1940's that the first successful antituberculous drug was available (streptomycin).

As for oxygen therapy, there is no reason to suppose that the intermittent inhalations this patient received were of any benefit. Oxygen was discovered in 1774 by Joseph Priestley and was employed for medical purposes shortly afterward. Nevertheless, it was not until well into the twentieth century that oxygen therapy was placed on a rational, scientific basis.

For almost the entire nineteenth century, oxygen was prescribed only for *intermittent* use. The first case report of continuous oxygen therapy was published in 1890 (Blodgett). If Dr. Mackey's patient was indeed hypoxic, oxygen delivered intermittently certainly did not help since the body does not store oxygen. Moreover, tuberculous organisms seem to favor lung regions with a high alveolar partial pressure of oxygen. After this fact became known and before the advent of antituberculous therapy, temporary pneumothorax was in vogue as a treatment for tuberculosis. An even more radical procedure was thoracoplasty, which entailed removal of part of the rib cage to permanently collapse the lung. The idea in both procedures was to make the tuberculous region of the lung airless to starve the tuberculous organisms from lack of oxygen. Although these techniques often did help, they also caused considerable morbidity; compared to modern day chemotherapy, lung collapse is primitive treatment.

Case III (Barach, 1927)

A man, aged 50, was sick with fever, cough and prostration of two weeks' duration. He was known to have had bronchiectasis for one year. On admission he was deeply cyanotic, dyspneic, and toxic. The lung signs gave evidence of bronchiectatic cavities and a diffuse bronchopneumonia. He was put in an oxygen tent with a concentration of 40 per cent of oxygen. At the end of seven days he was free from cyanosis, moderately dyspneic, very toxic and stuporous. The tent was removed. Four hours later, he was deeply cyanotic, the hands and face were both blue, he has gasping for breath, he was very restless and he was trying to get out of bed. His pulse had risen from 116 to 152 and the respiratory rate from 36 to 50. From a condition of comparative comfort he had passed into one of acute distress, restlessness and imminent collapse. He was transferred to the oxygen chamber, and in three hours after 40 per cent of oxygen had been established, his condition returned to that point before the removal of the tent.

The modern era of oxygen therapy is often said to have begun with the work of John Scott Haldane, the great English physiologist. He used oxygen therapy for victims of war gas injuries and published a brief paper in 1917 outlining the rationale for use of the gas (Haldane). Case III is from a paper on methods of oxygen treatment by Dr. Alvan Barach, another pioneer in the field. During the 1920's, Dr. Barach led in the development of oxygen tents for use in treating hypoxemic patients. Note that by this time oxygen was used on a continuous basis, a much more physiologic approach than the nineteenth century's intermittent technique.

Of interest is that no blood gas values were reported in Dr. Barach's case; even in the best hospitals, blood gas measurements were not routinely available. In fact it would take another 35 years for this test to enter the mainstream of clinical medicine. Today blood gas measurements are routine in cases of severe hypoxemia.

The first arterial puncture performed on humans was not done until 1912 by Hurter, a German physician. In 1919 arterial blood gas analysis was first used as a diagnostic procedure. Employing Hurter's radial artery puncture technique, W.C. Stadie (1919) measured oxygen saturation in patients with pneumonia and was able to show that cyanosis of critically ill patients was the result of incomplete oxygenation of hemoglobin.

Measurement of Po_2 and partial pressure of carbon dioxide (Pco_2) proved to be more difficult than measurement of oxygen saturation. It was not until the introduction of the Clark platinum electrode in 1953 that direct Po_2 measurement became routinely feasible (Clark, 1953). Later a Pco_2 electrode was developed, and by the 1960's the electrodes were commercially available.

Finally, it is of interest that Barach's patient did not receive artificial ventilation—it was also not available in 1927. Even though the oxygen tent relieved the patient's cyanosis, he remained "moderately dyspneic, very toxic and stuporous." The outcome is not reported.

Case IV (Louria, 1959)

A.Z. A 21 year old woman was admitted on Nov. 8, 1957, because of profound respiratory distress. Three days prior to admission she had developed a sore throat, myalgia, bifrontal headache, a dry cough and fever to 103° F (oral). She was seen by a physician who noted no respiratory distress or abnormalities on physical examination of the chest. The night prior to admission she developed pleuritic right chest pain, tachypnea and dyspnea. On the morning of admission her respiratory distress became increasingly severe. When seen by her physician she was markedly cyanotic and audible bubbling sounds could be heard at considerable distance from the patient.

Physical examination on admission revealed a critically ill, anxious dyspneic woman who was intensely cyanotic. Her temperature was 40.3° C., respiratory rate 60 per minute, pulse 160 per minute, and blood pressure 130/70 mm Hg. . . . Crackling inspiratory rales and harsh breath sounds were noted throughout both lung fields. Expiration was labored and appeared to be obstructed. There was evidence of consolidation of both lower lobes. . . . Initial laboratory studies showed the white blood cell count to be 2,000 cells per cu. mm. with 58 per cent lymphocytes, 8 per cent monocytes, 7 per cent polymorphonuclear cells, 9 per cent band forms, 13 per cent metamyelocytes and 5 per cent myelocytes. . . . The patient's arterial oxyhemoglobin saturation was reduced to 71.1 per cent.

Sputum was grossly bloody and contained large numbers of gram-positive cocci. Hemolytic *Staphylococcus aureus* was grown in pure culture from the sputum. This organism was sensitive to erythromycin, chloromycetin, streptomycin and novobiocin, but resistant to penicillin and the tetracyclines. The Asian strain of influenza A virus was recovered from throat washings. The admission chest roentgenogram revealed dense bilateral lower lobe infiltrates with scattered nodular densities present in the central areas of both lung fields.

The patient was given oxygen through a positive pressure oxygen mask, and administration of erythromycin, dihydrostreptomycin and chloromycetin, 2 Gm. each day, were started. Hydrocortisone, 100 mg. every 12 hours, was injected intravenously, and prednisone, 100 mg. daily, was given by mouth.

Over the first four days in the hospital the patient showed moderate improvement. Oxyhemoglobin saturation rose to 93.9 per cent with use of the IPPB mask. . . Nevertheless, signs of consolidation persisted, and she remained cyanotic and tachypneic when oxygen therapy was discontinued.

On the fifth hospital day the patient developed high tracheal obstruction which required tracheotomy and vigorous suctioning. Following this episode her condition worsened rapidly . . . A marked respiratory acidosis developed with the arterial P_{CO_2} rising to 78 mm Hg. The administration of acetazolamide, 1.0 Gm. daily, was associated with the return of arterial blood P_{CO_2} and pH to normal, but there was no improvement in the patient's clinical course. The onset of bloody diarrhea was associated with the recovery of hemolytic *Staphylococcus aureus* from stool cultures. On the sixth hospital day blood pressure fell to shock levels and the patient died.

Case IV is from a paper on the influenza pandemic of 1957-1958; by that time procedures for measuring blood gases were available in some hospitals. However, it is striking that there is no mention of artificial ventilation in this case. Today both Cases III and IV would undoubtedly receive artificial ventilation during their hospital courses.

When did artificial ventilation come about? According to Comroe (1977), artificial ventilation has been used in laboratory animals for centuries, with one report dating to 1667. By the nineteenth century, artificial ventilation was commonly employed in laboratory experiments. Despite the laboratory experience, artificial ventilation was not used when clearly indicated, such as in patients undergoing thoracic surgery in whom pneumothorax is always a major problem (pneumothorax is preventable with positive pressure insufflation of the lungs).

One factor holding back use of the technique of artificial ventilation was the use of negative pressure rooms for thoracic surgery. In 1904, the influential German surgeon Ernst Ferdinand Sauerbruch published his method of operating on a patient whose body, except for the head, was enclosed in a room kept at slightly negative air pressure; the surgeon and his assistants were also in the negative pressure room (Comroe, 1977). With this technique, the nonoperated lung stayed inflated throughout surgery, but the patient still breathed on his own (albeit under anesthesia), so there was no real artificial ventilation.

Because Sauerbruch's technique was inherently cumbersome, positive insufflation through an endotracheal tube gradually took over. This transition was aided by development of new technology, such as closed circuit anesthesia apparatus (Jackson, 1927).

Artificial ventilation outside of the operating room took a longer time to develop. Before World War II, artificial ventilators were usually negative pressure machines, with the best example being the iron lung (Drinker and Shaw, 1929; Drinker and McKhann, 1929). An iron lung surrounds the patient's body (except for the head) and alternates a negative atmospheric pressure with the ambient one, resulting in rhythmic expansion of the chest cage (and thus inhalation) in response to the negative extrathoracic pressure. During periods of ambient extrathoracic pressure, the lungs deflate. This type of machine is rarely used today (Drinker and McKhann, 1986).

A cuirass negative pressure respirator is designed to surround only a portion of the body, either the chest alone or the chest and abdomen together. For a while cuirass respirators were in vogue as an alternative to iron lungs (Collier and Affeldt, 1954). Today cuirass respirators are used occasionally for patients with neuromuscular problems who need artificial ventilation at home. Unfortunately, the cuirass respirator is often difficult to fit precisely to the patient. Also, it is not helpful in patients with significant lung or airway disease, a population for whom positive pressure ventilation is much more beneficial.

Positive pressure artificial ventilation was gradually phased in after World War II, but even by the late 1950's, positive pressure respirators were not routinely available outside the operating room. With the development throughout the 1960's of intensive care units, artificial positive pressure ventilation became a widely accepted technique. Today it is a standard therapy for respiratory failure in all hospitals.

FINAL COMMENT

The box below lists 15 major advances in medicine with emphasis on those advances that have profoundly influenced the practice of pulmonary medicine; several of the advances were touched

---

FIFTEEN GREAT ADVANCES IN MEDICINE*

1774	Discovery of oxygen (Priestley)
1816	Invention of stethoscope (Laennec)
1840	Invention of spirometry (Hutchinson)
1846	Introduction of general anesthesia (Morton, Wells, Jackson)
1882	Discovery of tuberculous bacillus (Koch)
†1895	Discovery of x-rays (Roentgen)
1897	Discovery of epinephrine (Abel, Takamine)
†1928	Discovery of penicillin (Fleming; later, Chain and Florey worked on development of the antibiotic, and all three shared in the 1945 Nobel Prize)
1929	Introduction of first workable iron lung (Drinker, Shaw, McKhann)
†1949	Introduction of corticosteroids to medicine (Hench, Kendall, Reichstein)
†1947	Introduction of antituberculous chemotherapy (Waksman)
1953	Invention of platinum P_{O_2} electrode (Clark)
†1955	Introduction of polio vaccine (Enders, Weller, Robinson; Salk and Sabin)
1966	Introduction of flexible fiberoptic bronchoscope (Ikeda)
1970	Introduction of flow-directed right heart catheter (Swan, Ganz)

*Date denotes when discovery or invention was announced, published, or introduced into clinical use, and parentheses enclose last names of the principal investigators.

†A Nobel Prize was awarded for these works (these awards began in 1901). In the case of polio vaccine, the Nobel Prize was awarded for successfully culturing the virus (Enders, Weller, Robbins) and not for implementing the vaccine (Salk, Sabin). In the case of antituberculous therapy, the Nobel Prize was awarded to Waksman for work on streptomycin; no Nobel Prize was awarded for work on isoniazid or other antituberculous drugs, which were all introduced later than streptomycin.

upon in this discussion. The advances chosen are necessarily arbitrary and are not meant to be comprehensive in any sense.

A paradox of modern medicine is that we know so much more than in years past and yet we practice in a way that often seems primitive against the forces of nature. Metastatic cancer, shock, brain hemorrhage, pneumonia in the immunocompromised patient—these and other conditions often pursue an inexorable downhill course no matter what we do. Yet consider medical practice without anesthetics, x-ray films, or antibiotics—a primitive state, no doubt. But these three advances only came to us in 1846, 1895, and the 1940's, respectively. What of medicine before then?

More to the point, what will our current practice look like 50, 100, or 150 years from now? Equally as backward as nineteenth century practice appears to us? Probably so. Barring some global catastrophe, there is no reason to doubt that our present state is anything but a transient phase in the continuing progress of medicine.

References

Barach, A.L.: Acute disturbance of lung function in pneumonia: methods of oxygen treatment, JAMA **89**:1865, 1927. Copyright 1927, American Medical Association.

Blodgett, A.N.: The continuous inhalation of oxygen in cases of pneumonia otherwise fatal and in other disease, Boston Med. Surg. J. **21**:481, 1890.

Clark, C., Wolf, R., Granger, D., et al.: Continuous recording of blood oxygen tensions by polarography, J. Appl. Physiol. **6**:189, 1953.

Collier, R., and Affeldt, J.E.: Ventilatory efficiency of the cuirass respirator in totally paralyzed chronic poliomyelitis patients, J. Appl. Physiol. **6**:531, 1954.

Comroe, J.H., Jr.: Retrospectroscope, Menlo Park, Cal., 1977, Von Gehr Press.

Drinker, P.A., and McKhann, C.F.: The iron lung. First practical means of respiratory support, JAMA **225**:1476, 1986.

Drinker, P., and McKhann, C.F.: The use of a new apparatus for the prolonged administration of artificial respiration. I. A fatal case of poliomyelitis, JAMA **92**:1658, 1929.

Drinker, P., and Shaw, L.A.: An apparatus for the prolonged administration of artificial respiration, J. Clin. Invest. **7**:229, 1929.

Haldane, J.S.: The therapeutic administration of oxygen, Br. Med. J. **1**:181, 1917.

Jackson, D.E.: A universal artificial respiration and closed anesthesia machine, J. Lab. Clin. Med. **12**:998, 1927.

Laennec, R.T.H.: A treatise on the diseases of the chest, London, 1821, T. & G. Underwood. (Translated by J. Forbes; originally published France, 1818.)

Louria, D.B., Blumenfeld, H.L., Ellis, J.T., et al.: Studies on influenza in the pandemic of 1957-58. II. Pulmonary complications of influenza, J. Clin. Invest. **38**:213, 1959.

Mackey, E.: On the therapeutical value of the inhalation of oxygen gas, Practitioner **2**:276, 1869.

Stadie, W.C.: The oxygen of the arterial and venous blood in pneumonia and its relation to cyanosis, J. Exp. Med. **30**:215, 1919.

Walsh, J.J.: Makers of modern medicine, New York, 1907, Fordham University Press.

chapter 1
Clinical approach

OUTLINE

Schema for diagnosis and management
History
Physical examination
Chest x-ray examination
Spirometry
Arterial blood gas analysis
Sputum examination
Other tests and procedures
Evaluation of dyspnea
Bedside vs. laboratory

The physiology in this book is presented from a clinical perspective—what is needed to understand and to manage respiratory patients. It is thus appropriate to begin with a chapter on the clinical approach to respiratory disease.

SCHEMA FOR DIAGNOSIS AND MANAGEMENT

A schema for diagnosing and managing respiratory disease is presented in Table 1-1. First, a data base is obtained. This information includes the patient's history, the results of a physical examination, and usually one or more tests to help make a diagnosis. Commonly ordered tests include chest x-ray, spirometry, arterial blood gas (ABG) analysis, blood count, serum electrolytes, and electrocardiogram; in addition, a variety of other procedures and examinations may be employed to complete the data base. There is enormous flexibility in obtaining this information. For example, data may be obtained within minutes, as during a cardiopulmonary arrest, or over a period of several months, as is done with many chronic conditions; the full evaluation may encompass only a single outpatient visit or may require several weeks in the hospital.

The next step is to determine the type of disorder. In respiratory medicine, the type can be divided into the physiologic disorder and the disease entity. A physiologic disorder can be subdivided into lung mechanics (normal, obstructive, or restrictive), gas exchange (assessment of ventilation, oxygenation, and acid-base balance), and hemodynamics (assessment of pulmonary pressures, flow, and resistance). Physiologic assessment is largely based on pulmonary function tests for lung mechanics, determination of ABGs for gas exchange, and catheterization of the right side of the heart for hemodynamics. The disease entity, which can range anywhere from asthma to Wegener's granulomatosis, encompasses the entire spectrum of respiratory disorders.

Patient management, the last step, depends on the entire data base and on the type of disorder and may range from the simple (e.g., telling the patient to stop smoking) to the complex (e.g., a combi-

Table 1-1. Approach to diagnosis and management of respiratory diseases

Data base →	Type of disorder →	Management

HISTORY
 PHYSICAL EXAMINATION
 CHEST X-RAY FILM
 PULMONARY FUNCTION TESTS (PFTs)
   Forced vital capacity (FVC)
   Forced expiratory volume in one second (FEV_1)
   FEV_1/FVC
   Peak flow
   Total lung capacity
   Diffusing capacity
 ARTERIAL BLOOD GASES (ABGs)
   pH, $Paco_2$ and Pao_2
   Percent saturation of hemoglobin with oxygen
 SPUTUM EXAMINATION
 OTHER TESTS AND PROCEDURES
   Electrolytes, ECG
   Renal and liver function tests
   Catheterization of the right side of the heart
   Exercise testing
	PHYSIOLOGIC
	 Mechanical (from PFTs)
	   Normal
	   Obstructive
	   Restrictive
	   Combination
	 Gas exchange (from ABGs)
	   Ventilation status
	   Oxygenation status
	   Acid-base balance
	 Hemodynamic (from catheterization of the right side of the heart)
	   Pulmonary pressures, flow, and resistance
	   Cardiac output
	 DISEASE ENTITY
	 Examples
	   Asthma
	   Bronchitis
	   Emphysema
	   Interstitial fibrosis
	   Lung cancer
	   Pneumonia
	   Respiratory failure
	   Sarcoidosis
		VARIABLE depending on problem—may include any combination of the following:
		   Removal from noxious environment
		   Stop smoking
		   Lose weight
		   Drugs—examples
		     Bronchodilators
		     Antibiotics
		     Oxygen
		     Steroids
		     Diuretics
		   Chest physiotherapy
		   Psychotherapy
		   Radiotherapy
		   Intubation and artificial ventilation
		   Bronchoscopy
		   Thoracentesis/pleural biopsy
		   Thoracic surgery

nation of drug therapy and chest physical therapy, fiberoptic bronchoscopy, and artificial ventilation).

This schema is the approach used for virtually every patient with respiratory disease. However, within this framework, variation is unlimited. Physiologic tests or blood gases may not be necessary, the physiologic disorder may not be characterized, and the specific disease may be unknown or obscure. Nonetheless, most respiratory patients sooner or later have some physiologic testing; therefore understanding pulmonary physiology is often integral to proper diagnosis and management.

Pulmonary physiology is a broad and complex subject. What is really essential for patient care and evaluation? Certainly one needs some understanding of physiologic tests, such as spirometry and blood gases. However, these tests are only means of obtaining information on lung mechanics and gas exchange. Better tests may someday replace spirometry and blood gases, so it is also important to learn some fundamentals of physiology; they will apply regardless of which tests are employed.

Chapters 2 to 15 cover the fundamentals of physiology most useful to clinical practice. In the remainder of this chapter, I will discuss selected aspects of the data base outlined in Table 1-1, in particular the history, physical examination, chest x-ray examination, and a few basic tests.

HISTORY

The history is simply the story of a patient's medical problem(s). History includes not only what the patient relates, but all other information relevant to the case. It has been stated that 90% of all diagnoses can be made from the medical history. This figure is likely an invented one, but it underscores the importance of a thorough history. Unfortunately, a patient rarely comes prepared to give the complete story; it often has to be elicited, found out, researched.

History taking encompasses far more than just talking to the patient. After all, many hospitalized patients are unable to talk because they suffer severe dyspnea, confusion, or coma. A complete history may require talking to family members, other physicians, or the patient's pharmacist; if the patient has been previously admitted to the same hospital, reviewing old records is certainly part of the history taking.

Acquiring a good patient history requires the physician to have a natural inquisitiveness, a curiosity that goes beyond filling in the blanks on a review of systems list. It also requires a caring and considerate attitude toward the patient. The skilled physician is one who can elicit a thorough history *and* takes the time to do so. Although teaching the art of history taking is beyond the scope of this book, at least one point must be strongly emphasized: *physiologic measurement is no substitute for a thorough history.*

The following three cases relate a few pitfalls frequently observed in history taking. They are presented in the form of brief scenarios. Think about the pitfall before reading the comments in the answer section.

Clinical problem 1

A 46-year-old man is seen because of weight loss and an abnormal lung mass visible in his chest x-ray film. The physician is in the middle of taking the patient's history.

 Physician: "Do you smoke?"
 Patient: "No, no, I don't smoke."
 Physician: "Do you drink?"
 PITFALL?

Clinical problem 2

A house officer is taking the history of a 56-year-old woman who came to the hospital because of progressive dyspnea.

 Patient: "I got this cold 3 days ago, and then I began to cough and couldn't catch my breath."
 Intern: "Did you see any doctor before coming to the hospital?"
 Patient: "No. I took my asthma medication, but it didn't seem to help."
 Intern: "What drugs do you take?"
 Patient: "I brought them all with me." (She gives several vials of drugs to the intern.)
 Intern: (He writes down list of drugs and dosages from prescription labels.) "Do you take anything else besides these drugs?"
 Patient: "No, just an occasional aspirin for headache."
 Intern: "Do you keep any pets or animals at home?"
 PITFALL?

Clinical problem 3

A 60-year-old man is admitted to the hospital because of progressive shortness of breath and a chest x-ray that shows interstitial infiltrates in both lungs.

 Intern: "What kind of work do you do?"
 Patient: "I'm retired now."
 Intern: "What work did you do?"
 Patient: "Oh, I worked for Automatic Motor Co. as a boiler man. I was with them for 30 years."
 Intern: "I see. Do you smoke?"
 PITFALL?

Everyone makes mistakes in history taking. But mistakes can be minimized by approaching each patient as someone with a unique story to tell, a story that may require digging and double checking, but one worth uncovering. In a sense it is like good newspaper reporting. As much information as possible must be obtained. The information must be accurate and must make sense to the reader. One can edit the reporting of it, but important or relevant information must not be left out.

How does one accomplish this information gathering? History taking is considered an art, partly because it cannot be measured or even easily taught. It is a skill that can be learned with practice. One must think about what the patient is saying. Is it complete? (Was the patient taking the drugs?) Is information being obtained, or is just a perfunctory answer being given to a routine question? ("Yes" or "no" questions often lead to the latter.) Is the occupational history complete? (A job title seldom explains one's job.) One must be probing, inquisitive, and caring. Remember that the patient has not been trained to give a history; one should train oneself to elicit the information.

PHYSICAL EXAMINATION

During the nineteenth century and the early twentieth century, before the advent of chest x-rays, chest physical examination reached its peak as a diagnostic skill. Diagnostic acumen was in part necessitated by the scourge of tuberculosis, then the number one killer in Europe and the United States. Today chest physical examination is less detailed in its performance and often is done with the knowledge that a chest x-ray may soon follow. In truth, the physical examination is no substitute for the information obtained from a routine chest x-ray (see the next section). Nonetheless, there are some basic aspects and pitfalls of the physical examination that bear emphasis.

Inspection

Inspection should begin the moment the patient is seen. Is his breathing obvious? Normal breathing is not obvious during inspection unless respiratory movement is specifically looked for. If a patient's breathing is immediately obvious, it is probably abnormal. Signs that make breathing obvious and that should draw attention include one or more of the following: (1) use of accessory muscles; (2) pursed lip breathing; (3) flaring of nostrils; (4) interrupted speech; and (5) a fast respiratory rate.

Accessory muscles are the neck and shoulder muscles that come into use during strenuous exercise. Patients frequently use these muscles to augment breathing when either diaphragm or lung function is severely compromised, such as occurs in asthma attacks, for example. Use of accessory muscles (e.g., the sternocleidomastoid muscles) during an acute asthma attack is one indication of its severity; the attack cannot be considered under control until the patient is no longer using accessory muscles.

Patients with severe emphysema often *purse (narrow) their lips* in order to increase airway pressure and aid expiration. *Flaring of nostrils,* like use of accessory muscles, is an attempt by dyspneic patients to bring in more air. *Interrupted speech* occurs when patients have little breathing reserve; they cannot hold their breath long enough to speak in sentences.

Respiratory rate is perhaps the simplest vital sign to measure since it requires no physical contact with the patient. Normal respiratory rate is approximately 8 to 16/min. In adults, a resting respiratory rate above 20/min is definitely abnormal (small children normally breathe much faster). An increase in respiratory rate is often the first sign of pulmonary edema or other acute pulmonary pathology. Respiratory rate in hospitalized patients should be monitored like body temperature is; any elevation has the same implication—an abnormal finding that needs to be explained.

Mental status evaluation

Assessment of the patient's mental status often takes place in the first few minutes of inspection. Clinical inspection and assessment of mental status are far more important, in most patients, than all the information obtained from the rest of the physical examination. Is the patient confused? Are questions answered appropriately? Is the patient oriented to his situation? If the patient is confused or obtunded, there is every reason to believe the diagnosis may be respiratory failure and blood gas analysis should be obtained.

Not only are inspection and evaluation of mental status critical for diagnosing suspected respiratory failure, but they are also important in deciding how to proceed once the problem is diagnosed. For example, the management of elevated carbon dioxide pressure (PCO_2) is far different for a confused or obtunded patient than for someone who is alert and comfortable.

Percussion and palpation

After inspection and mental status evaluation, percussion and palpation can be employed. Of the two procedures, percussion is more valuable; it is used to check for either dullness (as from pleural effusion or consolidation) or hyperresonance (as in emphysema or pneumothorax).

Auscultation

Auscultation with a stethoscope is the one physical diagnostic skill most physicians practice routinely. The principal adventitious or abnormal breath sounds can be divided into rales (synonymous with crackles) and wheezes (synonymous with rhonchi). Table 1-2 shows a graphic display

Table 1-2. Adventitious breath sounds

Acoustic characteristics	Waveform	Terms recommended by the ATS*	Other terms in some textbooks	British terms
Discontinuous, interrupted explosive sounds Loud, low in pitch		Coarse crackle	Coarse rale	Crackle
Discontinuous, interrupted explosive sounds Not as loud as above and of shorter duration; higher in pitch than coarse rales or crackles		Fine crackle	Fine rale	Crackle
Continuous sounds Longer than 250 ms, low pitched; dominant frequency about 200 Hz or more, a hissing sound		Wheeze	Sibilant rhonchus	High-pitched wheeze
Continuous sounds Longer than 250 ms, low pitched; dominant frequency about 200 Hz or more, a hissing sound		Rhonchus	Sonorous rhonchus	Low-pitched wheeze

From Rosman, J., and Murphy, R.: J. Respir. Dis. **3**(7):43, 1982; modified from Murphy, R.L.H., and Holford, S.H.: Basics of R.D. March, 1980, p. 3.)
*ATS = American Thoracic Society

of these lung sounds, along with their alternate terminology. Rales (crackles) are discontinuous sounds, usually heard on inspiration; they are simulated by the crinkling of cellophane. Rales are caused by the opening of small airways that contain fluid, mucus, or secretions or that are scarred, as in patients with pulmonary fibrosis.

Wheezes (rhonchi) are continuous sounds that can be simulated by closing the glottis and forcing out the air. Wheezes are caused by air moving through a narrowed air tube and are a common finding in obstructive airways disease. Like rales, the presence of wheezes does not imply any particular disease. Asthma, bronchitis, heart failure, and upper airways obstruction may all manifest wheezing. Stridor is a special type of wheeze: high-pitched, heard only on inspiration, and indicative of upper airways (above the main carina) obstruction. Since the sound can be transmitted to the lung bases, upper airway obstruction may mimic asthma.

Although space does not permit thorough discussion of the lung examination, the following cases illustrate some common pitfalls.

Clinical problem 4

A 34-year-old woman was being treated in the emergency room for asthma. After several hours of intravenous therapy, the treating physician listened to her chest and heard no wheezes. On the basis of this finding, the physician concluded that the patient was better and sent her out with a prescription for asthma medication.
PITFALL?

Clinical problem 5

A 61-year-old woman with episodic wheezing and dyspnea was treated for asthma over a 6-month period with no signs of improvement. She had never smoked and had no prior history of asthma. Five years earlier she had had surgery for removal of a thyroid goiter.
PITFALL?

Clinical problem 6

A 28-year-old man with a broken leg was being treated in the hospital. During his surgery, the patient received several units of blood and copious intravenous fluids. Over the next 2 days he frequently complained of pain and required several narcotic injections. The third postoperative day, the patient was noted to be tachypneic. He was afebrile, and chest auscultation revealed no rales or rhonchi. His tachypnea was attributed to anxiety and pain.
PITFALL?

CHEST X-RAY EXAMINATION

The chest x-ray examination is the most useful of all tests in pulmonary medicine. It has value in both diagnosing and ruling out parenchymal lung abnormality. Fig. 1-1 shows a woman receiving a routine posteroanterior chest x-ray, and Fig. 1-2 shows standard posteroanterior chest x-ray with labeling of some important structures. Figs. 1-3 and 1-4 show examples of abnormal x-rays. Many conditions invariably show up on the chest x-ray, such as pneumonia, pleural effusion, pneumothorax, pulmonary edema, and lung cancer. A clear chest film can thus be reassuring in some situations.

Anyone caring for respiratory patients should make a habit of looking at the chest x-ray and not waiting for the formal report. Only in this way can one fully appreciate the test's utility and feel comfortable in "reading" chest x-rays.

Apart from mistakes made in interpretation of chest x-rays, there are two common pitfalls to be avoided. The first pitfall is not ordering a chest x-ray when it can be helpful. The chest x-ray provides information not discernible from even the most compulsive history and physical examination. Since a single two-view study (posteroanterior and lateral) presents no risk to the patient and (as tests go) is relatively inexpensive, the chest x-ray should be obtained whenever it might help in diagnosis or treatment.

Clinical approach

Fig. 1-1. Schematic diagram of woman having a routine posteroanterior chest x-ray examination. She stands facing the x-ray film with arms above her head; the x-ray beams (represented by lines, but actually invisible) enter from the back and travel through her chest to hit the film. When the film is developed, the result is a standard posteroanterior view of the lungs and surrounding structures, shown in Fig. 1-2. (For a lateral chest x-ray, the subject stands with one side of her chest against the film plate.)

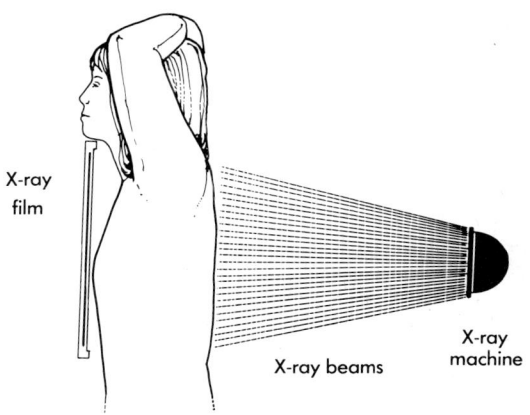

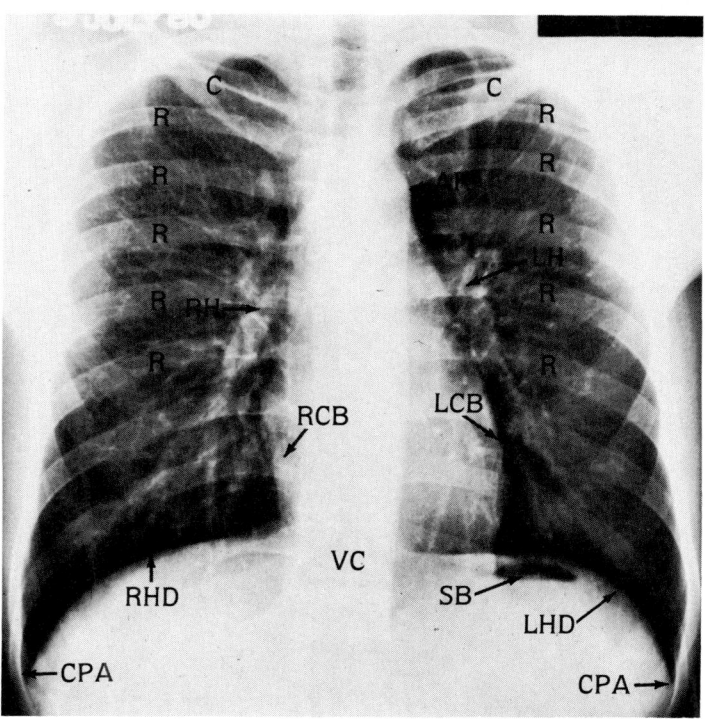

Fig. 1-2. Normal posteroanterior chest x-ray film, with labeling of important structures. The patient's right side is to the left and vice versa. (*RHD*, right hemidiaphragm; *LHD*, left hemidiaphragm; *CPA*, costophrenic angles; *LCB*, left cardiac border; *VC*, vertebral column; *AK*, aortic knob; *SB*, stomach bubble; *RH*, right hilum; *LH*, left hilum; *R*, rib; *C*, clavicle.) (From Wilkins, R.L., Sheldon, R.L., Krider, S.J.: Clinical assessment in respiratory care, St. Louis, 1985, The C.V. Mosby Co.)

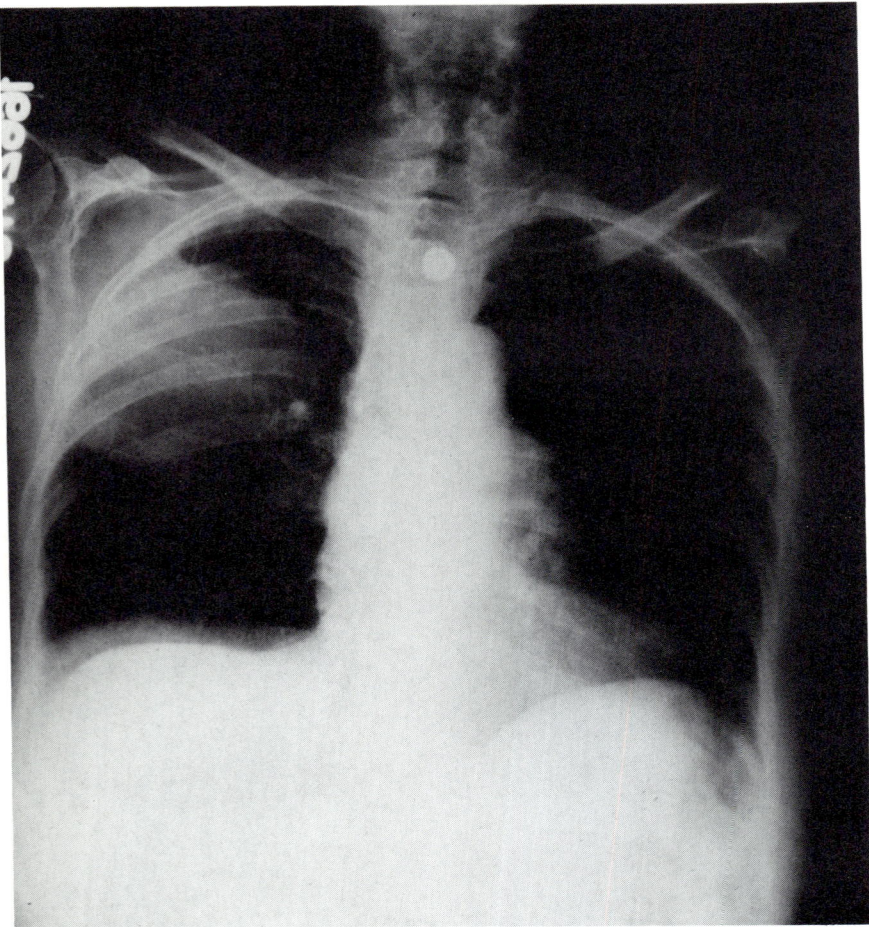

Fig. 1-3. Chest x-ray of a patient who claimed to be asymptomatic until he coughed up blood. It shows a huge right upper lobe mass that was diagnosed as inoperable lung carcinoma.

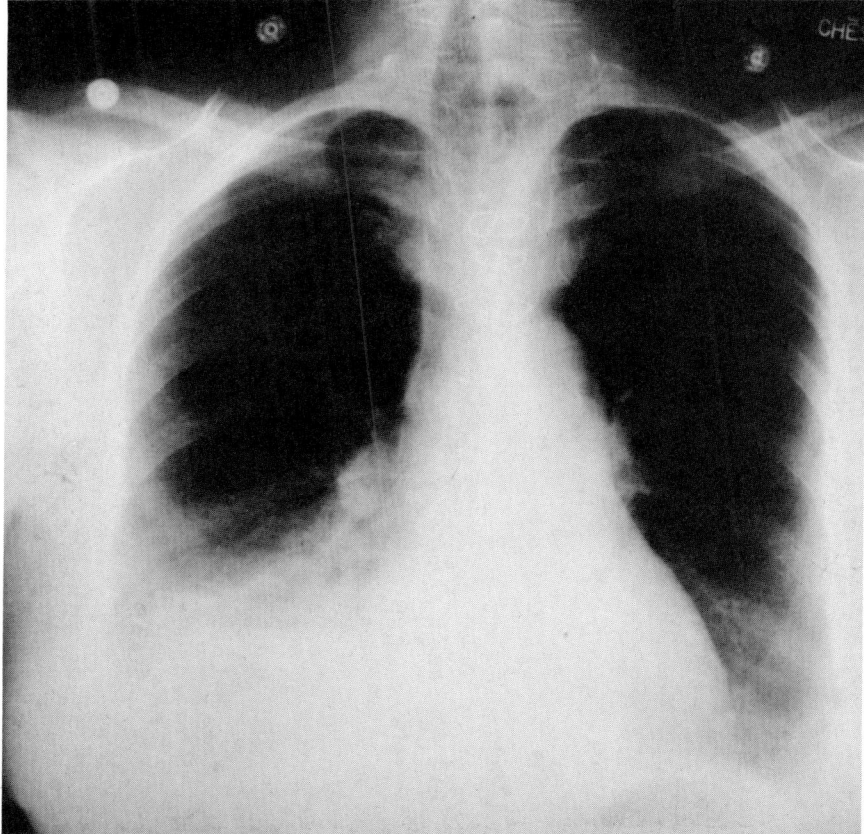

Fig. 1-4. Chest x-ray of the patient presented in Clinical Problem 5. Note the large mass surrounding the trachea. During surgery performed on this patient, a thyroid goiter was removed. Densities at the patient's right base are from chronic scarring and are unrelated to the goiter.

Clinical problem 7

For which of the following patients is a chest x-ray examination *least* indicated?

a. A 37-year-old woman, a nonsmoker, evaluated for cough of 3 days' duration has signs, including runny nose and sore throat, of an upper respiratory infection. Her lungs are clear to auscultation.
b. A 45-year-old cigarette smoker with a chronic cough of 3 weeks' duration has not yet received any treatment for his cough. Otherwise, he feels fine and has no other symptoms. Physical examination is normal.
c. A 26-year-old woman, a nonsmoker, with new onset of wheezing and dyspnea responds in the emergency room to inhalation treatment for asthma.
d. A 67-year-old man with formerly diagnosed emphysema has the clinical picture of congestive heart failure: leg edema, bilateral rales on auscultation, and abnormal third heart sound (S_3 gallop).

The second common mistake is not taking the time to compare a current x-ray with earlier ones. Previous x-rays may be available at once or may have to be obtained from other clinics or hospitals. The extra time it takes to retrieve and compare all films can often save the patient a procedure, a day in the hospital, or even a hospital admission.

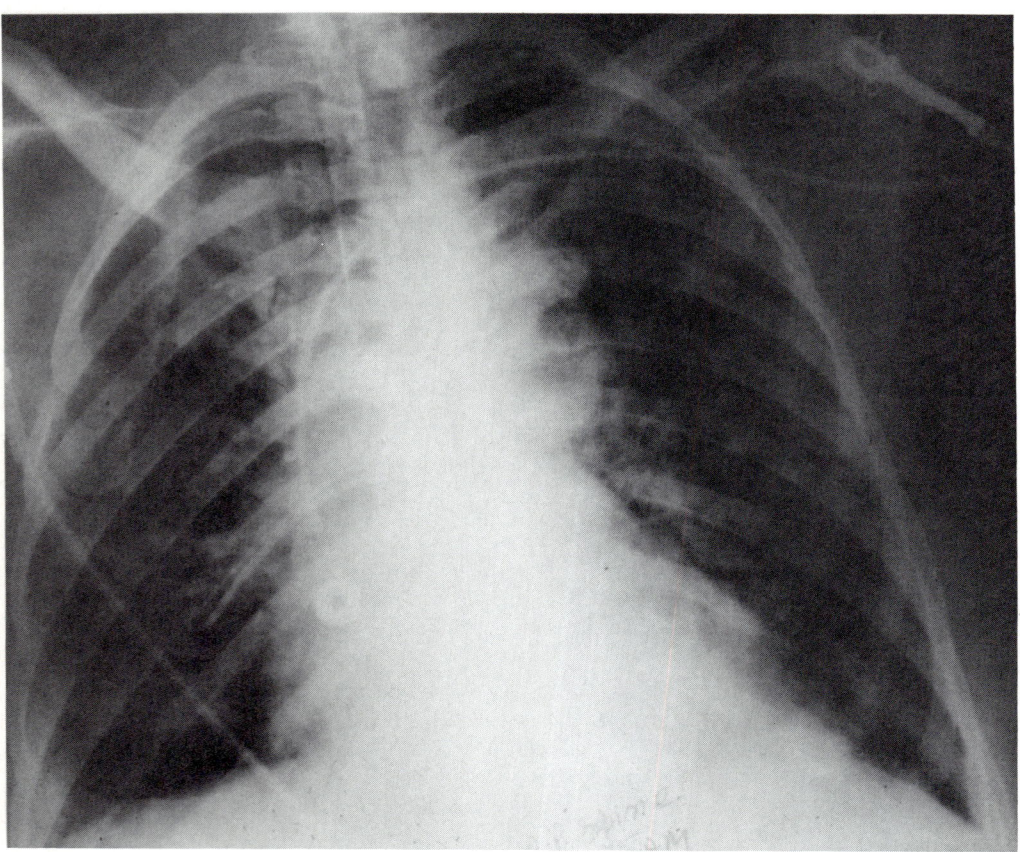

Fig. 1-5. An anteroposterior portable chest x-ray of a patient with pulmonary edema. Note the cardiac monitoring leads, endotracheal tube, and Swan-Ganz right heart catheter.

Clinical approach

For most intensive care patients, only an anteroposterior chest x-ray is obtained because they are not able to stand. Unlike the posteroanterior projection, anteroposterior films are not easily standardized. Anteroposterior films tend to show wide variation in technique and are more difficult to interpret (Fig. 1-5). The heart shown on an anteroposterior film usually appears larger than on a posteroanterior projection because the x-ray beam originates closer than 6 feet from the patient. Since the heart is an anterior structure and the beam covers a wider area as it strikes the film cassette, a slightly larger cardiac image results. Although anteroposterior films are usually marked as such, the x-ray itself often provides a clue to the technique; a cardiac catheter or endotracheal tube seen on the film is evidence enough that the technique is "anteroposterior portable."

Apart from the standard posteroanterior and lateral projections for ambulatory patients, other views are often helpful. Oblique projections are used to better reveal hilar structures and abnormalities near the heart borders. Decubitus views are useful in looking for free pleural fluid (see Chapter 13). An apical lordotic view is used to highlight lesions in or near the lung apices and in the right middle lobe.

In recent years, computerized axial tomography (CAT) scanning of the chest has been widely employed for diagnosing intrathoracic lesions (Fig. 1-6). CAT scanning is particularly valuable in demonstrating mediastinal and hilar masses and in dis-

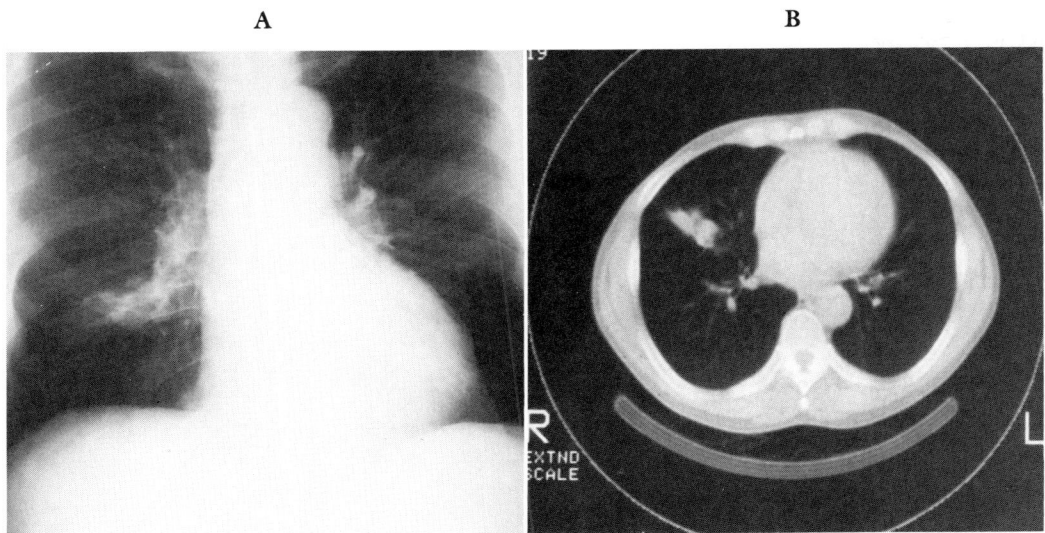

Fig. 1-6. A, Posteroanterior chest x-ray showing a right midlung field infiltrate. Another way of visualizing a chest lesion is with computerized axial tomography (CAT scan), which can provide a cross-sectional view at any level of the body. **B,** A CAT scan view showing that the infiltrate is a mass completely surrounded by air-containing lung. The mass was a lung carcinoma in the right middle lobe and was completely resected at surgery.

tinguishing vascular from nonvascular masses (using bolus injections of contrast material).

Other newer radiologic techniques are being investigated for their utility in diagnosing intrathoracic disease (e.g., magnetic resonance imaging and digital subtraction angiography). Although the improvements in radiologic technology are impressive, the fact is that the vast majority of respiratory patients can be diagnosed and managed with intelligent use of the ordinary chest x-ray examination.

SPIROMETRY

In clinical practice, pulmonary function tests are those procedures requiring patient effort; usually the patient comes to a central laboratory to have the tests performed. Pulmonary function tests are distinguished from tests done on a blood sample for which no patient effort is required. The patient's effort usually entails blowing air into an apparatus designed to measure lung volumes and flow rates. The simplest and most widely used pulmonary function test is that done on a spirometer and therefore called spirometry.

Although spirometry was first introduced in 1846 by J. Hutchinson, it was over a century before this test became a routine diagnostic tool. After World War II, the water-sealed spirometer gained favor as the standard instrument for measuring forced vital capacity (FVC). In the forced vital capacity maneuver, a patient inhales to total lung capacity and then exhales as forcefully and quickly as possible (Fig. 1-7). Exhaled air travels through the tube and displaces a movable bell, to which a pen is attached. As the bell moves, the pen traces a curve on a rotating drum; the curve is a time vs. volume plot of the forced vital capacity. The entire forced vital capacity curve does not have to be measured in all clinical situations. For example, the peak flow, which is obtained in the first second

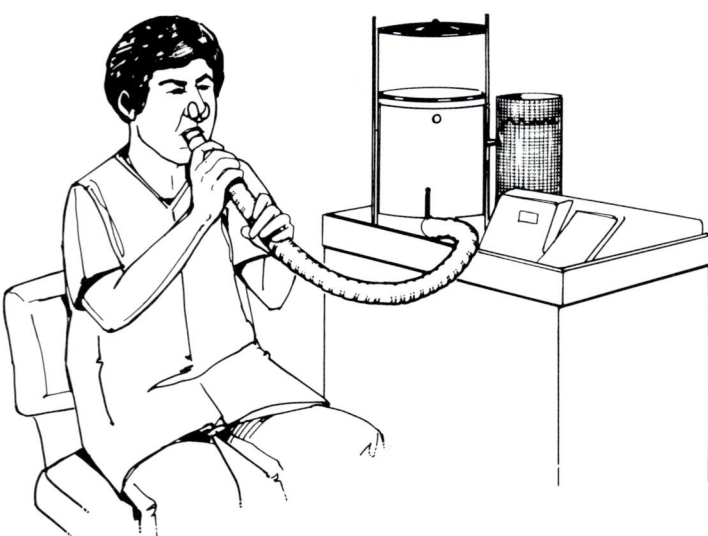

Fig. 1-7. Patient performing forced vital capacity maneuver. He takes in a full, deep breath, then exhales forcefully and rapidly into the tube that is connected to the bellows section of the spirometer. Movement of the spirometer bell deflects an attached pen that records a tracing of the expiratory effort on a rotating drum. Spirometry is discussed in Chapter 3.

of the forced vital capacity effort, gives sufficient information during an asthma attack. The physiology and utility of the forced vital capacity curve are discussed in Chapter 3.

ARTERIAL BLOOD GAS ANALYSIS

The first human arterial puncture was done in 1912 by Hurter. In 1919, Stadie became the first to obtain an arterial blood sample for gas analysis. Despite the early start, it was decades before arterial blood gases were routinely employed in patient care. The Clark platinum electrode for measuring oxygen pressure (PO_2) was introduced in 1953, and by the 1960's blood gas machines began to appear for the rapid analysis of arterial Po_2, carbon dioxide pressure (Pco_2), and pH. The blood gas test is now widely used in all acute care hospitals. In addition, separate machines (co-oximeters) are used to measure percent oxyhemoglobin (Sao_2), as well as percent carboxyhemoglobin and percent methemoglobin. From a single arterial sample, the blood gas machine and co-oximeter (Fig. 1-8) can provide valuable information about a patient's state of oxygenation, ventilation, and acid-base balance.

The box on p. 20 shows the basic information obtained from routine blood gas analysis, as well as the normal range for each test and the physiologic process assessed by these measurements. Oxygenation is assessed by the arterial oxygen pressure (Pao_2), oxygen saturation in arterial blood (Sao_2), and arterial carbon dioxide pressure ($Paco_2$); ventilation by the $Paco_2$ alone; and acid-base balance by the $Paco_2$, pH, and bicarbonate (HCO_3^-). Note that HCO_3^- is a calculation only and not a direct measurement from the blood gas laboratory.

Blood gas measurement is invasive in that it requires arterial puncture or an indwelling arterial line. There has been a trend in the past decade to develop noninvasive measurement of blood gases. Among the more popular measurements are trans-

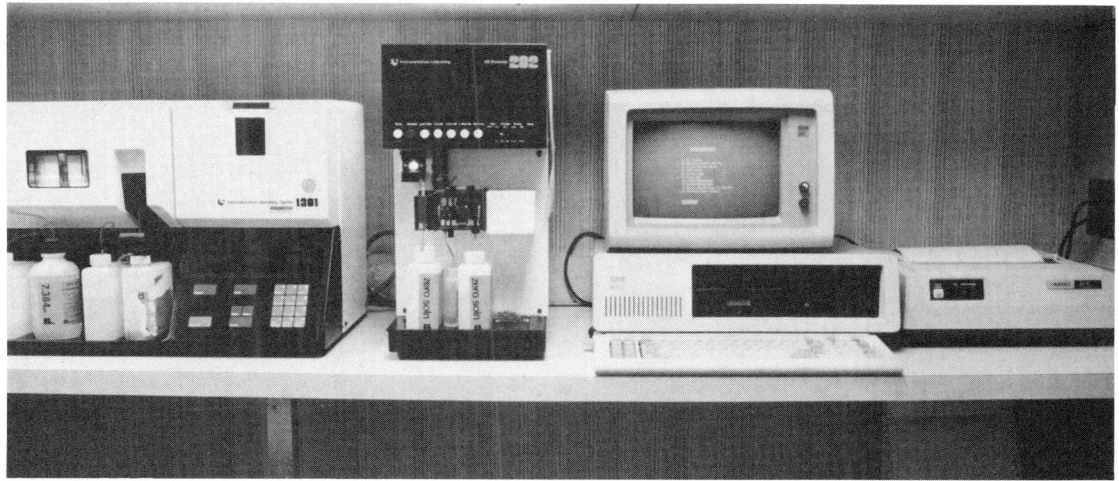

Fig. 1-8. Blood gas machines. The machine on the far left (Instrumental Laboratories' Model 1301) is used to measure Pao_2, $Paco_2$, and pH. The machine in the middle (Instrumental Laboratories' Model 282) is a co-oximeter and measures Sao_2 and percent carboxyhemoglobin. The computer (IBM XT) is connected to the blood gas machines and is used to store, retrieve, and interpret blood gas data. A small printer is shown on the extreme right.

	ARTERIAL BLOOD GASES*		
VENTILATION →	Pa_{O_2} Sa_{O_2} Pa_{CO_2} pH HCO_3^-	(70-100 mm Hg) (93%-98%) (36-44 mm Hg) (7.36-7.44) (22-26 mEq/L)	OXYGENATION ACID-BASE

*Normal range at sea level. Pa_{O_2} normal values are age-dependent; see Chapter 5 for further discussion of normal Pa_{O_2}.

cutaneous P_{O_2}, Sa_{O_2} by oximetry, and alveolar P_{CO_2} by expired gas analysis. Perhaps the major advantage of these tests over in vitro arterial blood analysis is their ability to provide *continuous physiologic monitoring*.

So far, these tests have not replaced arterial blood gas analysis for at least two reasons. First, each test measures only one thing at a time, such as P_{O_2} measured by the transcutaneous electrode or Sa_{O_2} measured by an oximeter used on an ear or a finger. Second, machines for noninvasive analysis can generally be used on only one patient at a time making each individual test much more expensive than a single arterial blood gas. For example, oximetry requires a machine that costs several thousand dollars, yet it measures only a single value (Sa_{O_2}) on one patient at a time. As of this writing, noninvasive tests must be significantly improved before they replace arterial puncture for blood gas analysis.

The physiologic processes assessed by blood gas measurement are discussed in Chapters 4 to 7.

SPUTUM EXAMINATION

Microscopic examination of sputum will often indicate the cause of acute pulmonary infections, especially bacterial pneumonia. The patient's sputum is stained with Gram's stain to look for the causative organism; if tuberculosis (TB) is suspected, a special acid-fast stain is used. If the sputum examination reveals only white blood cells and no bacteria, the causative organism is likely a virus or viruslike bacterium. In either case, the microscopic sputum examination is valuable. Sputum cultures take one to several days (longer for TB) and often serve only to confirm the results of initial staining.

Aside from the clear role of sputum examination in infections, other conditions can be diagnosed from the sputum examination. Patients with bronchogenic lung cancer often expectorate tumor cells; even a few tumor cells seen through the microscope can confirm the diagnosis of lung cancer. In some cases, a sputum examination will save the patient an invasive diagnostic procedure.

During a patient's asthma attack, his sputum usually contains large numbers of eosinophils, a type of white blood cell whose cytoplasmic granules stain a characteristic orange-red color. Sometimes the diagnosis of asthma is not obvious from the clinical examination, such as when heart failure is also a strong possibility. The presence of eosinophils strongly suggest asthma since the cells are absent in the sputum of heart failure patients. During successful treatment of an asthma attack, eosinophils will disappear from the sputum.

OTHER TESTS AND PROCEDURES

There is virtually an unlimited number of tests and procedures available in the modern hospital or clinic. Some are routine and available everywhere, such as the electrocardiogram and measurement of serum electrolytes. Others, such as catheterization of the right side of the heart and exercise testing, two tests that are discussed in Chapters 8 and 12, respectively, are done only in special situations.

Whatever tests and procedures are used to collect a data base, the goal is always the same—make an accurate diagnosis and treat the patient. The evaluation of dyspnea, a common respiratory complaint, provides a good example of the clinical approach outlined in this chapter.

EVALUATION OF DYSPNEA

Dyspnea is from the Greek words for "hard breathing." Patients often call it "shortness of breath" (see the box below). Since breathing is something people do automatically, it may be hard to appreciate how distressing it is when breathing is difficult. Everyone becomes dyspneic to some extent when exercising vigorously, and this response is appropriate. What is inappropriate is when patients feel short of breath at rest or with only slight exertion.

Dyspnea is usually taught as a symptom—something about which the patient complains. In clinical practice, it is also referred to as a sign—what is observed in a patient. One may say a patient "looks dyspneic" although he voices no complaint. This observation is usually based on the patient's respiratory rate or his use of accessory breathing muscles.

By far the most common clinical causes of dyspnea are cardiac and respiratory impairment, although other problems can lead to dyspnea (see the box below). Decreased hemoglobin content (anemia) and other blood disorders, such as abnormal hemoglobin (altered oxygen affinity, see Chapter 6) may also lead to dyspnea. Metabolic problems that may be associated with dyspnea include hyperthyroidism and ketoacidosis. Altitude causes dyspnea because of hypoxemia. Poor fitness is a common cause of dyspnea on exertion. Pregnancy is a common physiologic (i.e., normal) cause of dyspnea. Finally, dyspnea may be of purely psychogenic origin with no organ impairment. Such patients often sigh excessively and complain of inability to take in a satisfactory breath; their chest x-ray films, arterial blood gases, and spirometry are normal.

Clinically, dyspnea can be divided into two categories, acute and chronic. Patients with acute dyspnea are short of breath at rest and usually need immediate medical attention. Conditions commonly associated with acute dyspnea are pulmonary edema, asthma attack, pulmonary embolism, pneumothorax, pneumonia, and acute anxiety reaction.

Chronic dyspnea usually manifests as dyspnea

DYSPNEA

AS A SYMPTOM

"I feel short of breath."
"I can't catch my breath."
"My chest is tight."
"I can't get all my air in (or out)."

AS A SIGN

"The patient looks dyspneic."
"She's having trouble breathing."
"He's gasping for breath."

SYSTEM OR PROBLEM THAT MAY CAUSE DYSPNEA

Cardiac system (e.g., congestive heart failure)
Respiratory system
    —Central nervous system
    —Thoracic cage and muscles
    —Lungs
Hematologic disorders (e.g., anemia)
Metabolic disorders (e.g., hyperthyroidism)
Altitude (via hypoxemia)
Poor physical fitness
Pregnancy
Psychogenic disorders (no organic cause)

on exertion; such patients are seldom dyspneic at rest. Chronic dyspnea is commonly associated with chronic obstructive pulmonary disease (emphysema and chronic bronchitis), interstitial fibrosis, and chronic congestive heart failure.

Fig. 1-9 outlines a clinical approach to evaluating patients with dyspnea. This schema is a broad outline for the differential diagnosis and management of dyspnea.

The history is crucial in both suggesting a cause and assessing the severity of dyspnea. The division between acute and chronic is based on the history and the physician's perception of the problem. Is the patient in distress, gasping for air, diaphoretic, unable to talk in complete sentences? If so, the problem is acute. Evaluation is carried out on an emergent basis, and treatment is often given concurrently. For example, a patient suffering an acute asthma attack may receive bronchodilators while a chest x-ray film, spirometry, and blood gas analysis

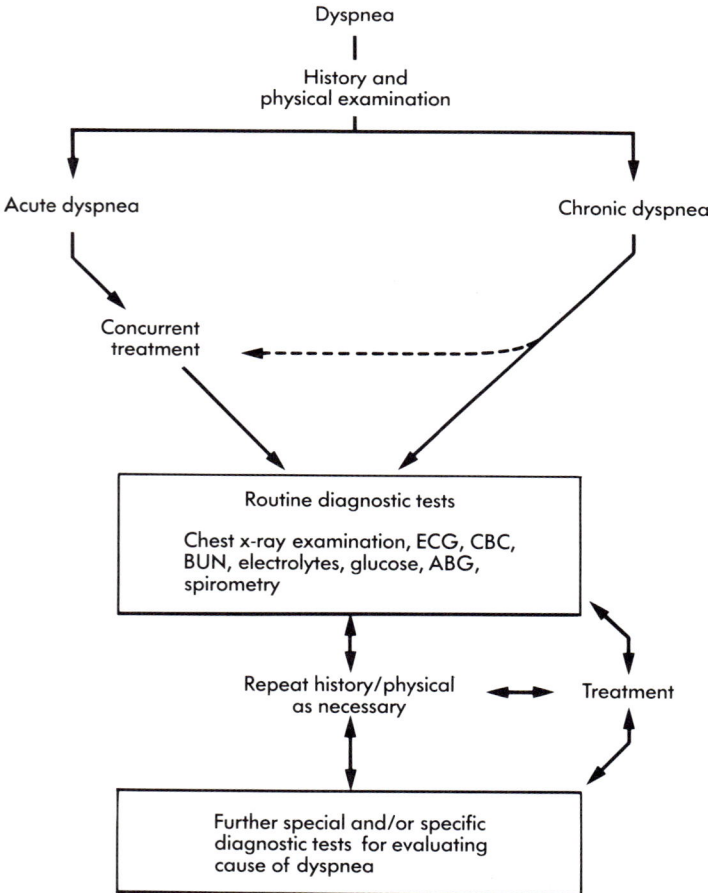

Fig. 1-9. Schema for evaluation and management of dyspnea.

Chronic dyspnea allows for a more leisurely approach, and concurrent treatment is not so imperative; more time can be spent obtaining the history and diagnostic tests (Fig. 1-9). When did the dyspnea begin? Is it present all the time or only on exertion? Is it worse any particular time of day? Does it wake the patient? The character of the dyspnea is seldom useful diagnostically, and the value of such questions lies more in understanding how dyspnea affects the patient than in pinpointing a diagnosis. For example, orthopnea and paroxysmal nocturnal dyspnea can occur from heart disease as well as from lung disease; episodic dyspnea associated with cough can occur from asthma as well as from emphysema.

Inspection is usually the most important part of the physical examination. Is there use of accessory muscles, or any of the other signs of dyspnea mentioned previously? What is the respiratory rate? On auscultation, are breath sounds of normal intensity or diminished? Are they equal from both lungs? Are wheezing or rales present? Is there an irregular heart rhythm or cardiac gallop?

Although the history and physical examination are of obvious importance, they seldom provide a definitive diagnosis without associated laboratory tests. Routine tests are listed in Fig. 1-9; as a group, these tests are relatively inexpensive and often provide valuable information for both diagnosis and therapy (see box below). The box on p. 24 lists additional tests that can further refine the diagnosis in difficult cases.

Exercise testing is one of the least understood

UTILITY OF ROUTINE DIAGNOSTIC TESTS IN EVALUATION OF DYSPNEA

CHEST X-RAY. If abnormal, the chest x-ray may suggest a specific diagnosis (e.g., pneumonia, lung cancer). Finding clear lungs on the chest x-ray helps rule out many diagnoses and suggests other causes (e.g., lungs are usually clear in asthma and chronic bronchitis).

ELECTROCARDIOGRAM (ECG). The electrocardiogram is useful for diagnosing myocardial ischemia and infarction and any cardiac arrhythmia. Sinus tachycardia, a common finding in many dyspneic patients, is nonspecific and therefore not helpful in diagnosis except in excluding a serious arrhythmia.

COMPLETE BLOOD COUNT (CBC). The complete blood count includes white blood cell count (WBC) and measurement of either hematocrit (Hct) or hemoglobin content (Hb). Hematocrit content or hemoglobin content is a diagnostic test for anemia; the lower the value, the more likely anemia is a cause or a contributor to dyspnea. An increased white blood count is usually found in the presence of infection, particularly of bacterial origin.

ELECTROLYTES. Electrolyte imbalance *per se* does not cause dyspnea, but many dyspneic conditions are accompanied by electrolyte abnormality. Sodium (Na^+), potassium (K^+), chloride (Cl^-), and bicarbonate (HCO_3^-) are usually measured at the same time, along with the blood urea nitrogen (BUN) and glucose. These six measurements are invaluable in diagnosing abnormal states of water balance (dehydration, overhydration), acid-base problems, and states of renal insufficiency.

ARTERIAL BLOOD GAS (ABG). Arterial blood gas is used to assess oxygenation, ventilation, and acid-base balance; this is discussed extensively in Chapters 4 to 7.

SPIROMETRY. Spirometry is invaluable for diagnosing obstructive airway problems. A normal forced vital capacity curve rules out clinically significant airway obstruction. Often, only one component of spirometry is measured (e.g., peak flow or one-second forced expiratory volume [FEV_1]). Spirometry is discussed extensively in Chapter 3.

SPECIAL AND/OR SPECIFIC DIAGNOSTIC TESTS FOR EVALUATING CAUSES OF DYSPNEA

CLINICAL TRIAL OF DIURETICS

TESTS OF PULMONARY FUNCTION

Spirometry before and after use of bronchodilators (to look for reversibility when baseline spirometry is abnormal)
Spirometry before and after bronchoprovocation (to look for airway obstruction when baseline spirometry is normal)
Diffusing capacity
Lung volumes
Physiologic exercise testing

TESTS OF PULMONARY CIRCULATION

Perfusion/ventilation lung scan
Pulmonary angiogram
Right heart catheterization

TESTS OF CARDIAC FUNCTION

Noninvasive: echocardiogram, nuclear studies, and exercise stress testing
Invasive: catheterization of the right and left side of the heart, and coronary angiography

BLOOD STUDIES, INCLUDING METABOLIC STUDIES

Hemoglobin electrophoresis
P_{50} measurement
Carboxyhemoglobin measurement
Methemoglobin measurement
Thyroid function tests
Drug analysis (e.g., cyanide levels)

MISCELLANEOUS

Sputum bacterial stains and culture
Thoracentesis and fluid examination (for pleural effusion)
Psychological evaluation
Allergy evaluation
Tensilon test
Electromyogram
Sleep study (measurement of respiratory rate, SaO_2, electroencephalogram [EEG], and other parameters during sleep)
Lung biopsy
Any other test that may help to evaluate cause of dyspnea

physiologic tests, mainly because it is not used nearly as often as spirometry or blood gas analysis. Exercise testing is helpful when a patient's complaint of dyspnea is not explained by other tests. Exercise stresses the whole body, not just one system at a time. The lungs must exchange extra oxygen and carbon dioxide, the heart must increase its output, and the circulatory system must deliver an augmented blood supply to the tissues. If any of these processes fail to function adequately, the patient may experience dyspnea or be unable to continue exercising. Chapter 12 discusses what to measure during exercise and how to interpret the results.

BEDSIDE VS. LABORATORY

Fig. 1-9 and the boxes on p. 23 and 24 present an outline for managing dyspnea, a common respiratory problem. Fig. 1-10 summarizes the essence of this clinical approach. Evaluation of dyspnea or any respiratory problem requires an artful integration of the history and physical examination with the laboratory tests, which are usually ones of physiologic function. Neither the history and the physical examination alone nor laboratory tests alone are sufficient to diagnose and manage most respiratory problems.

One must always guard against the misuse and overuse of laboratory tests. As pointed out previously and as will be emphasized throughout the remaining chapters, tests are no substitute for bedside evaluation. Physiologic measurement must *always* be evaluated in light of the patient's condition at the time the test was performed. Test results, whether from a blood gas analysis, spirometry, or catheterization of the right side of the heart, have different implications in different patients. Perhaps the best way to express this philosophy is the often heard bedside admonition, "Doctor, treat the patient, not the numbers."

SUMMARY

The clinical approach to respiratory diseases is conceptually the same as for any other branch of medicine: gather a data base, make a diagnosis, and treat the patient. Apart from the information gained from the history and the physical examination, important data may include results of the chest x-ray examination, pulmonary function tests, arterial blood gas analysis, and a few other basic tests. Diagnosis includes not only a specific disease entity but also assessment of the patient's physiologic status (mechanical, gas exchange, and hemodynamic). Patient management depends on the specific diagnosis and the degree of physiologic impairment.

Although physiologic measurement is often extremely valuable, it is no substitute for a thorough history. History taking requires time and a natural, inquisitive attitude. In addition, the physical examination is valuable for assessing severity of illness; tachypnea, use of accessory muscles, and flaring of nostrils are usually indicative of respiratory distress.

The chest x-ray examination is by far the single most valuable test for both diagnosing and ruling

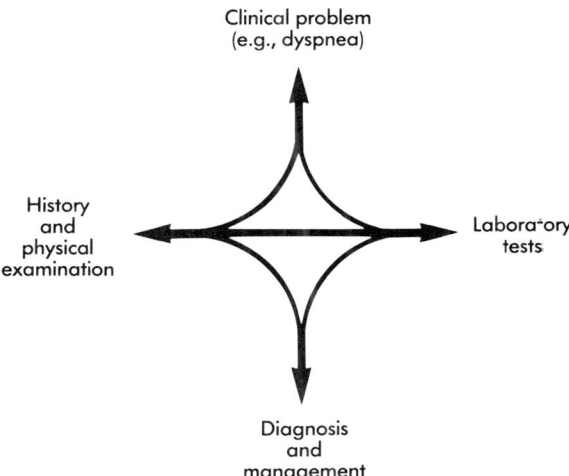

Fig. 1-10. Proper diagnosis and management of any clinical problem, such as dyspnea, requires the integration of the patient's history and physical examination with the appropriate laboratory tests.

out many pulmonary disorders. Arterial blood gases and spirometry provide information on gas exchange and lung mechanics, respectively. Along with the history and physical examination, these three tests are often all that are needed to assess patients with respiratory impairment.

Evaluation of dyspnea is used as an example of the clinical approach. Dyspnea, which means hard or difficult breathing, can be caused by a variety of medical problems, including cardiac, pulmonary, and hematologic ones. The clinical presentation can be acute (requiring immediate treatment) or chronic. Routine diagnostic tests include chest x-ray examination, ECG, blood count, electrolytes, blood gas, and spirometry, some or all of which may be performed on a given patient. The history, physical examination, and one or more of these tests are sufficient to diagnose and treat most patients with dyspnea. Many other special and specific diagnostic tests are available for difficult cases (e.g., physiologic exercise testing, lung scanning, and echocardiogram). Evaluation of dyspnea—or of any respiratory problem—requires an artful integration of the history and physical examination with laboratory tests.

REVIEW QUESTIONS

State whether each of the following is true or false.
1. Rales are discontinuous breath sounds that may signify fluid or fibrosis in the lungs.
2. Absence of cyanosis rules out clinically significant hypoxemia.
3. Stridor is a high-pitched wheeze characteristic of bronchial asthma.
4. Consolidation is manifested by hyperresonance to chest percussion.
5. In spirometry, the subject inhales to the maximum, then blows the air into a machine that can plot the volume and rate of flow.
6. The arterial blood gas test routinely includes measurement of the bicarbonate concentration.
7. Right middle lobe pneumonia can obscure the right heart border on a posteroanterior chest x-ray.
8. Hyponatremia commonly leads to dyspnea.
9. Computerized history taking has been shown helpful in diagnosing respiratory ailments in noncomatose patients.
10. Absence of wheezing rules out clinically significant asthma.

Reference

Rosman, J., and Cugell, D.: Chest physical examination: seeing what you hear, J. Respir. Dis. **3**(7):43, 1982.

Suggested readings

Felson, B., Weinstein, A.S., and Spitz, H.B.: Principles of chest roentgenology, Philadelphia, 1965, W.B. Saunders Co.

Heitzman, E.R.: The lung: radiologic-pathologic correlations, ed. 2, St. Louis, 1984, The C.V. Mosby Co.

Loudon, R., and Murphy, R.L.H., Jr.: Lung sounds: state of the art, Am. Rev. Respir. Dis. **130**:663, 1984.

Squire, L.F., Colaiace, W.M., and Strutynsky, N.: Exercises in diagnostic radiology, Philadelphia, 1981, W.B. Saunders Co.

The Occupational and Environmental Health Committee of the American Lung Association of San Diego and Imperial Counties: Taking the occupational history, Ann. Intern. Med. **59**:641, 1983.

See also General References in Appendix G.

chapter 2
Structure and function

OUTLINE

Gas properties
The atmosphere
Gas laws
ATPS, BTPS, and STPD
Gases in solution
Breathing—an overview of gas exchange
Lung disease and the respiratory system

GAS PROPERTIES

The main function of the respiratory system is gas exchange, which involves the transfer of oxygen (O_2) and carbon dioxide (CO_2) between the atmosphere and the blood. To understand gas exchange, some knowledge of gas properties and the basic gas laws is essential. Gas is a substance as is a solid or a liquid and thus is composed of molecules of definable mass. Since the molecules are in constant motion, they exert pressure and generate heat or temperature. Finally, gas molecules must take up space and thus have volume.

Mass is an intrinsic property of matter and exists irrespective of gravity. For a gas, mass is represented by the size and the number of its molecules. When acted on by gravity, the molecules have weight. An oxygen molecule on earth and in outer space have the same mass, but only the former has weight.

Temperature (T) is a physical property of all gases. The higher the temperature, the faster the gas molecules move. The temperature scale used in the gas laws is in degrees Kelvin (the centigrade temperature plus 273). In the Kelvin (K) scale, 0 degrees is absolute zero or $-273°$ Celsius (C); $0°$ C = $273°$ K; $37°$ C = $310°$ K.

Pressure (P) is determined by the frequency of random motion of gas molecules against a surface; in pulmonary physiology, gas pressures are given in millimeters of mercury (mm Hg). (Some texts use the term torr instead of mm Hg; one torr = 1 mm Hg.) At sea level, air pressure will support a column of mercury 760 mm high; hence the atmospheric pressure at sea level is 760 mm Hg (Fig. 2-1). Gases also exert a pressure when dissolved in liquid. Gas pressure in a liquid is sometimes called the gas *tension;* in this context pressure and tension are interchangeable terms.

Water vapor is water in its gas phase. Like any dry gas, water vapor exerts a pressure. The vapor pressure is a function of temperature only. The relationship between water vapor pressure and temperature is shown in Table 2-1.

Inspired air is fully saturated with water vapor in the upper airway; at $37°$ C (normal body temperature) water vapor pressure is approximately 47 mm Hg. Water vapor pressure must be subtracted from the total gas pressure before calculating the individual dry gas pressures. For example, dry air

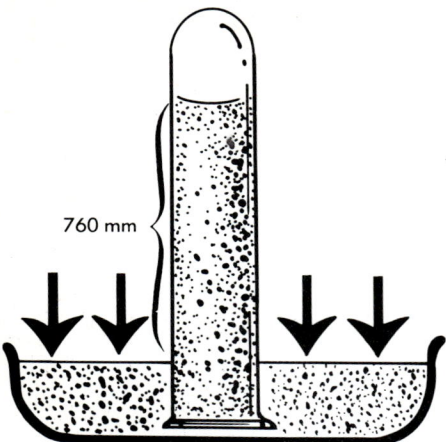

Fig. 2-1. Sea level air pressure will support a column of mercury 760 mm high. A long tube with one end closed is filled with mercury and is inverted over a pan of mercury. The height of the column of mercury equals the air pressure *(arrows)*. The space between the top of the column and the closed end of the tube is a vacuum that is created as the mercury falls to reach its equilibrium with the atmosphere.

Table 2-1. Water vapor pressure at various temperatures

Temperature (° C)	Water vapor pressure (mm Hg)*
20	17.54
21	18.65
22	19.83
23	21.07
24	22.38
25	23.76
26	25.21
27	26.74
28	28.35
29	30.04
30	31.82
31	33.70
32	35.66
33	37.73
34	39.90
35	42.18
36	44.56
37	47.07
38	49.69
39	52.44
40	55.32

*Fully saturated. In a completely dry environment, water vapor pressure is 0.

at sea level has a total pressure of 760 mm Hg. Since airways are open to the atmosphere, airway pressure also equals 760 mm Hg. As water vapor pressure is added to inspired air, the total dry gas pressure falls by a like amount. The final dry gas pressure in the airways is a result of the barometric pressure minus the water vapor pressure; at sea level this is 760 − 47 = 713 mm Hg.

Volume (V) is the space occupied by a gas. Unlike liquids and solids, gas is compressible; its volume is determined by whatever container it happens to occupy. Since gas molecules are in constant motion, a given mass of gas will expand to fill its container. As a mass of gas is expanded or contracted (i.e., as its volume changes), pressure and temperature will change according to the gas laws.

THE ATMOSPHERE

Earth is surrounded by a layer of atmosphere several hundred miles deep (Fig. 2-2). The atmosphere contains the earth's air, which is a mixture of gases. Nitrogen and oxygen are by far its most abundant gases; all other gases together make up less than 1% of the air. Certain laws govern the way these gases behave, whether the gases are free in the atmosphere or are contained within the lungs. Dalton's law of partial pressures states that each of the separate gases within a mixture exerts its own individual or *partial pressure* and that the total pressure of a gas mixture equals the sum of the individual or partial pressures.

According to Dalton's law, the sum of the individual gas pressures in the air equals the total atmospheric (barometric) pressure. Oxygen, which makes up almost 21% of the air, exerts a partial pressure of 159 mm Hg in dry air at sea level (Table

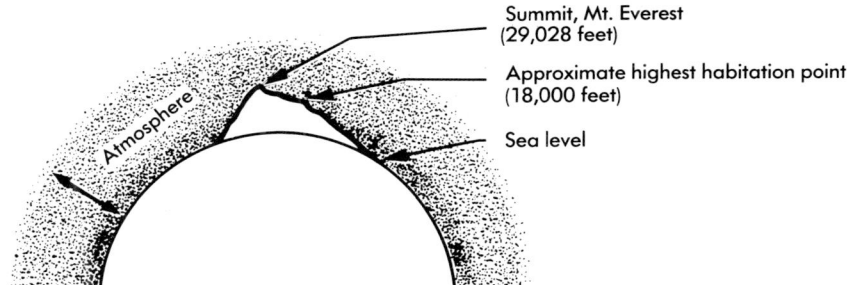

Fig. 2-2. The earth is surrounded by a layer of air, the atmosphere (not drawn to scale). Because of reduced oxygen pressure with increasing altitude, habitation is possible only within the first 18,000 feet of atmosphere. The closer air is to the surface of the earth, the more a given volume of air weighs and the greater the pressure it exerts. The greater the air pressure, the greater the pressure of its component gases, including oxygen.

Table 2-2. Composition of air

Gas	Percentage of dry gas*	Sea level partial pressure for dry air (mm Hg)	Sea level partial pressure when H_2O vapor is 47 mm Hg
Nitrogen	78.084	593.44	556.74
Oxygen	20.948	159.20	149.36
Argon	0.934	7.10	6.66
Carbon dioxide	0.031	0.24	0.22
Other gases†	0.003	0.02	0.02
Water vapor	0	0	47
Total percentage	100.00		
Total dry gas pressure		760	713
Total barometric pressure		760	760

*Percentage is the same throughout the breathable atmosphere.
†Neon, helium, krypton, xenon, hydrogen, ozone, nitrous oxide, and methane.

2-2). If nitrogen were removed from the atmosphere, the remaining oxygen would still exert 159 mm Hg pressure.

Since air is made up of matter, it is affected by gravity just like any solid or liquid. The closer air is to the surface of the earth, the more a given volume of air weighs. Air is also denser and exerts greater pressure the closer it is to earth. Conversely, with increasing altitude a given volume of air weighs less, exerts less pressure, and contains fewer gas molecules. In Denver (1 mile altitude) there is 1 mile less of the total atmosphere to press down on a surface; at this altitude atmospheric pressure is only 640 mm Hg, and oxygen pressure is 0.21(640) or 134 mm Hg (Fig. 2-3). At 18,000 feet, the highest altitude at which people have settled, atmospheric pressure is 380 mm Hg and oxygen pressure is 0.21(380) or 80 mm Hg.

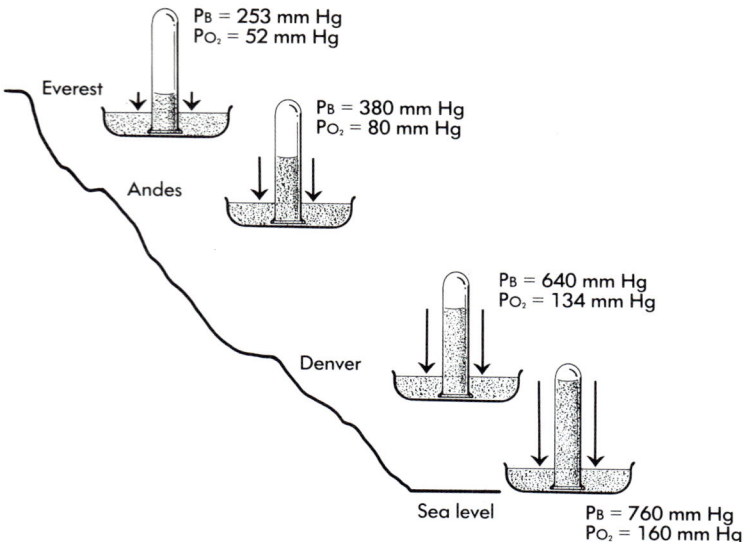

Fig. 2-3. Effects of altitude on barometric pressure. The height of the column of mercury that is supported by air decreases with increasing altitude, indicating a decreasing barometric pressure (P_B). P_{O_2} is the partial pressure of oxygen in dry air. Since $P_{O_2} = 0.21 \times P_B$, P_{O_2} also decreases with altitude.

The *fraction* of each gas in the air does not change with the altitude, at least throughout the breathable atmosphere. Since the atmospheric pressure decreases with altitude, each individual gas pressure must also decrease. The decrease in oxygen pressure with altitude explains why people can only live in the first few miles of the atmosphere (Fig. 2-3).

Clinical problem 1

What is the partial pressure of atmospheric oxygen at the top of Mt. Everest (29,028 ft), where barometric pressure equals 253 mm Hg? Could a person make it to the top of the mountain without supplemental oxygen?

In addition to fixed percentages of dry gases, air usually contains some water vapor. By definition, dry air contains no water vapor. Perfectly dry air is unusual and is confined mainly to desert areas. When air exposed to water is fully saturated, water vapor pressure is dependent only on temperature (Table 2-1). Water vapor pressure must be subtracted from the gas pressure before calculating partial pressure of dry gases (Table 2-2).

GAS LAWS*

One important gas law, that of Dalton, was presented previously. Mathematically, Dalton's law is expressed as:

$$P_T = P_1 + P_2 + P_3 + \ldots + P_n \quad (1)$$

where P_T is the total pressure of a gas mixture, and where P_1, P_2, P_3, and P_n are pressures of the

---

*These gas laws assume that the mass (number of molecules) of the gas remains constant and that temperature conditions are close to the physiologic range that encompasses room air (25° C) and body (37° C) conditions. Gas behavior deviates from these laws at extremes of temperature.

individual component gases. For the atmosphere, the total pressure is barometric pressure (P_B):

$$P_B = P_{N_2} + P_{O_2} + P_{H_2O} + P_{CO_2} \qquad (2)$$

where P_{N_2} represents nitrogen plus all other inert gases, and where P_{O_2}, P_{H_2O} and P_{CO_2} are the partial pressures of oxygen, water vapor, and carbon dioxide, respectively.

Another law relates to Avogadro's number, 6.02×10^{23}. This is the number of molecules in a mass of gas equal to its gram molecular weight. For example, since oxygen has a molecular weight of 32, 32 grams of oxygen contain 6.02×10^{23} oxygen molecules; nitrogen molecular weight is 28, so 28 grams of nitrogen contain 6.02×10^{23} nitrogen molecules. *Avogadro's law* states that equal volumes of gases at the same temperature and pressure contain the same number of molecules. At 273° K and 760 mm Hg pressure, this number of molecules will always occupy 22.4 L.

The next three laws relate the changes that occur in gas pressure, temperature, and volume.

Boyle's law.* If temperature is constant, pressure exerted by the gas varies inversely with the volume of the gas.

$$P \simeq \frac{1}{V} \qquad (3)$$

Result of Boyle's law: If either pressure or volume changes and if temperature remains constant, the product of pressure and volume remains constant,

$$P_1 V_1 = P_2 V_2 \qquad (4)$$

Charles' law. If pressure is constant, volume and temperature vary proportionately.

$$V \simeq T \qquad (5)$$

---

*$\simeq$, Is proportional to. In equation 4 and in subsequent equations, the number *1* after *P*, *V*, or *T* represents the initial pressure, volume, or temperature; the number *2* represents the final pressure, volume, or temperature.

Result of Charles' law: If either temperature or volume changes and pressure remains constant,

$$\frac{V_1}{T_1} = \frac{V_2}{T_2} \qquad (6)$$

General gas law. The two gas laws can be combined into the general gas law.

$$\frac{P_1 V_1}{T_1} = \frac{P_2 V_2}{T_2} \qquad (7)$$

ATPS, BTPS, AND STPD

The general gas law is useful for converting gas volumes collected under one set of conditions to a new volume for a different set of conditions. For example, when vital capacity is measured, the spirometer records volume under room air, not body, conditions. Body temperature and water vapor pressure are normally 37° C and 47 mm Hg, respectively; these conditions are referred to as *b*ody *t*emperature and *p*ressure *s*aturated (BTPS). Room air conditions are referred to as *a*mbient *t*emperature and *p*ressure *s*aturated (ATPS); typical ATPS conditions for temperature and water vapor pressure are 25° C and 24 mm Hg. The total air pressure under BTPS and ATPS is the same—the barometric pressure at the time the gas is collected.

To convert a volume of air collected in the spirometer to BTPS conditions, the general gas law (Equation 7) is used. Consider the collection of gas under ATPS conditions at sea level. By what factor is the collected gas volume converted to BTPS conditions?

ATPS conditions

V_1 = Volume of gas collected by spirometer
T_1 = 25° C + 273° = 298° K
P_1 = Barometric pressure minus water vapor pressure at T_1 (barometric pressure at sea level is 760 mm Hg; water vapor pressure at 25° C is 24 mm Hg)
   = 760 mm Hg − 24 mm Hg = 736 mm Hg

BTPS conditions

V_2 = Volume of gas to be determined
T_2 = 37° C + 273° = 310° K
P_2 = Barometric pressure minus water vapor pressure at T_2 (barometric pressure at sea level is 760 mm Hg; water vapor pressure at 37° C is 47 mm Hg)
  = 760 mm Hg − 47 mm Hg = 713 mm Hg

To calculate V_2, the BTPS volume, the known information is substituted into the general gas law (equation 7). Rearranging equation 7 to solve for V_2 is done as follows:

$$V_2 = \frac{V_1 P_1}{T_1} \times \frac{T_2}{P_2}$$
$$= V_1 \times \frac{T_2}{T_1} \times \frac{P_1}{P_2}$$
$$= V_1 \times \frac{310}{298} \times \frac{736}{713}$$
$$= V_1 \times 1.07$$

Since temperature and water vapor pressure values are generally less in a room than in the body, a given volume of gas collected *outside* the body will occupy a smaller volume than when it is *in the lungs*. Any spirometric volume collected under the conditions listed previously must be multiplied by 1.07 to obtain the corresponding BTPS volume.

In clinical practice, the exact conversion factor is not calculated every time a spirometric volume is collected unless a computer routine is used. If ATPS conditions do not vary greatly from day to day, the same factor (e.g., 1.07) can be used all the time. Whatever the practice in a particular laboratory, it is important to keep in mind the difference between ATPS and BTPS conditions as well as how gas volumes are affected by changes in temperature.

Clinical problem 2

A medical student has her vital capacity measured by a spirometer that provides a tracing of the effort plus a computer printout of the results. From the spirometric tracing, she calculates her vital capacity as 5.4 L. The computer printout states her vital capacity is 5.8 L. Which value is correct?

Gases that undergo a chemical reaction in the body, such as oxygen and carbon dioxide, are reported under conditions of *s*tandard *t*emperature and *p*ressure, *d*ry (STPD): 0° C, 760 mm Hg, and no water vapor pressure. For example, a normal resting oxygen uptake per minute is 250 ml, STPD. One can make conversions among STPD, BTPS, and ATPS using the same general gas law (Equation 7).

Clinical problem 3

A patient's oxygen uptake, when measured in a laboratory where the room temperature is 25° C and the barometric pressure is 747 mm Hg, is 327 ml/min. Assuming that the patient has normal body temperature, what is his oxygen uptake under STPD conditions?

GASES IN SOLUTION

The laws presented previously deal with dry gases or with gases saturated with water vapor. When a liquid is exposed to a gas and when there is no barrier to diffusion, gas molecules move into the liquid and exist in a dissolved state. A gas will dissolve into a liquid until the gas partial pressure in the liquid equals the gas partial pressure above the liquid, at which point equilibrium is established.

Henry's law states that, at equilibrium, the quantity of gas dissolved in a liquid at a given temperature is proportional to the partial pressure of the gas in the gas phase. This law does not state how much of the gas, in quantitative terms, will dissolve in solution, only that the quantity is proportional to the gas phase partial pressure. Henry's law also does not account for the chemical combination of the gas, e.g., oxygen with hemoglobin; oxygen that is chemically bound to hemoglobin no longer exerts a gas pressure.

The distinction between pressure and quantity is extremely important and is often a source of confusion. Consider a sample of blood with a P_{O_2} of

Table 2-3. Distinction between gas pressure and content

	Gas pressure	Gas content
Gas phase	Results from movement of gas molecules	Number of molecules per unit volume; directly proportional to gas pressure
Liquid phase	Equal to gas pressure in gas phase (at equilibrium)	Number of molecules, both dissolved in solution and chemically bound (if applicable); dissolved fraction depends on temperature and on gas solubility constant
Units	mm Hg (torr), for both gas and liquid	ml gas/unit gas volume (gas phase); ml gas/100 ml liquid (liquid phase)

100 mm Hg. How much oxygen is in the sample? To answer this question two other factors must be considered: the amount of gas dissolved in solution and the amount chemically bound. The amount of any gas dissolved in solution depends on the gas pressure *and* on the solubility of the gas in that particular liquid. Solubility, in turn, depends on the temperature and on the solubility constant of the gas in the liquid. These relationships can be expressed as:

$$\frac{\text{Volume of dissolved gas}}{\text{Volume of liquid}} = P \times K$$

where P is the partial pressure of the gas and K is the solubility constant. For example, the solubility of oxygen in plasma at normal body temperature is 0.003 ml O_2/100 ml plasma/mm Hg P_{O_2}.

Clinical problem 4

What is the partial pressure of oxygen and the oxygen content in 100 ml of plasma when exposed to air under the following conditions: barometric pressure, 760 mm Hg; water vapor pressure, 27 mm Hg; fraction of oxygen, 21%? If hemoglobin is added to the plasma to give a hemoglobin concentration of 10 grams%, what will the P_{O_2} be? Will the P_{O_2} change if the hemoglobin concentration is raised to 15 grams%?

Table 2-3 outlines the major differences between gas pressure and content for both the gas and the liquid phases.

BREATHING—AN OVERVIEW OF GAS EXCHANGE

Breathing is a physiologic function, and any disorder in this function is usually obvious. "Catch my breath," "out of breath," and "short of breath" are but a few phrases commonly used to indicate breathing trouble. Fortunately, the breathing process is automatic and does not have to be thought about. The respiratory system responds to meet the body's metabolic needs whether we are resting or exercising.

The body's metabolic needs include a continuous supply of oxygen and elimination of carbon dioxide. To accomplish this gas exchange, the respiratory system consists of three integrated components (Fig. 2-4): the control system that regulates breathing, including portions of the central nervous system plus peripheral receptors that send signals to the central nervous system; the chest bellows apparatus that contains the lungs and is responsible for their expansion and contraction; and the lungs and airways (Fig. 2-5).

The central nervous system area that regulates breathing is located in the brainstem, an area more

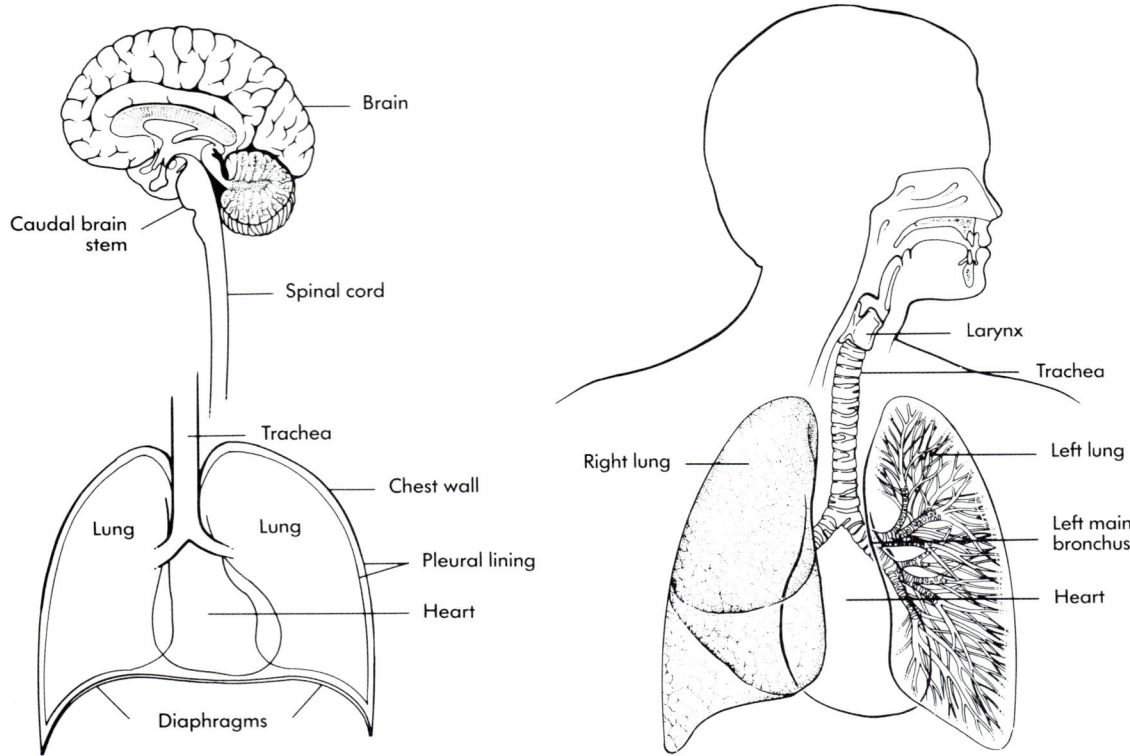

Fig. 2-4. The respiratory system components, which include the central nervous system structures that control ventilation; the chest bellows, including rib cage and respiratory muscles; and the lungs and airways.

Fig. 2-5. The structure of the airways. Air enters through the mouth and nose and then travels down the larynx and trachea into the bronchial airways. The bronchi terminate in alveoli, each of which is surrounded by capillaries. Views of an alveolar-capillary unit are shown in Fig. 2-10.

primitive than the cortex (Fig. 2-4). Although brainstem control of breathing is automatic, it may be altered by drugs or disease. For example, a relatively common cause of respiratory failure is narcotic or sedative overdose.

The chest bellows component of the respiratory system includes the *thoracic cage,* which contains the lungs; the diaphragm, which is the major muscle of breathing; and the pleural membranes, which cover the lungs and line the inside of the thoracic cage. The thoracic cage consists of the ribs, which protect the lungs from injury; the muscles and connective tissues, which connect the ribs together; and all the nerves and blood vessels, which serve the muscles. Fig. 2-6 shows the rib cage along with the muscles of inspiration and expiration.

The lungs are the site of gas exchange. Although the lungs have some metabolic and hormonal functions, these functions, unlike gas exchange, are apparently not vital. Because the body does not store oxygen, total respiratory failure is fatal within minutes.

Gas exchange takes place passively across pressure gradients. In one sense this passive exchange

Structure and function

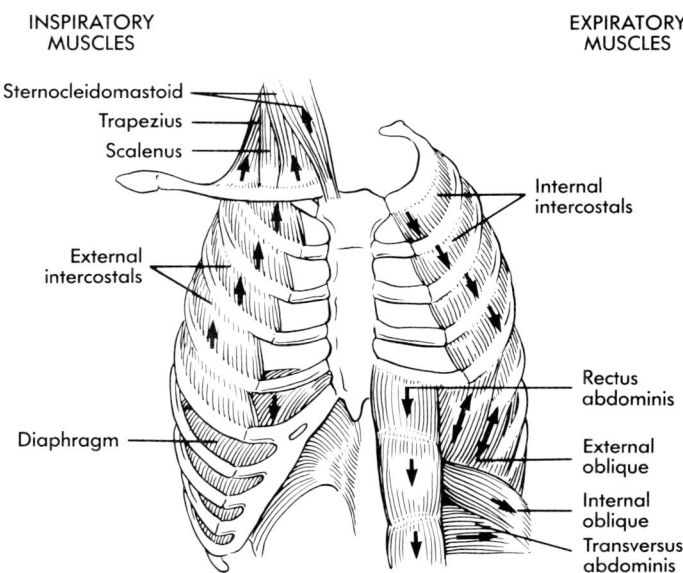

Fig. 2-6. Structure of the chest cage including the muscles of inspiration and expiration. In quiet breathing the diaphragm and the external intercostal muscles contract during inspiration and expand the rib cage and the lungs. Exhalation is passive. Heavy breathing uses the accessory muscles of inspiration: the sternocleidomastoid, trapezius, and scalenus muscles. Exhalation during heavy breathing employs the internal intercostal and abdominal muscles.

makes the physiology of gas exchange rather simple. But the lungs are not just two big bags connected to blood vessels. Gas exchange takes place across some 300,000,000 alveoli, with each one surrounded by a meshwork of pulmonary capillaries. The relationship of ventilation to perfusion in the millions of alveolar-capillary units determines the efficacy of gas exchange; when these units are diseased, ventilation-perfusion relationships, and hence gas exchange, can become greatly altered.

The following discussion divides the gas exchange function into its essential component parts: ventilation, diffusion, and circulation.

Ventilation

Approximately 10 to 16 times per minute while at rest, the midbrain control system sends impulses through the spinal cord to the diaphragm and the external intercostal muscles (Fig. 2-6); these muscles then contract. This contraction increases the volume of the thoracic cavity, an increase that, in turn, leads to expansion of the lungs. With lung expansion a breath of fresh air containing 21% oxygen and almost no carbon dioxide is inhaled (Fig. 2-7). Muscle contraction does not take place during quiet expiration (breathing that is unlabored and unforced); quiet expiration is a passive process in which the previously contracted muscles and expanded lungs relax into their resting position. (Other muscles come into play during forced inspiration and expiration; see Fig. 2-7).

To accomplish gas exchange the inhaled air is delivered through the branching airways (Fig. 2-5) to alveoli deep inside the lungs. The air first enters the mouth and nose, where many of the dust particles are filtered, purifying the air. Air from

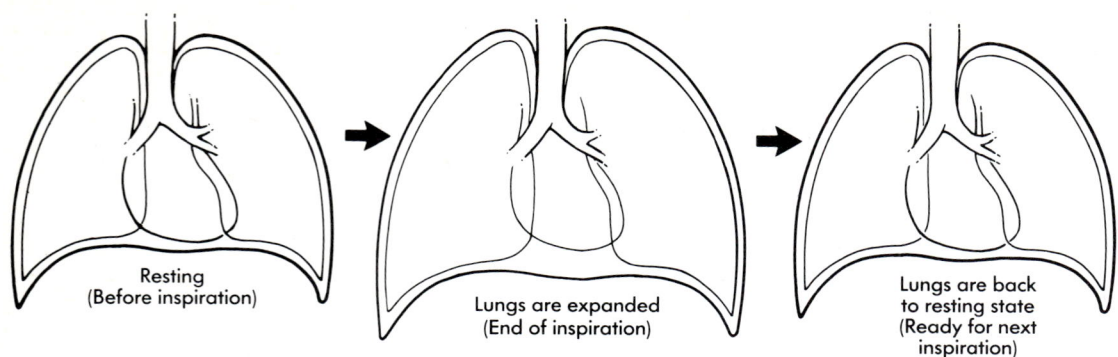

Fig. 2-7. Inspiration and expiration. A normal, quiet breathing cycle. This cycle is repeated approximately 10 to 16 times per minute. During inspiration fresh air, which is composed of 21% oxygen and negligible carbon dioxide, is inhaled. Muscles used include the diaphragm and the external intercostals. During expiration stale air, which is composed of approximately 17% oxygen and 4% carbon dioxide, is exhaled. Expiration is passive.

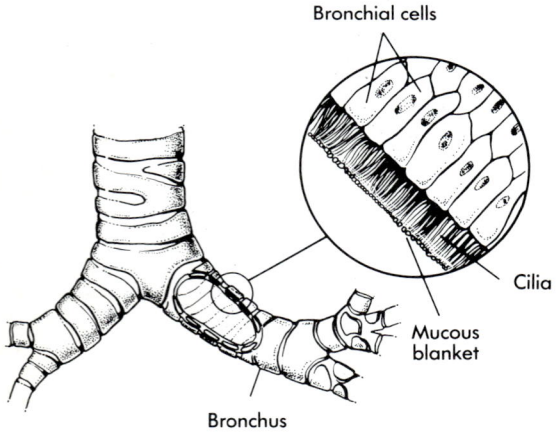

Fig. 2-8. Structure of the bronchus. Each bronchus is lined with tiny cilia that project into the airway lumen. The cilia are covered with a blanket of mucus that collects dust and other air pollutants. This mucous blanket, along with collected dust, is normally swept up and out of the airways by the cilia.

the mouth and nose come together in the throat and begin the journey toward the alveoli. The air first enters the larynx and then the trachea; the trachea then divides at the main carina into the right and left major bronchi. The trachea and major bronchi are lined with cartilage that provides a firm structure to keep the airways open during inspiration and expiration.

The airways above the carina are collectively called the upper airways or the upper respiratory system (Fig. 2-5). Air entering the upper airways is warmed to body temperature and is humidified with water vapor, which has a partial pressure of 47 mm Hg at normal body temperature (see Table 2-1).

The trachea and the main bronchi aid in keeping dust and other large particles from reaching the alveoli. Coughing is one way to clear the large airways of noxious material. In addition to the cough response, the bronchi function silently to mobilize dust and particles. A blanket of mucus lines the bronchi (Fig. 2-8); beneath this layer, rows of cilia constantly "sweep" the mucus, with its collected particles, out of the airways. When the mucus reaches the top of the trachea, it is usually swallowed.

Even if particles get past the airway defenses, alveolar macrophages can be mobilized to help digest foreign substances such as bacteria or tiny dust particles. All of these normal defense mechanisms may be damaged by chronic cigarette smoking, making smokers much more vulnerable to inhaled dusts. This damage is one reason why diseases such as asbestosis, silicosis, and pneumoconiosis tend to be much more severe in cigarette smokers. When disease affects airflow, diffusion, or pulmonary circulation, gas exchange may also be impaired.

The right and left major bronchi represent the first of over 20 divisions of airways (Fig. 2-5).

With each division the airways become narrower, but the total number of airways increases geometrically (Fig. 2-9). By the twentieth division, there is a huge number of individual airways. Also at the twentieth division, with the diameter of each airway less than 1 mm, alveoli begin to appear.

Each minute, an individual at rest breathes in (or out) approximately 6 L of fresh air, an amount known as the *minute ventilation*. About one third of this air stays in the mouth, throat, and large airways where no gas exchange takes place; collectively, this region is called the anatomic "dead space" because the air in the space does not transfer oxygen or carbon dioxide. The remaining 4 L of minute ventilation are distributed to the hundreds of millions of alveoli; the portion of this distribution that actually takes part in gas exchange is called the *alveolar ventilation*. Alveolar ventilation, a very important concept in clinical medicine, is discussed at length in Chapter 4.

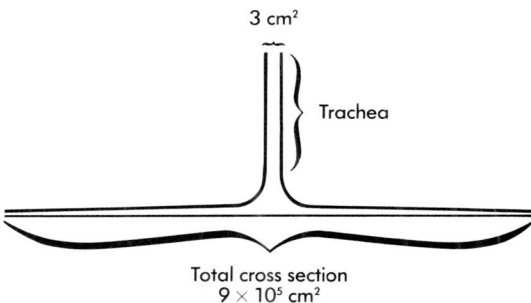

Fig. 2-9. Cross section of the airways. As the airways narrow with branching, the total cross-sectional area increases geometrically.

Pulmonary gas exchange takes place across the alveolar-capillary membrane where oxygen is delivered to, and carbon dioxide removed from, the capillary blood (Fig. 2-10, *A* and *B*). *Gas exchange converts the oxygen-poor blood entering the pulmonary capillary into oxygenated blood.*

At rest, approximately 250 ml of oxygen and 200 ml of carbon dioxide are exchanged per minute. The ratio of gas exchange is therefore 0.8. The

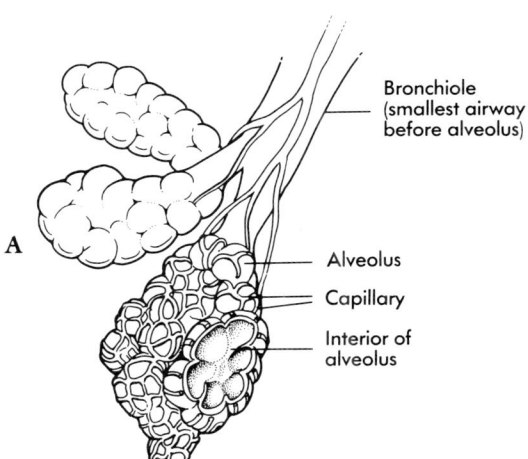

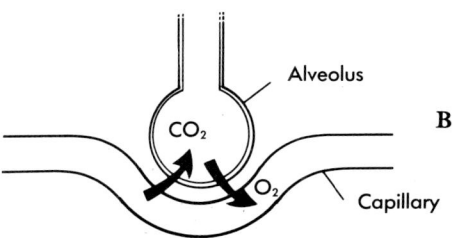

Fig. 2-10. **A**, Alveolar-capillary units. Each alveolar sac is surrounded by one or more pulmonary capillaries. This alveolar-capillary unit is where oxygen and carbon dioxide are exchanged with the atmosphere. **B**, A cross section of a single alveolus and capillary. As blood flows past the alveolus, carbon dioxide is given off and oxygen taken up.

amount of gas exchange and the ratio are dictated by the body's metabolic demands—how much oxygen the tissues need for metabolism and how much carbon dioxide is produced as a byproduct. The respiratory exchange ratio is an important consideration in pulmonary physiology and will come up again in later chapters.

Clinical problem 5

Suppose that at rest you have a minute ventilation of 6 L/min, an alveolar ventilation of 4 L/min, an oxygen uptake of 250 ml/min, and a carbon dioxide output of 200 ml/min. If you voluntarily hyperventilate to double your minute and alveolar ventilation, what will happen to your oxygen uptake and carbon dioxide output? Will they double?

After the lungs have expanded fully, the order from the central nervous system to inhale ceases, and the thoracic cage and the lungs passively return to their resting position. During this stage a breath of stale air is exhaled containing approximately 17% oxygen and 4% carbon dioxide (Fig. 2-7 and Table 2-4).

Diffusion

Oxygen from alveolar air diffuses across the alveolar-capillary membrane into capillaries surrounding the alveoli (Fig. 2-10). The combination of one alveolus (containing air) and its surrounding capillaries (containing blood) is the alveolar-capillary unit. In the capillary, oxygen enters first the plasma and then the red blood cell where it combines with hemoglobin (Fig. 2-11). At the same time carbon dioxide diffuses from the capillary blood into the alveoli and out of the lungs with each exhalation. The total surface area for diffusion is enormous (Fig. 2-9); flattened out and placed end to end, the alveolar membranes from two normal lungs would cover a tennis court.

Because gas molecules are in constant, random motion, as long as there is no physical impediment they always diffuse from a region of higher pressure to one of lower pressure. Diffusion is the only way oxygen and carbon dioxide are exchanged. There is no active transport of gases into or out of the blood. The gradient for diffusion changes along the capillary, being highest at the beginning (clos-

Table 2-4. Change in composition of inhaled dry air*

Gas	Atmosphere		Tracheal		Alveolar		Expired	
	Percent†	Pressure‡	Percent	Pressure	Percent	Pressure	Percent	Pressure
N_2§	79.02	600.6	79.02	563.4	80.1	571	79.0	584
O_2	20.95	159.2	20.95	149.4	14.3	102	17.2	127
CO_2	0.03	0.2	0.03	0.2	5.6	40	3.8	28
H_2O		0		47		47		21
Total Pressure		760		760		760		760

*Values in this table are approximations for a normal person at sea level. Actual values are dependent on barometric pressure, alveolar P_{CO_2}, water vapor pressure and, for expired air, the extent of the mix of alveolar air with inspired tracheal air.
†Percent of *dry* gas.
‡Partial pressure of gas, mm Hg.
§N_2, Argon and "Other gases" listed in Table 2-2.

est to a pulmonary artery) and lowest at the end (closest to a pulmonary vein). Initially, the oxygen gradient is: alveolar Po_2 − venous blood Po_2, or 102 − 40 = 60 mm Hg. The initial gradient for carbon dioxide is: venous blood Pco_2 − alveolar Pco_2, or 46 − 40 = 6 mm Hg.

Oxygen must traverse several barriers before gas exchange is completed: the alveolar cell, the interstitial tissue, the capillary membrane, the plasma, and finally the red blood cell (Fig. 2-11). Carbon dioxide must traverse the same structures but in the opposite direction. Carbon dioxide is approximately 20 times more diffusable than oxygen, and for practical purposes, it is never diffusion limited.

The following problem is based on blood gas measurements obtained from arterial and mixed venous blood; it can be solved by using the concept of gas diffusion discussed above.

Clinical problem 6

A series of blood gases is listed below. They are paired samples from both the radial artery (arterial oxygen pressure [Pao_2] and arterial carbon dioxide pressure [$Paco_2$]) and the pulmonary artery (venous oxygen pressure [Pvo_2] and venous carbon dioxide pressure [$Pvco_2$]), the latter representing mixed venous blood. Which of the three sets represents a measurement or technical error? (All values are in mm Hg.)
   a. Pao_2, 120; $Paco_2$, 40
      Pvo_2, 40; $Pvco_2$, 46
   b. Pao_2, 36; $Paco_2$, 33
      Pvo_2, 41; $Pvco_2$, 37
   c. Pao_2, 61; $Paco_2$, 40
      Pvo_2, 43; $Pvco_2$, 36

The diffusing capacity of the lungs for oxygen is also large and rarely limits capillary oxygenation. Thickening of any of the structures between the alveolar space and a capillary red blood cell can cause diffusion impairment, but not enough impairment to lower oxygen levels significantly. It is a common misconception that hypoxemia results from diffusion limitation. Studies have shown that this result does not occur in the resting state. During exercise, however, when blood flows through the lungs at a faster rate than normal, diffusion barrier can lead to significant hypoxemia. Nonetheless, at rest and during exercise, a much more common cause of hypoxemia is the mismatching of alveolar ventilation to capillary perfusion (see Chapter 5).

The pulmonary diffusing capacity can be measured in the laboratory using small amounts of inhaled carbon monoxide. This test and how it relates to oxygen diffusion is discussed in Chapter 5.

Circulation

The processes of bringing fresh air to the alveoli and transferring gases across the alveolar capillary membrane—alveolar ventilation and diffusion—are but two components of gas exchange. The other necessary component is pulmonary circulation.

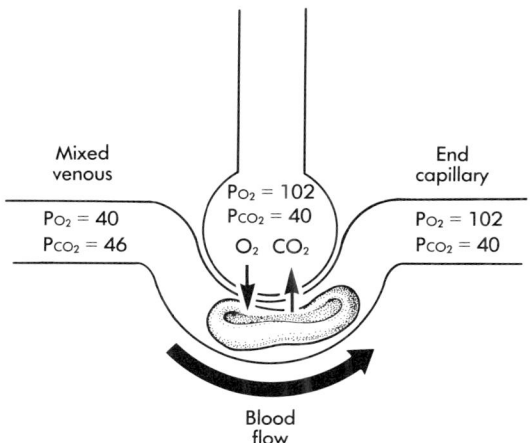

Fig. 2-11. Diffusion of oxygen and carbon dioxide. Gas exchange occurs solely by diffusion, from a region of relatively high gas pressure to one of relatively low gas pressure. For oxygen the initial diffusion gradient is 102 − 40 = 62 mm Hg; for carbon dioxide it is 46 − 40 = 6 mm Hg. The diffusion gradient for each gas decreases as blood moves along the capillary. Note that most of the oxygen that enters the capillary then enters the red cell to combine with hemoglobin. Most carbon dioxide is carried in the plasma either dissolved or as bicarbonate.

Each minute the heart pumps approximately 5 L of blood to the lungs, a cardiac output that is distributed among hundreds of millions of pulmonary capillaries. At any one time the total pulmonary capillary blood volume is only about 75 to 100 ml, roughly 2% of the cardiac output.

One alveolar sac is surrounded by many pulmonary capillaries in a meshwork arrangement (Fig. 2-10). The alveolus and its accompanying capillaries constitute the gas exchange unit. Not only must there be sufficient cardiac output to the lungs, but the output must be matched to the alveolar ventilation. Obviously, if there were no blood flow around the alveolus or if blood flow completely bypassed the alveolus, there could be no gas exchange. Lesser forms of mismatching are in fact the major cause of hypoxemia (see Chapter 5).

Circulation of the blood is, as its name indicates,

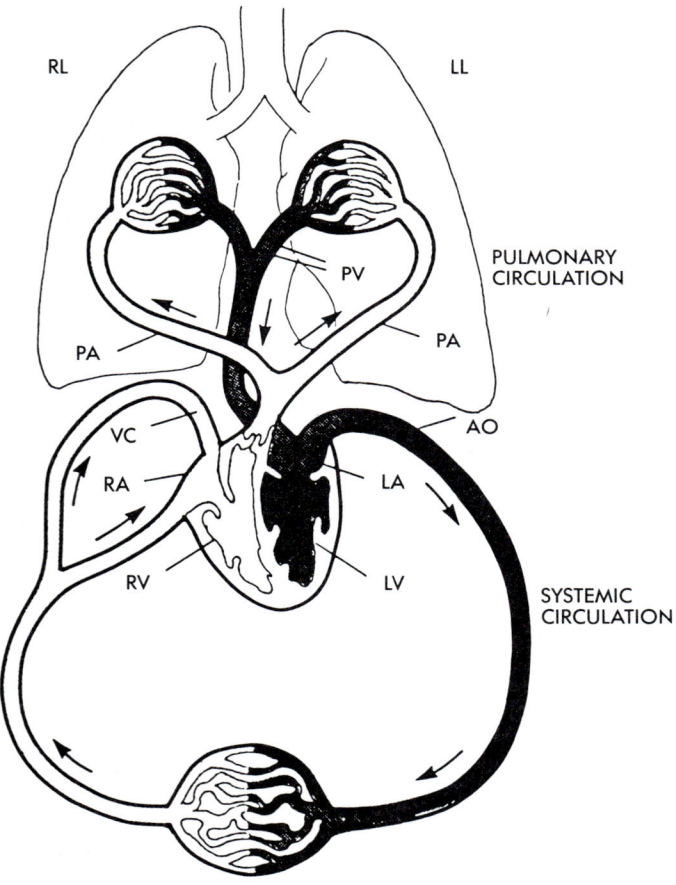

Fig. 2-12. Pulmonary and systemic circulation. Darkened portion of circulation represents arterial (oxygenated) blood and clear portion, venous (deoxygenated) blood. Arrows show direction of blood flow. (*RL*, right lung; *RV*, right ventricle; *RA*, right atrium; *VC*, vena cava; *PA*, pulmonary arteries; *PV*, pulmonary veins; *AO*, aorta; *LL*, left lung; *LV*, left ventricle; *LA*, left atrium.) (From Martin, L.,: Breathe easy: a guide to lung and respiratory diseases for patients and their families, © 1984, Prentice-Hall, Inc. Reprinted by permission of the publisher, Prentice-Hall, Inc., Englewood Cliffs, New Jersey.)

a circular affair (Fig. 2-12). Blood flowing to and from the lungs constitutes only one part of this circle. Arbitrarily, this discussion of the circle can start with one of the four heart chambers, the right atrium. From the right atrium venous blood goes to the right ventricle and then is pumped to the lungs where it receives a fresh supply of oxygen.

Right ventricular blood begins its journey to the lungs through the main pulmonary artery; this main artery then divides into two pulmonary arteries, with one going to each lung. Each of these arteries gives rise to many divisions, and in short order the blood is dispersed among the millions of pulmonary capillaries. The distance separating the alveolus from the capillary is very small so that oxygen is able to diffuse into the capillary while carbon dioxide is diffusing out (Fig. 2-11). The stale air is then exhaled, and fresh air is inhaled with the next breath (see Table 2-4).

Oxygenated blood from the millions of pulmonary capillaries travels through the pulmonary veins to the left atrium and then to the left ventricle. (Note that pulmonary *arteries* carry venous or deoxygenated blood and pulmonary *veins* carry oxygenated or arterial blood, a situation that is reversed in the systemic circulation.) Oxygenated blood is then pumped from the left ventricle through the arteries to all the muscles, tissues, and organs; this movement constitutes the systemic circulation (Fig. 2-12).

After entering the target organ or tissue, each systemic artery divides into thinner and thinner vessels, the smallest of which is the systemic capillary. These capillaries are structurally similar to the pulmonary capillaries and have the same function: to allow gas exchange to occur across a diffusion gradient. In the lung, oxygen diffuses into the capillaries and carbon dioxide diffuses out. In the systemic capillaries oxygen diffuses *out* of the capillary, and carbon dioxide diffuses *into* the capillary. In this way oxygen is delivered for cellular metabolism and carbon dioxide, a waste product of metabolism, is removed.

Blood entering the systemic (nonpulmonary) capillary is oxygenated. When blood leaves the systemic capillary it is relatively deoxygenated (venous). The venous blood vessels merge to form larger and larger veins; eventually all the systemic veins come together to form two great veins, the superior vena cava (carrying blood from the head and neck) and the inferior vena cava (carrying blood from the rest of the body). Both vena cavae enter the heart at the right atrium. Right atrial blood enters the right ventricle and is then pumped to the lungs to once again become saturated with oxygen. The circuit is complete.

Thus gas exchange occurs not only in the lungs but in all of the body's tissues. This exchange requires ventilation which is provided by breathing adequate amounts of fresh air, diffusion, which occurs by virtue of pressure gradients, and circulation, which is provided by the heart's pumping blood to the lungs and then throughout the body.

LUNG DISEASE AND THE RESPIRATORY SYSTEM

In good health this breathing cycle with its integration of alveolar ventilation, diffusion, and pulmonary circulation is silent, automatic, and effortless. In the process, oxygen is delivered from the atmosphere into the blood, and carbon dioxide is excreted from the blood into the atmosphere.

Although respiratory disease is often thought of as synonymous with lung disease, malfunction of any component of the system can cause a respiratory problem. For example, central nervous system depression can cause total system failure even though the lungs are functioning normally. In poliomyelitis (a common disease before the poliomyelitis vaccine), respiratory failure can result from involvement of the lower motor neurons serving the thoracic muscles; the brain and lungs can be intact, but the chest cage is paralyzed.

Thus all parts of the respiratory system must work correctly in order for normal breathing to occur. Despite the importance of all the respiratory system components, there is a good reason why the lungs are usually thought of when one hears about respiratory disease: lung disease does account for the vast majority of respiratory illness. Emphysema, bronchitis, asthma, pneumonia, and lung cancer all originate in the lungs. The lungs are the only internal organ in direct contact with the atmosphere, making them vulnerable to air pollutants, including cigarette smoke, airborne viruses, and bacteria. Almost all clinical cases of hypoxemia are caused by lung disease. Most respiratory illness is in fact *lung disease,* and most lung disease is accompanied by an altered physiology.

SUMMARY

The main function of the respiratory system is gas exchange, which is the transfer of oxygen and carbon dioxide between the atmosphere and the blood. The atmosphere is made up of approximately 78% nitrogen, 21% oxygen, and 1% miscellaneous gases. The fraction of each gas is the same throughout the breathable atmosphere, but the pressure of each gas falls with increasing altitude because of the fall in barometric pressure. Thus the inspired P_{O_2} is lower the higher one ascends, and humans can live up to an altitude of approximately 18,000 feet without receiving supplemental oxygen.

The gas laws define the behavior of gases under ideal conditions. The general gas law states that, for a given mass of gas, the product of pressure times volume over temperature is a constant value. Thus if pressure increases, the volume of the gas must decrease or its temperature must increase. This law is useful for converting a gas volume that is collected under one set of conditions to a new volume for a different set of conditions, e.g., converting the volume of air collected in a spirometer (ambient temperature and pressure) to the true volume of the gas in the subject's lungs (body temperature and pressure).

Gas pressure is distinguished from gas content. Gas content is the number of molecules per unit volume, whether in the gas or liquid phase, and it is measured in ml gas/unit volume. Gas pressure is caused by the movement of molecules and is measured in mm Hg. At equilibrium, the pressure of gas in a liquid equals the pressure of the gas overlying the liquid (in the gas phase).

The respiratory system consists of three integrated components: the control system that regulates breathing, the chest bellows apparatus, and the lungs. Dysfunction in any component can affect breathing and gas exchange. Gas exchange can be further divided into the physiologic processes of ventilation, diffusion, and circulation. In healthy people the normal breathing cycle, with its integration of these physiologic processes, is silent, automatic, and effortless.

REVIEW QUESTIONS

State whether each of the following is true or false.
1. A steady state exists when pulmonary gas exchange equals metabolic gas exchange.
2. Boyle's law states that when pressure is held constant, the volume and temperature of a fixed mass of gas are inversely related.
3. According to the law of partial pressures, the pressure of a gas in a mixture of gases is exerted independently from the other gases present.
4. Diffusion impairment is a common physiologic cause of hypoxemia.
5. The gas exchange unit consists of a single alveolus and its surrounding capillaries.
6. The higher the altitude, the lower the concentration of oxygen in inspired air.
7. The total surface area of the alveolar membranes is about 2 square meters.
8. Alveolar ventilation is defined as the volume of air that reaches the alveoli each minute.
9. The measured vital capacity must be multiplied by a factor greater than one to obtain the true vital capacity.
10. Under ATPS conditions, sea level barometric pressure is 760 mm Hg.

References

Pulmonary terms and symbols: a report of the ACCP-ATS Joint Committee on Pulmonary Nomenclature, Chest **67:**583, 1975.
See also General References (Physiology) in Appendix G.

chapter 3

Lung mechanics

OUTLINE

Breathing—a mechanical function
Pressure, volume, and flow
Generation of airway pressures
Lung compliance
Airway resistance
Lung volumes and capacities
Functional residual capacity
Forced vital capacity
Flow-volume curves and loops
Determinants of expiratory airflow
Small airways disease and dynamic compliance
Clinical value of using spirometry
Patterns of respiratory disease
Interpretation of spirometry
Mechanics and gas exchange—correlation?

BREATHING—A MECHANICAL FUNCTION

The previous chapter presented an overview of normal breathing with an emphasis on gas exchange. To bring in fresh air, the lungs and chest bellows must alternately expand and contract—the act of breathing. *Lung mechanics* is the study of this thoracic cage/lung movement and the resultant flow of air in and out of the lungs.

This discussion of lung mechanics begins with a review of respiration vis-à-vis the atmosphere.

The earth is surrounded by a sea of air that, for a given altitude, is at constant barometric pressure.* Because human airways are open to the atmosphere, average or mean airway pressure must equal the barometric or atmospheric pressure, e.g., 760 mm Hg at sea level. When airway pressure is more or less than barometric pressure, the lungs empty or fill, respectively, until airway pressure equalizes.

Air contains approximately 78% nitrogen and 21% oxygen, with its other 1% comprising a small amount of carbon dioxide plus some rare gases (see Table 2-2). The constant movement of the gas molecules is not sufficient to propel air into the lungs. Although there is an approximate 60 mm Hg difference between the atmospheric and the alveolar oxygen pressure, diffusion of oxygen down the airways does not occur to any appreciable extent. Air must reach the alveoli in some other manner.

Breathing is possible because of transient pressure changes in the airways. Unimpeded by a barrier, air will always move from a region of higher pressure to one of lower pressure; this movement occurs in the airways. During inspiration, airway and alveolar pressures are slightly less than atmospheric pressure, resulting in a net flow of air

---

*Minor fluctuations in barometric pressure at a given altitude are not clinically important.

into the lungs. During expiration, the opposite occurs—airway and alveolar pressures are slightly greater than atmospheric pressure, and air flows out of the lungs.

PRESSURE, VOLUME, AND FLOW

Reduced to basics, lung mechanics is the study of pressure, volume, and flow.

Pressure is the force per unit area acting against a surface. For gases, pressure is generated by the constant, random movement of gas molecules. At sea level air pressure is 760 mm Hg (see Fig. 2-1). Although air pressure is usually quoted in mm Hg, *airway pressures* are commonly recorded in centimeters of water. Because of potential confusion, the units should always be specified. Since the density of mercury is 13.6 × the density of water and since 1 cm = 10 × 1 mm, the conversion factor from mm Hg to cm H_2O is 1.36. Thus 760 mm Hg is equivalent to 1034 cm H_2O.

Volume in lung mechanics represents a quantity of air. The volume of a given mass of gas is dependent on its pressure and its temperature (general gas law; see Chapter 2). Lung volumes are generally measured under ATPS conditions and then are converted to either BTPS or STPD (see Chapter 2). Regardless of the conditions of measurement, the units for volume are milliliters (ml) or liters (L).

Flow is volume per time—the volume of air that flows past a given point in a specified time period. In pulmonary physiology the time frame is either seconds or minutes; units of flow are ml/sec, ml/min, L/sec, or L/min.

GENERATION OF AIRWAY PRESSURES

Atmospheric pressure in pulmonary physiology is assigned a value of 0; any pressure less than atmospheric pressure is then negative and any pressure greater is positive. By referencing all pressures to 0, much smaller numbers are possible than when

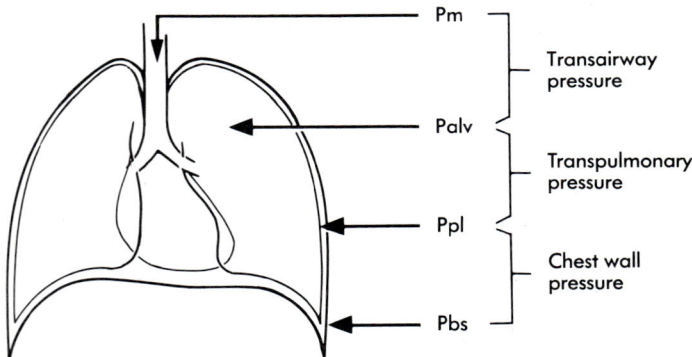

Fig. 3-1. Respiratory pressures—transmural pressures in chest. Transairway = Pm − Palv = pressure driving air into or out of the lungs. Transpulmonary = Palv − Ppl = pressure tending to inflate or deflate the lungs; under static conditions (no air flow), transpulmonary pressure is the same as elastic recoil pressure of the lungs. Chest wall = Ppl − Pbs = pressure tending to expand or contract the chest cavity. Transthoracic = Palv − Pbs = pressure tending to inflate or deflate the lungs and chest wall together. (*Pm*, pressure at the mouth [usually atmospheric pressure]; *Palv*, pressure in alveoli [intrapulmonary pressure]; *Ppl*, pressure in pleural space [intrapleural pressure]; *Pbs*, pressure at body surface [atmospheric pressure].)

Lung mechanics

pressures are recorded in absolute values (e.g., 10 mm Hg vs. 770 mm Hg).

Understanding lung mechanics requires some appreciation of pressure differences within the respiratory system; these differences are defined and diagramed in Fig. 3-1. Changes in pressure and in the resulting airflow during quiet breathing are shown in Fig. 3-2. During a single breathing interval (fresh air in, stale air out), oxygen and carbon dioxide are exchanged between the alveolus and pulmonary capillary.

During normal quiet breathing, alveolar pressure is slightly negative at midinspiration and is slightly positive at midexpiration (Fig. 3-2). The changes in alveolar pressure allow fresh air to enter during inspiration and stale air to exit during expiration.

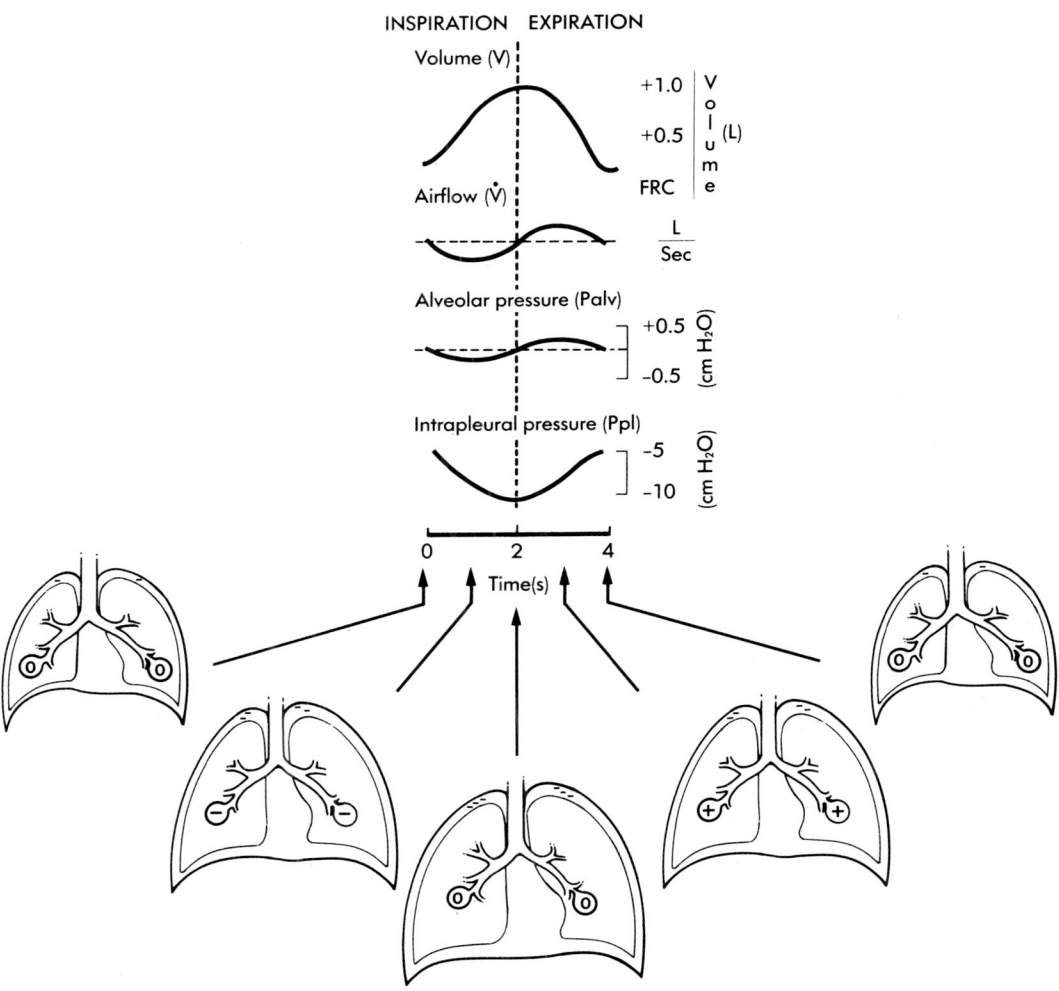

Fig. 3-2. Changes in pressure, volume, and flow during a single breath.

The changes in airway pressure are relatively small compared to total atmospheric pressure. No matter how large the changes in airway pressure are, the *average airway pressure* during spontaneous breathing always equals the atmospheric pressure.

The one area where airway pressure does not equal that of the atmosphere is in the pleural space.* The pleural space is not open to the atmosphere, and its pressure reflects the forces pulling on the pleural membranes. At rest the thoracic cage tends to expand and the lungs to contract. The result is that in normal quiet breathing, during both inspiration and expiration, intrapleural pressure is always negative, i.e., subatmospheric. Intrapleural pressure changes from approximately -5 cm H_2O at end-expiration to -10 cm H_2O at end-inspiration (Fig. 3-2). As intrapleural pressure becomes more negative and the lung expands, airway and alveolar pressures decrease, resulting in movement of air into the lungs.

LUNG COMPLIANCE

Pressure, volume, and flow are components of two important physiologic concepts: lung compliance (C_L) and airways resistance (R_{aw}). Their definitions are summarized in Table 3-1.

Lung compliance is the change in volume per change in distending pressure. C_L reflects the ease with which the lungs expand—their distensibility or, conversely, their stiffness. The higher the C_L, the greater the air volume that can be inhaled for a given change in distending pressure and the more distensible (less stiff) the lungs.

Lung compliance measurement

The volume of air needed for lung compliance measurement is simply the amount of air that is inhaled for a given change in distending pressure. The distending pressure is *transpulmonary*, i.e., the pressure difference *across* the lung, which is the difference between alveolar pressure and intrapleural pressure (Fig. 3-1). Compliance is determined at the point of zero airflow, i.e., during transient breathholding. When there is no airflow, alveolar pressure equals zero,* and transpulmonary pressure equals the absolute magnitude of intrapleural pressure. Thus under static conditions:

$$C_L = \frac{\text{Change in volume}}{\text{Change in intrapleural pressure}} \quad (1)$$

In the laboratory, intrapleural pressure is usually obtained indirectly, by measuring esophageal pressure. A balloon-tipped tube, which is swallowed by the patient and retained in his esophagus, is connected to a pressure transducer that records intraesophageal pressure; this pressure has been found to equal or closely approximate intrapleural pressure. Because the test is uncomfortable for most patients, it is rarely performed except for research purposes. A normal pressure-volume curve generated in this manner is shown in Fig. 3-3, *A*.

Fig. 3-3, *B* shows compliance curves from patients with emphysema and with lung fibrosis; these curves are compared with one from a healthy person. In the patient with emphysema, the lungs have lost some of their elastic recoil because of the destruction of alveolar-capillary membranes; as a result, the lungs are more easily expanded by a given amount of distending pressure. In the patient with pulmonary fibrosis, the lung interstitium is infiltrated with scar tissue; compared to normal lungs, fibrotic lungs are stiffer and hence bring in less air for a given change in pressure.

Clinical problem 1

A patient inhales 3 L of air and holds his breath for a second with his glottis open. At the beginning of inspiration, his esophageal pressure is -5 cm H_2O; during breath-holding his esophageal pressure is measured at -30 cm H_2O. What is his lung compliance? Is it normal?

---

*Actually, a potential space. The pleural membranes are separated by only a thin film of pleural fluid. To obtain pleural space measurements experimentally, a thin needle is inserted between the pleural membranes.

*The glottis must remain open during breath-holding.

Table 3-1. Lung compliance and airways resistance

Definition	Normal range	Measurement conditions	Measurements required
C_L: volume change produced by a change in air pressure	0.1-0.4 L/cm H_2O	Static: no air flow	Transpulmonary pressure Volume of air moved into the lungs
R_{aw}: pressure difference required for a change in air flow	0.5-2.5 cm H_2O/L/sec	Dynamic: during air flow	Transairway pressure Air flow

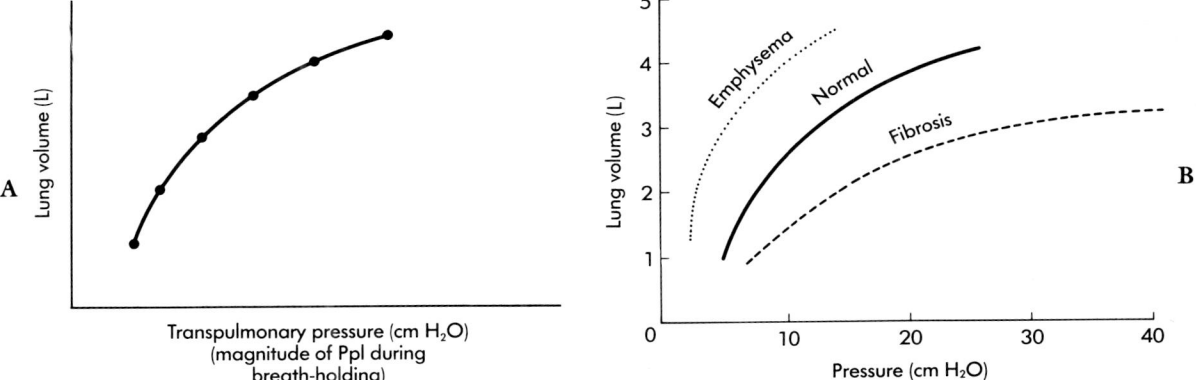

Fig. 3-3. **A,** Compliance measurement. After swallowing an esophageal tube, the patient inhales to a specified lung volume and holds his breath with the glottis open, assuring an alveolar pressure of zero. The amount of air inhaled (change in volume) divided by the change in esophageal pressure (read from a pressure meter) is the compliance at that point. Measurements are recorded at several different lung volumes, generating a compliance curve. **B,** Compliance curves. Normal lung compliance is approximately 0.2 L/cm H_2O (e.g., 2 L lung volume/10 cm H_2O distending pressure). Compliance is high in emphysema and low in pulmonary fibrosis.

Clinical problem 2

A patient with severe pulmonary fibrosis breathes 40 times per minute, with a minute ventilation of 10 L. Based on your knowledge concerning lung compliance, how do you explain this breathing pattern?

Despite the difficulty in measuring it, compliance is an important concept in understanding many clinical problems. Compliance is a quality of any distensible organ, not just of the lungs. For example, the chest wall is distensible, and its compliance is often a factor in cardiopulmonary disease. In artificially ventilated patients, changes in system compliance, which includes the ventilator tubing plus the patient's lungs and chest wall, may indicate improvement or worsening of the lung disease. System compliance is a feasible measurement since airway pressure and tidal volume can be obtained directly from the ventilator (see Chapter 10).

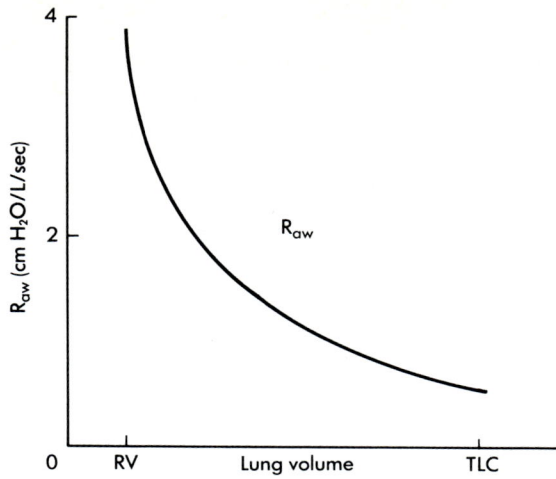

Fig. 3-4. Change in airways resistance (R_{aw}) with change in lung volume. See text for discussion.

AIRWAY RESISTANCE

In general terms, resistance is the driving pressure divided by the flow (see Table 3-1). The driving pressure in any tube is the pressure at the beginning of the tube minus the pressure at the end. The driving pressure in the lungs is the transairway pressure or the difference between mouth pressure (Pm) and alveolar pressure (Palv). The equation for airways resistance (R_{aw}) is

$$R_{aw} = \frac{Pm - Palv}{\dot{V}} \quad (2)$$

where $\dot{V}$ is gas volume per unit of time (airflow).

Because driving pressure is Pm − Palv, airflow will occur if either Pm is increased (as during artificial positive pressure ventilation; see Chapter 10) or Palv is reduced (as during normal breathing; see Fig. 3-2).

R_{aw} is a measure of the difficulty with which air flows through the airways. Adult R_{aw} ranges from 0.5 to 2.5 cm H_2O/L/sec. Normally, about half the R_{aw} occurs in the upper respiratory tract (nose, pharynx, and larynx). The nose has much greater resistance than the mouth; thus pure mouth breathing offers lower R_{aw} than does nasal breathing.

Resistance in any tube is directly proportional to the length of the tube and inversely proportional to the fourth power of the tube's radius; the wider the tube, the lower the resistance. This fact suggests that R_{aw} should *fall* as the lungs expand since expansion increases the diameter of the airways. Fig. 3-4 shows the inverse relationship of R_{aw} to lung volume. R_{aw} is lowest at high lung volumes where the airway diameter is largest; R_{aw} then rises hyperbolically as lung volume decreases.

The relationship of R_{aw} to airway radius also suggests that, at a given lung volume, R_{aw} is greater in the small airways than in the larger ones. A single bronchiole should have greater R_{aw} than a large bronchus of equal length. However, as the airways divide, they also become shorter. Furthermore, the total cross-sectional area of the branching airways increases geometrically with each division (see Fig. 2-9).

As airways branch, the individual airway diameter decreases, but the total pulmonary resistance increases very little. As a result, the smallest

Lung mechanics

airways, 2 mm diameter or less, account for only about 10% of total R_{aw}. This is an important concept in understanding small airways disease, the term for inflammation or narrowing that is confined to the small airways. Because small airways disease does not increase total R_{aw} very much, it is often difficult to detect. Small airways disease is discussed further in the section on spirometry.

Measurement of R_{aw}

Like lung compliance, R_{aw} is an important concept in pulmonary medicine, but it is not routinely measured in clinical practice. Measurement of R_{aw} requires a body plethysmograph or "body box," an expensive device not available in most hospitals. A body box consists of an airtight box the size of a telephone booth, in which the subject sits while breathing through a pneumotachometer (flow-measuring device). The body box operates on the principle of Boyle's law: $P_1V_1 = P_2V_2$. As the patient breathes, changes in air volume within the box cause reciprocal changes in pressure that provide the corresponding transairway pressure necessary for R_{aw} measurement.

Clinical problem 3

If the driving pressure (Pm − Palv) is 1 cm H_2O and airflow is 0.5 L/sec, what is R_{aw}? Is is normal? What is R_{aw} for the same airflow when driving pressure is 5 cm H_2O?

Clinical problem 4

The normal time span for inspiration and for expiration is approximately the same. In conditions of increased R_{aw} such as in a patient with asthma, what change would be expected in the ratio of inspiratory to expiratory time?

Instead of direct measurement, R_{aw} is usually quantitated indirectly by spirometry. When R_{aw} is increased enough to affect spirometric measurements, the patient is said to have airway obstruction. Airway obstruction (increased R_{aw}) can occur from a variety of pathologic causes and will be discussed later in this chapter.

LUNG VOLUMES AND CAPACITIES

Volume was earlier defined as a quantity of air. The term *lung volume* is used to describe specific quantities of air within both lungs (Fig. 3-5). The four named lung volumes are *tidal volume, expiratory reserve volume, residual volume,* and *inspiratory reserve volume.*

Lung capacity is the name for a quantity of air made up of two or more lung volumes; the four lung capacities are *total lung capacity, vital capacity, functional residual capacity,* and *inspiratory capacity.* Lung volumes and capacities are measured in milliliters (ml) or liters (L).

Before continuing, lung volumes and capacities and their relationship to one another should be reviewed (Fig. 3-5). It should be noted that lung volumes do not overlap.

Measurement of all the lung volumes and capacities requires two fundamentally different methods. The forced vital capacity (the quantity of air forcefully expired after maximal inhalation) and its subdivisions are measured with the relatively simple spirometer, which is standard equipment in every hospital and also in many physicians' offices (see Chapter 1).

The volume of air left in the lungs after maximal exhalation is called the *residual volume* (RV); RV *cannot* be measured by the spirometer, but it can be measured by inert gas dilution technique or by body plethysmography; either way requires a different and more sophisticated device than a spirometer. In practice, the functional residual capacity (FRC) is usually measured by the gas dilution or body plethysmograph technique, and the RV is obtained by subtracting expiratory reserve volume (ERV) from FRC (see Fig. 3-5). In any case, measurement of total lung capacity, which combines both the FVC and RV, requires more than spirometry.

Total lung capacity (TLC) is the total volume of air contained within the lungs at maximal inhalation. By definition, TLC includes all the lung volumes and capacities (Fig. 3-5). Total lung capacity is usually determined by adding the FRC, which

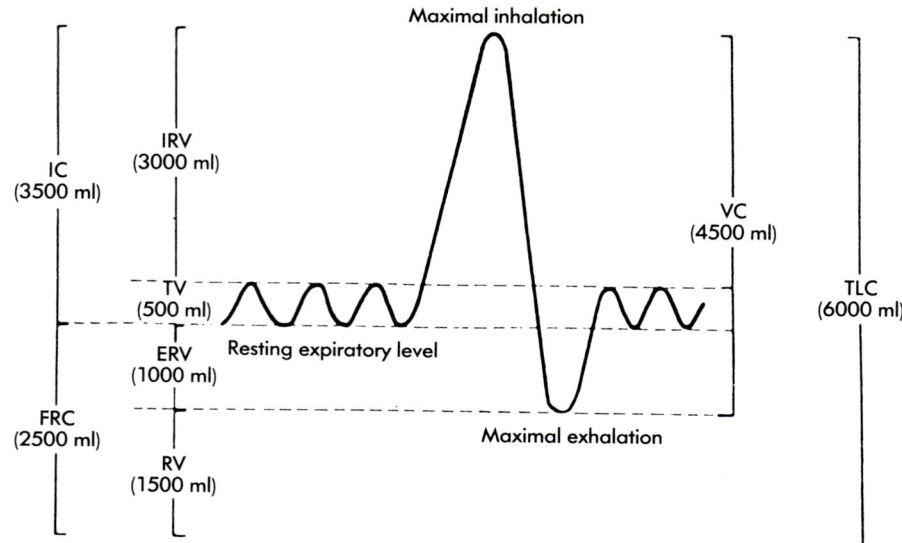

Fig. 3-5. Lung volumes and lung capacities. Lung volumes: tidal, expiratory reserve, residual, and inspiratory reserve. Lung capacities: functional residual, vital, inspiratory, and total lung. Values shown are for an average-size young adult. (From Spearman, C.B., Sheldon, R.L., and Egan, D.F.: Egan's fundamentals of respiratory therapy, ed. 4, St. Louis, 1982, The C.V. Mosby Co.)

is measured by inert gas dilution or by plethysmography, to the inspiratory capacity, which is measured by the spirometer. Any condition that limits or restricts lung expansion will reduce TLC. Pulmonary restriction is encountered in many diseases, ranging from interstitial lung fibrosis to chest muscle paralysis. A *sine qua non* of restrictive respiratory impairment is a reduced TLC. As a result of reduction in TLC, FVC is invariably reduced as well. Restrictive diseases are discussed later in this chapter.

FUNCTIONAL RESIDUAL CAPACITY

From the standpoint of understanding lung mechanics, the most important quantity of air is probably the functional residual capacity (FRC). FRC is the natural resting point of the lungs and chest cage and is determined by the interplay of forces that tend to expand the chest cage and contract the lungs. The opposing forces are shown in Fig. 3-6. The lungs normally adhere to the inner surface of the chest cage so that chest cage expansion or contraction leads to lung expansion or contraction, respectively.

Muscular structure of the chest cage is such that, at rest, the forces favor expansion; without the lungs as a counterbalance, the chest cage would be larger than it is at FRC. Conversely, the pulmonary interstitium contains much elastic tissue that gives the lungs a tendency to contract or recoil (elastic recoil) while at rest. (Lung elastic recoil pressure is measured as the transpulmonary pressure; see Fig. 3-1). The lungs would be far smaller than they are at FRC without the chest cage; at FRC the lung elastic recoil is exactly counterbalanced by the elastic recoil pressure of the chest wall.

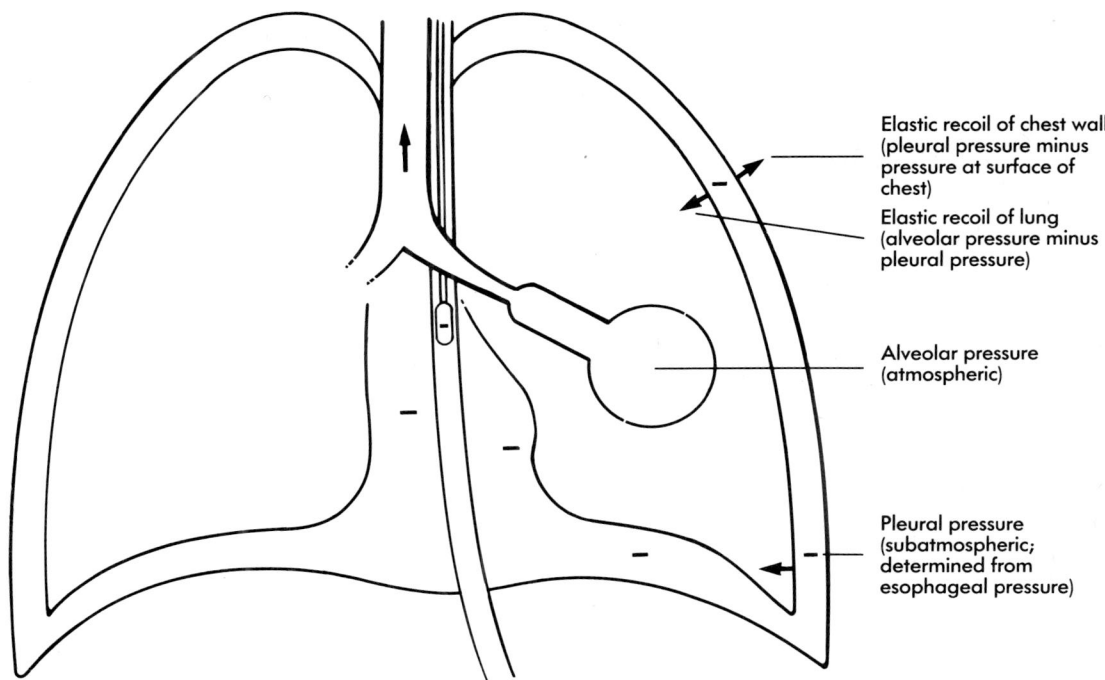

Fig. 3-6. Functional residual capacity (FRC). The lungs are at FRC at the beginning of inspiration or at the end of expiration (see Fig. 3-2). At FRC the respiratory muscles are at rest, and lung elastic recoil is exactly balanced by the outward recoil of the chest cage. At FRC the pressure in all the airways is atmospheric and there is no airflow. This diagram shows a balloon-tipped tube in the esophagus that is used to measure intraesophageal pressure, which in turn reflects intrapleural pressure.

The opposing recoil forces of the lung and the chest cage can be appreciated in a pneumothorax where one lung collapses from air leakage into the pleural space (Fig. 3-7). In a pneumothorax the pleural space is no longer sealed off from atmospheric pressure; as a result, chest cage pressure does not oppose lung elastic recoil pressure, and the lung collapses.

At FRC there is still considerable quantity of air in the lungs, approximately 2.5 L for an average-sized person. The FRC acts as a gas reservoir in that it contains far more oxygen than is actually taken up by the capillaries per breath and can absorb far more carbon dioxide than is excreted per breath. The FRC reservoir prevents large swings in blood oxygen and carbon dioxide concentration during breathing. Increase in FRC is one manifestation of improvement from severe pulmonary edema, in which FRC is invariably reduced.

Clinical problem 5

A patient with forced vital capacity of 3.5 L and total lung capacity of 5.4 L has what residual volume? What is this patient's FRC if the expiratory reserve volume is 1.3 L?

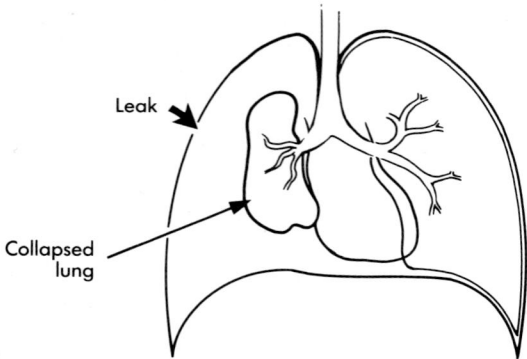

Fig. 3-7. Collapse of one lung from a pneumothorax. A pneumothorax may occur from a puncture of the chest wall (as diagramed here) or from a tear of the lung or of a mediastinal structure contiguous with the pleural space (e.g., the esophagus). In either case air will enter the pleural space, and the intrapleural pressure will change from subatmospheric to atmospheric. When this change occurs, the normal lung elastic recoil is unopposed, and the lung collapses. The right and left pleural cavities are physically separated by the mediastinum; thus an air leak on one side does not collapse the other lung.

Clinical problem 6

A patient's total lung capacity is 6 L and forced vital capacity is 4.2 L. If forced vital capacity decreases by one third with no change in total lung capacity, what will be the ratio of residual volume to total lung capacity? Does this change suggest a restrictive or obstructive problem?

FORCED VITAL CAPACITY

Forced vital capacity (FVC) is the volume of air that can be forcibly exhaled from the lungs after a full inhalation; in adults FVC ranges normally from approximately 3 to 5 L, depending on the individual's age, sex, and height. (See Appendix B for the range of normal values.) The FVC and its components, such as the peak flow, forced expiratory volume in one second (FEV_1), and FEV_1/FVC, are particularly valuable for diagnosing obstructive lung diseases. Forced vital capacity is measured with the spirometer and, including patient instruction, requires only a few minutes to perform. Spirometry, as measurement of FVC is called, is *the single most useful test of lung mechanics*.

Fig. 3-8 shows a normal FVC as a plot of volume vs. time. (Residual volume is not shown since it is not part of the FVC measurement.) Table 3-2 lists the commonly measured components of the FVC, which relate to volume, flow, and ratio of volumes.

The only commonly measured part of the FVC that is consistently reduced in both obstructive and restrictive respiratory disease is FEV_1 (Table 3-3). For this reason FEV_1 is an excellent screening test for respiratory impairment. A normal FEV_1 rules out clinically significant mechanical impairment; a reduced FEV_1, provided that the patient gave a satisfactory effort, indicates impairment, although

Table 3-2. FVC and its measured components

Component	Units
Volumes	
FVC	ml or L
FEV_1 second	ml or L
FEV_3 second	ml or L
Flows	
Peak flow	L/sec or L/min
Flow at 25%, 50%, and 75% of FVC	L/sec or L/min
MMF_{25-75}*	L/sec or L/min
Ratios of volumes	
FEV_1/FVC	Percent
FEV_3/FVC	Percent

*MMF_{25-75}, Maximal midflow between 25% and 75% of the FVC.

Lung mechanics

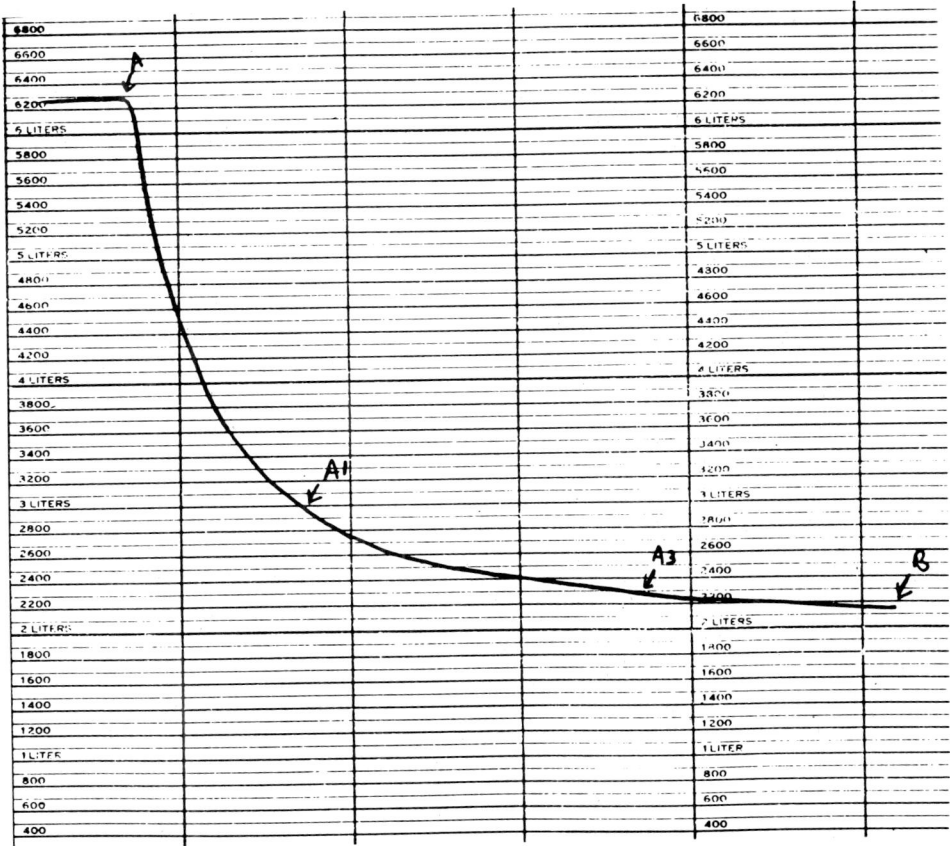

Fig. 3-8. Curve of normal forced vital capacity (FVC). The patient inhales to total lung capacity (A) and exhales as quickly and forcefully as possible. The curve is traced on standard spirometric paper, which rotates at 32 mm/sec. The time interval between vertical lines is 1 second. Volume is read from top to bottom. FVC is the volume from point A to point B (6300 − 2150 = 4.15 L). FEV_1 is the volume from point A to point A_1 (6200 − 3000 = 3.2 L). FEV_3 is the volume from point A to point A_3 (6200 − 2300 = 3.9 L). These volumes are uncorrected for BTPS. Under typical laboratory conditions BTPS values are obtained by multiplying the measured volumes by a factor of approximately 1.08. The ratios FEV_1/FVC and FEV_3/FVC are the same whether or not corrections are made for BTPS:

$FEV_1/FVC = 3.2/4.15 = 0.77$

$FEV_3/FVC = 3.9/4.15 = 0.94$

Measurement of flows from the time-volume plot are discussed in a later section.

Table 3-3. Utility of FEV_1 as screening test for respiratory impairment*

Impairment	FVC	FEV_1	Peak flow	MMF_{25-75}	FEV_1/FVC
Restrictive	D	D	D, N, or I	D, N, or I	N to I
Obstructive	D or N	D	D or N	D	D

*FEV_1 is the only commonly measured FVC component consistently reduced in either pattern of impairment. (D, decreased; N, normal; I, increased.)

---

it does not distinguish between restriction and obstruction. The FEV_3 requires greater effort than the FEV_1 and is no more helpful than the entire FVC.

The peak flow is the most useful FVC *flow* parameter. Peak flow is the preferred test of lung mechanics during an asthma attack for several reasons. Since peak flow occurs within the first second of the FVC, it requires only an initial patient effort and not the longer effort needed to generate the entire FVC curve. This is an important consideration when a test must be repeated in patients who already suffer shortness of breath. Peak flow can also be measured with an easily portable device, the peak flow meter (Fig. 3-9); the standard spirometer is usually bulkier and not as portable. Finally, peak flow correlates well with the other parameters of the FVC, particularly the FEV_1; in asthmatics, for example, a low FEV_1 usually predicts a low peak flow and vice versa.

Clinical problem 7

Using a pencil and ruler, estimate the peak flow from the FVC curve shown in Fig. 3-8.

Of the other flow parameters, reduced maximal midflow between 25% and 75% of FVC (MMF_{25-75}) may be an indicator of small airways disease in certain situations; it is discussed in a later section. The flow at 25%, 50% and 75% of the vital capacity is reported only when a flow-volume curve is obtained; this is also discussed later.

The ratio of FEV_1 to FVC is the best indicator of airways obstruction. Normally, this ratio should be approximately 70% or higher (it is age-dependent). FEV_1/FVC may, on occasion, be normal in severe airways obstruction when the FEV_1 and FVC are reduced proportionately.* Also, FEV_1/FVC can be normal in the presence of small airways disease when the alteration in R_{aw} is not enough to change this spirometric ratio. However, reduced FEV_1/FVC is a sure sign of airways obstruction.

Clinical problem 8

Which of the following patients is the most likely to have airways obstruction? (All volumes are in liters).
Patient A: FVC = 5.5; FEV_1 = 4.0
Patient B: FVC = 4.6; FEV_1 = 1.4
Patient C: FVC = 2.3; FEV_1 = 2.0

---

*Presence of obstructed air flow under these circumstances can be determined in several ways: (1) measurement of total lung capacity, which is increased in asthmatics and in other states of hyperinflation; (2) chest x-ray films, which can provide a good qualitative assessment of total lung capacity (an x-ray film showing hyperinflation in the presence of very low FVC and FEV_1 with normal FEV_1/FVC suggests severe airways obstruction); (3) a pattern of response to inhalation of a bronchodilator whereby FVC and FEV_1 increase disproportionately so that FEV_1/FVC falls (when this occurs the bronchodilator has "unmasked" the underlying airways obstruction).

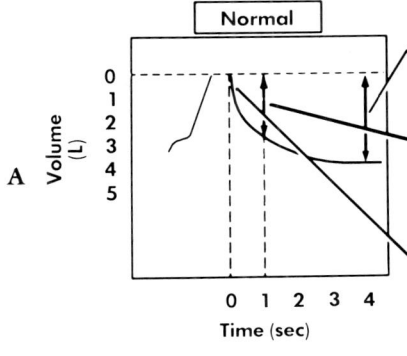

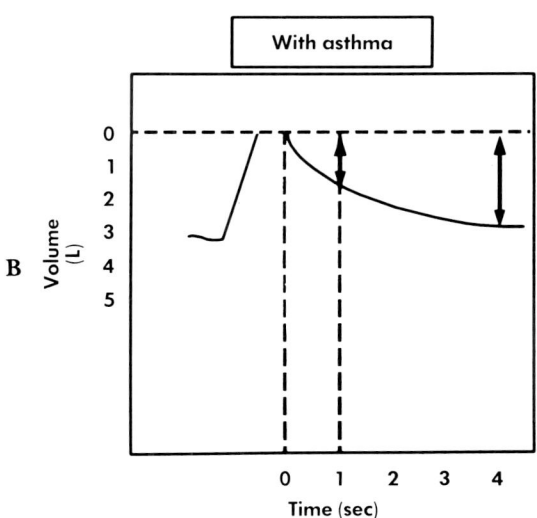

Fig. 3-9. Peak flow and its measurement. **A,** Forced vital capacity (FVC) curve from a healthy person. **B,** Forced vital capacity curve from a person with asthma. Peak flow, the steepest slope of the FVC curve, is normally between 400 and 700 L/min. Although peak flow can be measured from the curve, it is more easily obtained with a portable peak flow meter.

Continued

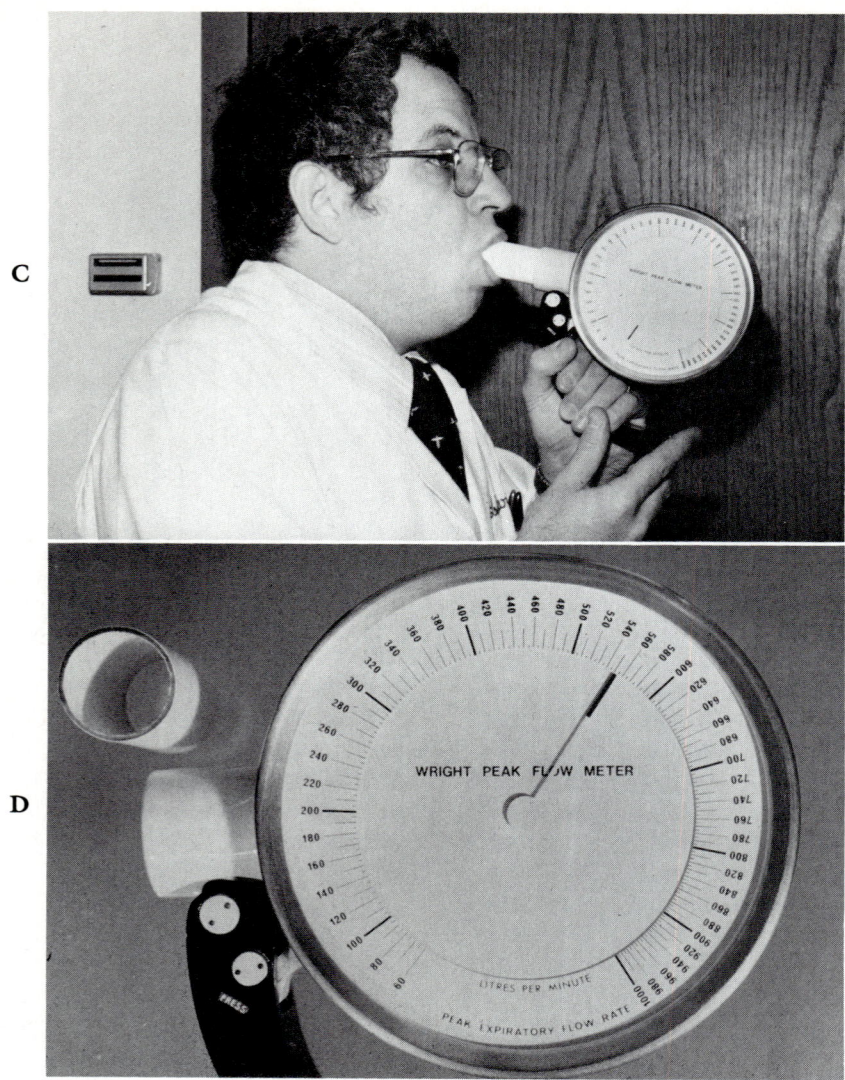

Fig. 3-9, cont'd. **C,** Individual performing peak flow using a portable meter. He inhales to total lung capacity and then exhales through the cardboard tube as forcefully and quickly as possible. Just before exhalation the meter needle registers zero. **D,** After exhalation the needle registers 550 L/min, this person's peak flow.

Lung mechanics

FLOW-VOLUME CURVES AND LOOPS

The standard spirometric curve is a plot of volume vs. time (Fig. 3-8). Inherent in this time-volume plot is a *flow* for each point of the curve (Fig. 3-10, A). For example, the change in volume per change in time at any point in Fig. 3-10, A, is the flow at that point; it can be measured by drawing a tangent to the curve at any given point.

The change in flow can be appreciated by placing an index finger in front of your mouth and performing the forced vital capacity (FVC) maneuver. For descriptive purposes, various points in Fig. 3-10, A, are labeled A, B, C, and D. At point A, just before exhalation begins, the flow is zero (there is no air flowing past your finger). Shortly afterward, well within the first second, the flow rate is maximal (point B); the air is flowing past your finger at the fastest rate of the entire FVC maneuver. The flow rate rapidly declines after point B. Near the end of the vital capacity maneuver, after at least 2 seconds, air flow is considerably slowed; this is point C. Finally, at the end of FVC (point D), flow is again zero.

Although flow is an inherent part of the FVC curve, it is not easy to visualize or measure from the time-volume plot. For this reason an alternative way of visualizing the FVC maneuver has gained popularity—plotting the actual flow (in L/sec) vs. the volume exhaled. This is the expiratory flow-volume curve (Fig. 3-10, B). The patient goes through the same maneuver, but the result is plotted on a different device, e.g., an X-Y recorder or a graphics plotter. (Some spirometers can simultaneously plot both time and flow vs. volume from the same effort.) Note that the flow-volume curve contains no new information but is only another

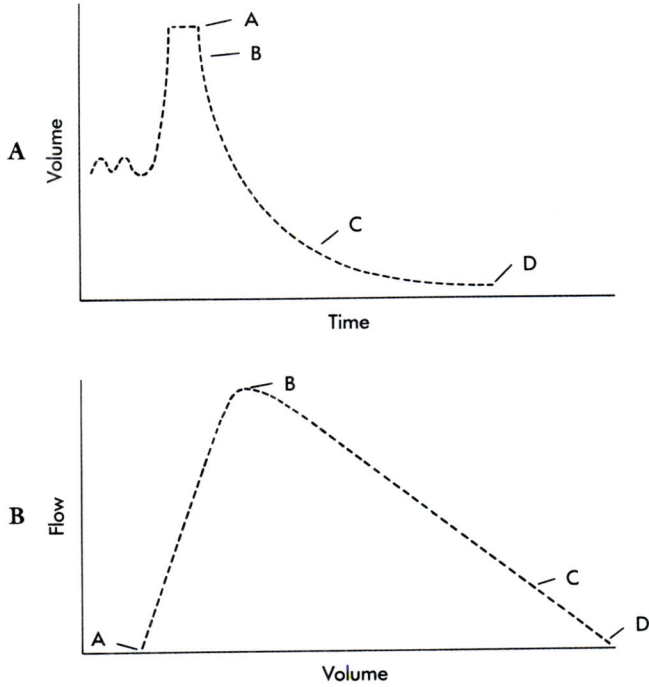

Fig. 3-10. Normal forced vital capacity. **A,** Plotted as volume vs. time. **B,** Plotted as volume vs. flow. See text for discussion.

way of visualizing the FVC curve.

A flow-volume loop includes both the forced expiratory and forced inspiratory effort. At the end of the FVC maneuver (i.e., at RV), the subject inhales as rapidly and forcefully as possible. The result is an *inspiratory* vital capacity curve; the expiratory and inspiratory curves together describe a flow-volume loop (Fig. 3-11).

Flow-volume curves and loops are useful for diagnosing upper airways obstruction, i.e., obstruction in or above the trachea. Depending on the obstruction's location in the upper airways, there is a characteristic pattern for the flow-volume curves; examples are shown in Fig. 3-12. These are idealized patterns in the sense that actual tracings do not usually have such straight lines. Flow-volume curves obtained from the patient described in Clinical Problem 5, Chapter 1, are shown in Fig. 3-13. During the patient's surgery a huge goiter involving both the intrathoracic and extrathoracic trachea was found and removed.

In practice, the exact type of upper airways obstruction is not diagnosed from flow-volume curves but from exhaustive investigation that may include x-ray films, bronchoscopy, and, in many cases, surgery. Nonetheless, flow-volume curves are valuable for finding upper airways obstruction or confirming its presence once suspected.

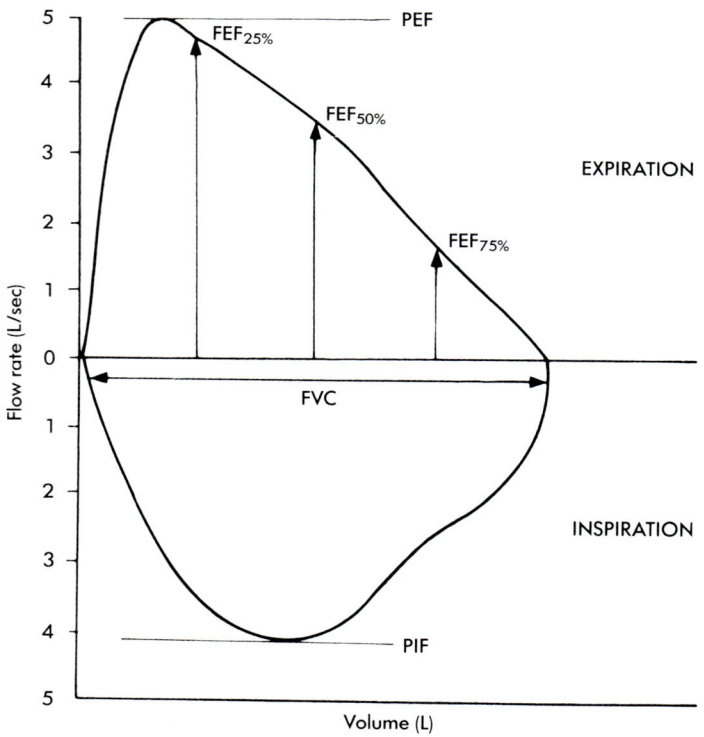

Fig. 3-11. Normal flow-volume loop. The flow-volume loop includes both expiratory and inspiratory flow-volume curves. The FVC can be read directly on the horizontal axis. The peak and other flows can be read directly on the vertical axis. (*PEF,* peak expiratory flow; *PIF,* peak inspiratory flow; *$FEF_{25\%}$, $FEF_{50\%}$,* and *$FEF_{75\%}$,* forced expiratory flow at 25%, 50%, and 75% of the FVC.) (From Spearman, C.B., Sheldon, R.L., and Egan, D.F.: Egan's fundamentals of respiratory therapy, ed. 4, St. Louis, 1982, The C.V. Mosby Co.)

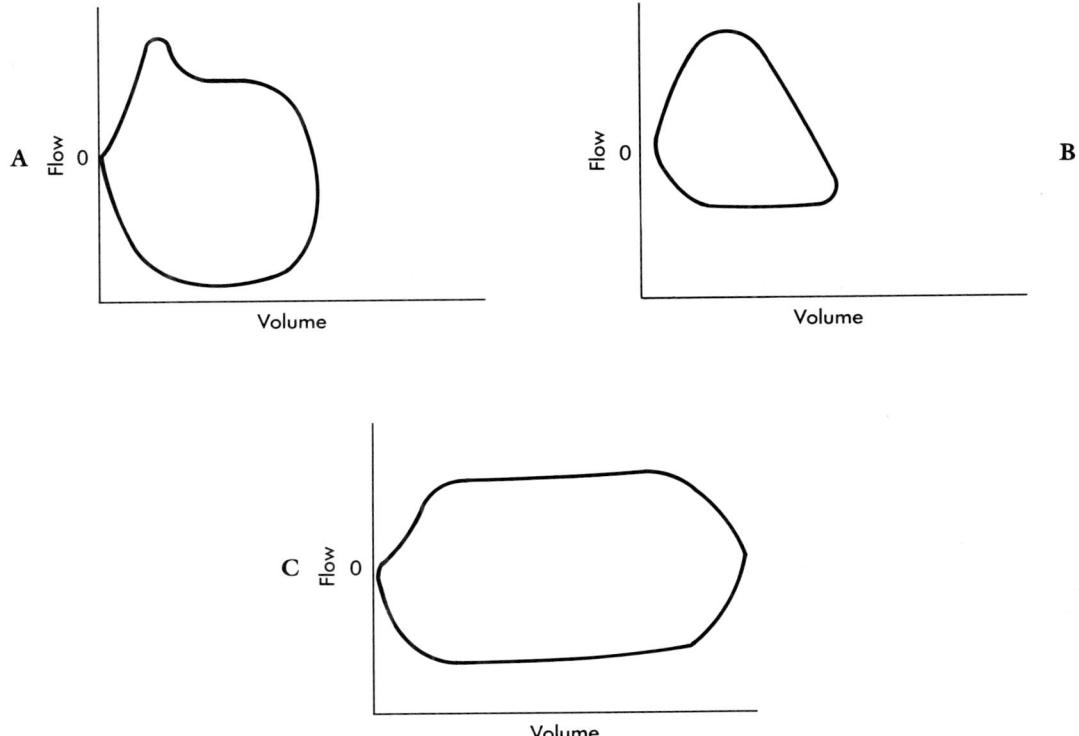

Fig. 3-12. Flow-volume loops in upper airways obstruction (idealized). In each flow-volume loop, expiration is shown above the line of "0" flow; inspiration is shown below. **A,** Variable intrathoracic upper airways obstruction. **B,** Variable extrathoracic upper airways obstruction. **C,** Fixed extrathoracic upper airways obstruction.

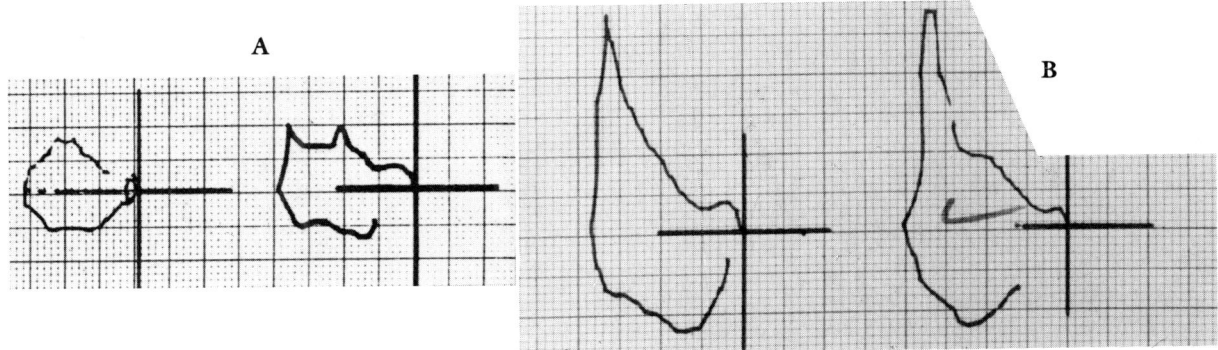

Fig. 3-13. Expiratory flow-volume curves from patient in Chapter 1 (Clinical Problem 5). **A,** Before removal of thyroid goiter; **B,** After removal of thyroid goiter.

DETERMINANTS OF EXPIRATORY AIRFLOW

Obstruction of airflow is a major cause of respiratory morbidity. Airways obstruction is a cardinal manifestation of asthma, chronic bronchitis, and emphysema. In this section the determinants of expiratory airflow are examined.

Fig. 3-14, *A*, shows the change in pressures during a *forced* expiratory maneuver. These pressures are all *positive;* this is in distinct contrast to normal quiet breathing (Fig. 3-2), in which the intrapleural pressure is always negative and the alveolar pressure is negative during inspiration.

The initial alveolar pressure is the sum of two pressures: the intrapleural pressure (Ppl) of +20 cm H_2O and the elastic recoil pressure of +10 cm H_2O. Together, Ppl and lung elastic recoil pressure give an initial airway driving pressure of +30 cm H_2O. Pressure in the airways drops as air flows from the alveolus to the mouth where the pressure is atmospheric (0). The point at which the pressure inside the airways equals the outside pressure is the *equal pressure point* (EPP). Toward the mouth Ppl exceeds the airway pressure, tending to compress or collapse the airways. The tendency of airways to collapse is aided by the narrowing of the airways as the lung volume shrinks. Airways collapse is resisted by the airways' rigidity, which is

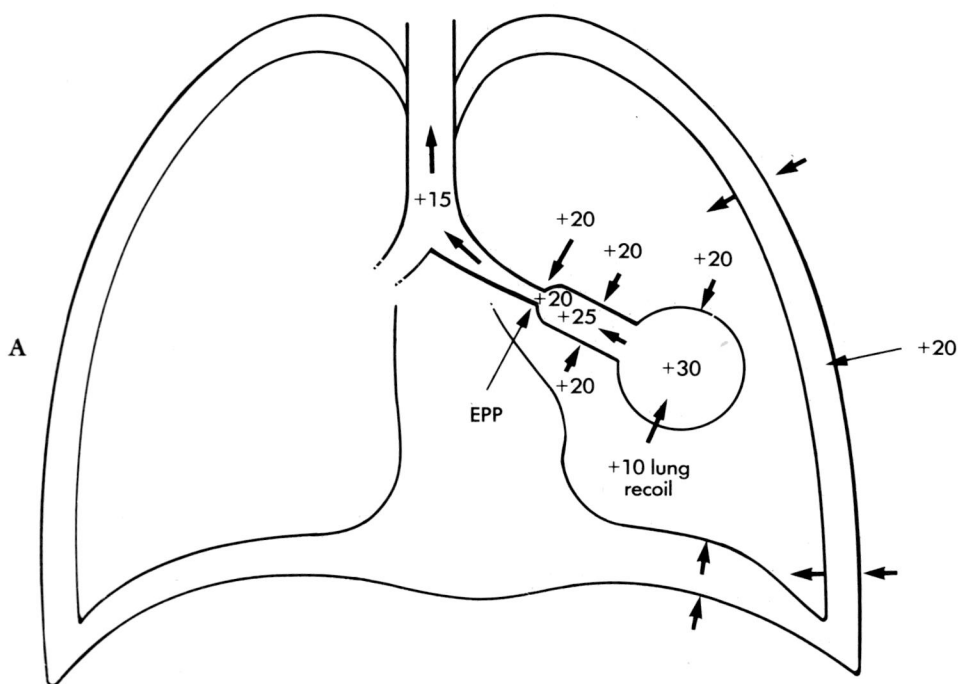

Fig. 3-14. **A,** Generation of equal pressure point (EPP) in normal lungs: pleural pressure (Ppl) 20 cm H_2O. This figure shows generation of the EPP when Ppl is 20 cm H_2O during forced exhalation. Alveolar pressure is the sum of Ppl (20 cm H_2O) plus lung elastic recoil pressure (10 cm H_2O), or 30 cm H_2O. Airways pressure falls continually from the alveolus to the mouth. At the EPP airway pressure within the airways equals Ppl. Further toward the mouth, airway pressure falls below Ppl, resulting in a narrowed airway and limitation of airflow.

Continued

provided by the cartilage and other supporting structures.

With increasing expiratory effort, Ppl increases (Fig. 3-14, *B*). Since elastic recoil pressure is unchanged, the decrease in airway pressure from the alveolar pressure to the EPP *and* the location of the EPP are the same. However, as a result of the increase in Ppl, the airway is narrowed even further and the flow is limited. Thus once the EPP has limited airflow in a segment, increasing the forced effort will not increase the flow in that segment.

The EPP exists only during forced expiration; it does not occur during quiet breathing. Also, in healthy subjects, the EPP only occurs at a lung volume below functional residual capacity and is not seen during normal tidal volume breathing.

In some conditions, particularly emphysema where elastic recoil pressures are reduced, the EPP may occur in the tidal volume region (Fig. 3-15). Partly for this reason, airways tend to collapse much earlier in a patient with emphysema. The reason for early airways collapse in emphysema is the loss of lung elastic recoil caused by destruction of the elastic supporting tissue. Because recoil pressure is reduced, airway driving pressure is reduced. At the same time, large airways in emphysematous lungs may be weakened from loss of supporting elastic tissue. As a result of both decreased

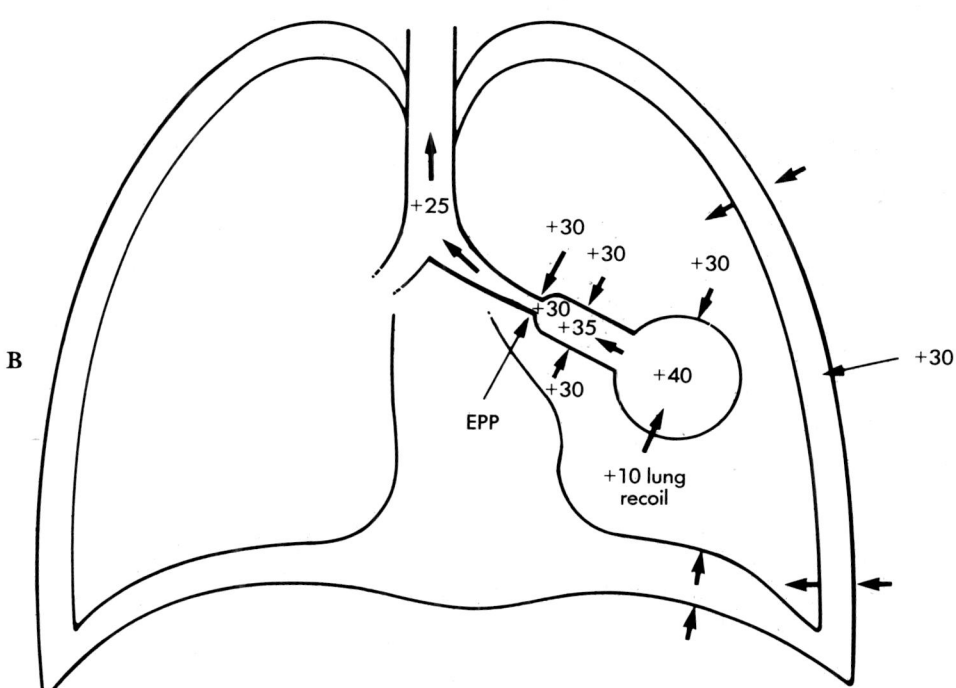

Fig. 3-14, cont'd. **B,** Generation of EPP in normal lungs: Ppl 30 cm H_2O. EPP is generated when Ppl is increased to 30 cm H_2O during forced exhalation. Alveolar pressure is now 40 cm H_2O (Ppl of 30 cm H_2O plus lung elastic recoil pressure of 10 cm H_2O). Although alveolar pressure is higher than in **A,** location of the EPP is unchanged.

driving pressure and weakened airways, the EPP occurs further toward the alveolus than normal, and the patient closes off some airways while there is still a relatively large amount of air in the thorax. (This is only one of several potential mechanisms causing airways obstruction in patients with emphysema.)

Clinical problem 9

Patients with severe emphysema frequently purse their lips to aid breathing. This spontaneous maneuver, done only during expiration, consists of bringing the lips close together to narrow the mouth opening. How is this maneuver explained in light of the EPP theory?

The EPP theory helps to explain another important aspect of forced expiration—effort-dependence. Fig. 3-16 shows pressure-flow curves during *forced* expiration. The pleural pressure is initially negative, but it becomes positive as flow rates increase (in contrast, pleural pressure is always negative during quiet breathing; see Fig. 3-2). Percent of vital capacity (VC) is relative to the patient's own VC and represents the lung volume inhaled before forced expiration begins. The expiratory flow (L/sec) is that generated by the forced expiratory effort.

For efforts beginning at 25% and 50% of the VC, flow generated by forced expiration reaches a

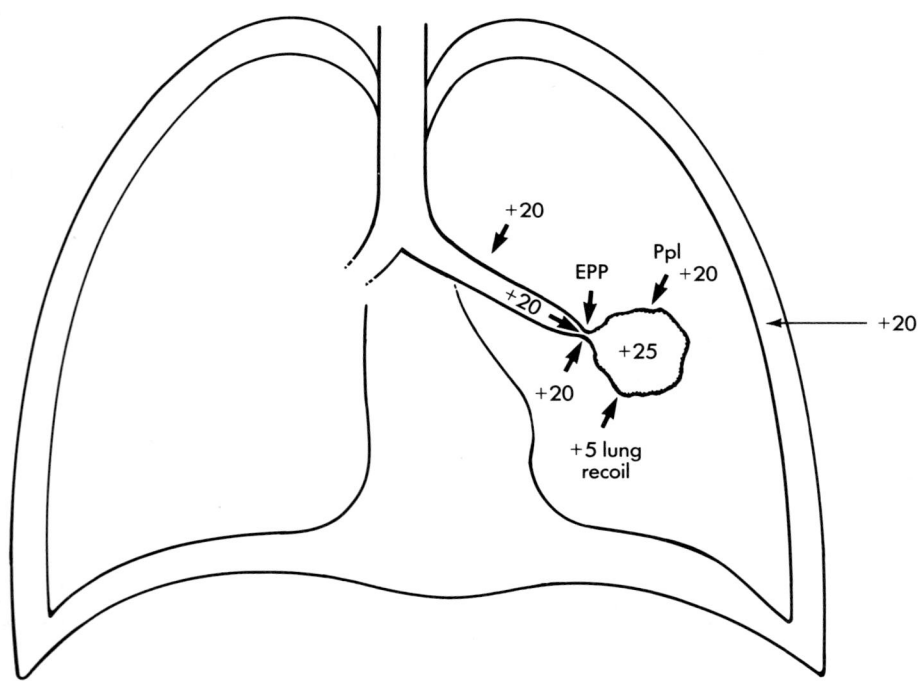

Fig. 3-15. EPP in emphysematous lungs. Despite maximal expiratory effort from total lung capacity, Ppl is 20 cm H₂O but lung elastic recoil pressure is only 5 cm H₂O (compare with Fig. 3-14, *A*). As a result, airway driving pressure in the emphysematous lungs is only 25 cm H₂O. Airway driving pressure dissipates further down the airway and equals the Ppl (EPP) at a point earlier than it is reached in healthy lungs. As a result the airways narrow or collapse at a larger lung volume than is normal. In patients with emphysema, airway collapse is contributed to by the weakened bronchial walls.

plateau as pleural pressure increases. For example, if one starts to exhale at 25% of VC and blows out hard enough to generate a positive pleural pressure of 15 cm H_2O, a flow rate of approximately 2.5 L/sec will be achieved. Repeating the maneuver from *the same lung volume* but increasing pleural pressure to 25 cm H_2O (i.e., a much harder effort) will not give a greater flow rate. Similarly, forced exhalation from 50% of VC produces a plateau of expiratory flow after a pleural pressure of approximately 15 cm H_2O is reached.

The curves in Fig. 3-16 show that at low lung volumes, after a certain pleural pressure is reached, flow rate is *effort-independent;* harder effort generates higher pleural pressure but no greater air flow. This is because the positive pleural pressure that tends to collapse the airways exceeds the airway pressure that tends to keep the airways open; as a result, the airways narrow, preventing any further increase in air flow despite greater effort.

Unfortunately, the term effort-independent, often used to describe the phenomenon of flow limitation, can be confusing; obviously, some effort is required to reach the plateau, and the flow is only effort-independent once the plateau is reached.

At 75% of VC, the greater the pleural pressure generated (the harder one forces the air out), the *greater* the air flow. Thus flows generated near the total lung capacity (above 75% of VC) are said to be effort-dependent—the greater one can raise pleural pressure the greater the resulting air flow.

Fig. 3-17 shows the result of varying lung volume and degree of effort on the expiratory flow-

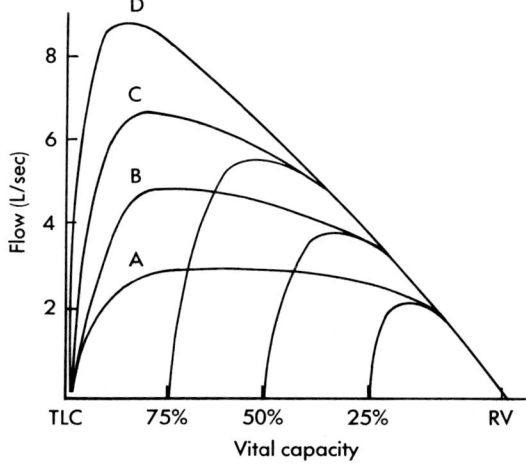

Fig. 3-17. Flow-volume curves generated at various lung volumes and degrees of effort. The three pressure-volume curves from Fig. 3-16 are shown here as the initial flow-volume curves beginning at 25%, 50%, and 75% of the FVC. For each higher lung volume the flow rate in the beginning of FVC increases, but as lung volume diminishes the flow rate falls to the level of the smaller curve. Four curves are also shown that begin at the total lung capacity (TLC), *A-D*. The patient has inhaled to TLC and then exhaled the entire FVC, but he has done so with varying effort, ranging from minimal *(curve A)* to maximal *(curve D)*. Again note that, with increasing effort, flows increase in the early portion of the FVC, but that, as lung volume decreases, the flow rate does not go any higher than it was with submaximal effort.

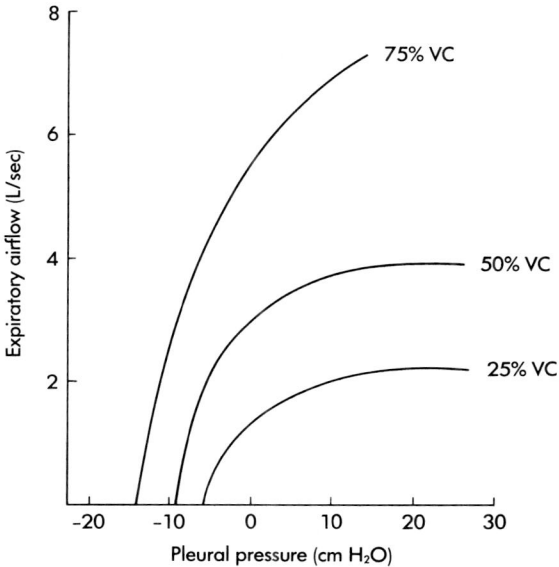

Fig. 3-16. Pressure-flow curves. See text for discussion.

volume curve. From a practical standpoint, respiratory muscle training and exercise can increase the early flow rates (those achieved close to total lung capacity). Because of airway dynamics, flow rates at low lung volumes will not increase with training. Thus approximately the first quarter of the forced vital capacity maneuver is said to be effort-dependent, and the last three-quarters, effort-independent.

SMALL AIRWAYS DISEASE AND DYNAMIC COMPLIANCE

As stated previously, the small airways (2 mm diameter or less) account for approximately 10% of total airways resistance (R_{aw}). If a patient's normal R_{aw} is 1 cm H_2O/L/sec, small airways disease can, at most, increase R_{aw} approximately 0.1 cm H_2O/L/sec, to 1.1 cm H_2O/L/sec, a value still well within the normal range.

The question of small airways disease arises only when the usual parameters of airways obstruction are *normal*. If the forced vital capacity (FVC), FEV_1, and FEV_1/FVC are reduced, airways resistance is definitely increased, and there is little concern about the contribution from the small airways. In most obstructive lung diseases, e.g., asthma, bronchitis, and emphysema, *all* the airways are involved, large and small, and there is no clinical reason to separate out the slight contribution of the smaller airways to the patient's airway obstruction.

The problem of detecting small airways disease arises only in patients whose FVC, FEV_1, and FEV_1/FVC are in the normal range. How can small airways disease be detected? Physiologically, there are several methods. One method, called frequency dependence of compliance, is a research technique. Another, the most widely used method in clinical practice, is the calculation of the maximal midflow between 25% and 50% of FVC (MMF_{25-75}) from spirometry.

Frequency dependence of compliance

Compliance is a static measurement, i.e., it is measured at points of no airflow. However, the

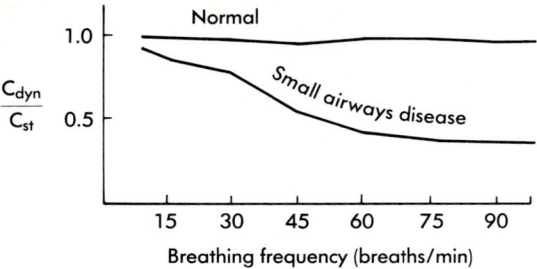

Fig. 3-18. Dynamic compliance. Normally, dynamic compliance is approximately the same as static compliance when the respiratory rate increases. In the presence of small airways disease, dynamic compliance falls relative to static compliance. See text for discussion.

change in lung volume per change in distending pressure *during breathing* gives a "dynamic" compliance. Dynamic compliance is obtained by dividing the tidal volume by the transpulmonary pressure, which is measured while the subject is breathing. This is not a true compliance since measurement is made during airflow, but it does represent a volume/pressure relationship; hence dynamic compliance is a useful term.

Dynamic compliance does not normally change during breathing, even up to respiratory rates as high as 60 breaths/min. When dynamic compliance decreases at respiratory rates below 60/min, it is called frequency-dependent and is a marker for small airways disease (Fig. 3-18).

Frequency dependence is a sensitive test for small airways disease. Presumably, as breathing frequency increases, the tidal volume does not have enough time to equilibrate throughout the diseased smaller airways. Thus for a given change in distending airway pressure, the tidal volume is lower than normal and the dynamic compliance is reduced. This phenomenon does not occur in healthy lungs since the small airways are open and the tidal volume can equilibrate in a very short time.

Maximal midflow

Measurement of dynamic compliance, like that of static compliance, is not common in clinical practice because of the need for using an esophageal balloon. A useful correlate of dynamic compliance is the maximal midflow (MMF_{25-75}), which is obtained from the FVC curve (Fig. 3-19). A reduced MMF_{25-75} in the presence of otherwise normal spirometry is a marker for small airways disease.

This spirometric pattern (normal FVC, FEV_1 and FEV_1/FVC, along with a reduced MMF_{25-75}) is found most commonly in people who smoke cigarettes and in people with asymptomatic asthma (asthma in remission). These patients may also have a mild reduction in arterial oxygen pressure (PaO_2), reflecting altered ventilation-perfusion relationships in the small airways (see Chapter 5).

It is not known if people who smoke cigarettes and have small airways disease (as an isolated finding) are at risk of later developing severe airways obstruction. Given the known harmful effects of cigarettes (e.g., lung cancer and coronary artery disease), detection of small airways disease should not be needed to convince a patient to quit smoking.

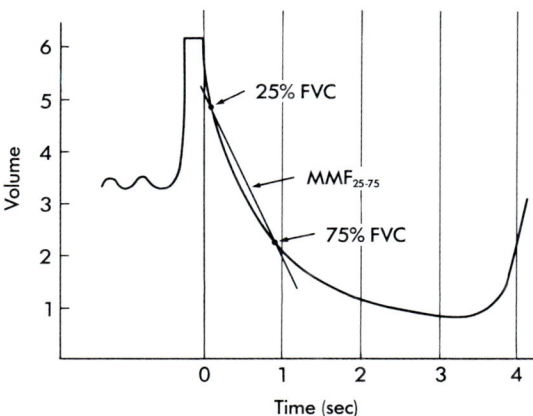

Fig. 3-19. Maximal midflow (MMF_{25-75}) is measured from the time-volume plot of the FVC. A line is drawn between the 25% and 75% points of the FVC. The slope of this line (measured in L/sec) is the MMF_{25-75}. In this example MMF_{25-75} is approximately 3.2 L/sec.

Clinical problem 10

Calculate the MMF_{25-75} from the spirometry curve in Fig. 3-8.

CLINICAL VALUE OF USING SPIROMETRY

Spirometry is in many ways analogous to the electrocardiogram (ECG). Both tests are noninvasive, relatively inexpensive, capable of yielding valuable information, and can be performed by machines that are relatively portable and easily operated by skilled technicians. These tests generally do not diagnose specific diseases as much as they suggest a pattern of dysfunction. The spirometric curve is as useful to the pulmonologist as the ECG is to the cardiologist.

Perhaps the biggest difference in this analogy is that the ECG requires no real effort on the patient's part, whereas the spirometric measurement is critically dependent on patient effort and good patient-technician interaction.

The spirometer measures a time-volume plot of the forced vital capacity. Although the same information can be obtained by plotting flow versus volume, in practice the time-volume plot is more commonly obtained. Volume vs. time is a more traditional way of looking at the FVC, and the apparatus tends to be less expensive than that needed to plot flow vs. volume.

The effort of forcing out air is recorded on graph paper, which is attached to a drum that is set at a standardized paper speed; with the standard "water-seal" spirometer, the drum rotates at 32 mm/sec (see Fig. 1-7). While the paper is rotating, the patient blows through a hose that displaces a bell; the bell sits in a barrel of water—hence, water-seal. The bell is attached to an ink pen that traces the patient's breathing effort on the rotating paper.

There are several different kinds of spirometers besides the water-seal variety (e.g., electronic, wedge), but they all provide the same information. As long as the spirometer is reasonably accurate and the test is performed properly, the type of spirometer is not important.

PATTERNS OF RESPIRATORY DISEASE

Pulmonary physicians often speak of many lung diseases as representing one of two patterns of breathing: *restrictive* or *obstructive*. These terms refer only to how a respiratory problem affects a patient's breathing pattern; they say nothing about cause, symptoms, chest x-ray findings, treatment, or prognosis. Furthermore, the two breathing patterns can be found together in one patient (e.g., a patient with severe pulmonary fibrosis). For the individual patient, the terms restrictive and obstructive are merely descriptive. Nevertheless, the terms have spirometric and physiologic correlates and are used pervasively in pulmonary medicine.

Restrictive respiratory disease

Any respiratory condition in which the patient is unable to take in a full, deep breath is considered restrictive. This condition can arise from the lungs, from the chest bellows, or from a nervous system disease. By way of an analogy, imagine a steel hoop placed around someone's chest so that he can breathe in a little but cannot take a full, deep breath. His breathing is then restricted. The closer the steel hoop comes to his resting breathing level at the end of quiet expiration (functional residual capacity), the less he can inspire and the more severe is the pulmonary restriction.

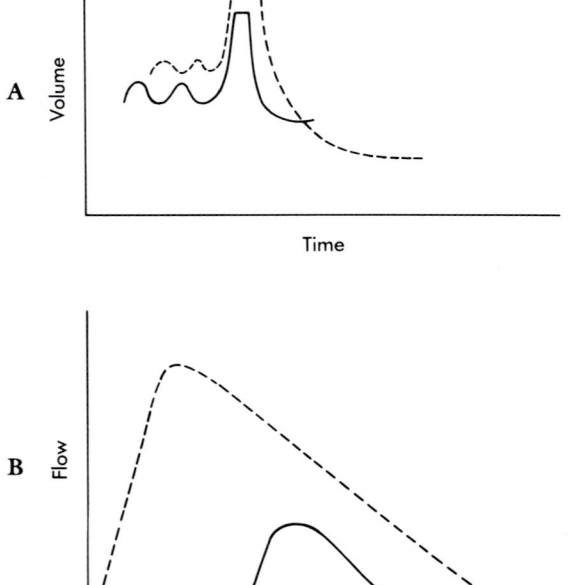

Fig. 3-20. Spirometric pattern seen in restrictive respiratory disease. **A,** Time-volume plot of the FVC. **B,** Flow-volume plot of the FVC. (*Dotted line,* the normal curve; *solid line,* the abnormal curve.)

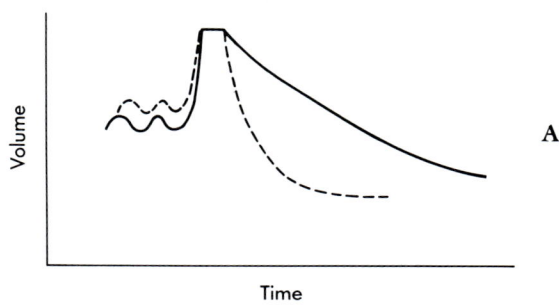
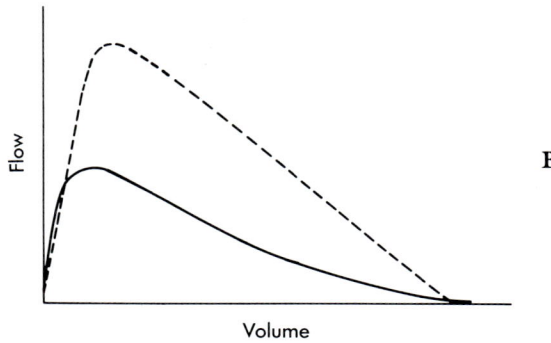

Fig. 3-21. Spirometric pattern seen in obstructive respiratory disease. **A,** Time-volume plot of the FVC. **B,** Flow-volume plot of the FVC. (*Dotted line,* the normal curve; *solid line,* the abnormal curve.)

Any respiratory condition resulting in an inability to fully expand the lungs is a restrictive problem. Once the air is inhaled, patients with restrictive disorders can usually exhale without any impediment or obstruction; the ratio FEV_1/FVC is usually normal or above normal. Hence, a major distinction between restrictive and obstructive lung disease is between the difficulty breathing in all the air (restrictive) and breathing out all the air (obstructive). Spirometric patterns for each condition are shown in Figs. 3-20 and 3-21.

Respiratory diseases and conditions commonly associated with a restrictive breathing pattern are listed in Table 3-4. Although some of these conditions may also be associated with airways obstruction, restriction is usually predominant.

Obstructive respiratory disease

Asthma, chronic bronchitis, and emphysema are examples of obstructive respiratory disease. As a group, obstructive lung diseases are the greatest cause of respiratory morbidity in the United States. The severity of obstructive lung disease is assessed by the forced vital capacity and its measured components (Table 3-2). As shown in Fig. 3-21, the patient with obstructed airways can take a deep breath, but his air flow during forced expiration is slowed. This breathing pattern differs from that of a patient with restricted air flow who cannot inhale as much air but who can readily exhale it.

Table 3-5 lists clinical examples of airways ob-

Table 3-4. Respiratory conditions commonly associated with a restrictive breathing pattern

Involving the chest bellows	Involving the lungs
Myasthenia gravis	
Guillain Barré syndrome	Atelectasis
Pleural effusion and pleural disease	Pulmonary sarcoidosis
	Pulmonary fibrosis
Flail chest (multiple broken ribs)	Pulmonary edema
	Pneumonia
Massive obesity	Congestive heart failure
Diaphragm paralysis	

Table 3-5. Conditions associated with obstruction to airflow

Location of airways obstruction	Associated pathology
Upper (above the main carina)	
Foreign body	Mechanical obstruction of airways
Croup and tracheitis	Mucosal edema of upper airways
Epiglottitis	Swelling of epiglottis
Various tumors and foreign bodies involving the airways	Mechanical obstruction of airways
Neuromuscular disease, e.g., Parkinson's disease	Weakness of upper airways' muscles
Lower (below the main carina)	
Asthma	Bronchoconstriction, mucosal edema, and mucous plugging
Chronic bronchitis	Mucosal edema and mucous plugging; bronchoconstriction if there is an asthmatic component
Cystic fibrosis	Same as chronic bronchitis
Emphysema	Loss of elastic recoil
Sarcoidosis	Sarcoid granulomas in airways
Foreign body	Mechanical obstruction of airways

Table 3-6. Spirometric and physiologic correlates of restrictive and obstructive lung disease

Clinical example	Spirometric measurements	Nonspirometric lung volumes	Lung compliance	Airway resistance
Restrictive				
Pulmonary fibrosis	Decreased FVC Decreased FEV_1 Increased $\frac{FEV_1}{FVC}$	Decreased TLC Decreased FRC Decreased RV	Decreased	Decreased
Neuromuscular disease	Decreased FVC Decreased FEV_1 Normal $\frac{FEV_1}{FVC}$	Decreased TLC Normal FRC Increased RV	Normal	Normal
Obstructive				
Asthma (during attack)	Decreased FVC Decreased FEV_1 Decreased $\frac{FEV_1}{FVC}$	Increased TLC Increased FRC	Normal	Increased
Emphysema	Same as asthma	Same as asthma	Increased	Increased

struction along with their underlying pathologies. Most causes of airways obstruction are caused by bronchospasm, mucous plugging, or mucosal edema, which are the main pathologic findings in asthma and chronic bronchitis. Another important cause of obstruction is the loss of elastic recoil from destruction of lung tissue, a process commonly found in severe emphysema. Table 3-6, using some common clinical conditions as examples, lists spirometric and physiologic correlates of the two breathing patterns.

INTERPRETATION OF SPIROMETRY

Spirometry is the most important test of lung mechanics. Although many laboratories also routinely measure nonspirometric lung volumes and lung capacities (TLC, FRC, RV), spirometry is the bedrock of lung function testing.

Interpretation of spirometry is different from interpreting most other tests in one important aspect: the test is effort-dependent. The patient must be cooperative, comfortable, and able to give forth his or her best effort. Equally important, the technician performing the test must establish good rapport with the patient and must be able to elicit a maximal response. Proper interpretation should always take into account the intangible "quality" of the test. Without patient motivation and good patient-technician interaction, tests of lung mechanics are apt to be invalid.

Interpretation is also sometimes difficult because the normal range for any given test is large, e.g., + or −20% for lung volumes. Furthermore, normal ranges are dependent on the patient's age, sex, height, and race (see Appendix B). Thus one must be careful to compare a given patient's effort

Table 3-7. Spirometric criteria for assigning pulmonary impairment*

Test	Normal	Mild	Moderate	Severe
		Percent of predicted value		
FVC	>80%	61%-80%	50%-60%	<50%
FEV_1	>80%	61%-80%	50%-60%	<50%
Peak flow	>80%	61%-80%	50%-60%	<50%
		Percent		
FEV_1/FVC†	70%-75%	60%-69%	50%-59%	<50%

Normal, mild, moderate, and *severe* refer to degree of impairment. The criteria for FVC, FEV_1, and peak flow are based on a percent predicted value. Criteria for FEV_1/FVC are based on an absolute percentage.
†FEV_1/FVC decreases slightly with increasing age.

against the normal values of a population closely matched to that patient.

Pulmonary physicians often use the terms *mild, moderate,* and *severe* to describe the degrees of impairment shown by pulmonary function tests. Unfortunately, these terms are not standardized; thus one physician's adjectives for a given set of values are apt to differ from another's. Table 3-7 presents arbitrary criteria for assigning the degree of impairment, recognizing that other physicians may choose different values.

Note that lung volumes and flows are based on percent of predicted value. By contrast, the adjectives describing ratio of FEV_1/FVC are based on the actual minimal value; normally, one should be able to exhale 70% to 75% of the FVC in 1 second. This is the accepted convention, but unfortunately it is often confusing. For example, an FVC that is 90% of the predicted FVC is within normal limits. Likewise, an FEV_1/FVC reported as 75% is also within normal limits; in this case the 75% is not a percent predicted value but is an absolute value (the FEV_1 is 75% of the FVC).

If a patient's predicted ratio of FEV_1 to FVC is 75% and his actual FEV_1/FVC is 65%, then his FEV_1/FVC is 65/75 or 87% *of predicted value;* this is an abnormal value since the predicted value of 75% *is a minimal value.* When interpreting spirometry, one should always keep in mind the difference between a simple ratio expressed as a percent (e.g., FEV_1/FVC = 75%) and a result expressed as a percent of predicted value (e.g., FEV_1 = 75% of predicted value). To avoid unnecessary confusion, the percent predicted value for FEV_1/FVC is omitted from Clinical Problems 12 and 13.

Clinical problem 11

Fig. 3-22, *A,* shows a normal spirometric pattern; Fig. 3-22, *B,* shows a tracing from an asthmatic patient before and after inhaling a bronchodilator. Without correcting to BTPS conditions, calculate the following values from the normal curve, from the before-bronchodilator curve, and from the after-bronchodilator curve: FVC, FEV_1, FEV_1/FVC, and peak expiratory flow rate.

Clinical problem 12

A 46-year-old man is evaluated for episodic dyspnea and coughing of several weeks duration. He can no longer function at his job and has recently quit playing racquetball because of dyspnea during exertion. He frequently awakens during the night because of coughing, wheezing, and dyspnea. For 1 week he has used an over-the-counter asthma inhaler. It gives some relief but has not helped his dyspnea during exercise.
An examination shows that he is mildly short of breath at rest, and there is expiratory wheezing bilaterally. A chest x-ray shows only slight hyperinflation.
Spirometry results are shown at the top of p. 70. *Pre-drug* and *post-drug* refer to spirometry done before and after inhalation of a bronchodilator; there is a 10 to 15 minute interval between pre- and post-drug tests. (*%PRED,* Percent of predicted value; *PRED,* predicted.)

Continued

Clinical problem 12, cont'd.

Measurement	Pre-drug			Post-drug	
	Actual	Pred	%Pred	Actual	%Pred
FVC (L)	2.07	4.67	44	3.12	67
FEV_1 (L)	1.23	3.52	35	1.70	48
FEV_1/FVC (%)	60	75		54	
MMF_{25-75} (L/sec)	0.67	3.64	18	0.77	21
Peak flow (L/min)	216	535	40	368	69

How do you interpret these pulmonary function tests?

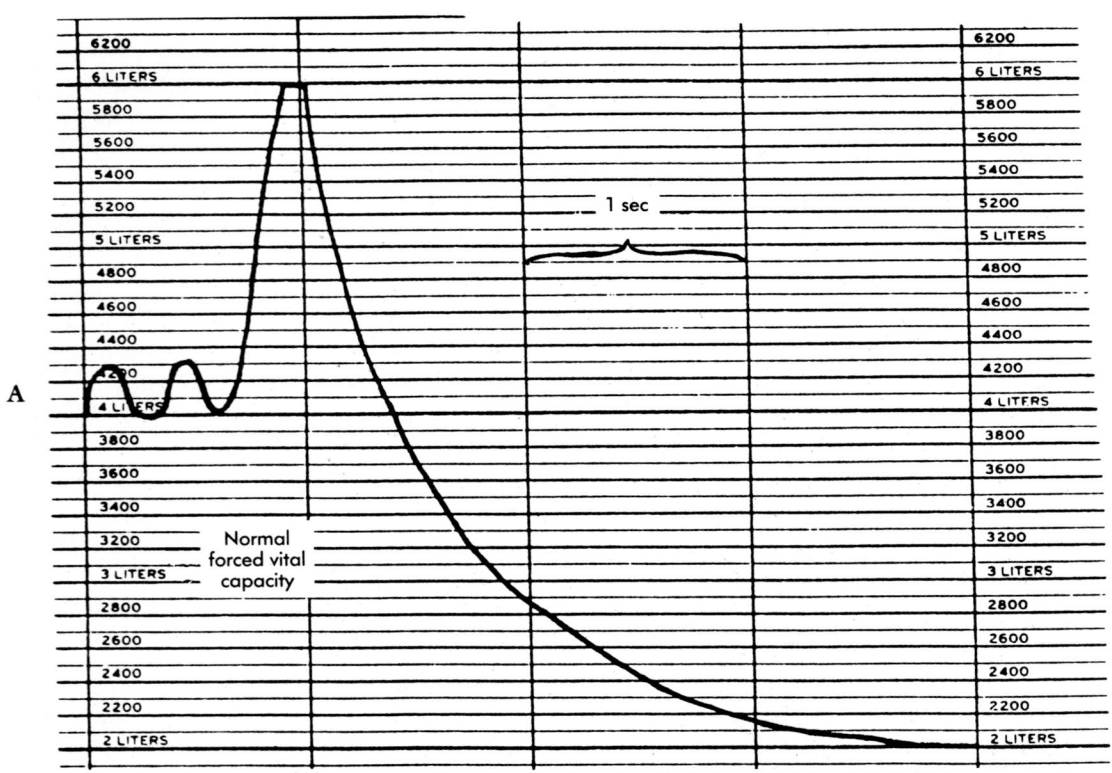

Fig. 3-22. Spirometric curves. **A,** From asthmatic patient in remission; spirometry is normal.

Continued

Lung mechanics

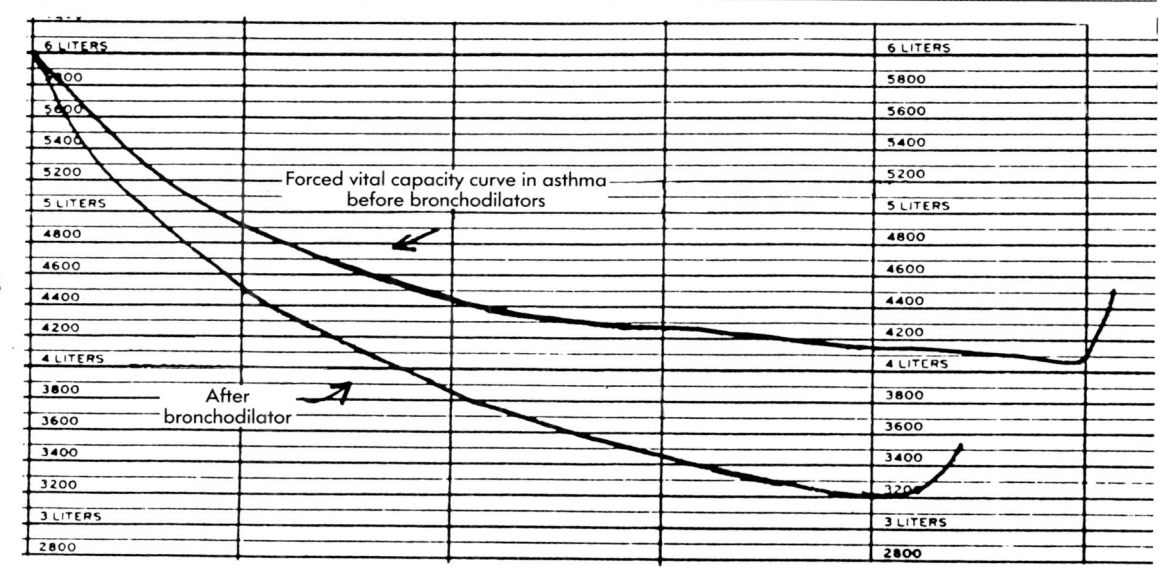

Fig. 3-22, cont'd. **B,** From patient during asthma attack, before and after use of bronchodilators.

Clinical problem 13

Two weeks after treatment, the patient from Clinical Problem 12 feels much better. Spirometry shows the following:

Measurement	Pre-drug			Post-drug	
	Actual	Pred	%Pred	Actual	%Pred
FVC (L)	4.73	4.67	101	4.81	103
FEV_1 (L)	3.28	3.52	93	3.54	100
FEV_1/FVC (%)	69	75		73	
MMF_{25-75} (L/sec)	2.06	3.64	56	2.54	70
Peak flow (L/min)	589	535	110	611	114

How do you interpret these tests?

MECHANICS AND GAS EXCHANGE—CORRELATION?

The next three chapters discuss gas exchange and the physiologic processes of alveolar ventilation and oxygenation. One might wonder if there is a correlation between mechanical impairment, as determined by the forced vital capacity, and gas exchange abnormality, as found by arterial blood gas analysis. For example, if FEV_1 is 50% of the predicted value, will partial pressure of oxygen be similarly reduced?

For the individual patient there is no useful correlation between tests of mechanics and gas exchange. Tests of mechanics cannot be used to infer any information regarding gas exchange and vice versa. Fig. 3-23 shows a plot of 100 patients referred consecutively to the pulmonary laboratory for lung function testing. Note that FEV_1 does not correlate with abnormal arterial oxygen pressure or arterial carbon dioxide pressure until it falls to less than 40% of the predicted value, and even then the correlation is weak. Diseases that impair lung mechanics do not necessarily affect gas exchange to the same extent; conversely, gas exchange can be markedly impaired without similar impairment of lung mechanics.

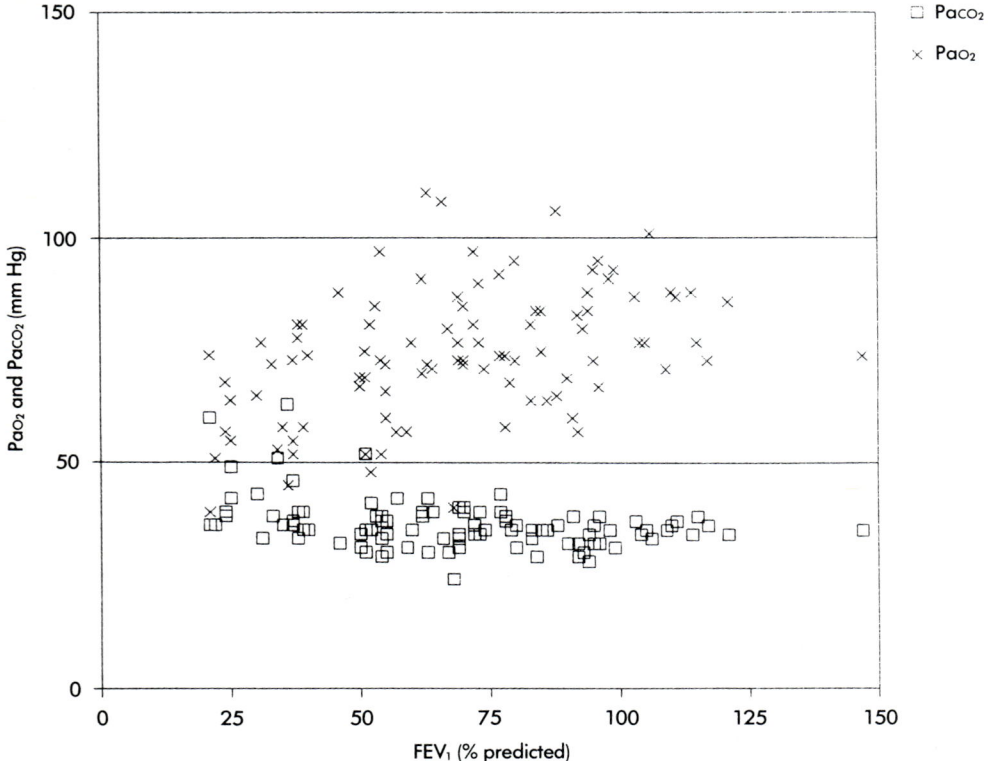

Fig. 3-23. Lack of clinically useful correlation between measurements of lung mechanics (% predicted FEV_1) and gas exchange (Pa_{O_2} and Pa_{CO_2}). Data are from 100 patients referred for pulmonary function testing. The abscissa represents the range of values for FEV_1 (% predicted). Above each measured FEV_1 (% predicted) value is a corresponding Pa_{O_2} *(X)* and Pa_{CO_2} *(box)* value. All blood gas values were obtained on room air at a barometric pressure of approximately 747 mm Hg. As the FEV_1 (% predicted) declines, there is a slight decline in Pa_{O_2}, but the variation is large. Thus for FEV_1 between 50% and 52% predicted, Pa_{O_2} ranges from 48 to 81 mm Hg; for FEV_1 between 21% and 25% predicted, Pa_{O_2} ranges from 39 to 74 mm Hg. There is no significant change in Pa_{CO_2} until the FEV_1 is severely reduced; with FEV_1 values below 40% of predicted there is a slight tendency for carbon dioxide retention, again with wide variation among patients. Based on these data, one cannot reliably infer an individual patient's mechanical function from blood gas data, or vice versa. A patient with a low FEV_1 may or may not be retaining carbon dioxide and may or may not be hypoxemic.

SUMMARY

Lung mechanics deals with the movement of air into and out of the lungs and the changes in pressure, volume, and flow during breathing. During quiet breathing intrapleural pressure is always negative (subatmospheric). During inspiration the chest cage expands making the intrapleural pressure more negative and creating transient negative airway pressure; as a result, fresh air moves into the lungs. During expiration the chest cage contracts, intrapleural pressure becomes less negative, and airway pressure becomes slightly positive; as a result, air moves out of the lungs.

Compliance is a measurement of a change in volume over a change in pressure. Compared to the action of normal lungs, lungs with high compliance (e.g., ones with emphysema) are easier to expand (less stiff); lungs with low compliance (e.g., ones with pulmonary fibrosis) are harder to expand (more stiff).

Airway resistance is a measurement of a change in pressure over a change in air flow. Airway resistance is increased in obstructive lung diseases such as asthma. Although compliance and airway resistance are not routinely measured in clinical laboratories, they are nonetheless important concepts in understanding many lung disorders.

Air within the thorax is conveniently divided into several lung volumes and capacities. The forced vital capacity (FVC) is the amount of air one can forcefully exhale after a maximal inhalation. FVC is routinely measured as part of spirometry, the most useful test of lung mechanics. FVC can be plotted as volume vs. time or as flow vs. volume, depending on the particular recording apparatus used; the effort by the patient is identical.

Subdivisions of the FVC, such as the FEV_1, FEV_1/FVC, and peak flow can give information about the pattern of respiratory impairment. Normally, one should be able to exhale approximately 70% to 75% of the FVC in the first second. An FEV_1/FVC less than the predicted value indicates airways obstruction. A reduction in both FVC and FEV_1, with an increase in FEV_1/FVC, suggests restrictive respiratory impairment.

REVIEW QUESTIONS

State whether each of the following is true or false.

1. The forced vital capacity is the total volume of air held by the lungs and airways.
2. During normal, resting breathing, intrapleural pressure is always less than atmospheric pressure.
3. Lung compliance is a measure of expired volume divided by air flow.
4. Residual volume is the resting volume of the lungs, the point at which the chest cage and lung elastic recoil balance.
5. As the airway diameter increases, airway resistance decreases.
6. The best single test of airways obstruction is the FEV_1.
7. The only difference between a flow-volume curve and a time-volume curve is in the way they are plotted.
8. Small airways disease is diagnosed by finding a reduced maximal midflow (flow between 25% and 75% of the vital capacity).
9. The best single spirometric measurement for revealing respiratory impairment is the FEV_1.
10. Peak expiratory flow rate is dependent on the lung volume at which exhalation begins.

References

American Thoracic Society: ATS statement: snowbird workshop on standardization of spirometry, Am. Rev. Respir. Dis. **119**:831, 1979.

Robinson, D.R., Chaudhary, B.A., and Speir, W.S.: Expiratory flow limitation in large and small airways, Arch. Intern. Med. **144**:1457, 1984.

Ruppel, G.: Manual of pulmonary function testing, ed. 3, St. Louis, 1982, The C.V. Mosby Co.

Zamel, N., Altose, M.D., and Speir, W.A.: ACCP scientific section recommendations. Statement on spirometry: a report of the section on respiratory pathophysiology, Chest **83**:547, 1983.

See also General References (Physiology) in Appendix G.

chapter 4
P_{CO_2} and alveolar ventilation

OUTLINE

Ventilation—minute, alveolar, and dead space
P_{CO_2}—its relation to alveolar ventilation and carbon dioxide production
P_{CO_2} and the respiratory quotient
Hyperventilation and hypoventilation
Clinical importance of the P_{CO_2} equation
P_{CO_2} in the clinical setting
Physiologic basis for hypercapnia
V_D/V_T and the Bohr dead space equation
Dangers of hypercapnia
Pa_{CO_2} and need for ventilatory assistance
Noninvasive measurement of P_{CO_2}
Pa_{CO_2}—its relation to oxygenation and acid-base balance

VENTILATION—MINUTE, ALVEOLAR, AND DEAD SPACE

In casual conversation, the word ventilation is often used by different people to mean different things. This ambiguity is often confusing for the listener, especially when terms like "hyperventilation" and "hypoventilation" are mentioned. To prevent any such confusion, it is necessary to define certain terms at the outset.

Ventilation is a general term for the movement of air into and out of the lungs; without a preceding adjective, such as alveolar or minute, the term does not have any more specific meaning. The symbol for ventilation is $\dot{V}$; V stands for volume and the dot for "per unit time."

Minute or *total ventilation* is the amount of air moved in or out of the lungs per minute. Quantitatively, the amount of air breathed in per minute ($\dot{V}_I$) is slightly greater than the amount expired per minute ($\dot{V}_E$). Clinically this difference is not important, and by convention minute ventilation is always measured on an expired sample and symbolized $\dot{V}_E$. It is useful to remember that $\dot{V}_E$ is the breathing frequency (f) per minute times the tidal volume (V_T, volume of tidal breath):

$$\dot{V}_E = f \times V_T \qquad (1)$$

$\dot{V}_E$ is also the sum of two other ventilations, alveolar ventilation and dead space ventilation. These and other relationships are diagrammed in Fig. 4-1, along with representative normal values.

Alveolar ventilation ($\dot{V}_A$) is the volume of air breathed in per minute that (1) reaches the alveoli *and* (2) takes part in gas exchange. Alveolar ventilation is often misunderstood as representing only the volume of air that reaches the alveoli. Physiologically, $\dot{V}_A$ is the volume of alveolar air/minute that takes part in gas exchange (transfer of oxygen and carbon dioxide) with the pulmonary capillaries. Air that reaches the alveoli, but for one reason or other does not take part in gas exchange, is not considered part of $\dot{V}_A$ (for example, air that goes to an unperfused alveolus). Such alveolar regions lacking gas exchange constitute alveolar dead

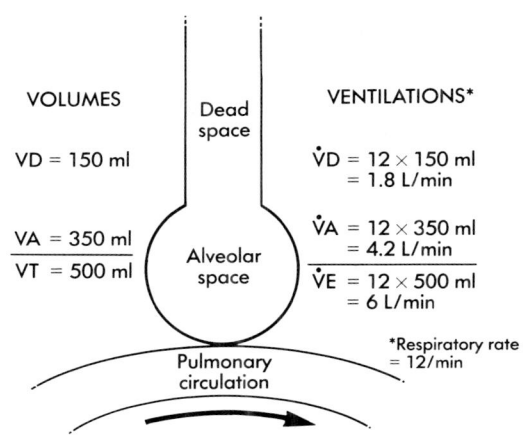

Fig. 4-1. Lung volumes and ventilations. Representation of lungs and pulmonary circulation. See text for discussion.

space. Clinically, the terms hyperventilation and hypoventilation apply to alveolar ventilation only (see below).

Dead space ventilation is that part of minute ventilation that does not take part in gas exchange; it is also referred to as "wasted ventilation." Dead space (wasted) ventilation ($\dot{V}_D$) includes (1) air that enters only conducting airways (referred to as anatomic dead space), *and* (2) air that reaches alveoli but does not exchange carbon dioxide or oxygen with the capillary blood. The combined volume of these two areas is often referred to as *physiologic dead space*.

Based on these definitions,

$$\dot{V}_E = \dot{V}_A + \dot{V}_D \text{ or,} \quad (2)$$
$$\dot{V}_A = \dot{V}_E - \dot{V}_D$$

In actual practice, $\dot{V}_E$ is relatively easy to measure with a spirometer (or any device that can measure tidal volume). However, neither $\dot{V}_A$ nor $\dot{V}_D$ is usually measured in the clinical setting; they are difficult to measure, and knowing their absolute value is not all that helpful.

PCO_2—ITS RELATION TO ALVEOLAR VENTILATION AND CARBON DIOXIDE PRODUCTION

Although minute ventilation ($\dot{V}_E$) is easily measured, it does not provide sufficient information for assessing the adequacy of alveolar ventilation ($\dot{V}_A$), the component that affects gas exchange. The tidal volume and the respiratory rate do not give any clue as to how much air is ventilating dead space vs. alveolar space. Even if dead space ventilation ($\dot{V}_D$) and $\dot{V}_A$ were measurable, the measurements would not indicate how much carbon dioxide was being produced in the body or how much $\dot{V}_A$ would be sufficient to eliminate the carbon dioxide that is produced.

The needed information can be obtained by measuring the partial pressure of carbon dioxide in the arterial blood ($PaCO_2$), which is the only blood gas measurement that provides information on $\dot{V}_A$. Furthermore, $PaCO_2$ states directly, with one number, the *relationship of $\dot{V}_A$ to carbon dioxide production,* at least at the time the sample is taken.

To understand why this is so, consider what happens to carbon dioxide in the body (Fig. 4-2). Carbon dioxide is a by-product of food metabolism. Toxic in large amounts, carbon dioxide is literally a waste product that must be eliminated for the body to function normally. However, carbon dioxide is also a component of the bicarbonate buffer system, the largest of the blood buffers, and hence is an important determinant of acid-base balance. Furthermore, $PaCO_2$ is one determinant of arterial oxygen pressure (PaO_2) and hence plays a role in oxygenation (shown by the alveolar air equation, discussed in Chapter 5). Not only must carbon dioxide from metabolism be continually eliminated, but the body must also maintain a certain level of carbon dioxide in the blood.

The total amount of carbon dioxide transported in the body is approximately 49 ml/100 ml for arterial blood and 54 ml/100 ml for venous blood (Fig. 4-2). Carbon dioxide is transported in the blood in three forms: as bicarbonate (the greatest amount), combined with hemoglobin and other

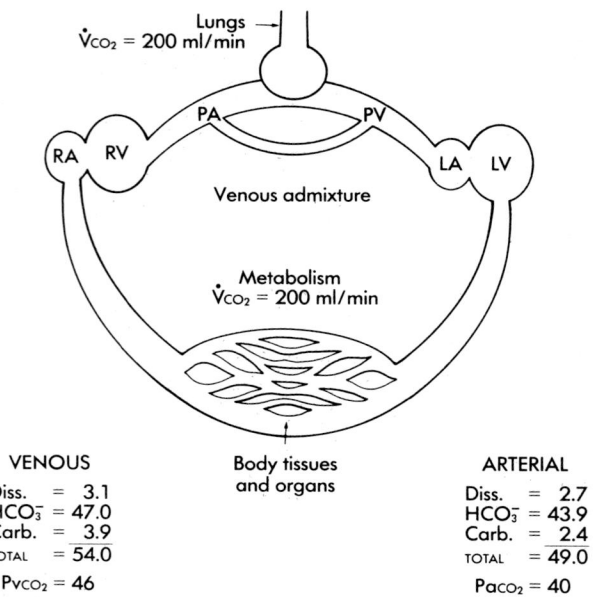

Fig. 4-2. Production, transport, and excretion of carbon dioxide in the lungs and circulation. Carbon dioxide, a by-product of metabolism, is transported in three forms: dissolved *(Diss.)*, bound to hemoglobin and other proteins *(Carb.)*, and as bicarbonate (HCO_3^-). Only the dissolved fraction exerts a partial pressure. Partial pressure of carbon dioxide (P_{CO_2}) values are in mm Hg; all other values represent the volume of carbon dioxide in whole blood (ml CO_2/100 ml). Approximately 5 ml CO_2/100 ml are excreted per minute. Venous admixture represents all normal physiologic shunting. (P_{VCO_2} and P_{aCO_2}, mixed venous and arterial P_{CO_2}, respectively; RA, right atrium; RV, right ventricle; PA, pulmonary arteries; PV, pulmonary veins; LA, left atrium; LV, left ventricle.)

proteins (carbamino compounds), and dissolved. These forms are in equilibrium with one another, and it is the dissolved fraction in plasma that exerts the partial pressure measured as P_{aCO_2}. Normal P_{aCO_2} ranges between 36 and 44 mm Hg; mixed venous partial pressure of carbon dioxide (P_{VCO_2}) is approximately 6 mm Hg higher.

At rest, the average-sized person produces approximately 200 ml of carbon dioxide per minute (Fig. 4-2). Carbon dioxide production ($\dot{V}_{CO_2}$) is of course a continuous process, as is oxygen consumption. During exercise $\dot{V}_{CO_2}$ increases, and it declines slightly during sleep; on the average, 288 L of carbon dioxide are produced per day (1440 min × 200 ml CO_2/min). That's a lot of CO_2! How is this huge load eliminated while a normal P_{aCO_2} is maintained?

Carbon dioxide elimination is accomplished by bringing fresh air into the lungs; there is no other way to excrete it. (A miniscule amount of carbon dioxide, less than 1%, is excreted by the kidneys as bicarbonate.)

In the lungs, fresh air is brought next to the pulmonary capillaries where it is separated from mixed venous blood by only a thin, gas-permeable alveolar-capillary membrane (see Chapter 1). Fresh air contains almost no carbon dioxide when it is first inhaled. In the alveoli, the partial pressure of carbon dioxide (P_{ACO_2}) is practically the same as P_{aCO_2}, whatever the value. Carbon dioxide is transferred across the alveolar-capillary membrane by virtue of a pressure gradient that exists between mixed venous P_{CO_2} and alveolar P_{CO_2} (normally 46 and 40 mm Hg, respectively). Carbon dioxide that enters the alveolar spaces is exhaled during breathing. In a steady state, the amount of carbon dioxide produced from metabolism equals the amount eliminated by the lungs.

One of the most important physiologic relationships in all of clinical medicine can now be derived: that between P_{CO_2} and $\dot{V}_A$.

Because dead space does not take part in gas exchange, all of the expired carbon dioxide comes from the alveolar gas. Thus the amount of $\dot{V}_{CO_2}$ excreted by the lungs equals $\dot{V}_A$ times the fraction of alveolar carbon dioxide (F_{ACO_2}):

$$\dot{V}_{CO_2} = \dot{V}_A \times F_{ACO_2} \quad (3)$$

Since $P_{ACO_2} = F_{ACO_2}$ times total alveolar gas pressure,

$$\dot{V}_{CO_2} = \dot{V}_A \times P_{ACO_2} \times K \quad (4)$$

where K is a constant that takes into account the different units as well as the conversion of F_{ACO_2} to P_{ACO_2}; 1/K has the value 0.863. Rearranging,

$$P_{ACO_2} = \frac{\dot{V}_{CO_2} \times 0.863}{\dot{V}_A} \quad (5)*$$

Equation 5 expresses the relationship between alveolar P_{CO_2} and $\dot{V}_A$. Because carbon dioxide is a highly diffusable gas, alveolar P_{CO_2} is assumed to be equal to arterial P_{CO_2}. Also, in the steady state, carbon dioxide excreted by the lungs equals that produced from metabolism. With these relationships in mind, it will be useful to conceptually derive Equation 5 for arterial P_{CO_2}.

Assume that carbon dioxide production is constant at 200 ml/min. Without alveolar ventilation, carbon dioxide will build up in the blood since there is no other way to eliminate it; as a result, severe acidity and death will quickly follow. The same thing will happen if there is just a small amount of $\dot{V}_A$; carbon dioxide builds up, although not quite as fast as when there is no $\dot{V}_A$.

Conversely, if $\dot{V}_A$ exceeds its normal amount, excessive carbon dioxide is eliminated from the blood and P_{aCO_2} falls. Thus as long as $\dot{V}_{CO_2}$ is constant, P_{aCO_2} is *inversely* related to the amount of $\dot{V}_A$:

$$P_{aCO_2} \simeq \frac{1}{\dot{V}_A} \quad (6)$$

Now assume that the level of $\dot{V}_A$ is constant at 4 L/min. If metabolism increases during exercise, for example, carbon dioxide enters the circulation at a rate greater than normal. Without a concomitant increase in $\dot{V}_A$, P_{aCO_2} will rise. Conversely, if metabolism is slowed but $\dot{V}_A$ remains unchanged, P_{aCO_2} will fall. Thus P_{aCO_2} is *directly* proportional to $\dot{V}_{CO_2}$. Combining this observation with the one in Equation 6:

$$P_{aCO_2} \simeq \frac{\dot{V}_{CO_2}}{\dot{V}_A} \quad (7)$$

P_{aCO_2} is measured in mm Hg, $\dot{V}_{CO_2}$ in ml/min (STPD), and $\dot{V}_A$ in L/min (BTPS); hence the units must be converted to mm Hg. This conversion is achieved by the constant, 0.863. Thus

$$P_{aCO_2} = \frac{\dot{V}_{CO_2} \times 0.863}{\dot{V}_A} \quad (8)$$

where

$$\dot{V}_A = \dot{V}_E - \dot{V}_D. \quad (2)$$

Of all the relationships in this book, the one expressed by Equation 8 is among the most important.

P_{CO_2} AND THE RESPIRATORY QUOTIENT

P_{CO_2} is determined by the ratio of carbon dioxide production ($\dot{V}_{CO_2}$) over alveolar ventilation (see the previous section). Carbon dioxide production is determined by several factors, including the type of foods ingested, level of exercise, body temperature, and hormonal activity (e.g., that of the thyroid hormone). Basal $\dot{V}_{CO_2}$, approximately 200 ml/min

---

*The complete derivation of this equation, including the constant 0.863, is given in Appendix C.

for the average-sized adult, can increase severalfold during exercise (see Chapter 12).

The ratio of oxygen consumption ($\dot{V}O_2$) to $\dot{V}CO_2$ is called the respiratory quotient (RQ).

$$RQ = \frac{\dot{V}CO_2}{\dot{V}O_2} \qquad (9)$$

In a person at rest who consumes a normal diet (mixture of fats, carbohydrates, and proteins), $\dot{V}O_2$ is approximately 250 ml/min, for an RQ of approximately 0.80. When the diet consists of only carbohydrates, RQ increases to 1.0—the quantity of carbon dioxide produced equals the quantity of oxygen consumed. If only fats are eaten, the RQ is 0.71.

There is an RQ for both metabolism in the tissues and gas exchange in the lungs. In the steady state, *metabolic RQ* (production of carbon dioxide and consumption of oxygen by the tissues) is exactly matched by the *pulmonary RQ* (output of carbon dioxide and uptake of oxygen by the lungs). In fact,

$$RQ\ (metabolic) = RQ\ (pulmonary) \qquad (10)$$

defines a steady state for the respiratory system.*

Normal ventilation is governed by the body's metabolic demands. For example, during exercise the body consumes far more oxygen and produces more carbon dioxide than at rest; as a result, minute (and alveolar) ventilation increase to meet the increase in metabolic demand.

From Equation 8 it can be seen that if $\dot{V}CO_2$ rises proportionately more than $\dot{V}A$, $PaCO_2$ will increase. Does this ever happen in a healthy person? For example, can one exercise to such a point that $\dot{V}CO_2$ exceeds the capacity of the respiratory system to excrete carbon dioxide? Apparently not. In fact the more a healthy person exercises, the more likely his $PaCO_2$ will *fall* because of compensatory hyperventilation in response to developing metabolic acidosis (see Chapter 12).

If $\dot{V}CO_2$ increases and if $\dot{V}A$ cannot rise proportionately, $PaCO_2$ will increase. In such cases the cause of hypercapnia is inadequate $\dot{V}A$ for the amount of carbon dioxide presented to the lungs for excretion. This inadequacy is discussed in the section on hypercapnia.

HYPERVENTILATION AND HYPOVENTILATION

Hyperventilation and hypoventilation are defined by $PaCO_2$. Low $PaCO_2$ (hypocapnia) defines a state of hyperventilation, high $PaCO_2$ (hypercapnia), a state of hypoventilation. This terminology is often confusing to neophytes for two reasons. First, the prefixes are opposite to the level of $PaCO_2$: *hyper*ventilation for hypocapnia or low $PaCO_2$, *hypo*ventilation for hypercapnia or high $PaCO_2$.

Second, the terms seem (at first glance) to state something about rate and depth of breathing. After all, is not someone who is breathing fast and deep "hyperventilating"? Such a person may be hyperventilating in the physiologic sense (i.e., has a low $PaCO_2$) but then again *may also be hypoventilating* (has a high $PaCO_2$). The latter could come about if most of the minute ventilation were going to dead space with very little left over for $\dot{V}A$; this situation may arise in severe chronic obstructive pulmonary disease when there is a large amount of dead space from ventilation-perfusion imbalance (see Chapter 5).

Thus hyperventilation and hypoventilation refer to the state of $\dot{V}A$ in relation to carbon dioxide production, a relationship that can only be known by measuring $PaCO_2$. As used in pulmonary medicine, the terms do not relate to rate or depth of breathing or to any aspect of a patient's effort to breathe. Perhaps better terms are hyper*alveolar*ventilation and hypo*alveolar*ventilation, but the shorter terms seem firmly entrenched in clinical practice.

---

*The fact that there is both a metabolic and a pulmonary RQ can be confusing because of nonspecific terminology. *R* is sometimes used to denote the metabolic RQ and *RQ* to denote the pulmonary RQ; however, this convention is not universal. It is always best to specify which RQ is being discussed and not to assume an understanding based on any abbreviation. In clinical practice the term R or RQ is found most frequently in the alveolar air equation (see Chapter 5) where it refers to pulmonary gas exchange.

Clinical problem 1

You are called to the bedside of a patient who appears anxious and short of breath. Her respiratory rate is 24/min, and she seems to be moving a lot of air with each breath. Is she hyperventilating?

Clinical problem 2

A patient is brought to the emergency room after being found comatose in his apartment. His respirations appear shallow, approximately 10/min, and blood pressure and pulse are stable. He remains comatose. Is he hypoventilating?

Clinical problem 3

A well-conditioned student decides to jog around the block. Assuming she has normal resting values for carbon dioxide production ($\dot{V}_{CO_2}$) of 200 ml/min and for alveolar ventilation ($\dot{V}_A$) of 4.3 L/min, what would be her most likely values just before she finishes running?
a. Pa_{CO_2} 25 mm Hg; $\dot{V}_A$ 8.6 L/min; $\dot{V}_{CO_2}$ 400 ml/min
b. Pa_{CO_2} 40 mm Hg; $\dot{V}_A$ 8.6 L/min; $\dot{V}_{CO_2}$ 400 ml/min
c. Pa_{CO_2} 40 mm Hg; $\dot{V}_A$ 4.3 L/min; $\dot{V}_{CO_2}$ 400 ml/min
d. Pa_{CO_2} 40 mm Hg; $\dot{V}_A$ 8.6 L/min; $\dot{V}_{CO_2}$ 200 ml/min
e. Pa_{CO_2} 50 mm Hg; $\dot{V}_A$ 8.6 L/min; $\dot{V}_{CO_2}$ 400 ml/min

CLINICAL IMPORTANCE OF THE P_{CO_2} EQUATION

The simple relationships expressed by the Pa_{CO_2} equation (Equation 8) are key to understanding patients with respiratory problems.

By defining Pa_{CO_2}, Equation 8 demonstrates both what determines Pa_{CO_2} and what does not. Pa_{CO_2} equals the level of carbon dioxide production over alveolar ventilation (times a constant) and nothing more. Pa_{CO_2} is *not* equated to such clinically apparent factors as rate and depth of breathing, level of anxiety, mental status, or sensation of dyspnea.

True, $\dot{V}_A = \dot{V}_E - \dot{V}_D$,* and $\dot{V}_E$ is the breathing frequency times the tidal volume, but these variables do not define Pa_{CO_2}. One cannot infer the Pa_{CO_2} from the $\dot{V}_E$ alone since $\dot{V}_E$ gives no information on either $\dot{V}_A$ or $\dot{V}_{CO_2}$. In addition, since neither $\dot{V}_A$ nor $\dot{V}_{CO_2}$ can be determined clinically, one cannot reliably determine Pa_{CO_2} on clinical grounds alone. If one is concerned about the status of a patient's $\dot{V}_A$, there is no clinical substitute for measuring Pa_{CO_2}.

The importance of this observation in patient care cannot be overstated. For years, before arterial blood gas analysis became widely available, many physicians thought that the level of $\dot{V}_A$ (and hence Pa_{CO_2}) could be reliably estimated at the bedside. With the advent of blood gas analysis, clinical assessment has been shown unreliable both by formal study (Mithoefer, Bossman, Thibeault, et al., 1968) and by everyday experience. The physiologic reason is apparent—one cannot estimate $\dot{V}_A$ reliably nor know a given patient's $\dot{V}_{CO_2}$.

Clinical problem 4

Two patients have the following respiratory and P_{CO_2} measurements:
Patient A: Respiratory rate = 10/min
Tidal volume = 600 ml
Pa_{CO_2} = 35 mm Hg
Patient B: Respiratory rate = 10/min
Tidal volume = 600 ml
Pa_{CO_2} = 45 mm Hg
The reason these two patients have different Pa_{CO_2} values is best explained by which of the following statements:
a. They are different ages, and Pa_{CO_2} is age-dependent.
b. One is a man, one a woman, and Pa_{CO_2} is sex-dependent.
c. Their rate of oxygen consumption is different.
d. They have a difference in dead-space ventilation.
e. Their minute ventilation is different.

P_{CO_2} IN THE CLINICAL SETTING

Knowing the Pa_{CO_2} is not enough, of course, to fully evaluate alveolar ventilation. Pa_{CO_2} must be explained and understood in light of the full clinical picture.

For example, a patient with asthma, who is using his accessory muscles during an acute broncho-

---

*$\dot{V}_E$, minute ventilation; $\dot{V}_D$, dead space ventilation.

spasm attack, is trying to *hyperventilate* and thus blow off carbon dioxide (the respiratory stimulus is not hypoxemia but an irritation of lung receptors in the narrowed bronchi). If such a patient has a "normal" Pa_{CO_2}, e.g., 40 mm Hg, then $\dot{V}_A$ is adequate for carbon dioxide production (by definition). However, Pa_{CO_2} in the "normal" range during an acute asthma attack is indicative of a very severe airways obstruction and an inability to hyperventilate despite the respiratory effort. It may signify impending respiratory failure and an imminent need for intubation and artificial ventilation. In this setting, Pa_{CO_2} of 40 mm Hg is not "normal" and is certainly not reassuring.

As another example, a patient with diabetic ketoacidosis should hyperventilate in response to the acidemia. Finding a Pa_{CO_2} of 40 mm Hg and a pH of 7.25 in a patient with acidosis suggests that an additional *primary respiratory problem* is inhibiting the ventilatory response to acidemia. Although the patient's Pa_{CO_2} is adequate for carbon dioxide production, it is far from optimal considering the metabolic acidosis.

Interpreting Pa_{CO_2} in light of the clinical picture (and not just as a number) is essential for good patient management whenever a blood gas analysis is obtained. Such assessment will often determine major management decisions, such as the use of intubation and artificial ventilation.

Clinical problem 5

All of the following factors, except one, are important in assessing whether or not $\dot{V}_A$ is appropriate for the clinical situation; which one is the exception?
a. Mental status of the patient
b. Rate and depth of respiration
c. Carbon dioxide production/min
d. Arterial P_{O_2}
e. Arterial pH

Clinical problem 6

Below are five descriptions of patients. State if the patient in each case is hyperventilating, hypoventilating, or normally ventilating with respect to carbon dioxide production. Explain the Pa_{CO_2} value in each situation.
a. A patient with diabetic ketoacidosis (blood sugar markedly elevated at 830 mgm%); arterial pH 7.27; Pa_{CO_2} 25 mm Hg; serum bicarbonate (HCO_3^-) 11 mEq/L.
b. A patient suffering from an acute asthma attack and using accessory muscles of respiration; forced expiratory volume, 1 second (FEV_1) is 30% of predicted; Pa_{CO_2} 38 mm Hg.
c. A patient with severe chronic obstructive pulmonary disease (COPD) who appears comfortable at rest; forced vital capacity (FVC) only 25% of predicted; blood gas analysis shows pH 7.34 and Pa_{CO_2} 55 mm Hg.
d. A patient with severe COPD is acutely short of breath and cyanotic but appears to be moving a lot of air as judged by chest excursions; arterial blood gas, obtained on room air, shows pH 7.25; Pa_{CO_2} 68 mm Hg; and Pa_{O_2} 29 mm Hg.
e. A patient appearing lethargic but in no visible distress, with Pa_{CO_2} 38 mm Hg; pH 7.42; Pa_{O_2} 40 mm Hg; 75% oxygen saturation.

PHYSIOLOGIC BASIS FOR HYPERCAPNIA

Failure to bring in enough fresh air to adequately eliminate carbon dioxide is one type of respiratory failure and is called ventilatory failure (see Chapter 11). Thus the hallmark of ventilatory failure is hypercapnia—elevated Pa_{CO_2}.

It can now be appreciated that there is only one fundamental reason for hypercapnia in clinical medicine: decreased alveolar ventilation ($\dot{V}_A$) relative to carbon dioxide production. This can be viewed as *the* physiologic basis for all carbon dioxide retention.* Under this broad physiologic umbrella can be classified every clinical case of hypercapnia (see box on p. 81). This categorization derives directly from the physiologic relationships expressed in Equations 2 and 8.

---

*Hypercapnia will also occur inhaling carbon dioxide, but this situation is outside the realm of clinical medicine.

PHYSIOLOGIC BASIS FOR CARBON DIOXIDE RETENTION—DECREASED $\dot{V}_A$ RELATIVE TO $\dot{V}_{CO_2}$

This decrease is always explained by one of three situations:
1. Decreased $\dot{V}_A$ caused by decreased or inadequate minute ventilation ($\dot{V}_E$);
2. Decreased $\dot{V}_A$ caused by increased dead space ventilation ($\dot{V}_D$); or
3. A combination of 1 and 2

Decreased alveolar ventilation caused by decreased or inadequate minute ventilation

Decreased $\dot{V}_A$ may occur from anything that decreases $\dot{V}_E$, e.g., respiratory center depression (drug overdose) or chest wall dysfunction (paralysis from neuromuscular disease). Whatever the actual clinical cause, $\dot{V}_E$ is reduced enough to lower $\dot{V}_A$ and raise arterial carbon dioxide pressure (Pa_{CO_2}). The decrease in $\dot{V}_E$ may be manifested by an alteration in tidal volume and/or breathing frequency (Equation 1).

Clinical problem 7

A 38-year-old woman is admitted to the hospital following an overdose of sleeping pills. She is comatose and is breathing approximately 10 times per minute. After blood gas analysis is obtained, she is intubated and connected to a volume-cycled ventilator. If her carbon dioxide production were 200 ml/min and her Pa_{CO_2} were 80 mm Hg, what was her probable $\dot{V}_E$ before intubation?

$\dot{V}_A$ can also be decreased (relative to carbon dioxide production) because of inadequate $\dot{V}_E$; in such cases $\dot{V}_E$ does not actually decrease from the patient's normal resting value, but instead it *does not increase appropriately*. For example, if, during exercise, carbon dioxide production ($\dot{V}_{CO_2}$) increases but $\dot{V}_E$ does not, Pa_{CO_2} will increase. This occurrence is sometimes seen in patients with severe emphysema who simply cannot augment $\dot{V}_E$ above their resting level. In such cases the fundamental cause is still inadequate $\dot{V}_A$ for the level of $\dot{V}_{CO_2}$. In the most extreme cases of increased carbon dioxide production (during very heavy exercise), healthy people increase their $\dot{V}_E$ and $\dot{V}_A$ appropriately and Pa_{CO_2} does not increase.

Clinical problem 8

A patient in the intensive care unit is receiving artificial ventilation at 10 breaths/min, 700 cc/breath; he has no spontaneous breathing. His Pa_{CO_2} is 38 mm Hg. If metabolic $\dot{V}_{CO_2}$ is 200 ml/min, what will Pa_{CO_2} be if $\dot{V}_{CO_2}$ increases to 300 ml/min? What might cause such an increase in $\dot{V}_{CO_2}$?

Decreased alveolar ventilation caused by increased dead space ventilation

Increased physiologic dead space is a more common cause of hypercapnia than decreased minute ventilation. In fact, increased dead space ventilation ($\dot{V}_D$) is an underlying mechanism in virtually all cases of obstructive and restrictive lung disease that lead to carbon dioxide retention. Increased $\dot{V}_D$ may occur in two ways. The most common way is from an imbalance in ventilation-perfusion (V/Q) relationships; this is the same V/Q imbalance responsible for most clinical hypoxemia (discussed in Chapter 5).

The V/Q imbalance may so alter the architecture of the lungs that there is more dead space and less alveolar (gas-exchanging) space than normal. For such a patient to have sufficient alveolar ventilation, he must either take deeper breaths or breathe more frequently to compensate for the increased dead space and to deliver enough air to the gas-exchanging alveoli; although many patients are able to do this, some are not, either because of fatigue, muscle weakness, or a decreased "drive" to breathe (see Chapter 5 for further discussion).

Clinical problem 9

A patient with severe chronic obstructive pulmonary disease has the following resting pulmonary function and blood gas values: FEV_1 37% of predicted; FVC 43% predicted; $Paco_2$ 62 mm Hg; Pao_2 67 mm Hg; pH 7.36 (while breathing room air). Tidal volume is 550 ml; respiratory rate 16/min. How do you explain the patient's hypercapnia?

The second way increased $\dot{V}D$ can occur is occasionally seen in patients with severe restrictive lung disease; these patients breathe shallowly and rapidly. With their small tidal volume, the dead space volume is *proportionately* higher even though the anatomic dead space may be unchanged. Since anatomic dead space comes *before* alveolar space, $\dot{V}A$ will be lower.

Note that in both of these examples (severe obstructive disease and severe restrictive disease), the $\dot{V}E$ may be normal or even above normal, but the *distribution* of $\dot{V}E$ is abnormal. In other words, the ratio of dead space to tidal volume (VD/VT) is abnormally high and is the reason for hypercapnia.

Decreased alveolar ventilation from combined causes

Finally, patients may have a combination of both processes: diminished $\dot{V}E$ *and* increased $\dot{V}D$. This may occur, for example, in patients with severe lung disease who become "tired out" and cannot maintain $\dot{V}E$ because of muscle fatigue or chest bellows impairment.

Clinical problem 10

A 49-year-old, 350 lb, 5 ft 1 in woman, has normal pulmonary function except for a slight restrictive defect caused by her obesity. When breathing room air, her $Paco_2$ is 39 mm Hg, Pao_2 74 mm Hg, and pH 7.39. Tidal volume is 750 ml, respiratory rate 21 per min, and oxygen consumption 500 ml/min (approximately twice the normal amount).

One year later, she is admitted to the hospital in a state of respiratory failure. Her weight is now 470 lbs. Arterial blood gas analysis while breathing nasal oxygen shows pH 7.30, $Paco_2$ 60 mm Hg, and Pao_2 58 mm Hg. Average tidal volume is now 300 ml, and her respiratory rate is 28 per min. A chest x-ray shows cardiomegaly and a pleural effusion.
How would you explain her hypoventilation?

Table 4-1. Ventilatory adaptations to increased VD/VT

Physiologic parameter	Normal	Increased VD/VT		
		Decreased VT	Normal VT	Increased VT
VD/VT	0.33	0.60	0.60	0.60
VT	500 ml	300	500	700
VD	150 ml	180	300	420
VA	350 ml	120	200	280
f*	10	30	18	13
$\dot{V}A$	3.50 L/min	3.60	3.60	3.64
$Paco_2$	40 mm Hg	39	39	39

*f, frequency.

VD/VT AND THE BOHR DEAD SPACE EQUATION

The normal ratio of dead space to tidal volume (VD/VT or $\dot{V}D/\dot{V}E$, which is the same thing) is approximately 150 ml VD/500 ml VT, or 0.3. Normal VD/VT ranges from approximately 0.28 to 0.33.

As pointed out previously, VD/VT can be elevated from either a reduction of VT or an actual increase in VD. Either cause of increased VD/VT can cause a decrease in alveolar volume (VA) and hence in alveolar ventilation ($\dot{V}A$).

When the cause of increased VD/VT is lung disease, ventilatory adaptations will try to keep $\dot{V}A$ and $Paco_2$ normal (Table 4-1). These adjustments of course require an intact central nervous system and intact chest bellows. When ventilatory adaptations fail, $\dot{V}A$ will fall and $Paco_2$ will rise.

On occasion it is useful to quantitate the VD/VT. This can be done using the Bohr dead space equation:

$$\frac{VD}{VT} = \frac{Paco_2 - Peco_2}{Paco_2} \quad (11)$$

where $Peco_2$ is the mean expired carbon dioxide pressure, which is obtained from an expired air sample that is collected over a few minutes time.

Normal P_{ECO_2} is approximately 28 mm Hg. Thus $40 - 28/40 = 0.30$.

Clinical problem 11

During an attempt to wean a patient from the use of artificial ventilation, her P_{aCO_2} and P_{ECO_2} are measured with the following results: P_{aCO_2}, 56 mm Hg; P_{ECO_2}, 26 mm Hg. What is the V_D/V_T? Apart from any other factors, does this ratio indicate the patient can be removed from the ventilator?

DANGERS OF HYPERCAPNIA

The dangers from an elevated P_{aCO_2} are usually not from the excess carbon dioxide per se. In fact carbon dioxide is a respiratory stimulant until very high P_{aCO_2} values are reached (90 mm Hg or greater), at which time carbon dioxide may depress breathing. In addition to indicating a state of respiratory failure, there are three distinct dangers associated with an elevated P_{aCO_2}.

Low P_{aO_2} from high P_{aCO_2}. For a constant fraction of inspired oxygen (F_{IO_2}), as the P_{aCO_2} rises, the alveolar oxygen pressure (P_{AO_2}) falls, roughly on a mm Hg-for-mm Hg basis. This change can be appreciated from the relationship of P_{aCO_2} to P_{AO_2} in the alveolar air equation (discussed extensively in Chapter 5); in addition a fall in P_{AO_2} results in a corresponding drop in P_{aO_2}. Although this cause of hypoxemia can often be corrected by judicious use of supplemental oxygen, there are situations in which a further rise in P_{aCO_2} will cause P_{aO_2} to fall to a dangerous level.

Low pH from high P_{aCO_2}. A rise in P_{aCO_2} will lead to a fall in pH; this can be seen in the relationship of P_{aCO_2} to pH (Henderson-Hasselbalch equation; see Fig. 4-5 and Chapter 7). Acidemia is a potential trigger of cardiac arrhythmias. Although the critical level for hydrogen ion concentration varies in each situation, an arterial pH below 7.30 that is not improving should be considered potentially life-threatening.

Decreased ventilatory reserve. Finally, a high P_{aCO_2} represents a precarious situation in terms of ventilatory reserve. Small changes in alveolar ventilation ($\dot{V}_A$) that would be inconsequential in a healthy individual can be disastrous in someone retaining carbon dioxide. The reason why can be seen in the hyperbolic relationship when $\dot{V}_A$ is plotted against P_{aCO_2} (Fig. 4-3). For example, when carbon dioxide production ($\dot{V}_{CO_2}$) is 200 ml/min, a 500 ml/min decrease in $\dot{V}_A$ (which may

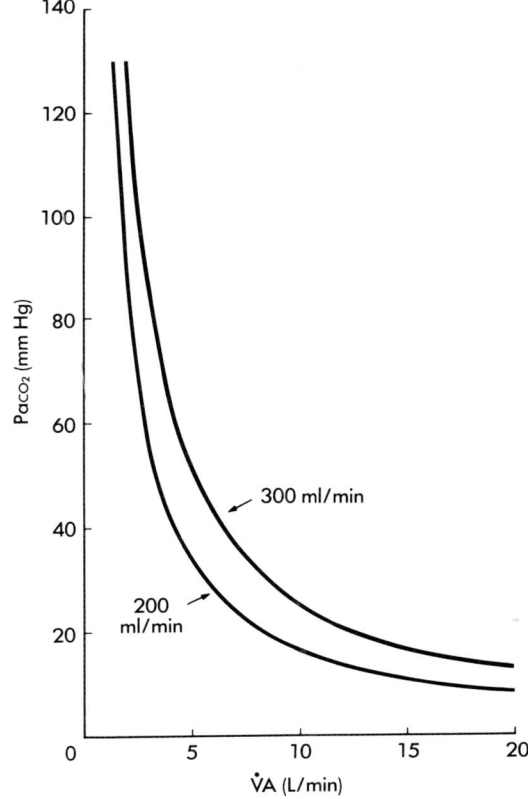

Fig. 4-3. P_{aCO_2} vs. alveolar ventilation ($\dot{V}_A$). The relationship is shown for carbon dioxide production rates of 200 ml/min and 300 ml/min. A decrease in alveolar ventilation ($\dot{V}_A$) in the hypercapnic patient will result in a greater rise in P_{aCO_2} than will the same $\dot{V}_A$ change when P_{aCO_2} is low or normal. Also, an increase in carbon dioxide production when $\dot{V}_A$ is fixed will result in an increase in P_{aCO_2}.

occur during central nervous system depression) will increase Pa_{CO_2} only 5 mm Hg, from a normal baseline Pa_{CO_2} of 40 mm Hg ($\dot{V}A$ = 4.3 L/min) to 45 mm Hg ($\dot{V}A$ = 3.8 L/min). When the baseline Pa_{CO_2} is 60 mm Hg ($\dot{V}A$ = 2.9 L/min), the same 500 ml/min decrease will elevate Pa_{CO_2} by 12.5 mm Hg to 72.5 mm Hg ($\dot{V}A$ = 2.4 L/min). The resultant changes in Pa_{O_2} and pH will also be amplified.

Clinical problem 12

For the following two patients, an initial $\dot{V}A$ and Pa_{CO_2} are given. Assuming constant $\dot{V}_{CO_2}$ of 200 ml/min, what is the new Pa_{CO_2} after the described change in $\dot{V}A$?

Patient A:
$\dot{V}A$ = 6 L/min Pa_{CO_2} = 29 mm Hg $\dot{V}A$ decreases by 1 L/min because of administration of anesthesia

Patient B:
$\dot{V}A$ = 3 L/min Pa_{CO_2} = 57.5 mm Hg $\dot{V}A$ decreases by 1 L/min because of pulmonary edema

Pa_{CO_2} AND NEED FOR VENTILATORY ASSISTANCE

Because hyperventilation represents an excess of alveolar ventilation ($\dot{V}A$), intubation to increase $\dot{V}A$ is never needed if the Pa_{CO_2} is low. (Patients with low Pa_{CO_2} may need artificial ventilation to help correct other problems, e.g. hypoxemia or severe alkalosis.)

Ventilatory assistance is used only for patients with elevated Pa_{CO_2} or in those unusual situations where Pa_{CO_2} is in the normal range but the patient is in imminent danger of life-threatening hypoventilation.* Ventilatory assistance usually requires tracheal intubation and connection to an artificial respirator. Alternate methods of directly augmenting $\dot{V}A$, such as by using a tight-fitting face mask and intermittent positive pressure breathing, are almost never satisfactory in adults needing ventilatory assistance.

Given an elevated Pa_{CO_2}, a good clinical rule is *never intubate for hypercapnia alone*. Different durations of hypercapnia, different buffering capacities, oxygen levels, and a host of other variables influence the need for ventilatory assistance. In the presence of hypercapnia, intubation and artificial ventilation are indicated only if one or more of the following are also present and judged to be life threatening:

1. Decreased mental status, not improving and potentially worsening
2. Increased fatigue, not improving and potentially worsening
3. Low pH (usually less than 7.30), not improving and potentially worsening
4. Low arterial oxygen pressure (Pa_{O_2}) that cannot otherwise be improved except by lowering the Pa_{CO_2}
5. Secretions or mucus that is threatening upper airways patency

Obviously, a great deal of clinical judgment must enter into the decision to intubate a patient. Once a patient is intubated, Pa_{CO_2} can only be followed by specific measurement for the reasons given previously. Even though the tidal volume and the respiratory rate are set by the ventilator and minute ventilation is therefore known, $\dot{V}A$ and carbon dioxide production remain unknown. Furthermore, in the nonstable patient, one cannot assume a constant dead space ventilation ($\dot{V}D$) since changing tidal volume, respiratory rate, and the time course of acute parenchymal disease (changing V/Q relationships) may influence $\dot{V}D$ throughout a patient's course.

Weaning a patient from the ventilator also involves careful observation of his arterial blood gases and, on occasion, measurements of lung mechanics (see Chapter 10). It is impossible to give specific guidelines about how often to obtain blood gas analysis; this decision has to be individualized for each patient's course. A single blood gas measurement following intubation may not reflect a stable Pa_{CO_2}; generally at least two or more blood gas measurements should be obtained in the first

---

*Another indication for ventilatory assistance is the use of general anesthesia. Patients receiving general anesthesia are routinely ventilated to prevent hypercapnia and hypoxemia.

few hours after intubation to help assure that the patient has reached a ventilatory steady state.

NONINVASIVE MEASUREMENT OF P_{CO_2}

Because carbon dioxide is never diffusion limited, alveolar carbon dioxide pressure (P_{ACO_2}) is assumed equal to arterial carbon dioxide pressure (P_{aCO_2}). In theory, measurement of P_{ACO_2} could substitute for P_{aCO_2}, although in practice this is not always the case.

Fig. 4-4 *A*, shows a normal tracing of partial pressure of carbon dioxide (P_{CO_2}) measured during a single expired tidal volume with an infrared carbon dioxide analyzer. The first part of the expired air is the same as the last part that was *inspired* on

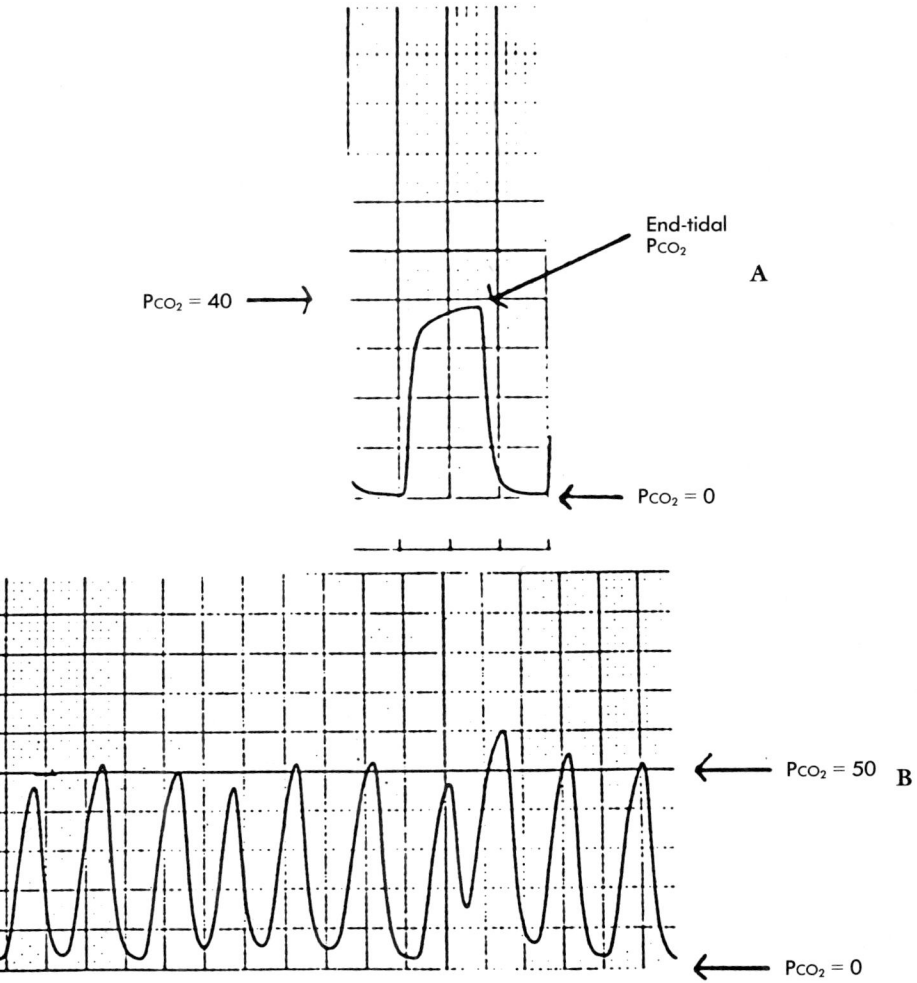

Fig. 4-4. **A,** Carbon dioxide measurement during a single expired breath. In this example from a healthy patient, the end-tidal point reflects alveolar, and hence arterial, partial pressure of carbon dioxide. **B,** Continuous monitoring of end-tidal carbon dioxide (P_{etCO_2}). This patient has severe chronic obstructive pulmonary disease. Some variation is seen during quiet breathing, but average P_{etCO_2} is approximately 50 mm/Hg. The P_{aCO_2} measured at the same time was 74 mm Hg.

the previous breath; (it is dead-space air from the upper airways and will contain almost no carbon dioxide). Gradually, air from some of the alveoli begins to join this dead-space air, and the P_{CO_2} rises. By the very end of exhalation all the dead-space air has left the lungs, and the last few milliliters of air are from the alveoli only. This tracing shows that the end-tidal P_{CO_2} (Pet_{CO_2}) is approximately 38 mm Hg, which indicates a normal Pa_{CO_2}.

Pet_{CO_2} can be measured on a continuous basis (Fig. 4-4, *B*), but the measurement has limitations. One has to assure that the carbon dioxide cannula, which delivers the expired air to the carbon dioxide analyzer, is not contaminated with room air. This is not so much of a problem with intubated patients for whom the cannula is inserted in the ventilator's expiratory circuit as it is in other patients.

Perhaps the major pitfall is the difficulty of obtaining true Pa_{CO_2} in patients with severe lung disease. In such cases Pet_{CO_2} may not reflect alveolar and arterial P_{CO_2} because of severe ventilation-perfusion imbalance and a resulting large increase in physiologic dead space (see Chapter 5). In the example shown in Fig. 4-4, *B*, from a patient with severe chronic obstructive pulmonary disease, the Pet_{CO_2} averaged approximately 50 mm Hg, but Pa_{CO_2} was 74 mm Hg, resulting in a Pa_{CO_2}-Pet_{CO_2} difference of 24 mm Hg. In this situation the diseased alveoli do not empty evenly, and the end-tidal sample still reflects considerable dead space air.

A Pa_{CO_2}-Pet_{CO_2} difference does not obviate the value of the end-tidal measurement for physiologic monitoring; a rise in Pet_{CO_2} still suggests a rise in Pa_{CO_2}, but one cannot equate the measured Pet_{CO_2} with Pa_{CO_2}. For physiologic monitoring of critically ill patients, one or two comparisons should be made of Pet_{CO_2} with Pa_{CO_2} before following the Pet_{CO_2} trend.

The absolute value of the Pa_{CO_2}-Pet_{CO_2} difference has also been advocated for diagnostic purposes, especially in acute pulmonary embolism where the value is often much higher than in chronic lung conditions. The pulmonary embolus creates extra dead space by blocking perfusion to a group of alveoli. However, because of a lack of specificity, this measurement is not widely used in clinical practice.

Pa_{CO_2}—ITS RELATIONSHIP TO OXYGENATION AND ACID-BASE BALANCE

Any discussion of gas exchange should begin with Pa_{CO_2} since it is the only blood gas value that provides information on ventilation, oxygenation, and acid-base balance. Fig. 4-5 shows the relationship of Pa_{CO_2} to alveolar ventilation (the Pa_{CO_2} equation), alveolar partial pressure of oxygen (the alveolar-air equation; see Chapter 5), and pH (Henderson-Hasselbalch equation; see Chapter 7).

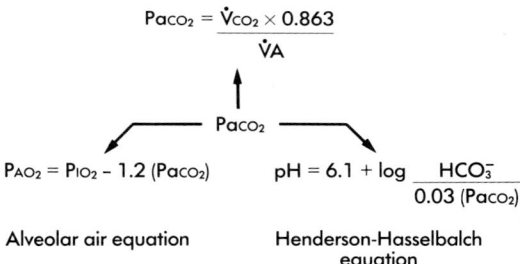

Fig. 4-5. Arterial carbon dioxide pressure (Pa_{CO_2}) in ventilation, oxygenation, and acid-base equations. A rise in Pa_{CO_2} indicates diminished $\dot{V}_A$ in relation to $\dot{V}_{CO_2}$ and will result in a fall in Pa_{O_2} and pH. See Chapters 5 and 7.

SUMMARY

For gas exchange to occur fresh air must be brought into the alveoli. Alveolar ventilation ($\dot{V}_A$) is defined as the amount of fresh air that enters the alveoli *and* takes part in gas exchange; it is the difference between total or minute ventilation ($\dot{V}_E$) and the amount of air that does not take part in gas exchange—the dead-space ventilation ($\dot{V}_D$).

$\dot{V}_A$ is inversely related to the partial pressure of carbon dioxide in arterial blood (Pa_{CO_2}) and is directly related to metabolic carbon dioxide production ($\dot{V}_{CO_2}$). When $\dot{V}_A$ rises proportionately higher than $\dot{V}_{CO_2}$, Pa_{CO_2} is reduced, a condition known as hyperventilation; conversely, a level of $\dot{V}_A$ proportionately lower than normal will raise Pa_{CO_2} (hypoventilation).

By employing a constant (0.863) to equate the different units for Pa_{CO_2}, $\dot{V}_A$, and $\dot{V}_{CO_2}$, the three variables can be related thus: $Pa_{CO_2} = \dot{V}_{CO_2} \times 0.863/\dot{V}_A$. Normally, $\dot{V}_A$ will rise to match any increase in $\dot{V}_{CO_2}$. During mild to moderate exercise, both $\dot{V}_A$ and $\dot{V}_{CO_2}$ increase proportionately, so that Pa_{CO_2} stays the same; the exercising person neither hyperventilates nor hypoventilates.

Based on this equation, it follows that hypercapnia is always caused by a level of $\dot{V}_A$ that is inadequate for $\dot{V}_{CO_2}$. Furthermore, since $\dot{V}_A = \dot{V}_E - \dot{V}_D$, all cases of hypercapnia can be seen as caused by a reduced or inadequate $\dot{V}_E$, or an elevated $\dot{V}_D$ (or a combination of the two). Hypercapnia caused by drug overdose, for example, can be explained by a reduction in $\dot{V}_E$. Hypercapnia in chronic obstructive lung disease can be explained by an elevation of $\dot{V}_D$.

The most common cause of elevated $\dot{V}_D$ is ventilation-perfusion imbalance. Dead-space ventilation can also be elevated in states of rapid shallow breathing, in which a larger-than-normal proportion of each tidal volume goes to satisfy anatomic dead space.

Pa_{CO_2} is a key blood gas measurement. Not only does it help assess adequacy of $\dot{V}_A$, but it is also a component of the alveolar air equation and the Henderson-Hasselbalch equation.

REVIEW QUESTIONS

State whether each of the following are true or false.

1. To estimate Pa_{CO_2} at the bedside, one can start with a measurement of 40 mm Hg, then subtract 2 mm Hg for every breath above 10/min.
2. Pa_{CO_2} is inversely related to alveolar ventilation.
3. Pa_{CO_2} is directly related to level of carbon dioxide production.
4. Pa_{CO_2} is always low if the alveolar ventilation is twice the resting level.
5. Normally, one can voluntarily hyperventilate to lower Pa_{CO_2} more than 10 mm Hg.
6. Normally, one can voluntarily hypoventilate to raise Pa_{CO_2} more than 10 mm Hg.
7. Dead-space ventilation can rise solely from a change in the pattern of breathing, i.e., without a change in the lung architecture.
8. Most of the blood carbon dioxide is carried in the form of bicarbonate.
9. To calculate the ratio of dead space to tidal volume using the Bohr equation, one need measure only tidal volume and Pa_{CO_2}.
10. As Pa_{CO_2} goes up, alveolar P_{O_2} goes down.

References

Mithoefer, J.C., Bossman, O.G., Thibeault, D.W., et al.: The clinical estimation of alveolar ventilation, Am. Rev. Resp. Dis. **98**:868, 1968.

Suggested readings

Goldring, R.M., Heinemann, H.O., and Turino, G.M.: Regulation of alveolar ventilation in respiratory failure, Am. J. Med. Sci. **269**:160, 1975.

Javaheri, S., Blum, J., and Kazemi, H.: Pattern of breathing and carbon dioxide rentention in chronic obstructive lung disease, Am. J. Med. **71**:228, 1981.

Thomas, H.M.: Ventilation and P_{CO_2}: make the distinction, Chest **79**:617, 1981.

See also General References (Physiology) in Appendix G.

chapter 5

Oxygen transfer

OUTLINE

Clinical questions
Lung oxygen transfer
Oxygen diffusion and diffusing capacity
Alveolar oxygen pressure
Arterial oxygen pressure
Alveolar-arterial oxygen pressure difference
Pa_{O_2}/PA_{O_2} and Pa_{O_2}/FI_{O_2}
Causes of low Pa_{O_2}
Nonrespiratory causes of low Pa_{O_2}
Respiratory causes of low Pa_{O_2}
Ventilation-perfusion imbalance
Shunts and venous admixture
How V/Q imbalance reduces Pa_{O_2} and increases Pa_{CO_2}
Low mixed venous oxygen—effect on Pa_{O_2}
V/Q imbalance in patients—variable effect on oxygen and carbon dioxide

CLINICAL QUESTIONS

There are two broad clinical questions concerning the physiology of oxygenation. One question asks if oxygenation is adequate for the patient; it encompasses the patient's history and physical examination, plus measurement of his blood oxygen content, cardiac output, and oxygen delivery and uptake. This question is discussed in Chapter 6.

The other question asks if the lungs are properly transferring oxygen into the blood; it is answered simply by comparing the patient's alveolar-arterial P_{O_2} difference with the expected difference.* If this difference is elevated, the answer is *no*. Understanding why this is so is the subject of this chapter.

LUNG OXYGEN TRANSFER

In Chapter 4 one gas exchange function of the respiratory system was examined: elimination of carbon dioxide. The other component of gas exchange is the delivery of oxygen from the atmosphere, through the lungs, and into the blood. Gas exchange is a passive process; there is no active transport of oxygen by the lungs.

Gas exchange is accomplished solely by diffusion of gas from a region of higher, to one of lower, gas pressure. Fig. 5-1 shows the change in oxygen pressure as oxygen moves from the atmosphere to the arterial blood (when breathing ambient air at sea level). Note the following (see Fig. 5-1):

1. The partial pressure of oxygen in dry air is the fraction of inspired oxygen (FI_{O_2}) times the barometric pressure; at sea level this is $0.21(760) = 160$ mm Hg. With increasing altitude, the barometric pressure falls and FI_{O_2} remains constant.

---

*Some refer to the alveolar-arterial oxygen pressure difference as the "A-a gradient"; strictly speaking, this terminology is incorrect since the overall difference is not caused by any pressure gradient, but rather by normal anatomic shunting and ventilation-perfusion imbalance. In this book the term *difference* is used rather than *gradient*.

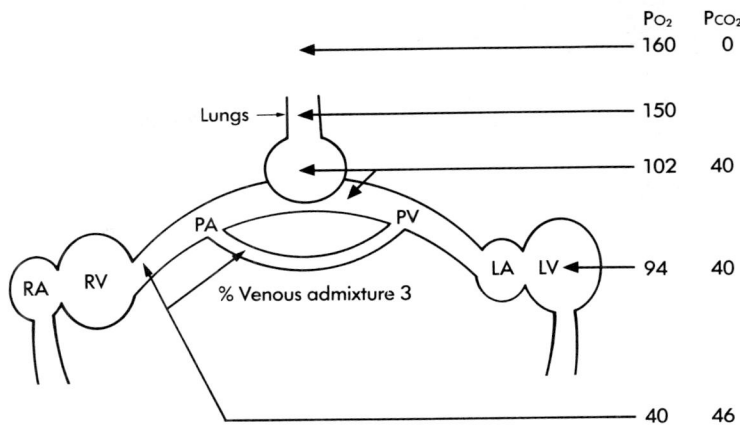

Fig. 5-1. Changes in P_{O_2} and P_{CO_2} as oxygen moves from the atmosphere to the arterial blood. All pressures are in mm Hg. The P_{O_2} and P_{CO_2} are calculated using an FI_{O_2} of 0.21 and a barometric pressure of 760 mm Hg. (*RA*, right atrium; *RV*, right ventricle; *PA*, pulmonary arteries; *PV*, pulmonary veins; *LA*, left atrium; *LV*, left ventricle.)

2. In the upper airways (nose, larynx, trachea), water vapor is added to the inspired air. Water vapor pressure is 47 mm Hg at normal body temperature; this pressure affects all dry (nonvapor) gas pressures (oxygen, nitrogen, carbon dioxide). Thus tracheal $P_{O_2} = 0.21(760-47) = 150$ mm Hg.
3. Inhaled carbon dioxide is negligible and can be considered zero for clinical purposes. As air travels toward the alveoli, carbon dioxide increases; P_{CO_2} at the alveolar level = arterial P_{CO_2} = 40 mm Hg (normal alveolar ventilation).
4. Since the lungs are an open system in continuous contact with the atmosphere, total alveolar pressure equals barometric pressure. But since inspired P_{CO_2} is zero and alveolar P_{CO_2} equals 40 mm Hg, the partial pressure of some other gas must fall. Water vapor does not change since it is a function of body temperature. What about nitrogen and oxygen? Nitrogen is inert—it is not metabolized, and there is no net uptake or excretion. Oxygen, on the other hand, is transported into the pulmonary capillary blood *at the same time* carbon dioxide is entering the alveoli. The result is a fall in inspired oxygen pressure commensurate with the addition of carbon dioxide to alveolar air.
5. The fall in P_{O_2} from the trachea to the alveoli is almost all accounted for by the alveolar P_{CO_2} (PA_{CO_2}). However, the change in P_{O_2} does not quite equal PA_{CO_2} since more oxygen is taken up as carbon dioxide is eliminated. Under normal steady state conditions, approximately 250 ml of oxygen are added to the pulmonary circulation per minute (the $\dot{V}_{O_2}$), while 200 ml of carbon dioxide are removed (the $\dot{V}_{CO_2}$). The ratio of $\dot{V}_{CO_2}/\dot{V}_{O_2}$ is the respiratory quotient (R or RQ), so the normal R is approximately 0.8. Thus, as air moves from the trachea to the alveoli, P_{O_2} will fall 1.2 mm Hg for every 1 mm Hg increase in PA_{CO_2}. If tracheal P_{O_2} is 150 mm Hg and if PA_{CO_2} is 40 mm Hg, alveolar partial pressure of oxygen (PA_{O_2}) is 102 mm Hg.
6. The initial diffusing gradient for oxygen is PA_{O_2} minus mixed venous P_{O_2} ($P\bar{v}_{O_2}$) = 102 − 40 = 62 mm Hg. This large gradient, plus the rapidity with which oxygen diffuses across the alveolar-capillary membrane, assures that end-capillary P_{O_2} is almost equal to PA_{O_2} (Fig. 5-2).
7. If the lungs were ideal organs, arterial P_{O_2} would equal end-capillary P_{O_2} and PA_{O_2}. Normally, however, a small fraction of the cardiac output bypasses the alveoli, either anatomically or physiologically.

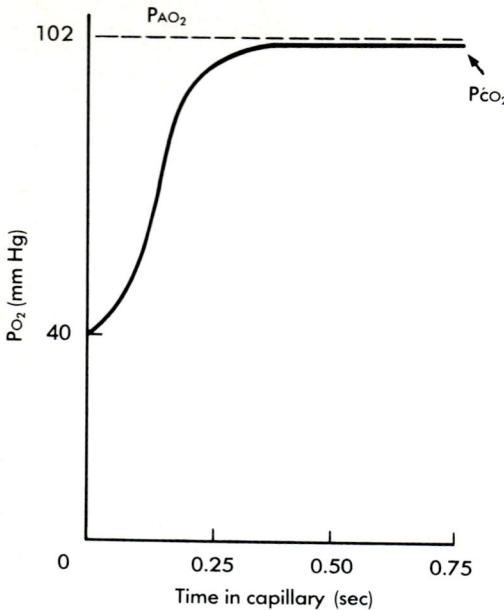

Fig. 5-2. Alveolar-capillary P_{O_2} gradient. Normal transit time for a red blood cell in the pulmonary capillary is approximately 0.75 seconds. Blood P_{O_2} when entering the pulmonary capillary is 40 mm Hg. Diffusion of oxygen is rapid so that capillary P_{O_2} reaches near equilibrium with alveolar P_{O_2} (P_{AO_2}) well before the end of capillary transit time. Although there remains a very small difference between end-capillary P_{O_2} ($P\dot{c}_{O_2}$) and P_{AO_2}, for practical purposes, such as when calculating shunt percentage, one can assume $P\dot{c}_{O_2} = P_{AO_2}$.

This shunted blood, unoxygenated, mixes with the oxygenated blood so that arterial oxygen pressure is always *lower* than end-capillary P_{O_2}. In Fig. 5-1, Pa_{O_2} is 8 mm Hg lower than end-capillary P_{O_2}.

Based on the physiologic changes in oxygen pressure outlined above, the following observation can be made: the adequacy of overall lung oxygen transfer can be determined by comparing the oxygen pressure both in the alveolar air and in the blood entering the left atrium to normal oxygen pressure values. Since oxygen enters the blood only through the lungs, an increase in the alveolar-left atrial P_{O_2} *difference* must indicate either an impairment of oxygen diffusion or an increase in pulmonary venous admixture.

It is not practical to measure oxygen pressure in blood entering the left atrium. Instead, the difference between alveolar (P_{AO_2}) and *arterial* oxygen pressure (Pa_{O_2}) must be used to assess the adequacy of oxygen transfer. Except for the situation where some unoxygenated blood enters the left side of the heart without passing through the lungs, the P_{AO_2}-Pa_{O_2} difference will indicate the adequacy of pulmonary oxygen transfer. This difference is notated $P(A-a)O_2$. Since Pa_{O_2} is a basic blood gas measurement and P_{AO_2} can be calculated from the alveolar air equation (discussed later in this chapter), $P(A-a)O_2$ is easily determined. If $P(A-a)O_2$ is elevated above the normal range, the lungs are not transferring oxygen properly.*

OXYGEN DIFFUSION AND DIFFUSING CAPACITY

Before discussing alveolar and arterial partial pressure of oxygen, it will be helpful to clarify the concept of *oxygen diffusing capacity.* Oxygen enters the blood by diffusion from the alveoli into the pulmonary capillaries. Diffusing capacity of the lung for oxygen (DL_{O_2}) is the quantitative amount of oxygen the lungs can transfer from the alveoli into the blood; units for DL_{O_2} are ml O_2/min/mm Hg driving pressure. If 250 ml of oxygen are trans-

---

*The only exception to this statement is the uncommon situation of a patient with a right-to-left anatomic, extrapulmonary shunt. Normally, less than 3% of the cardiac output is anatomically shunted. This shunting occurs in the Thebesian vessels, which enter the left ventricular myocardium carrying oxygenated blood and drain back into the left ventricle with deoxygenated blood, and in the bronchial arteries, which supply the main bronchi with oxygenated blood and then drain deoxygenated blood into the left atrium. This shunted blood accounts for part of the normal $P(A-a)O_2$. Apart from this occurrence, right-to-left anatomic shunting is uncommon in adults but can occur through a patent foramen ovale or a ventricular septal defect. With either cardiac defect however, a *left-to-right* shunt is more common since the pressure in the left ventricle is greater than in the right ventricle. A pure left-to-right shunt will not reduce Pa_{O_2}.

ferred per minute and if the average alveolar-capillary P_{O_2} difference is 25 mm Hg, then DL_{O_2} is 10 ml O_2/min/mm Hg.

Measurement of DL_{O_2} is technically difficult since the gradient for diffusion changes constantly along the capillary. Using the values presented in the previous section, the initial gradient for oxygen diffusion is 62 mm Hg and the final gradient is almost zero. The decrease in diffusion gradient along the capillary is nonlinear, and the average gradient can be determined only by a complicated method employing calculus.

In practice the pulmonary diffusing capacity is measured by having the patient inhale carbon monoxide (CO) in a small enough amount that the test is harmless. The normal diffusing capacity of the lung for carbon monoxide (DL_{CO}) is age-, sex-, and height-dependent and ranges from approximately 20 to 30 ml CO/min/mm Hg. The reason for using carbon monoxide is based on its properties as a gas. It is taken up so readily by hemoglobin that it is not perfusion limited; that is, no matter how fast blood flows past the lungs, carbon monoxide will combine with the available hemoglobin. On the other hand, carbon monoxide is *diffusion limited* so that a thickened alveolar membrane will delay its transfer into the blood.

An additional reason for using inhaled carbon monoxide is that normally very little of it is in the blood (less than 1.5% carboxyhemoglobin). Since virtually all inhaled carbon monoxide is taken up by hemoglobin, the plasma concentration and hence partial pressure of carbon monoxide remain very low (once a gas chemically combines with hemoglobin it no longer exerts a partial pressure).

For test purposes the partial pressure of plasma carbon monoxide along the entire capillary is considered zero so that CO alveolar pressure is, in effect, the pressure gradient for CO diffusion. By knowing the amount of inhaled and exhaled carbon monoxide, the mean alveolar CO pressure and the amount of carbon monoxide transferred into the blood can be calculated. Since the mean alveolar CO pressure is the gradient for diffusion, it becomes relatively easy to calculate the diffusing capacity of the lung for carbon monoxide.*

There are several problems and potential pitfalls in interpretation of the DL_{CO} test:
1. The diffusing capacity for carbon monoxide is not the same thing as DL_{O_2}, and one cannot infer any specific value for DL_{O_2} from measurement of DL_{CO}.
2. The diffusing capacity for carbon monoxide can be reduced by conditions other than a thickened alveolar membrane. Anemia will lower a patient's DL_{CO} since carbon monoxide needs hemoglobin for maximal diffusion; without hemoglobin the plasma concentration would rise quickly and prevent further diffusion. Loss of alveolar membrane will also lower DL_{CO}, and for this reason the DL_{CO} is often reduced in emphysematous patients. Excess blood carbon monoxide, common in smokers, will also inhibit CO diffusion. Finally, ventilation-perfusion imbalance can lead to a reduced DL_{CO}.
3. A reduced DL_{CO} does not account for clinically significant hypoxemia at rest. The diffusion reserve of the lungs is so great that DL_{CO} (or DL_{O_2}) can be markedly reduced without lowering Pa_{O_2} very much. Diseases leading to low DL_{CO}, such as interstitial fibrosis, cause hypoxemia by the mechanism of ventilation-perfusion imbalance, not by impaired diffusion.

---

*There are several ways of performing the DL_{CO} test. The simplest and most widely used is the "single breath" method. The patient inhales to his total lung capacity a single breath of a gas mixture containing 0.3% carbon monoxide and 10% helium; he is instructed to hold his breath for 10 seconds and then forcefully exhale. During this 10-second interval carbon monoxide is taken up in the capillary blood, but helium, being inert and insoluble, is not. By measuring the concentration of carbon monoxide and helium at the beginning of inhalation and again at exhalation, the amount of carbon monoxide taken up and its alveolar concentration (or pressure) can be determined. The change in helium concentration provides the volume of CO distribution. By entering these gas measurements into the appropriate equation, DL_{CO} can be readily calculated.

In practice, DLCO is helpful if it is normal, since a normal DLCO implies a normal diffusing capacity for oxygen. If the DLCO is reduced, the possible reasons mentioned previously must be considered, and one must avoid any premature conclusion about the lungs' intrinsic diffusing capacity for oxygen.

Since reduced pulmonary diffusing capacity does not cause significant resting hypoxemia, the DLCO test is not helpful in evaluating most abnormalities of gas exchange. There is simply no useful correlation between DLCO and resting arterial blood gas values. Nonetheless, the DLCO test is widely performed in hospital pulmonary function laboratories and is considered routine when "complete pulmonary function tests" are requested. Properly performed and interpreted, the DLCO test can provide useful information. The test is useful when treating patients with interstitial lung disease, either as a sign of disease progression or as a sign of response to treatment. Also, DLCO correlates with oxygen desaturation during exercise, an application discussed in Chapter 12.

ALVEOLAR OXYGEN PRESSURE

The partial pressure of oxygen in alveolar gas (P_{AO_2}) represents an average of all the individual alveolar oxygen pressures throughout the lungs. It depends on the fraction of inspired oxygen (FI_{O_2}), barometric pressure (P_B), respiratory quotient (R), and alveolar carbon dioxide pressure (P_{ACO_2}). By calculating P_{AO_2}, one can obtain a good idea of what the resulting arterial P_{O_2} *should* be if the lungs were functioning *normally*. If the difference between *calculated P_{AO_2}* and *measured P_{aO_2}* is increased, the lungs are not transferring oxygen properly.

Alveolar oxygen pressure is calculated using the alveolar air equation:

$$P_{AO_2} = P_{IO_2} - P_{ACO_2}\left(FI_{O_2} + \frac{(1-FI_{O_2})}{R}\right) \quad (1)$$

where PI_{O_2} is the FI_{O_2} times the barometric pressure after water vapor pressure (47 mm Hg) has been subtracted; P_{ACO_2} is alveolar partial pressure of carbon dioxide (assumed equal to P_{aCO_2}); and R is the lung respiratory quotient (normally 0.8). Breathing ambient air ($FI_{O_2} = 0.21$), Equation 1 can be abbreviated to

$$P_{AO_2} = FI_{O_2}(P_B - 47) - 1.2(P_{aCO_2}) \quad (2)$$

Physicians make several assumptions in the clinical application of Equation 1 (see box below). For this reason, plus the fact that there are no precise normal values for $P(A-a)O_2$ when FI_{O_2} is above 0.21, Equation 2 is sufficient for clinical purposes (Martin, 1986).

The assumptions listed in the box, which are

ASSUMPTIONS IN CLINICAL APPLICATION OF ALVEOLAR AIR EQUATION

FI_{O_2} is accurately known. In fact, this is not always the case since face masks and other methods of oxygen delivery do not always deliver a precise FI_{O_2}.

Barometric pressure is precisely known. More often barometric pressure is approximated and is not measured.

Water vapor pressure is 47 mm Hg. This value is temperature dependent and is not usually adjusted for febrile patients.

P_{aCO_2} equals P_{ACO_2}. This may not always be so, especially in states of severe ventilation-perfusion imbalance.

R value is 0.8. Respiratory quotient may vary widely from 0.8, e.g., in patients who are hyperventilating or who have high carbohydrate diets.

routinely made in clinical practice, render the P_{AO_2} calculation no more than a useful approximation; reporting PaO_2 as more than a simple integer is false precision.*

ARTERIAL OXYGEN PRESSURE

Arterial PO_2 can be looked at both for what it *effects* or causes, and what it *reflects* or results from. It *effects* the percent saturation of hemoglobin with oxygen and thus is a major determinant of oxygen content (Chapter 6). But to look at PaO_2 only in this way is to miss other important information.

Arterial oxygen pressure is a result of, and therefore *reflects*, alveolar oxygen pressure (P_{AO_2}) and the alveolar air–pulmonary capillary interface. This interface is determined by the ratios of ventilation to perfusion in the millions of alveolar-capillary units. Oxygen enters the blood only by passive diffusion across a pressure gradient; hence, if the distribution of alveolar air and capillary perfusion is unchanged, then as P_{AO_2} increases, so will PaO_2; conversely, as P_{AO_2} decreases, so will PaO_2. PaO_2 alone is insufficient to indicate the adequacy of oxygen transfer. Without reference to P_{AO_2} it is not known if PaO_2 reflects an abnormal ratio of alveolar ventilation to capillary perfusion or simply a reduction in P_{AO_2}.

ALVEOLAR-ARTERIAL OXYGEN PRESSURE DIFFERENCE

The normal PaO_2 is age-dependent, declining slightly over the years (Fig. 5-3). This decline reflects shifts in ventilation/perfusion (V/Q) ratios in the aging lung. In contrast, alveolar partial pressure of oxygen (P_{AO_2}) depends only on the pressure of inspired oxygen (P_{IO_2}), respiratory quotient (R), and alveolar partial pressure of carbon dioxide (P_{ACO_2}). Since none of these values is age-depen-

*At F_{IO_2} values above 0.60, somewhat greater accuracy can be obtained by eliminating the value 1.2 from Equation 2. This is because the correction factor (in brackets, Equation 1) decreases as F_{IO_2} increases and goes to 1.0 when breathing 100% oxygen, at which point $P_{AO_2} = P_{IO_2} - P_{ACO_2}$ (Martin, 1986).

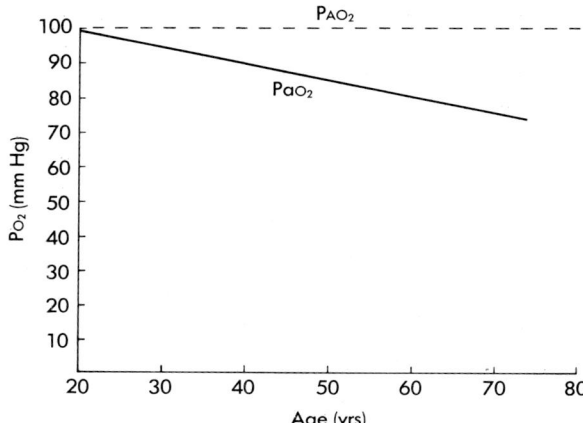

Fig. 5-3. Changes in PaO_2 and $P(A-a)O_2$ with age. The line for PaO_2 is based on the regression equation, $PaO_2 = 109 - 0.43$ (age in years), for PaO_2 measured at P_B 760 mm Hg. (From Sorbini, C.A., Grassi, V., Solinas, E., et al.: Respiration **25**:3, 1968.)

dent, P_{AO_2} does not change as we age. The horizontal line in Fig. 5-3 shows normal P_{AO_2} breathing ambient air ($F_{IO_2} = 0.21$) at sea level; the difference between the diagonal band and the horizontal P_{AO_2} line is the alveolar-arterial oxygen pressure difference ($P(A-a)O_2$). Note that normal $P(A-a)O_2$ breathing ambient air can reach approximately 30 mm Hg in elderly people.

Studies defining normal $P(A-a)O_2$ for increments of F_{IO_2} above 0.21 show that it increases as F_{IO_2} increases, at least up to an F_{IO_2} near 0.6 (Fig. 5-4). Thus both age and F_{IO_2} affect the normal $P(A-a)O_2$. Whatever the normal value, with the exception of a right-to-left extrapulmonary shunt, an elevated $P(A-a)O_2$ indicates either lung disease or an abnormal lung condition interfering with oxygen transfer. A $P(A-a)O_2$ determination is most useful when F_{IO_2} is 0.21 (Fig. 5-4).

Clinical problem 1

A 35-year-old patient has a PaO_2 of 90 mm Hg. Are his lungs working properly to transfer oxygen? Is more information needed?

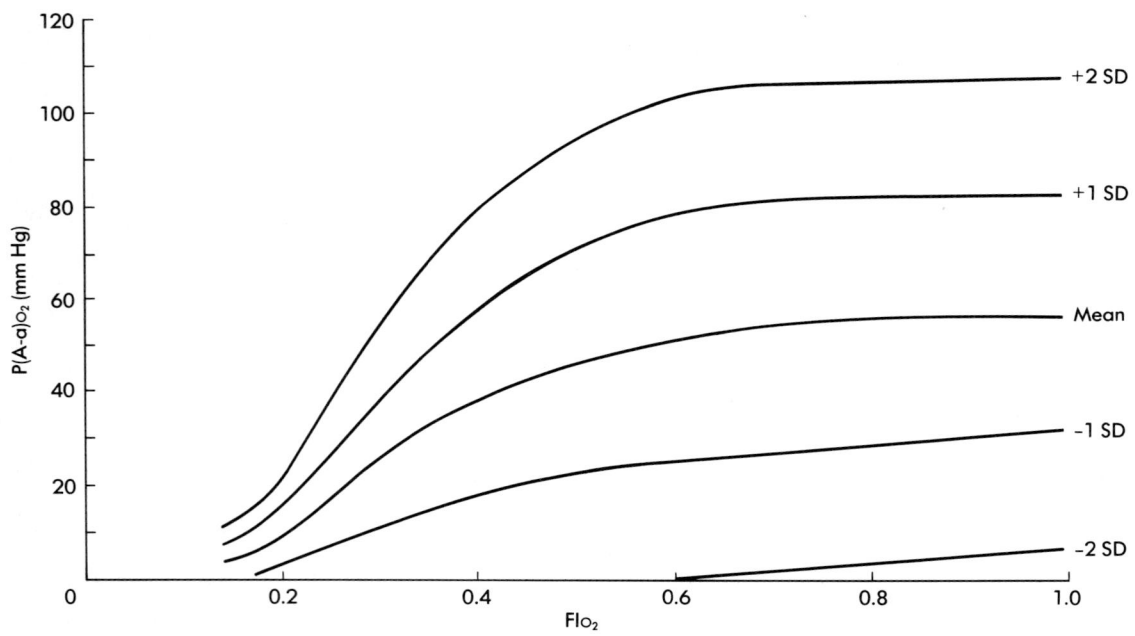

Fig. 5-4. Normal range of P(A-a)o_2 from FIO_2 of 0.21 to 1.00, based on data obtained from 16 healthy subjects aged 40 to 50 years. Lines represent mean values and + or − 2 SD (standard deviations). The P(A-a)o_2 increases up to 0.6 and then plateaus with increasing FIO_2. Note that P(A-a)o_2 may normally exceed 100 mm Hg on an FIO_2 of 1.00. (Redrawn based on data from Harris, E.A., et al. Reprinted by permission from Clin. Sci. Mol. Med., vol. 46, pp. 89-104, copyright (c) 1974, The Biochemical Society, London.)

Clinical problem 2

A 35-year-old patient has an arterial Po_2 at sea level of 85 mm Hg. For each of the following FIO_2 and $Paco_2$ values, state if his lungs are transferring oxygen properly. Assume R = 0.8.
a. FIO_2 = 0.21, $Paco_2$ = 25 mm Hg
b. FIO_2 = 0.21, $Paco_2$ = 40 mm Hg
c. FIO_2 = 0.21, $Paco_2$ = 50 mm Hg
d. FIO_2 = 0.40, $Paco_2$ = 30 mm Hg

Clinical problem 3

Which of the following are potential causes of increased P(A-a)o_2 in a patient who is healthy except for the indicated physiologic condition?

a. Thickening of alveolar-capillary membrane
b. Elevated $Paco_2$
c. Ventilation-perfusion imbalance
d. Anemia
e. Right-to-left intrapulmonary shunting
f. Right-to-left intracardiac shunting
g. High altitude
h. Carbon monoxide inhalation

Clinical problem 4

For each of the following patients, calculate P(A-a)o_2, assuming an R of 0.8 and barometric pressure of 760 mm Hg. Which of these patients is most likely to have lung disease? Do any of the values represent a measurement or recording error?

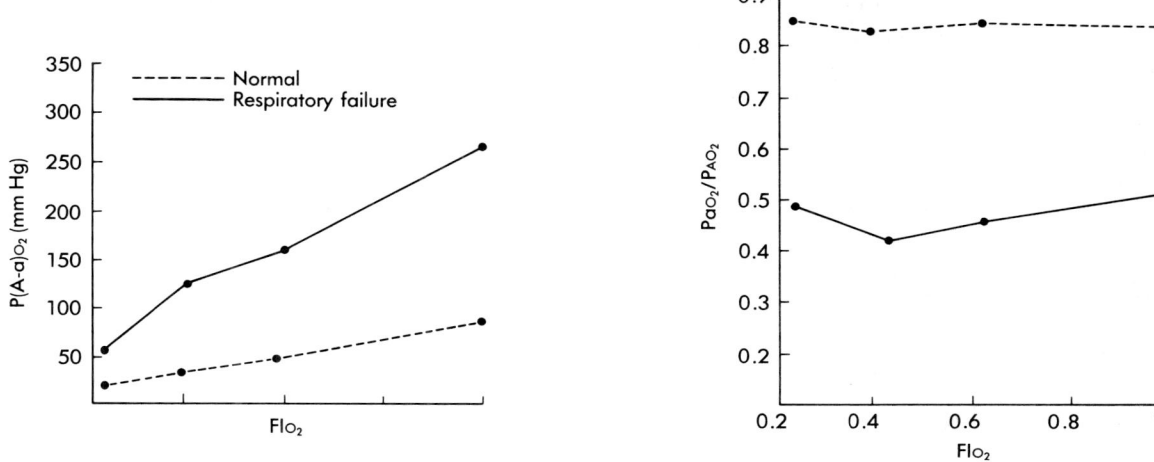

Fig. 5-5. Changes in $P(A-a)O_2$ and PaO_2/PAO_2 with increasing FIO_2, in a healthy subject and in a patient with respiratory failure. With increasing FIO_2, PaO_2/PAO_2 varies much less than $P(A-a)O_2$.

a. A 35-year-old patient with $PaCO_2$ of 50 mm Hg, PaO_2 of 150 mm Hg, and FIO_2 of 0.40

b. A 44-year-old patient with $PaCO_2$ of 75 mm Hg, PaO_2 of 95 mm Hg, and FIO_2 of 0.28

c. A young, anxious patient with PaO_2 of 120 mm Hg, $PaCO_2$ of 15 mm Hg, and FIO_2 of 0.21

d. A patient in the intensive care unit with PaO_2 of 350 mm Hg, $PaCO_2$ of 40 mm Hg, and FIO_2 of 0.80

e. A patient with PaO_2 of 80 mm Hg, $PaCO_2$ of 72 mm Hg, and FIO_2 of 0.21

PaO_2/PAO_2 AND PaO_2/FIO_2

Since the normal $P(A-a)O_2$ increases with increasing FIO_2, it is not a useful test to follow a patient's course when FIO_2 changes. A more stable parameter is PaO_2/PAO_2, the ratio of arterial to alveolar partial pressure of oxygen (Gilbert and Keighley, 1974). In contrast to $P(A-a)O_2$, PaO_2/PAO_2 remains fairly constant with increasing FIO_2, *as long as the underlying lung condition is stable;* the reason is that both PaO_2 and PAO_2 increase by the same factor when FIO_2 is raised.

Normal PaO_2/PAO_2 ranges from 0.74 in elderly people to approximately 0.9 in young subjects. If FIO_2 changes for a given patient, PaO_2/PAO_2 should not change much unless there is a change in V/Q relationships. The effect of an increasing FIO_2 on $P(A-a)O_2$ and on PaO_2/PAO_2 is shown in Fig. 5-5.

Recently some investigators have used PaO_2/FIO_2 as an index of oxygenation (Hess and Maxwell, 1985). This ratio has the advantage of avoiding the calculation of PAO_2, but it also ignores changes in arterial carbon dioxide pressure. There is no evidence that PaO_2/FIO_2 is any better than PaO_2/PAO_2 as an index of oxygenation.

CAUSES OF LOW PaO_2

Table 5-1 lists the physiologic causes, which are classified as respiratory or nonrespiratory, of a low arterial PO_2. For completeness, artifactual causes are also listed, and these will be discussed before the nonrespiratory and respiratory causes.

When the white blood cell count (WBC) is over 100,000 (e.g., in leukemia), the excess cells in the

Table 5-1. Physiologic causes of a low PaO_2

Causes	Effect on $P(A-a)O_2$
Nonrespiratory	
Right-to-left intracardiac shunt	Increased
Decreased PIO_2	Normal
Low barometric pressure	
Low FIO_2	
Decreased R value	Normal
Low mixed venous oxygen content*	Increased
Respiratory	
Diffusion barrier	Increased
Hypoventilation (increased $PaCO_2$)	Normal
Right-to-left intrapulmonary shunt	Increased
Pulmonary parenchymal	
Pulmonary vascular	
V/Q imbalance	Increased
Artifact	
Very high white blood cell count	Increased
Patient hyperthermia	Increased

*Only in presence of increased venous admixture

blood may consume enough oxygen between the time the blood is drawn and the PaO_2 is measured to cause a very low PaO_2 measurement. The true (in vivo) PaO_2 is not affected by the high WBC count since oxygen is continuously replenished from the atmosphere.

In patients with hyperthermia, the in vivo PaO_2 is higher than what is measured. Hyperthermia raises the in vivo PaO_2, but the blood sample is always measured using a water bath that is maintained at normal body temperature, 37° C. For example, if a patient's temperature is 39° C, the measured PaO_2 (at 37° C) will be approximately 8 mm Hg lower than the in vivo PaO_2. For this reason, some laboratories correct for body temperature when reporting blood gas results.

NONRESPIRATORY CAUSES OF LOW PaO_2 (Table 5-1)

Right-to-left intracardiac shunt is rare in adult medical practice; its presence is usually suggested by the patient's history, physical examination, and chest x-ray, although its confirmation may require cardiac catheterization.

Decreased inspired oxygen pressure (PIO_2) is rarely, if ever, a cause of hypoxemia in hospitalized patients. The PIO_2 is a function of both fraction of inspired oxygen (FIO_2) and barometric pressure. A decrease in FIO_2 may occur during administration of an anesthetic (as from improper installation of oxygen supply lines) or from being in a sealed chamber cut off from adequate ventilation. Low barometric pressure is the cause of decreased PIO_2

Table 5-2. Inspired and alveolar oxygen pressure at various altitudes*

Location	Altitude (feet)	P_B (mm Hg)	PI_{O_2} (mm Hg)	P_{AO_2}† (mm Hg)
Miami	0	760	160	102
Denver	5,280	629	132	74
Airplane—passenger cabin	6,000	608	128	70
Mexico City	7,347	578	121	64
Leadville, Colorado	10,200	517	109	51
Top of Mt. Everest‡	29,028	253	53	−5
Air outside plane while cruising	35,000	160	34	−24

*At all altitudes, FI_{O_2}, 0.21; P_B, barometric pressure; PI_{O_2}, partial pressure of oxygen in atmosphere (dry air); P_{AO_2}, alveolar P_{O_2}.
†P_{AO_2} is calculated using the formula $P_{AO_2} = FI_{O_2}(P_B - 47) - 1.2(P_{CO_2})$, where $P_{CO_2} = 40$ mm Hg. Normally there is compensatory hyperventilation with increasing altitude so that the actual P_{AO_2} will be higher than is shown, depending on the degree of hyperventilation.
‡Calculations for Mt. Everest are based on data from West, J.B., Hackett, P.H., and Maret, K.H., et al.: J. Appl. Physiol. **55**:678, 1983. On the top of Mt. Everest alveolar P_{CO_2} was measured as 7.5 mm Hg, and P_{AO_2} measured as 35 mm Hg; the calculated P_{AO_2} without supplemental oxygen is 28 mm Hg.

at a high altitude, and low alveolar P_{O_2} has been implicated in high-altitude pulmonary edema. Note that FI_{O_2} does not change with increasing altitude (Table 5-2).

Clinical problem 5

An unacclimatized, 40-year-old man went hiking in the Colorado mountains. After 6 hours he became acutely short of breath and was taken to a hospital in Leadville, Colorado (see Table 5-2). The patient's initial arterial blood gas revealed Pa_{CO_2} 27 mm Hg, Pa_{O_2} 40 mm Hg, and pH 7.52 (room air). How should these values be interpreted? Is $P(A-a)_{O_2}$ increased?

Decreased respiratory quotient (R) ($\dot{V}_{CO_2}/\dot{V}_{O_2}$) has been described in patients undergoing hemodialysis and is a result of the diffusion of carbon dioxide from the patient's blood directly into the dialysis solution (Aurigemma, Feldman, Gottlieb, et al., 1977; Martin, 1980; Hunt, Chappell, Henrich, et al., 1984; Quebbeman, Maierhofer, and Piering, 1984). This carbon dioxide diffusion occurs when the dialysis is performed against an acetate bath but not when bicarbonate dialysate is used. Because some carbon dioxide diffuses from the patient's blood into the acetate bath, less carbon dioxide is delivered to the lungs for excretion; as a result alveolar ventilation declines. However, arterial partial pressure of carbon dioxide does not change (alveolar ventilation is still matched to the amount of carbon dioxide brought to the lungs for elimination). The alveolar-arterial oxygen pressure difference ($P(A-a)_{O_2}$) also does not change.*

The *metabolic* exchange of carbon dioxide and oxygen does not change during dialysis; thus the lungs must bring in the normal (predialysis) oxygen consumption ($\dot{V}_{O_2}$). However, because the amount of carbon dioxide brought to the lungs for elimination (the $\dot{V}_{CO_2}$) is reduced, the R value decreases. The result is a reduced alveolar (and hence arterial) P_{O_2}. Calculate the new R value in the following problem to see how this reduction occurs.

---

*The $P(A-a)_{O_2}$ *can* increase during dialysis as a result of other mechanisms, such as stasis of white blood cells within the pulmonary capillaries.

Clinical problem 6

A patient is being dialyzed against an acetate dialysis solution. Before dialysis his Pa_{O_2} is 84 mm Hg, Pa_{CO_2} is 38 mm Hg, and pH is 7.36. If predialysis carbon dioxide production and oxygen consumption are 200 and 250 ml/min, respectively, and if 50 ml of carbon dioxide enters the dialysate per minute, what is his Pa_{O_2} during dialysis? Assume the patient is breathing room air (FI_{O_2} 0.21) and that Pa_{CO_2}, pH, and $P(A-a)_{O_2}$ are unchanged during dialysis.

Low mixed venous oxygen content will aggravate hypoxemia only in the presence of venous admixture. This is of some importance in patients with pulmonary edema or with other causes of large venous admixture. The reserve for oxygen diffusion is so great that mixed venous blood with a P_{O_2} of zero would be fully oxygenated after one pass through normally ventilating alveoli. This important cause of hypoxemia is discussed on p. 106.

RESPIRATORY CAUSES OF LOW Pa_{O_2}

Compared to nonrespiratory causes, respiratory causes of low Pa_{O_2} are far more common. Of the four physiologic respiratory causes (Table 5-1), *diffusion barrier* is rarely, if ever, a cause of low Pa_{O_2} in patients at rest. It can, however, account for hypoxemia during exercise (see Chapter 12). This leaves ventilation-perfusion imbalance, right-to-left pulmonary shunt, and hypoventilation as the physiologic respiratory causes of low Pa_{O_2} at rest.

Hypoventilation (elevated Pa_{CO_2}) does not, per se, lead to an increase in the $P(A-a)_{O_2}$. This is because increased Pa_{CO_2} lowers PA_{O_2} and Pa_{O_2} together. Hence one can always determine whether or not hypoventilation is a cause of low Pa_{O_2}—simply check the Pa_{CO_2}; if it is elevated, hypoventilation is one reason for the decrease in Pa_{O_2}. If $P(A-a)_{O_2}$ is normal when Pa_{CO_2} is elevated, then hypoventilation is the sole cause of any reduction in Pa_{O_2}. This hypoventilation can occur from nonpulmonary conditions such as brainstem depression or chest muscle paralysis. On the other hand, hypercapnia accompanied by an elevated $P(A-a)_{O_2}$ invariably indicates lung disease or an abnormal lung condition affecting oxygen transfer.

Clinical problem 7

A 73-year-old woman is brought to the emergency room in a comatose state. The family states she had become confused and had swallowed an excess number of sleeping pills. Blood gas analysis obtained with the patient breathing room air ($FI_{O_2} = 0.21$) shows the Pa_{O_2} is 42 mm Hg, the Pa_{CO_2} is 74 mm Hg, and the pH is 7.10. Why is her Pa_{O_2} reduced?

A *right-to-left pulmonary shunt* can occur from an alteration in normal lung parenchyma or through abnormal vascular channels within the lungs. In either case the shunt represents one extreme of ventilation-perfusion imbalance. Such areas of the lung have a ventilation to perfusion ratio of 0.

VENTILATION-PERFUSION IMBALANCE

Ventilation-perfusion (V/Q) imbalance is by far the most common physiologic explanation for reduced Pa_{O_2}. It is the physiologic mechanism in virtually all parenchymal lung diseases, such as asthma, atelectasis, bronchitis, emphysema, pneumonia, and pulmonary embolism. Just what is V/Q imbalance?

Ventilation-perfusion imbalance is a disturbance of the normal distribution of V/Q ratios among the millions of alveolar-capillary units. Normally, most lung units receive an amount of ventilation equal to or close to the amount of their blood flow (e.g., 1 ml air for 1 ml blood flow); such units are "balanced" with a V/Q ratio of 1 or close to 1. When an alveolar-capillary unit has more air than blood flow, the ratio of that unit is greater than 1; if more blood flow than air is present, the ratio is less than 1.

Fig. 5-6 shows the range of V/Q ratios. To the extent that ventilation is greater than perfusion, as shown in the top two units, there is wasted ventilation or alveolar dead space. To the extent that ventilation is less than perfusion, the mixed venous

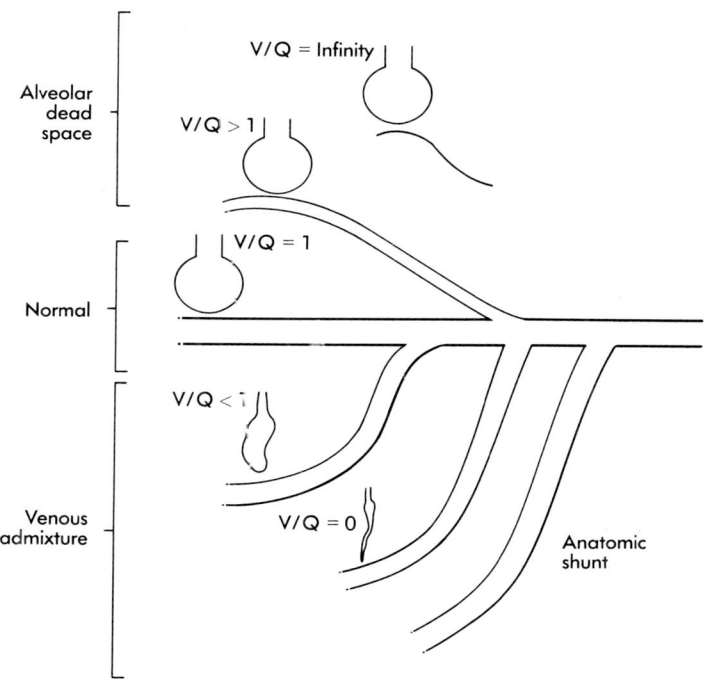

Fig. 5-6. The range of V/Q ratios. See text for discussion.

blood is unventilated and therefore unoxygenated; when the mixed venous blood mixes with blood that has been normally ventilated and oxygenated, the result is reduced arterial oxygen content and reduced PaO_2.

When lung disease creates a deviation from the normal distribution of ventilation to perfusion so that there is both excess wasted ventilation and excess venous admixture, *V/Q imbalance* is present. As a consequence, PaO_2 will be reduced—V/Q imbalance makes the lung a less efficient organ for exchanging oxygen. In fact V/Q imbalance also impairs carbon dioxide exchange. Although V/Q imbalance impairs overall gas exchange (both oxygen and carbon dioxide), the effect on PaO_2 is usually more profound than on partial pressure of arterial carbon dioxide $PaCO_2$; the reason why is discussed later in this chapter.

As used in clinical medicine, the term V/Q imbalance refers to an abnormal state: the deviation from the normal distribution of ventilation to perfusion among the millions of alveolar capillary units. However, the normal distribution represents *some* V/Q mismatch. Normally *some* lung units are overventilated or overperfused, a result mainly of the effect of gravity. In the upright lung, both ventilation and perfusion increase toward the bottom of the lung (Fig. 5-7). However, because perfusion increases more than ventilation, there is a change in V/Q ratios from less than 1 at the bottom to more than 3 at the top of the lung.

It is easy to see how gravity favors blood flow to the dependent lung. Blood has weight; thus the heart must pump blood *against* gravity in order for the blood to reach the apices of the lung. For blood traveling *down* from the heart, the hydrostatic pres-

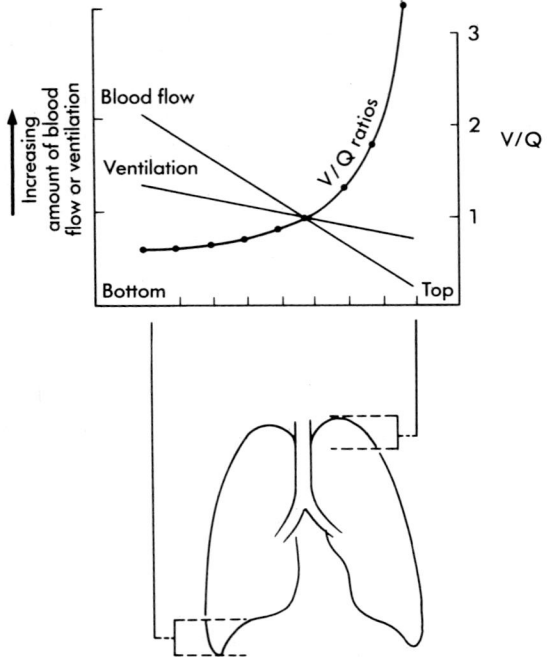

Fig. 5-7. Changes in V/Q ratios in the upright lung. At the top of the lung, ventilation is greater than perfusion, resulting in high V/Q ratios. From the top to the bottom of the lung, there is a progressive increase in both ventilation and perfusion. Since blood flow increases more than ventilation, the V/Q ratios decrease and are lowest at the bottom of the lung. (Modified from West, J.B.: Ventilation/blood flow and gas exchange, Oxford, 1980, Blackwell Scientific Publications, Ltd.)

sure is aided by gravity; thus the lung bases receive most of the blood flow when a person stands or sits. Gravitational effect can be used to predict pulmonary blood flow distribution regardless of a person's position; for example, the posterior (dorsal) portions of the lung receive the greatest blood flow when in the supine position.

The reason why gravity favors ventilation toward the bases is more complex. In Fig. 5-8, *A*, the lung is represented by a coiled spring suspended vertically and shows greater separation of the upper coils than of the lower coils. The upright lung is also "tethered" in this manner; thus the apical alveoli are stretched more than those at the bases (Fig. 5-8, *C*). Because of the difference in stretch, the compliance of lung regions varies from apex to base. Alveoli at the apex are actually less compliant than alveoli at the base. Even though apical alveoli have a larger volume, the amount of air they can exchange per breath is less than the amount for basilar alveoli. From Fig. 5-8, *B*, it can be seen that the same change in transpulmonary (recoil) pressure will cause a greater volume *change* for basilar than for apical alveoli. As a result, during normal tidal breathing more air is exchanged in the bases than in the apices.

These gravity-dependent differences in regional ventilation have been shown to definitely affect gas exchange in patients with unilateral lung disease (Remolina, Khan, Santiago, et al., 1981).

Clinical problem 8

A 54-year-old man is admitted to the hospital following a stroke that has left him partially paralyzed and comatose. He is severely hypoxemic. His chest x-ray shows pneumonia in the right lung and a clear left lung. He has been intubated and artificially ventilated, and an arterial line is inserted to allow monitoring of his blood gases. After several adjustments are made, he is found to require 70% inspired oxygen.

To help prevent bed sores, the patient is turned every 2 hours. During a period in which the ventilator settings are not changed, the following blood gas values are obtained:

1 PM Patient lying on his right side: pH 7.45; $Paco_2$ 30 mm Hg; Pao_2 76 mm Hg
2 PM Patient lying on his left side: pH 7.43; $Paco_2$ 32 mm Hg; Pao_2 123 mm Hg
How do you explain these blood gas values?

West and his colleagues have done studies to plot the distribution of ventilation and perfusion in healthy and abnormal lungs, and their figures are useful for visualizing V/Q distribution (see Fig. 5-9, which shows V/Q distribution in two subjects, one age 22 and the other age 44). Most of the ventilation and perfusion goes to lung units with

Oxygen transfer

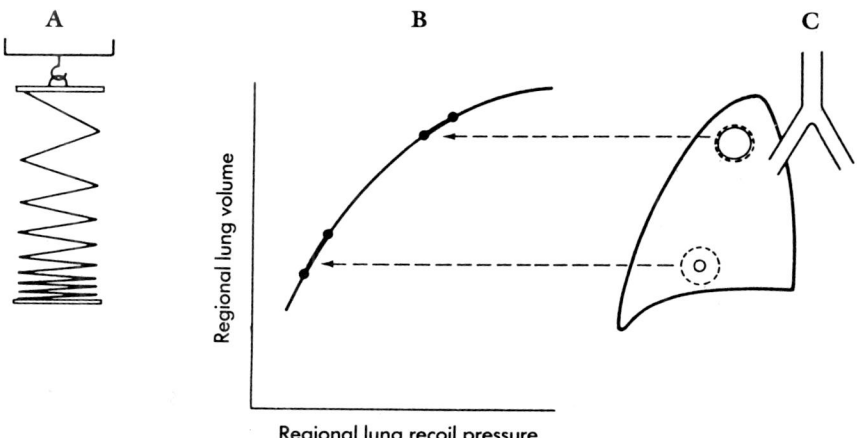

Fig. 5-8. Effect of gravity on regional ventilation in the lung. **A**, A coiled spring suspended vertically; the greatest separation between coils is at the top of the spring, the least separation is at the bottom. This is the same situation with alveoli in the upright lung. **B**, The pressure-volume curve of the lung demonstrating the relative position of apical and basilar alveoli. (Lung recoil pressure, transpulmonary pressure or Ppl [see Fig. 3-3].) **C**, Apical and basilar alveoli in the upright lung. *Dotted circle,* the end of inspiration; *solid circle,* end of expiration. For a given change in lung recoil pressure, the basilar alveoli have a larger change in volume and therefore a larger ventilation. (From Gibson, G.J.: Clinical tests of respiratory function, New York, 1984, Raven Press.)

V/Q ratios around 1. Contrast this distribution to the abnormal curves in Fig. 5-10.

Fig. 5-10 shows the V/Q curves obtained from two patients with chronic obstructive pulmonary disease. The curve in Fig. 5-10, *A,* is from a patient with pulmonary emphysema. His V/Q problem is a result of unperfused or underperfused alveoli and a resulting large amount of alveolar dead space. His pulmonary blood flow is matched by adequate alveolar ventilation, so his blood gas readings are normal or nearly so. However, so much extra air has to be brought in to fill the increased alveolar dead space that, although hypoxemia is not present, dyspnea is marked. Clinically this type of patient is often called a "pink puffer" because he has plenty of oxygen (is therefore not cyanotic), yet he has to labor to breathe. Typical blood gas values might be a Pa_{O_2} of 79 mm Hg, Pa_{CO_2} of 38 mm Hg, and pH of 7.43, with a respiratory rate of 30/min.

The curve in Fig. 5-10, *B,* is from a patient with chronic bronchitis who is hypoxemic, cyanotic, and perhaps in right-sided heart failure—the so-called "blue bloater." He is bloated (often manifested by leg edema and ascites) because of failure of the right side of the heart. Note that a large amount of perfusion goes to areas that are underventilated. As a result, relatively unoxygenated blood passes through the lungs and mixes with the blood in the left side of the heart, thus severely depressing Pa_{O_2}. Typical blood gas readings from such a patient are: Pa_{O_2} of 45 mm Hg, Pa_{CO_2} of 48 mm Hg, and pH of 7.36. (For reasons that are poorly understood, blue bloaters tend to be much less dyspneic at rest than are emphysema patients.)

Although V/Q imbalance can explain most cases of hypoxemia, exactly how the clinical disorder causes the imbalance is not always clear.

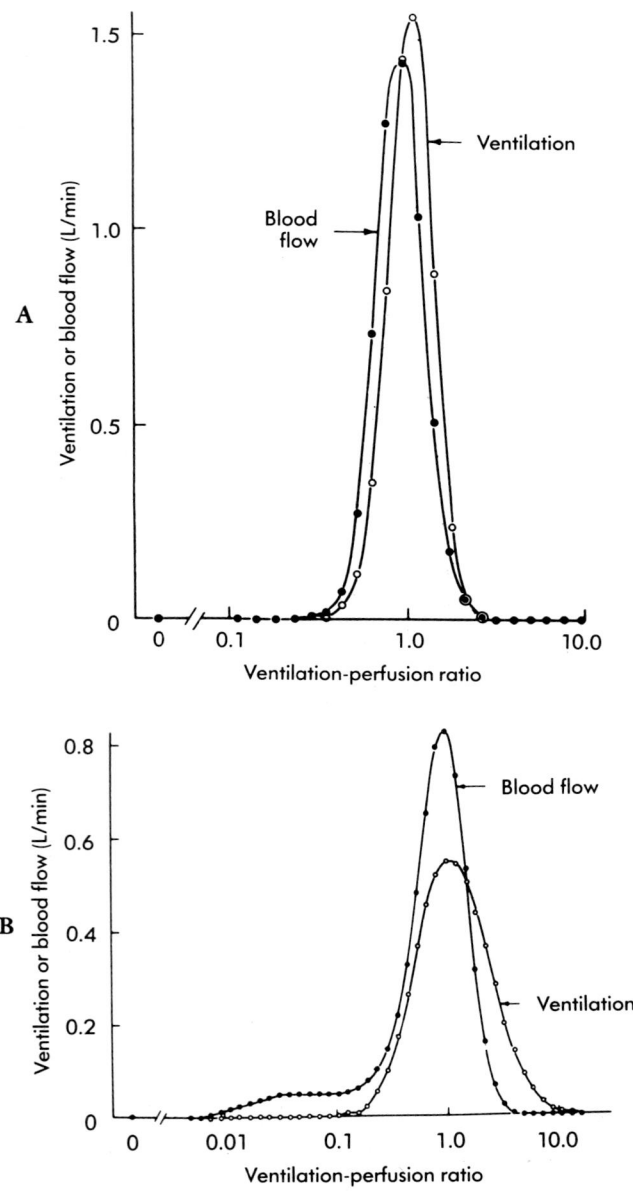

Fig. 5-9. Distribution of ventilation to perfusion in healthy people. **A**, V/Q distribution for a 22-year-old man; **B**, V/Q distribution for a 44-year-old man. In the older man 10% of the blood flow is to regions with V/Q ratios less than 0.1. (Reprinted from West, J.B., and Wagner, P.D.: Bioengineering aspects of the lung, p. 405, N.Y., 1977, by courtesy of Marcel Dekker, Inc.)

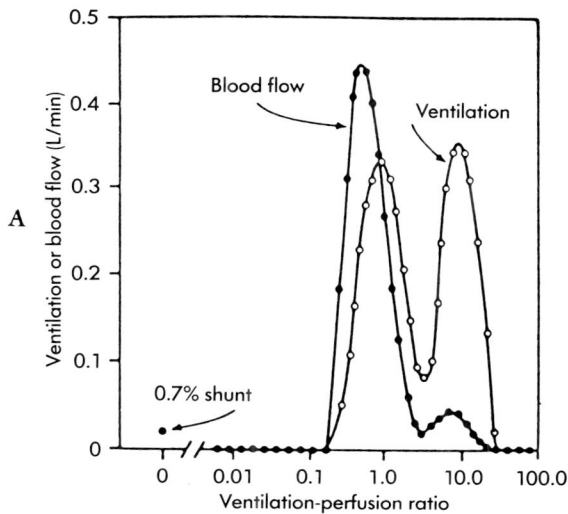

Clinical problem 9

A patient with severe chest pain is admitted to the hospital's coronary care unit. A few rales are heard in his chest, and an arterial blood gas is obtained while he is receiving 2 L/min nasal oxygen with the following results: Pao$_2$ 77 mm Hg, Paco$_2$ 36 mm Hg, and pH 7.45. A chest x-ray is normal.

For the first 24 hours he is stable. He then develops severe pain on the right side of his chest. A repeat chest x-ray reveals slightly elevated lung diaphragms but no infiltrates or other abnormality. A repeat blood gas while on 2 L/min nasal oxygen shows a Pao$_2$ of 45 mm Hg, Paco$_2$ of 28 mm Hg, and pH of 7.51. A perfusion lung scan reveals markedly decreased perfusion in the right lower lung field.

How do you explain these blood gas values?

SHUNTS AND VENOUS ADMIXTURE

Shunt is an overused word in pulmonary physiology and often means different things to different people.

In its simplest definition, a shunt occurs whenever one thing bypasses another. In the lungs, a *shunt* can be thought of as an extreme form of venous admixture, i.e., a mixing of totally unventilated, unoxygenated blood with ventilated, oxygenated blood.*

Venous admixture can occur in one of three situations, only two of which are traditionally called "shunt."

1. An *anatomic shunt* occurs when blood bypasses the lungs through an anatomic channel, such as from the right to the left ventricle through a ventricular septal defect or from a branch of the pulmonary artery directly to a pulmonary vein.
2. A *physiologic shunt* occurs when a portion of the cardiac output goes through the regular pulmonary vasculature without coming into

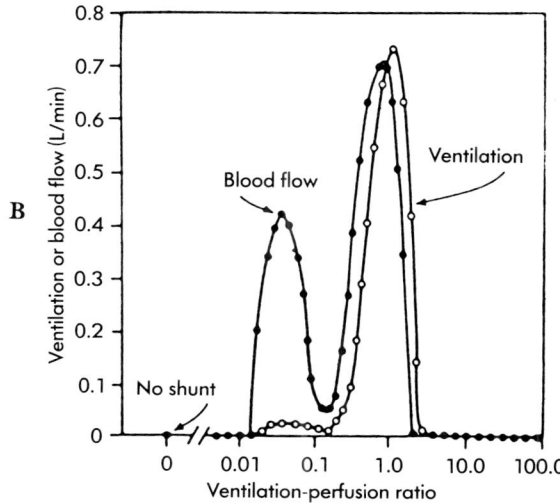

Fig. 5-10. Distribution of ventilation to perfusion in patients with chronic obstructive pulmonary disease. **A,** V/Q distribution for a patient with emphysema. **B,** V/Q distribution for a patient with chronic bronchitis. (From Wagner, P.D., et al.: J. Clin. Invest. **59:**203-206, 1977.)

---

*Technically, this is a *blood* shunt. One can also consider air that enters unperfused alveoli as being shunted since it bypasses the pulmonary circulation. However, when the term shunt is used without qualification, it refers to blood that is being shunted.

any contact with alveolar air. There is no abnormal connection between the blood vessels; rather, there is a severe redistribution of pulmonary blood flow. Physiologic shunting is often seen in conditions such as pulmonary edema, pneumonia, and lobar atelectasis.

3. *Low ventilation-perfusion ratios* occur when there is relatively more blood in the pulmonary capillary than can be fully oxygenated by the alveolar air. Although blood flow is to some extent redistributed, the blood is still exposed to *some* alveolar air. Low V/Q ratios account for most cases of hypoxemia seen clinically.

In terms of its effect on oxygenation, a physiologic shunt is not different from an anatomic shunt. In both, some unoxygenated blood bypasses the alveoli and mixes with oxygenated blood. Although both types of shunt represent venous admixture, they differ in one important aspect from venous admixture that occurs from low V/Q ratios. Since shunted blood contacts no air, increasing the fraction of inspired oxygen (FIO_2) will not improve oxygenation (except by adding more dissolved oxygen to the normally oxygenated blood). In contrast, oxygenation of the blood from low V/Q areas will definitely be improved by increasing FIO_2 because blood in low V/Q units is in contact with *some* air. Increasing the FIO_2 should eventually denitrogenate the alveolar air in the low V/Q units and completely oxygenate the blood that serves these units; 100% oxygen should accomplish this exchange completely.

Administration of 100% oxygen was recommended in the past to determine whether hypoxemia was from low V/Q areas or from a shunt. It is now known that 100% oxygen can *cause* shunting by converting areas of low V/Q to *0* V/Q. This conversion happens when the pure oxygen in the poorly ventilated alveoli is fully absorbed by the capillary blood and the alveoli collapse. Well-ventilated alveoli (normal or high V/Q) are anatomically larger, and their collapse is less likely. Even if 100% oxygen gave an accurate measure of the percent shunt, the calculation would not ordinarily affect therapy. (Shunts and their calculation are discussed further in Chapter 11.)

HOW V/Q IMBALANCE REDUCES PaO_2 AND INCREASES $PaCO_2$

PaO_2. It has been stated that V/Q imbalance is the most common cause of hypoxemia, a result of lung units with low V/Q ratios. The mechanism of hypoxemia can now be examined more closely. In Fig. 5-11, arterial partial pressure of oxygen (PaO_2) is plotted against the arterial oxygen content; this is the oxygen dissociation curve for a hemoglobin content of 15 grams%. The shape of the curve is the same as when PaO_2 is plotted against the percent oxygen saturation of hemoglobin (see Chapter 6). Note that the curve is nearly flat in the range of physiologic PaO_2 values (above 70 mm Hg) and falls steeply below 60 mm Hg. Points representing oxygen contents from three separate alveolar-capillary units are also shown. These units have V/Q ratios of 0.1, 1.0, and 10.0. Note that the decrement in capillary oxygenation caused by the low V/Q unit is not compensated for by the high V/Q unit.

Units with low V/Q ratios have low alveolar PO_2 values. Blood perfusing these units has a low end-capillary PO_2 (PcO_2) and hence a low end-capillary oxygen content. If there were a range of V/Q units from 1.0 (normal) down to 0, the result could only be hypoxemia since low oxygen contents would be mixing with normal oxygen contents. In fact, V/Q imbalance implies that at least some units are overventilated (high V/Q ratios) while others are underventilated (low V/Q ratios). The shape of the oxygen dissociation curve (Fig. 5-11) shows that high V/Q ratios will not balance out the low V/Q units.

The final PaO_2 is determined *not* by an average of oxygen partial pressures but by an average of the *oxygen contents*. This may seem confusing at first, especially since the point was already made that PaO_2 determines oxygen saturation and that oxygen saturation is a determinant of oxygen con-

Oxygen transfer

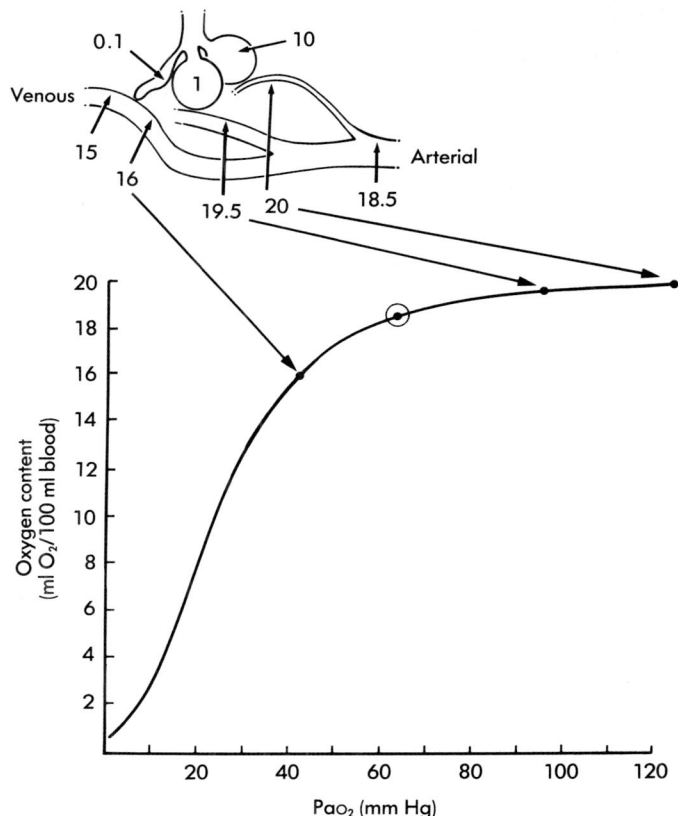

Fig. 5-11. Oxygen dissociation curve: Pa_{O_2} vs. oxygen content. Oxygen content from alveolar-capillary units with V/Q ratios of 0.1, 1, and 10 are, respectively, 16, 19.5, and 20.0 ml O_2/100 ml blood. Lines are drawn for each content to its point on the dissociation curve. The average oxygen content, 18.5 ml O_2/100 ml, is represented by a circle on the dissociation curve. Note that the arterial oxygen content after all the blood is mixed (18.5 ml O_2/100 ml) is lower than the oxygen content from the normal unit (19.5 ml O_2/100 ml).

tent. However, the oxygen dissociation curve shows that when aliquots of unequal oxygen content mix, the resulting P_{O_2} is *not* an average of the mixing P_{O_2}s, but instead is an average of the mixing *oxygen contents*. Partial pressures of gases *do not* average out when equal aliquots of blood mix. It is the gas *contents* (in this case, oxygen and carbon dioxide) that mix and average out.

Think of it this way. Alveolar P_{O_2} determines P_{O_2} and percent oxygen saturation in the pulmonary capillary; the percent oxygen saturation and the hemoglobin content determine the oxygen content (this is discussed further in Chapter 6). When a range of capillary oxygen contents mix, the average oxygen content will determine Pa_{O_2}. Careful study of the dissociation curve will help clarify this important point.

Hyperventilation of some units does not add

enough oxygen to balance out the low oxygen content from the hypoventilated units. Hyperventilation will increase Pa_{O_2} in high V/Q units, but above a Pa_{O_2} of 70 mm Hg, there is not much increase in the oxygen content of blood perfusing these units. The result is a final *oxygen content* determined mainly by the low V/Q areas and a resulting Pa_{O_2} that is lower than would be predicted by averaging the P_{O_2} values from each pulmonary capillary.

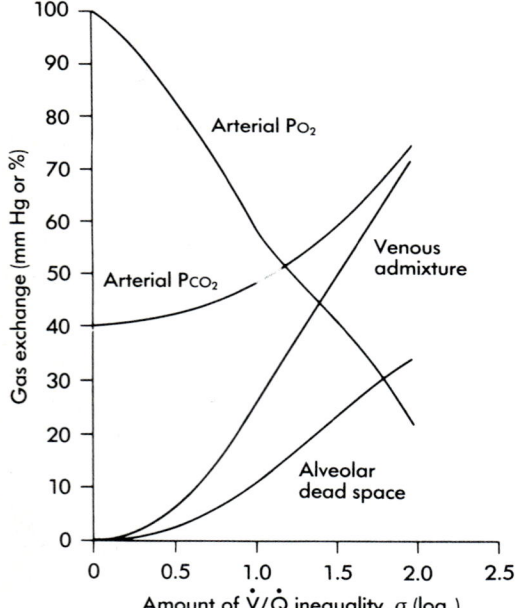

Fig. 5-12. Gas exchange effects from progressive V/Q imbalance. Ventilation-perfusion inequality and overall gas exchange in computer model of the lung. For this model, oxygen uptake and carbon dioxide output were kept constant. As the amount of V/Q inequality increases (represented by a log scale on the abscissa), Pa_{O_2} decreases and Pa_{CO_2} increases; this change is because V/Q inequality causes increases in *both* venous admixture and alveolar dead space. (From Murray, J.F.: The normal lung, Philadelphia, 1976, W.B. Saunders Co.; modified from West, J.B.: Respir. Physiol. **7:**88-110, 1969.)

The decrease in Pa_{O_2} and the increase in venous admixture from progressive V/Q imbalance are shown in Fig. 5-12. This figure represents a computer lung model in which cardiac output, minute ventilation, and oxygen uptake are kept constant, and the effects of increasing V/Q imbalance on gas exchange are analyzed.

Pa_{CO_2}. For many years it was taught that V/Q imbalance does not lead to elevated Pa_{CO_2} (hypercapnia) and that a patient had to hypoventilate to have carbon dioxide retention. No mention was made of the possible role of V/Q imbalance in carbon dioxide retention (West, 1971). In fact, "hypoventilation" and "elevated Pa_{CO_2}" mean the same thing: *decreased alveolar ventilation relative to carbon dioxide production*, which can result from either decreased minute ventilation ($\dot{V}_E$) or increased dead space ventilation ($\dot{V}_D$) (see Chapter 4).

The most common cause of increased $\dot{V}_D$ is V/Q imbalance. That V/Q imbalance can increase Pa_{CO_2} may not be intuitively obvious. Computer simulation (Fig. 5-12) also shows a progressive increase in alveolar dead space and in Pa_{CO_2} as V/Q imbalance decreases and when other factors are held constant.

Clinically, V/Q imbalance has a different effect on Pa_{O_2} and Pa_{CO_2} than that predicted in the computer model. The reason is that "other factors" are almost never kept constant in a real patient. The variable effect of V/Q imbalance is discussed in the last section of this chapter.

LOW MIXED VENOUS OXYGEN—EFFECT ON Pa_{O_2}

Low mixed venous oxygen was earlier listed as one of the nonrespiratory factors that may lower arterial oxygen pressure (Pa_{O_2}) (Table 5-1). Discussion of this mechanism was purposely delayed until the concept of shunt and venous admixture was covered. It is only in the presence of shunting and/or low V/Q ratios that low mixed venous oxygen will depress the Pa_{O_2}.

Factors that affect mixed venous oxygen content

(Cvo_2) include cardiac output, hemoglobin content, and oxygen consumption. When the cardiac output or the hemoglobin content is reduced, the amount of oxygen delivered to the systemic capillaries will be reduced; if the body's oxygen consumption stays the same, it follows that the oxygen content of the blood returning to the right side of the heart will be reduced. This reduction will also be the case when the amount of oxygen delivered to the tissues is fixed and total oxygen consumption increases.

If there is no venous admixture, mixed venous blood will be fully oxygenated on one pass through the lungs. In the presence of venous admixture (low V/Q ratios or shunt), some of the mixed venous blood will not be oxygenated but will pass through the lungs and will join with the oxygenated blood in the pulmonary veins. The resulting oxygen content will be determined by the relative contribution of the amount of shunted blood that is poor in oxygen and the amount of nonshunted blood that is rich in oxygen. Given a certain amount of venous admixture, the *lower* the Cvo_2 (and hence the mixed venous oxygen pressure [Pvo_2]) the more will the arterial oxygen content (and Pao_2) be reduced.

Reduction in Pao_2 from low Cvo_2 is shown in Table 5-3, where the effect of anemia on Pao_2 is calculated. In this example, the following are held constant: percent venous admixture, inspired oxygen pressure, $Paco_2$, cardiac output, and oxygen uptake. The result is a progressive fall in Pao_2 as the hemoglobin is reduced—solely because the anemia leads to reduced arterial oxygen delivery. Since oxygen uptake is unchanged, the amount of venous oxygen transport is reduced and hence Cvo_2 (and Pvo_2) is reduced. Low Cvo_2 depresses the oxygen content (and hence Pao_2) of the normally oxygenated blood. If there were *no* venous admixture, pulmonary venous blood would be completely oxygenated on one pass through the lungs and hemoglobin content would not affect Pao_2.

A real patient with reduced mixed venous oxygen resulting from anemia would try to compensate, mainly by increasing cardiac output and hyperventilating; this compensation would either prevent or ameliorate the fall in Pao_2. Effects of reduced Cvo_2 are discussed further in Chapter 6.

V/Q IMBALANCE IN PATIENTS— VARIABLE EFFECT ON OXYGEN AND CARBON DIOXIDE

Fig. 5-12 demonstrates that increasing degrees of V/Q imbalance should cause both low Pao_2 and elevated $Paco_2$. Clinically, however, most patients who are hypoxemic from V/Q imbalance have low Pao_2 but *also* low or normal $Paco_2$. Why this apparent contradiction?

The reason is *not*, as some often think, the greater diffusability of carbon dioxide as compared to oxygen. (Diffusion impairment is not a limiting factor for transfer of carbon dioxide or oxygen, at least with the patient at rest.) The main reason is the *physiologic difference* between the oxygen and carbon dioxide dissociation curves (Fig. 5-13).

Table 5-3. Effect of anemia on Pao_2 in the presence of venous admixture*

Hemoglobin content (gm%)	Mixed venous oxygen content (ml O_2/100 ml)	Mixed venous Po_2 (mm Hg)	Arterial Po_2 (mm Hg)
15	13.9	36	70
12	10.0	32	67
10	7.4	29	64
7.5	4.1	24	59
5	0.9	14	52

*The above values are kept constant for these calculations: percent venous admixture, 15%; Flo_2, 0.21; $Paco_2$, 40 mm Hg; cardiac output, 5 L/min; oxygen consumption, 250 ml/min; arterial-venous oxygen content difference, 5 ml/100 ml blood.

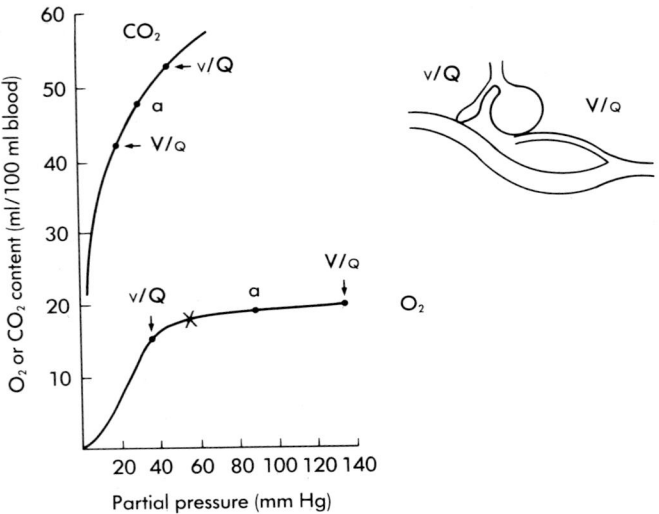

Fig. 5-13. V/Q imbalance and the dissociation curves for carbon dioxide and oxygen. v/Q represents low V/Q units and V/q represents high V/Q units. See text for discussion.

The different shape and position of the two curves allows increased alveolar ventilation to lower partial pressure of carbon dioxide (P_{CO_2}), but not raise partial pressure of oxygen (P_{O_2}).

With V/Q imbalance, some alveolar-capillary units are relatively overventilated and others relatively underventilated. Blood leaving the various units mixes in the pulmonary veins. As already pointed out, hyperventilation of some units does not add enough oxygen to balance the low oxygen contents from low V/Q areas.

Fig. 5-13 shows the oxygen and carbon dioxide dissociation curves plotted on the same scale. The upper curve is for carbon dioxide; note that it is diagonal in the physiologic range. The lower curve is for oxygen; it is almost flat in the physiologic range. (This is the same oxygen dissociation curve shown in Fig. 5-11.) On the abscissa is the partial pressure of either oxygen or carbon dioxide; on the ordinate is the content of either oxygen or carbon dioxide. Point *a* on each curve is the normal arterial point for content and partial pressure.

To the right of the graph are two lung units, one representing low V/Q and one high V/Q. The content of oxygen and carbon dioxide in the blood from each type of unit is represented on the dissociation curves.

Note that the effect of low V/Q units is to lower P_{O_2} *and* raise P_{CO_2}; the shape of the dissociation curves dictates that the respective *contents* will also change in the same direction. The effect of high V/Q units is to raise P_{O_2} *and* lower P_{CO_2}; the shape of the dissociation curves dictates that this high V/Q unit can reverse the high P_{CO_2} but not the low P_{O_2}. Thus any elevation in P_{CO_2} from low V/Q units can be compensated for by P_{CO_2} reduction in high V/Q units. These high V/Q units *cannot* compensate for the reduction in oxygen content since the oxygen dissociation curve is nearly flat in the range of high P_{O_2} values.

The final carbon dioxide content in Fig. 5-13 is point *a* on the carbon dioxide dissociation curve, arrived at by averaging the high and low V/Q points on the carbon dioxide curve. The final oxygen con-

Oxygen transfer

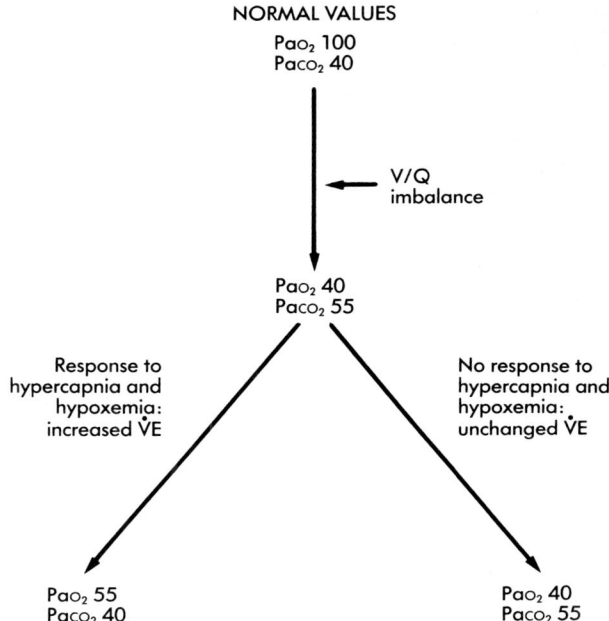

Fig. 5-14. Changes in Pa_{O_2} and Pa_{CO_2} from V/Q imbalance. All values are mm Hg. See text for discussion.

tent is point *x*, arrived at by averaging the high and low V/Q points on the oxygen curve. Point *x* is between the low V/Q and arterial points on the oxygen curve and represents a P_{O_2} considerably reduced from normal.

The important point is that hyperventilation in some units *can* compensate for the tendency of hypoventilated units to increase the P_{CO_2}. Thus if P_{CO_2} is increased in the blood draining the hypoventilated units, hyperventilation of other units can compensate *because* the carbon dioxide dissociation curve (carbon dioxide content vs. P_{CO_2}) is almost linear and diagonal in the range of physiologic P_{CO_2} values. To take advantage of this mechanism, the patient has to augment his minute ventilation and alveolar ventilation (Fig. 5-14). Patients who are able to increase their minute ventilation in the face of V/Q imbalance will usually manifest hypoxemia along with normal or low Pa_{CO_2}.

Although the majority of patients with V/Q imbalance do not manifest hypercapnia, some do, particularly when V/Q imbalance is severe and chronic. Such patients are unable to sustain the necessary increase in minute ventilation. The most common example clinically is the patient with severe chronic obstructive pulmonary disease whose V/Q imbalance has resulted in large amounts of alveolar dead space. Such a patient must maintain an increased minute ventilation to maintain a normal Pa_{CO_2}. However, if the work of breathing that is required to keep a high minute ventilation is too great, the patient will opt for less work and hence an elevated Pa_{CO_2}; this occurs in many patients with severe chronic lung disease. Even so, in such cases the basic cause of hypercapnia is increased dead space from V/Q imbalance. *V/Q imbalance is the most common cause, not only of reduced Pa_{O_2}, but, by the mechanism just explained, also of elevated Pa_{CO_2}.*

SUMMARY

The physiologic process of oxygenation involves (1) delivering oxygen from the atmosphere to the lungs where it is taken up by the pulmonary capillaries, and (2) transporting oxygen from the pulmonary circulation to all the body's tissues. Understanding the basic physiology of these two steps helps answer two important clinical questions: (1) Are the lungs properly transferring oxygen into the blood? and (2) Is the patient adequately oxygenated?

The first question can be answered yes or no by determining the alveolar-arterial oxygen pressure difference ($P(A-a)O_2$), also referred to as the "A-a gradient." The $P(A-a)O_2$ is determined by subtracting the measured arterial partial pressure of oxygen (PaO_2) from the calculated alveolar partial pressure of oxygen (PAO_2), with the latter obtained from the equation $PAO_2 = PIO_2 - (1.2 \times PaCO_2)$. For a patient breathing room air, normal $P(A-a)O_2$ is age-dependent, ranging from approximately 5 to 30 mm Hg. Normal $P(A-a)O_2$ increases as the fraction of inspired oxygen (FIO_2) increases and can go up to approximately 100 mm Hg on 100% oxygen. If $P(A-a)O_2$ is elevated above normal, the lungs are not transferring oxygen properly. An elevated $P(A-a)O_2$ represents a parenchymal lung problem and is almost always caused by ventilation-perfusion (V/Q) imbalance.

V/Q imbalance is an imbalance of the normal distribution of ventilation to perfusion among the millions of alveolar capillary units. Gas exchange (the transfer of oxygen and carbon dioxide between the alveolar air and the pulmonary capillary blood) is always disturbed in the presence of V/Q imbalance. Hypoxemia results when areas of the lung are relatively overperfused (or underventilated), a common occurrence in parenchymal lung diseases.

Graphic representation of V/Q relationships helps explain the pattern of gas exchange abnormality seen clinically. For example, patients with predominant chronic bronchitis are hypoxemic because they have relatively large areas of underventilated (overperfused) lung. Patients with predominant emphysema have large areas of overventilated (underperfused) lung representing extra dead space that they must ventilate with each breath; as long as they can augment their total ventilation to satisfy the extra dead space, hypoxemia does not occur.

REVIEW QUESTIONS

State whether each of the following is true or false.

1. The most common physiologic cause of hypoxemia is diffusion barrier.
2. An increase in the alveolar-arterial PO_2 difference most commonly arises from a ventilation-perfusion imbalance within the lungs.
3. Thebesian vessels supply the myocardium and drain the venous blood directly into the ventricles.
4. Alveolar PO_2 is a function of, among other factors, PCO_2, respiratory quotient, and altitude.
5. The alveolar-arterial PO_2 difference may normally be as high as 50 mm Hg when breathing 100% oxygen.
6. Both the PaO_2 and $PaCO_2$ are age-dependent, the former decreasing and the latter slightly increasing with age.
7. The reason why patients with ventilation-perfusion imbalance commonly manifest hypoxemia but not hypercapnia is the greater diffusability of carbon dioxide compared to oxygen.
8. While breathing 100% oxygen, a patient's respiratory quotient becomes unity.
9. Hemodialysis can lead to hypoxemia by reducing alveolar ventilation.
10. Alveolar units that receive ventilation but no perfusion have a ventilation-perfusion ratio of infinity.

References

Aurigemma, N.M., Feldman, N., Gottlieb, M., et al.: Arterial oxygenation during hemodialysis, N. Engl. J. Med. **297**:871, 1977.

Gibson, G.J.: Clinical tests of respiratory function, New York, 1984, Raven Press.

Gilbert, R., Keighley, J.F.: The arterial/alveolar oxygen tension ratio: an index of gas exchange applicable to varying inspired oxygen concentrations, Am. Rev. Respir. Dis. **109**:142, 1974.

Harris, E.A., Kenyon, A.M., Nisbet, H.D., et al.: The normal alveolar-arterial oxygen-tension gradient in man, Clin. Sci. Mol. Med. **46**:89, 1974.

Hess, D., and Maxwell, C.: Which is the best index of oxygenation—$P(A-a)O_2$, PaO_2/PAO_2, or PaO_2/FIO_2? Respir. Care **30**:961, 1985.

Hunt, J.M., Chappell, T.R., Henrich, W.L., et al.: Gas exchange during dialysis: contrasting mechanisms contributing to comparable alterations with acetate and bicarbonate buffers, Am. J. Med. **77**:255, 1984.

Martin, L.: Abbreviating the alveolar gas equation: an argument for simplicity, Respir. Care **31**:40, 1986.

Martin, L.: Hypoventilation without CO_2 retention, Chest **77**:720, 1980.

Quebbman, E.J., Maierhofer, W.J., and Piering, W.F.: Mechanisms producing hypoxemia during hemodialysis, Crit. Care Med. **12**:359, 1984.

Remolina, C., Khan, A.U., Santiago, T.V., et al.: Positional hypoxemia in unilateral lung disease, N. Engl. J. Med. **304**:523, 1981.

Sorbini, C.A., Grassi, V., Solinas, E., et al.: Arterial oxygen tension in relation to age in healthy subjects, Respiration **25**:3, 1968.

West, J.B.: Ventilation-perfusion inequality and overall gas exchange in computer models of the lung, Respir. Physiol. **7**:88, 1969.

West, J.B.: Causes of carbon dioxide retention in lung disease, N. Engl. J. Med. **284**:1232, 1971.

West, J.B.: Ventilation/blood flow and gas exchange, Oxford, 1980, Blackwell Scientific Publications, Ltd.

West, J.B., and Wagner, P.D.: Bioengineering aspects of the lung, New York, 1977, Marcel Dekker, Inc.

West, J.B., Hackett, P.H., Maret, K.H., et al.: Pulmonary gas exchange on the summit of Mt. Everest, J. Appl. Physiol. **55**:678, 1983.

Suggested readings

Begin, R., and Renzetti, A.D.: Alveolar-arterial oxygen pressure gradient. I. Comparison between an assumed and actual respiratory quotient in stable chronic pulmonary disease. II. Relationship to aging and closing volume in normal subjects, Respir. Care **22**(5):491, 1977.

Burrows, B., Fletcher, C.M., Heard, B.E., et al.: The emphysematous and bronchial types of chronic airways obstruction: a clinicopathological study of patients in London and Chicago, Lancet **1**:830, 1966.

Huet, Y., Lemaire, F., Brun-Buisson, C., et al.: Hypoxemia in acute pulmonary embolism, Chest **88**:829, 1985.

Mellemgaard, K.: The alveolar-arterial oxygen difference: its size and components in normal man, Acta. Physiol. Scand. **67**:10, 1966.

Wagner, P.D., Saltzman, H.A., and West, J.B.: Measurement of continuous distributions of ventilation-perfusion ratios: theory, J. Appl. Physiol. **36**(5):588, 1974.

West, J.: Ventilation-perfusion relationships, Am. Rev. Resp. Dis. **116**:919, 1977.

See also General References (Physiology) in Appendix G.

chapter 6
Is the patient adequately oxygenated?

OUTLINE

Clinical assessment
Hypoxemia vs. hypoxia
The oxygenation cycle
Sao_2 and oxygen content
Shifts of oxygen dissociation curve and P_{50}
Carbon monoxide
Carbon monoxide exposure and its effects
Methemoglobinemia and sulfhemoglobinemia
Causes of reduced Sao_2
Oxygen delivery
Fick equation
Mixed venous oxygen saturation

CLINICAL ASSESSMENT

Adequacy of oxygenation is deceptively difficult to assess in patients. Certainly if someone appears healthy, has no respiratory symptoms, and is being evaluated for a problem unrelated to the cardiopulmonary system (e.g., an orthopedic injury), there may be no concern about oxygenation.

In respiratory patients the situation is different. There is often a history of respiratory illness, or the patient may appear dyspneic or mentally confused or may manifest other signs suggesting a lack of oxygen. Given a clinical suspicion, there is no reliable way to assess the adequacy of oxygenation without some measurement of blood oxygen. Mental status, pulse rate, breathing pattern, and a number of other clinical signs are unreliable guides to oxygenation. Physicians who practiced before the era of blood gas analysis had to make an educated guess about a patient's oxygenation status. Except for the most obvious case of cyanosis, this guess was as apt to be wrong as to be correct.

As has been pointed out by Comroe (1947), even the assessment of cyanosis is unreliable. Too much depends on the patient's skin pigment, the available light, and interobserver variation. Also, since cyanosis does not occur until 5 gm of hemoglobin are desaturated in the skin capillaries, anemic patients may never appear cyanotic *even when severely hypoxemic*.

The patient's history and physical examination are not to be slighted, however. How else would one know when to worry about a patient's level of oxygenation? Certainly if a healthy athlete breaks a toe, his oxygenation is not questioned. Conversely, oxygenation is an obvious concern in a patient suffering from pulmonary edema and shock. But what about the vast number of patients between these extremes—the ones who initially have shortness of breath only on exertion, who are confused, or who have cardiomegaly of unknown cause? These and many other clinical signs and symptoms shown in the following box should result in questioning the level of oxygenation. In clinical practice, this questioning should lead to measurement of arterial partial pressure of oxygen (PaO_2) and percent saturation of hemoglobin with oxygen (SaO_2).

Blood gas machines provide measurement of both PaO_2 and SaO_2, but neither measurement tells how much oxygen is in the blood, a quantity that is provided by the *oxygen content*. Oxygen content takes into account the amount of hemoglobin available to carry the oxygen and is the minimal laboratory information needed to assess oxygenation. But even oxygen content may not be sufficient information about oxygenation in patients with compromised cardiac function.

HYPOXEMIA VS. HYPOXIA

Although the terms hypoxemia and hypoxia are often used interchangeably, they are not synonymous. Hypoxemia means low oxygen *(hypox)* in the blood *(emia)* and refers to either low arterial pressure of oxygen (PaO_2) or low arterial oxygen content (CaO_2). Patients can have low PaO_2 without much reduction in oxygen content (i.e., PaO_2 of 60 to 70 mm Hg), but nonetheless such patients are considered hypoxemic. Ideally the term should either be qualified or clearly understood in its context.

Hypoxia is a more general term and signifies general lack of oxygen in the whole body. It thus includes hypoxemia (low oxygen in the blood), as well as those conditions in which the oxygen content is adequate but the circulation is impaired or in which insufficient oxygen is taken up by the tissues. The box below gives a general classification of hypoxia.

CLUES TO SUGGEST INADEQUATE OXYGENATION

Dyspnea, either at rest or on exertion
Any state of confusion, lethargy, or obtundation
Persistent dizziness or lightheadedness
Any unexplained state of anxiety, irritability, or restlessness
Any unexplained headache, especially if severe and chronic
Cardiomegaly or heart failure of unknown cause

CAUSES OF HYPOXIA—A GENERAL CLASSIFICATION

1. **Hypoxemia** (reduced arterial oxygen content)
   a. Reduced PaO_2*
   b. Reduced SaO_2†
   c. Reduced hemoglobin content (anemia)
2. **Reduced oxygen delivery**
   a. Reduced cardiac output
   b. Left-to-right systemic shunt (e.g., septic shock)
3. **Decreased tissue oxygen uptake**
   a. Mitochondrial poisoning (e.g., cyanide)
   b. Left-shifted hemoglobin dissociation curve (e.g., abnormal hemoglobin structure)

*See Table 5-1
†See Table 6-3

The whole process of oxygenation is, like all physiologic processes, dynamic; one thing affects another, and changes happen very quickly. Oxygen is a necessary element for life, and lack of it leads to death in a few minutes. The process of getting oxygen from the atmosphere into the blood and then to all the tissues involves not only the respiratory system, but also the heart and the circulatory system. It is helpful to review the entire cycle of human oxygenation and then discuss its components one at a time.

THE OXYGENATION CYCLE (Fig. 6-1)

Oxygen enters the blood by diffusion across the alveolar capillary membranes; the overall relationship of alveolar ventilation to capillary perfusion results in the arterial partial pressure of oxygen (PaO_2) (see Chapter 5) and a percent saturation of the available hemoglobin (SaO_2). For a PaO_2 of 100 mm Hg, SaO_2 is approximately 97% at normal pH. (SaO_2 for a given PaO_2 also depends on other factors, which are discussed in a later section.) The vast majority of oxygen is carried by hemoglobin,

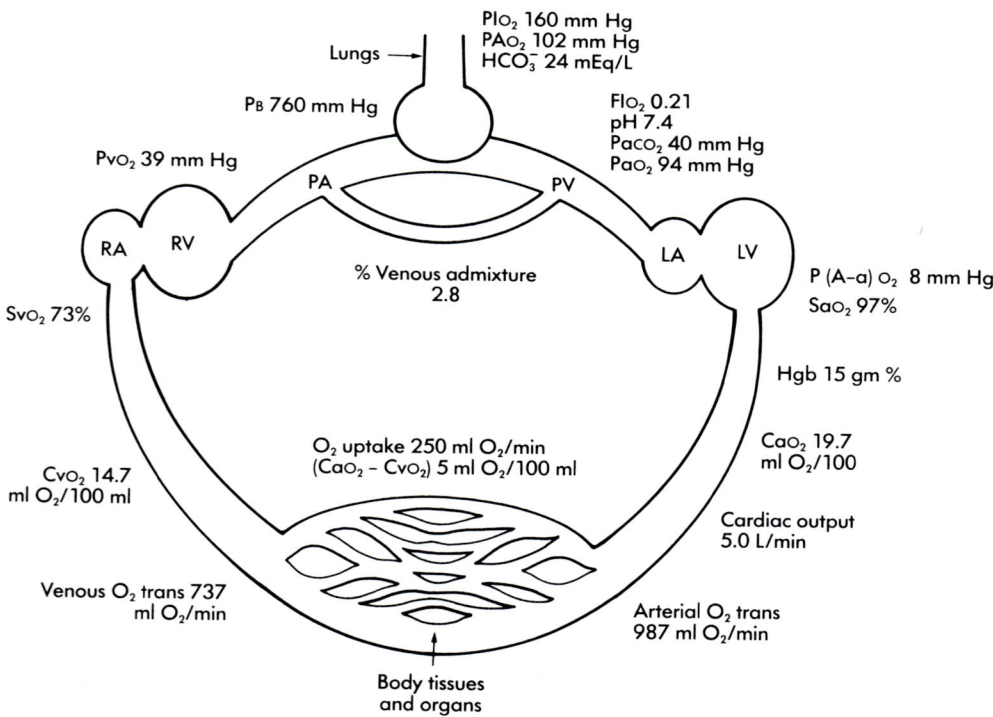

Fig. 6-1. The oxygenation cycle. Using representative normal values for barometric pressure, cardiac output, hemoglobin content, venous admixture, and oxygen uptake, the changes in oxygen pressure and oxygen content are shown from the arterial blood to the mixed venous blood. (*PA*, pulmonary arteries; *PV*, pulmonary veins; *LA*, left atrium; *LV*, left ventricle; *RV*, right ventricle; *P(A-a)O_2*, alveolar-arterial PO_2 difference; *($CaO_2 - CvO_2$)*, arterial-venous oxygen content difference; *Hgb*, hemoglobin; *RA*, right atrium; *Trans*, transport; *PB*, barometric pressure.)

Is the patient adequately oxygenated?

with only a small amount dissolved in plasma. Thus arterial oxygen content (CaO_2) is largely determined by the SaO_2 and the hemoglobin content; when the latter is 15 gm%, CaO_2 is approximately 20 ml O_2/100 ml blood.

Oxygen delivery to the tissues requires adequate cardiac output and arterial circulation. Cardiac output times the CaO_2 gives the amount of oxygen delivered to all tissues per minute; in an average person this amount is approximately 1000 ml O_2/min at rest. Normally, the body uses approximately one quarter of the oxygen that is delivered, or 250 ml O_2/min; this measurement is the metabolic oxygen consumption ($\dot{V}O_2$). (At the same time, metabolism produces approximately 200 ml CO_2/min.)

A disturbance in the oxygen cycle at any point up to and including oxygen consumption can result in hypoxemia or hypoxia, as shown in the box on p. 113.

Oxygen transport in the venous system is determined by the arterial oxygen delivery minus the oxygen uptake; using the values given previously, venous oxygen transport is 750 ml O_2/min. Venous oxygen contents in blood from the various organs and tissues vary widely, so venous oxygen levels are usually measured only in the pulmonary artery where the values are sure to represent mixed venous blood and thus the body as a whole. Normal mixed venous oxygen content, percent saturation, and partial pressure are, respectively, 15 ml O_2/100 ml blood, 75%, and 40 mm Hg.

Mixed venous blood, regardless of its partial pressure of oxygen, is fully oxygenated after passing through normal alveolar-capillary units. Mixed venous blood that does not pass through normal units, such as the small amount shunted past the lungs, mixes with oxygenated blood either in the pulmonary veins, the left atrium, or the left ventricle; this venous admixture results in some reduction of arterial oxygen content. Normal venous admixture accounts for the normal alveolar-arterial PO_2 difference (see Chapter 5).

SaO_2 AND OXYGEN CONTENT

Arterial partial pressure of oxygen (PaO_2) determines the percent saturation of hemoglobin with oxygen (SaO_2), which, along with available hemoglobin, largely determines the oxygen content. Fig. 6-2 shows PaO_2 vs. SaO_2 (the oxygen dissociation curve) and PaO_2 vs. oxygen content when the hemoglobin content is 10 gm% (anemia) and 15 gm% (normal).

Arterial oxygen content equals:

Amount of oxygen bound to hemoglobin +
    Amount of oxygen dissolved in plasma = **(1)**
        ($SaO_2 \times Hgb \times 1.34$) + ($0.003 \times PaO_2$)

where SaO_2 is the percent saturation of hemoglobin with oxygen, Hgb is the hemoglobin content in gm%, 1.34 is the oxygen binding capacity of hemoglobin (ml O_2/gm Hgb), and 0.003 is the milliliters of oxygen that dissolve in 100 ml plasma per mm Hg PaO_2. Normal arterial oxygen content is approximately 16 to 20 ml O_2/100 ml blood. Note that the amount of dissolved oxygen is not clinically significant at a normal PaO_2. Most of the oxygen is carried bound to hemoglobin, hence the importance of oxygen content, rather than just SaO_2 or PaO_2, as a gauge of oxygenation.

Note also that anemia does not affect SaO_2, only oxygen content. Thus the oxygen dissociation curve (PaO_2 vs. SaO_2) is unaffected by hemoglobin content.

Clinical problem 1

What is the arterial oxygen content if PaO_2 is 92 mm Hg, SaO_2 is 98%, and hemoglobin is 15 gm%?

Clinical problem 2

Which patient is more hypoxemic?

Test	Patient A	Patient B
PaO_2	50 mm Hg	80 mm Hg
SaO_2	85%	94%
Hemoglobin	15 gm%	8 gm%

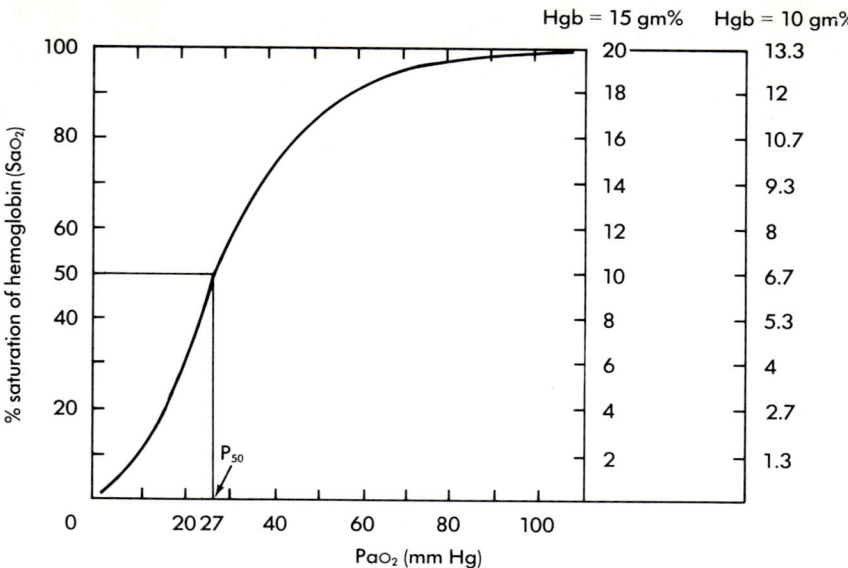

Fig. 6-2. Pa_{O_2} vs. Sa_{O_2} and oxygen content. The oxygen dissociation curve relates Pa_{O_2} to Sa_{O_2}. The shape and the position of the curve are the same regardless of hemoglobin content. The right ordinate shows arterial oxygen contents for two different concentrations of hemoglobin: 15 gm% and 10 gm%. Normal P_{50} is approximately 27 mm Hg. If this were the partial pressure of oxygen in arterial blood (a very sick patient), the oxygen content would be 10 ml O_2/100 ml blood for a hemoglobin content of 15 gm% and 6.7 ml O_2/100 ml blood for a hemoglobin content of 10 gm%. (The P_{50} is the Pa_{O_2} at which hemoglobin is 50% saturated with oxygen.)

SHIFTS OF OXYGEN DISSOCIATION CURVE AND P_{50}

The partial pressure of oxygen is not affected by changes in hemoglobin or percent saturation. As discussed in Chapter 5, the arterial P_{O_2} is determined by the alveolar air–pulmonary capillary interface and is not affected by the chemical makeup of the blood. The solubility of oxygen in plasma is a physical constant and does not change with alterations of hemoglobin. However, the percent saturation of hemoglobin with oxygen (Sa_{O_2}) for a given Pa_{O_2} can change.

The oxygen dissociation curve shown in Fig. 6-2 is the standard curve for when the pH, arterial partial pressure of carbon dioxide (Pa_{CO_2}), body temperature, and concentration of 2,3-diphosphoglycerate (DPG) are normal. Alteration of these and other factors (e.g., the presence of carboxyhemoglobin) can shift the dissociation curve from its normal position (Fig. 6-3). Both the direction and the degree of shift are measured by the P_{50}, which is the Pa_{O_2} at which 50% of the hemoglobin is saturated with oxygen; it is normally approximately 27 mm Hg.

To determine P_{50}, a sample of blood (venous or arterial) is exposed to two different samples of air containing low concentrations of oxygen, usually 3% and 4%. (In effect, the blood is exposed to a fraction of inspired oxygen (FI_{O_2}) of 0.03 and 0.04; ambient air has 21% oxygen or an FI_{O_2} of 0.21.) This exposure will give two saturation points, one above and one below the usual range of P_{50}. A line

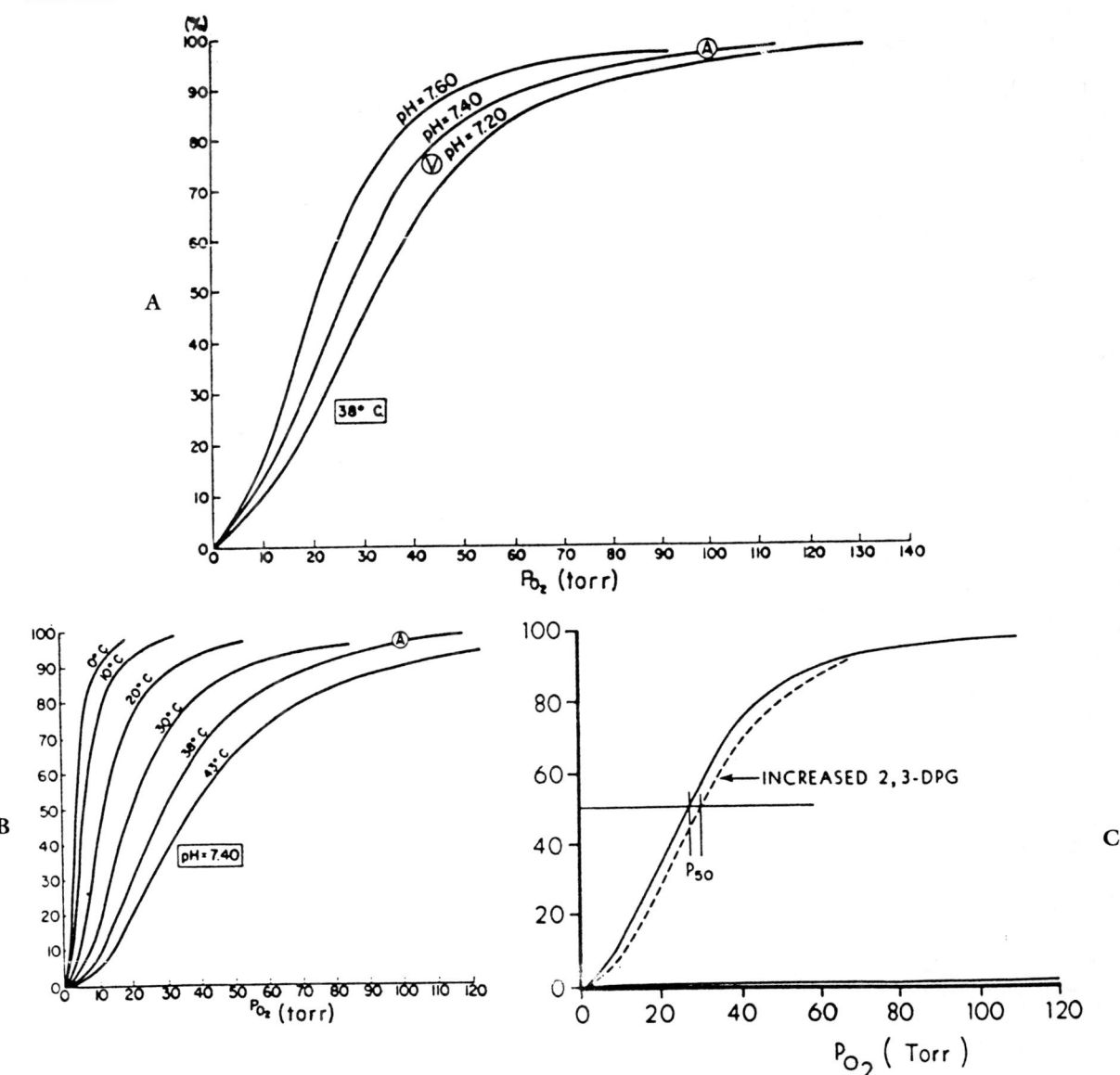

Fig. 6-3. Effects of pH, temperature, and 2,3-diphosphoglycerate (DPG) on the oxygen dissociation curve. **A,** Effect of pH on position of the curve. A high pH shifts the curve to the left, a low pH, to the right. **B,** Effect of temperature on position of the curve. A high temperature shifts the curve to the right, a low temperature to the left. **C,** Effect of 2,3-DPG on position of the curve. Increased 2,3-DPG shifts the curve to the right. (From Slonim, N.B., and Hamilton, L.H.: Respiratory physiology, ed. 4, St. Louis, 1981, The C.V. Mosby Co.)

is then drawn connecting the two saturations, and the 50% saturation point is identified. The P_{O_2} corresponding to this point is the P_{50}.

A P_{50} higher than 27 mm Hg represents a *rightward* shift of the oxygen dissociation curve; less than 27 mm Hg represents a *leftward* shift. What happens when the curve is shifted? In a rightward shift, blood picks up less oxygen at the pulmonary capillary level but delivers relatively more oxygen at the tissue level (Fig. 6-3). A curve shifted to the right causes a reduction in Sa_{O_2} for a given Pa_{O_2} (see Table 6-3).

When the oxygen dissociation curve is shifted to the left, blood picks up more oxygen at the pulmonary capillary but delivers relatively less to the systemic capillary, where the P_{O_2} is normally very low. A curve shifted to the left causes an increase in Sa_{O_2} for a given Pa_{O_2}.

In terms of oxygen delivery, a right shift is considered a helpful adaptation. Attempts have been made to artificially shift the curve and improve oxygen delivery, but such an attempt is generally not a useful therapeutic maneuver. Factors affecting the curve's position are complex, and altering one or two of them does not guarantee that the patient will benefit. Instead, an attempt should be made to maintain the patient's pH and body temperature within normal limits, and the exact position of the oxygen dissociation curve should not be a cause for concern.

CARBON MONOXIDE

Carbon monoxide (CO) combines avidly with hemoglobin, displacing oxygen and thereby lowering the percent saturation of hemoglobin with oxygen (Sa_{O_2}). Small amounts of carbon monoxide are normally present in the blood (from the breakdown of hemoglobin), and less than 2% *carboxyhemoglobin* (HbCO) is generally acceptable. To the extent that the carboxyhemoglobin is increased, the percentage of *oxyhemoglobin,* and thus the oxygen content, is decreased. Carbon monoxide does not directly affect Pa_{O_2}, so the Sa_{O_2} must be measured to appreciate a reduction in oxygen content.

Fig. 6-4 plots Pa_{O_2} vs. oxygen content when no carbon monoxide is present and when the blood is 20%, 40%, and 60% saturated with carbon monoxide. For comparison a curve is also shown for an anemic patient (40% of normal hemoglobin). Note that the normal curve for Pa_{O_2} vs. oxygen content has the same sigmoid shape as the curves of Pa_{O_2} vs. Sa_{O_2}. This similarity exists because the only difference between Sa_{O_2} and oxygen content for a given amount of hemoglobin is a constant (1.34 ml O_2/gm hemoglobin).

Most people who smoke cigarettes or cigars have an HbCO level between 5% and 10%. This amount is not usually clinically significant when cardiopulmonary function and the hemoglobin content are normal. However, small increases of HbCO can be harmful in the presence of angina, anemia, or pulmonary impairment.

Besides lowering the total oxygen content, carbon monoxide also shifts the oxygen dissociation curve to the left; this movement is best appreciated by comparing the oxygen dissociation curve in the presence of HbCO with the curve for anemia and identical arterial oxygen content (Fig. 6-4). At the capillary level, where the P_{O_2} is much lower than in the arteries, hemoglobin holds onto oxygen more strongly in the presence of carbon monoxide. This added effect (the first

---

Clinical problem 3

A semicomatose patient is brought to the emergency room and has the following blood gas values: Pa_{O_2}, 85 mm Hg; pH, 7.40; Sa_{O_2}, 50%; (fraction of inspired oxygen, 0.21). Which of the conditions listed below could explain these blood gas values?
   a. Anemia
   b. Carbon monoxide poisoning
   c. Hypothermia
   d. Severe parenchymal lung disease
   e. Normal values for a middle-aged patient

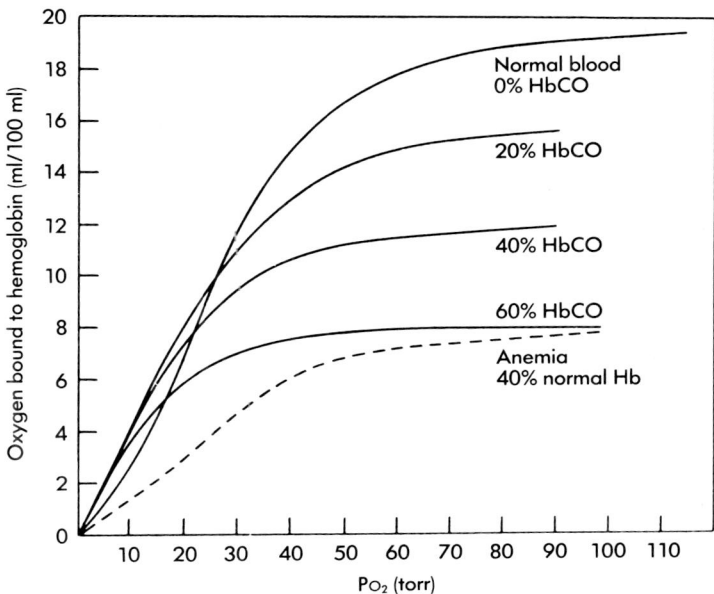

Fig. 6-4. Effects of carbon monoxide on oxygen dissociation curve. ([Redrawn from Roughton, F.J.W., and Darling, R.C.: Am. J. Physiol. **141**:17-31, 1944.] and reproduced with permission from Comroe, J.H., Jr.: Physiology of respiration, 2nd edition. Copyright © 1974 by Year Book Medical Publishers, Inc., Chicago.)

Clinical problem 4

If the patient in Clinical Problem 3 has a hemoglobin content of 13 gm%, the approximate oxygen content is:
    a. 5.6 ml O_2/100 ml blood
    b. 9.0 ml O_2/100 ml blood
    c. 10.6 ml O_2/100 ml blood
    d. 14.3 ml O_2/100 ml blood
    e. 18.2 ml O_2/100 ml blood

---

effect is reduction of arterial content) further aggravates the patient's hypoxia.

Arterial blood gas measurement may or may not be helpful when carbon monoxide poisoning is suspected, depending on what is actually measured. All blood gas instruments *measure* Po_2, and from this measurement the Sao_2 can be *estimated*, but it is always better to *measure* the Sao_2. This measurement is obtained with an instrument called a *co-oximeter*.*

An estimate of Sao_2, based on a standard oxygen dissociation curve, will be incorrect if carbon monoxide is present in any excess. It is important to always know what was measured when blood gas results are reported. The Pao_2 is unaffected by carbon monoxide and may be normal in the presence of carbon monoxide poisoning. It is the Sao_2 that

---

*The modern blood gas laboratory contains both a *blood gas machine*, which measures Po_2, Pco_2, and pH, and a *co-oximeter* (see Fig. 1-8). Both machines are often called blood gas machines, although the co-oximeter does not technically measure a blood gas.

is always reduced from excess carbon monoxide.

Thus if the SaO_2 is *estimated* from the arterial PO_2, it may be *falsely* reported as normal. The clue to a diagnosis of carbon monoxide poisoning (without direct measurement of %HbCO) is a measured SaO_2 *inappropriately low* for the PaO_2, e.g., a PaO_2 of 80 mm Hg and a SaO_2 of 50%. The definitive diagnosis of carbon monoxide poisoning is made by measuring %HbCO directly, a measurement that can also be done with some co-oximeters.

CARBON MONOXIDE EXPOSURE AND ITS EFFECTS

People breathing carbon monoxide-free air will have a percent carboxyhemoglobin (%HbCO) of less than 2%. Exposure to heavy downtown traffic for 8 hours can produce %HbCO between 3% and 5%, and heavy cigarette smokers may have up to 10% HbCO. Although these levels should not produce symptoms in otherwise healthy people, they can have long-term harmful effects in some groups. For example:
 a. Chronic lung disease patients show decreased exercise tolerance at approximately 4% HbCO.
 b. Excess HbCO results in an increase in coronary artery blood flow to compensate for the decreased oxygen content; in the presence of fixed coronary artery obstruction, this increase may not occur. The result can be a decrease in the aerobic capacity of the myocardium and, in severe cases, actual anaerobic metabolism. This effect has been shown to occur at levels of 5% to 8% HbCO.
 c. There is a decrease in the threshold for ventricular fibrillation, which may relate to the sudden death of smokers with coronary artery disease, and there is a possible role for carbon monoxide in the initiation or the acceleration of atherosclerosis itself.
 d. Finally, the low birth weight seen in the newborns of mothers who smoke is probably caused by chronic maternal carboxyhemoglobinemia.

Automobile exhaust in closed spaces and fires are the most common causes of acute carbon monoxide poisoning. In treating fire victims, it is important not to let the presence of burns or smoke inhalation hide the less obvious but more immediate danger of carbon monoxide poisoning. There are other sources of carbon monoxide poisoning—malfunctioning fireplaces, wood stoves, and space heaters, as well as charcoal grills or hibachis that are used in closed spaces.

When they are conscious, victims of carbon monoxide poisoning initially have *headache;* in more severe cases, *lethargy* or *coma* can be the initial symptoms. Shortness of breath is *not* a typical symptom of carbon monoxide poisoning. There is a rough correlation of the symptoms with the level of HbCO (Table 6-1). Any patient complaining of a chronic headache, especially during the winter months, should: (1) be asked if anyone else in the home is having headaches; (2) be asked about the use of space heaters and charcoal fires; and (3) have his %HbCO level measured, a measurement that can be done on venous blood. An alternative to HbCO analysis is the measurement of PaO_2 and SaO_2.

The physical examination is usually not helpful in assessing carbon monoxide poisoning other than in assessing alertness. "Cherry-red coloration" in carbon monoxide poisoning is usually *not* present. Because the PaO_2 is not reduced, the patients do not hyperventilate and do not appear dyspneic. The chest x-ray film is often normal, and the arterial blood gas values suggest the diagnosis only if *measured* SaO_2 is inappropriately low for the PaO_2. To make the diagnosis of carbon monoxide poisoning, it must first be suspected; then laboratory confirmation must be obtained. Failure to consider this diagnosis can result in a preventable tragedy.

The treatment of carbon monoxide poisoning is based on the fact that high oxygen pressures compete with carbon monoxide for the Fe^{++} binding site of hemoglobin and thus speed the dissociation of HbCO and the excretion of carbon monoxide. Treatment is discussed further in Chapter 9.

Table 6-1. Correlation of symptoms and signs with carbon monoxide level

Percent of carbon monoxide in inspired air	Percent of HbCO in blood	Signs and symptoms
0.007	10	Common in cigarette smokers; dyspnea during vigorous exertion; occasional tightness in forehead; dilation of cutaneous blood vessels
0.012	20	Dyspnea during moderate exertion; occasional throbbing headache in temples
0.022	30	Severe headache; irritability; easy fatigability; disturbed judgment; possible dizziness and possible dimness of vision
0.035-0.052	40-50	Headache; confusion; fainting on exertion
0.080-0.122	60-70	Unconsciousness; intermittent convulsions; respiratory failure; death if exposure prolonged
0.195	80	Fatal

Modified from Winter, P.M., and Miller, J.N.: JAMA **236**:1503, 1976, Copyright 1976, American Medical Association.

METHEMOGLOBINEMIA AND SULFHEMOGLOBINEMIA

Aside from carbon monoxide, other factors can affect the affinity of hemoglobin for oxygen. Methemoglobin (metHb) occurs when the Fe^{++} of hemoglobin is oxidized to Fe^{+++}; oxidized hemoglobin is then unable to carry oxygen. Normally, about 1.5% of hemoglobin is in the oxidized state; an amount greater than 1.5% defines a state of methemoglobinemia.

As with carboxyhemoglobin (HbCO), each one percent increase of metHb means 1% less oxyhemoglobin (HbO_2). In addition, metHb strengthens the affinity of normal hemoglobin (Fe^{++}) for oxygen. Thus, as with HbCO, metHb causes hypoxia in two ways: (1) it reduces the amount of oxygen that hemoglobin can bind at the pulmonary capillary, causing a reduction in arterial oxygen content; and (2) it causes the hemoglobin that does bind with oxygen to hold the oxygen more tightly so that it is less available at the tissue level. This last effect represents a leftward shift of the oxygen dissociation curve since, for a given PaO_2, oxygen is more tightly bound to hemoglobin than when metHb is not present.

In contrast to HbCO, metHb causes profound cyanosis because of the color of oxidized hemoglobin. Patients with only 1.5 gm% metHb (10% metHb with a hemoglobin content of 15 gm%) will appear cyanotic, but they may not be particularly hypoxic or symptomatic. (By contrast, cyanosis from hypoxemia requires at least 5 gm% of desaturated hemoglobin in the systemic capillaries.)

Clinical problem 5

A patient has the following blood gas values, obtained while he was breathing room air: PaO_2, 85 mm Hg; SaO_2, 60%; $PaCO_2$, 37 mm Hg; pH, 7.39; and hemoglobin content, 14.8 gm%. Explain each of the following terms as they might apply to these blood gas values: reduced hemoglobin; oxidized hemoglobin; oxyhemoglobin; deoxygenated hemoglobin; carboxyhemoglobin; and methemoglobin. Would you expect the patient to appear cyanotic?

Although methemoglobinemia can occur as an inherited defect, in adults it most commonly occurs as an idiosyncratic reaction to certain oxidant drugs, particularly nitrites and sulfonamides. Several drugs that have been implicated in causing methemoglobinemia are listed in Table 6-2.

Treatment of methemoglobinemia depends on its severity; in mild to moderate cases, e.g. %metHb less than 30%, use of supplemental oxygen and removal of the offending drug may be all that are necessary. The oxidized hemoglobin will convert to normal over a period of 1 to 3 days. In severe or symptomatic cases for which a quick conversion is necessary, the drug of choice is methylene blue.

Table 6-2. Some drugs implicated in causing methemoglobinemia

Generic name	Use
Dapsone	Skin protectant
Benzocaine	Local anesthetic
Metoclopramide	Gastric stasis
Nitroglycerin	Angina
Phenazopyridine	Urinary tract analgesic
Prilocaine	Local anesthetic
Primaquine	Malaria prophylaxis and treatment
Trimethoprim	Urinary antibacterial
Amyl nitrite	Rarely used clinically; often used by drug abusers

Methylene blue acts as a reducing agent, converting Fe^{+++} to Fe^{++} so that hemoglobin can again carry oxygen. The dose is 1 mg/kg intravenously over a 5-minute period.

Sulfhemoglobin (SuHb) is produced when a sulfur atom is incorporated into the hemoglobin molecule; like metHb, SuHb occurs most commonly as a drug reaction and results in a deep bluish skin color. Unlike metHb, SuHb is not reversible and does not respond to methylene blue. Also in contrast to metHb, SuHb causes a *rightward* shift of the oxygen dissociation curve, thus ameliorating the arterial hypoxemia. In the presence of excess SuHb, oxygenated hemoglobin gives up its oxygen more readily at the tissue level.

CAUSES OF REDUCED SaO_2

Except for patients whose primary problem is anemia, all cases of hypoxemia manifest a reduction in SaO_2 (see Causes of Hypoxia, p. 113). Causes of reduced SaO_2 are listed in Table 6-3; this table should be compared and contrasted with Table 5-1.

Included in Table 6-3 are two categories that require further explanation. *Abnormal hemoglobin*

Table 6-3. Causes of reduced SaO_2

Cause	PaO_2	Oxygen dissociation curve	Clinical*	Treatment
Reduced PaO_2	Low	Normal	1, 2	Increase PIO_2† Correct pulmonary problem
HbCO excess	Normal	Left shift	1, 3	Increase PIO_2 Remove from carbon monoxide
MetHb excess	Normal	Left shift	1, 2	Increase PIO_2 Methylene blue Remove offending drug
SuHb excess	Normal	Right shift	1, 2	Increase PIO_2 Remove offending drug
Abnormal Hgb	Normal	Right shift	1, 3	Increase PIO_2 Exchange transfusion
Plasma factors	Normal	Right shift	1, 3	Increase PIO_2 Correct factor(s)

*1, symptoms of hypoxemia; 2, cyanosis; 3, no cyanosis. For effects of excess carbon monoxide, see also Table 6-1.
†PIO_2, pressure of inspired oxygen.

Is the patient adequately oxygenated?

refers to a hemoglobin molecule composed of an amino acid sequence that differs from the normal sequence. These hemoglobinopathies are inherited defects. Several abnormal hemoglobins are known to cause a rightward shift of the oxygen dissociation curve, resulting in arterial desaturation. (Some abnormal hemoglobins result in a leftward shift, which increases arterial saturation for a given PaO_2.)

Plasma factors refer to those physical and biochemical changes that may shift the oxygen dissociation curve to the right: increased 2,3-diphosphoglycerate (DPG), increased body temperature, and acid pH (see Fig. 6-3).

As noted in Chapter 5, unless the alveolar air–pulmonary capillary interface is altered, changes in hemoglobin should not affect PaO_2. For this reason SaO_2 must always be measured if its value is to be used for clinical purpose. Treatment based on only a calculated SaO_2 may be misdirected.

OXYGEN DELIVERY

Knowing just the oxygen content of a patient's blood may not be sufficient to assess the adequacy of oxygenation. Low or inadequate cardiac output may impair oxygen delivery, which is the total cardiac output (QT) times arterial oxygen content (CaO_2):

$$\text{Oxygen delivery} = QT \times CaO_2 \quad (2)$$

For example, assuming a normal QT and a normal CaO_2:

Oxygen delivery = 5000 ml/min × 20 ml O_2/100 ml blood = 1000 ml O_2/min

Patients in shock can have a normal CaO_2 but still suffer severe hypoxia because of decreased cardiac output and inadequate oxygen delivery. In such patients CaO_2 measurement is not sufficient to assess adequacy of oxygenation, and cardiac output or other measurements must be obtained.

Normal resting cardiac output ranges between 4 and 7 L/min, and a normal CaO_2 between 16 and 20 ml O_2/100 ml blood. Hence, normal oxygen delivery for a given individual may range between 640* and 1400† ml O_2/min.

Clinical problem 6

If the patient in Clinical Problem 4 has a cardiac output of 5 L/min, the approximate oxygen delivery is:
 a. 385 ml O_2/min
 b. 448 ml O_2/min
 c. 580 ml O_2/min
 d. 756 ml O_2/min
 e. 840 ml O_2/min

FICK EQUATION

The Fick equation expresses the important relationship of tissue oxygen uptake ($\dot{V}O_2$) to cardiac output (QT) and the arterial-venous oxygen content difference ($CaO_2 - C\bar{v}O_2$):

$$\dot{V}O_2 = QT \times (CaO_2 - C\bar{v}O_2) \quad (3)$$

where CaO_2 is the arterial oxygen content, and $C\bar{v}O_2$ is the mixed venous oxygen content.

This equation can be conceptually derived by thinking about oxygen delivery as follows: the amount of oxygen delivered to the tissues per minute equals the cardiac output (QT) times the arterial oxygen content (CaO_2) (see Fig. 6-1). The total amount of venous oxygen delivered to the right side of the heart is the cardiac output times the venous oxygen content, or $QT \times C\bar{v}O_2$. The total venous oxygen delivery must also equal the arterial oxygen delivery minus the amount of oxygen extracted by the tissues ($\dot{V}O_2$).

Hence,

$$(QT \times C\bar{v}O_2) = (QT \times CaO_2) - \dot{V}O_2 \quad (4)$$

Rearranging,

$$\dot{V}O_2 = (QT \times CaO_2) - (QT \times C\bar{v}O_2) \quad (5)$$

$$\dot{V}O_2 = QT \times (CaO_2 - C\bar{v}O_2) \quad (3)$$

---

* $\dfrac{16 \text{ ml } O_2}{100 \text{ ml blood}} \times 4$ L/min

† $\dfrac{20 \text{ ml } O_2}{100 \text{ ml blood}} \times 7$ L/min

Average resting values for a normal subject are QT, 5000 ml/min; CaO_2, 20 ml/100 ml blood; CvO_2, 15 ml/100 ml blood; and $\dot{V}O_2$, 250 ml/min.

Substituting these values into Equations 4 and 3:

$$750 \text{ ml } O_2/\text{min} = 1000 \text{ ml } O_2/\text{min} - 250 \text{ ml } O_2/\text{min} \quad (4)$$

and,

$$250 \text{ ml } O_2/\text{min} = \underset{(\dot{V}O_2)}{\underbrace{\underset{\text{(Cardiac output)}}{5000 \text{ ml blood/min}} \times \underset{(CaO_2 - CvO_2)}{5 \text{ ml } O_2/100 \text{ ml blood}}}} \quad (3)$$

Clinical problem 7

What is the oxygen uptake in the following situation: hemoglobin content, 15 Gm%; pH, 7.5; $PaCO_2$, 30 mm Hg; PaO_2, 80 mm Hg; SvO_2, 75%; and cardiac output, 5.2 L/min? Assume the patient has a normal body temperature.

Clinical problem 8

A 49-year-old man is admitted to the hospital with a massive gastrointestinal hemorrhage. Because of his persistent bleeding and his low hemoglobin level of 6 gm% despite receiving a transfusion, he is taken to the operating room for surgery. Before the operation, a Swan-Ganz catheter is placed, and cardiac output is measured at 7.5 L/min. At the same time his arterial PO_2 is 125 mm Hg, and SaO_2 is 97%. Assuming his oxygen requirement of 250 ml/min is being met, what is his (CaO_2-CvO_2)?

MIXED VENOUS OXYGEN SATURATION

At the present time our ability to assess oxygenation is limited to the whole patient and does not extend to assessment of the individual organs. Specific organ hypoxia is usually recognized only after damage has occurred. This situation is unfortunate since some clinical conditions (e.g., septic shock) may cause selective organ hypoxia even though the global oxygen supply is adequate.

For patients with a normal mental status and a normal or near-normal cardiac output (determined by the history, physical examination, and chest x-ray), knowledge of their arterial oxygen content (CaO_2) is usually sufficient to assess the adequacy of oxygen delivery. This is often *not* true for patients with impaired cardiac output or hemodynamic instability (e.g., shock); in this group the single best measurement to assess oxygenation is usually the mixed venous oxygen saturation (SvO_2). Why is this so?

Equation 3 helps to explain the importance of SvO_2 in assessing oxygen adequacy. Arterial oxygen delivery is the product of cardiac output (QT) and arterial oxygen content (CaO_2); reduction in either QT or CaO_2 threatens the adequacy of oxygen delivery. In either case (reduced QT or reduced CaO_2), lactic acidosis and death will ensue if tissue oxygen uptake ($\dot{V}O_2$) is not maintained by the product of QT times the ($CaO_2 - CvO_2$).

From Equation 3, the compensatory mechanisms for any decrease in oxygen delivery can be deduced; these mechanisms are outlined in Table 6-4.

When cardiac output is decreased or when cardiac output cannot compensate for a decrease in CaO_2, the mixed venous oxygen content (and thus SvO_2 and PvO_2) *will fall*. Normally both the cardiac output and the ($CaO_2 - CvO_2$) can increase up to threefold as compensation: up to 15 L/min for QT and 15 ml O_2/100 ml for ($CaO_2 - CvO_2$). Increasing ($CaO_2 - CvO_2$) is almost always at the expense of lowering CvO_2*; thus SvO_2 is a barometer of the adequacy of oxygen delivery (QT × CaO_2) for the body's oxygen needs.

When the SvO_2 falls to 40% or less (roughly corresponding to a PvO_2 of 27 mm Hg at pH 7.36),

---

*Compensatory mechanisms to improve CaO_2 are limited; hyperventilation barely raises SaO_2, and any increase in hemoglobin concentration takes a long time to occur.

Table 6-4. Compensatory mechanisms for decrease in oxygen delivery

Problem	Compensatory mechanism	Effect on Cvo_2, Svo_2, and Pvo_2*
Decreased QT	Increase in (Cao_2-Cvo_2)	All reduced
Decreased Cao_2 (low Sao_2 or anemia)	Increase in QT and/or	All normal
	Maintenance of (Cao_2-Cvo_2)	All reduced

*Pvo_2, partial pressure of oxygen in mixed venous blood.

the limits of compensation are such that any further fall will likely result in lactic acidosis. This condition should be considered preterminal unless reversal is fairly rapid.

The problems in using Svo_2 to assess global oxygenation are both technical and theoretical. Technical problems in obtaining a pulmonary artery sample are discussed in Chapter 8. Assuming that a proper sample is obtained and that the measurement is accurate, the following statement appears valid in patients at rest: *a low Svo_2 indicates inadequate oxygen delivery for the body's needs; the lower the Svo_2, the more severe is the derangement.*

Conversely, *a normal Svo_2 does not assure that oxygenation is adequate;* this is so for several reasons.

1. Regional hypoperfusion may be masked by an adequate blood flow to the rest of the body; thus one organ could be oxygen deficient, yet its oxygen-poor venous blood flow may not be enough to cause significant reduction in the mixed venous oxygen content.
2. Left-to-right systemic shunts may have the same effect as regional hypoperfusion. These shunts have been described in both septic and hemodynamic shock. If oxygenated blood is shunted from the arteries to the veins (thus bypassing capillaries), a normal (or even elevated) Svo_2 may result. This measurement could be falsely reassuring since selective tissues or organs may be critically hypoxic and on the verge of irreversible damage.
3. In some conditions, such as cyanide poisoning, oxygen delivery is adequate but the mitochondria are poisoned; thus oxygen transfer between systemic capillaries and the tissue cells does not take place. Again, Svo_2 may be normal or above normal.

In summary, Svo_2 is the best single measurement to use in assessing the adequacy of oxygenation in critically ill patients. If Svo_2 is reduced, the patient's ability to efficiently oxygenate the tissues is either impaired or severely strained. If Svo_2 is normal, oxygenation is probably adequate as long as there is no problem with regional hypoperfusion, left-to-right shunts, or mitochondrial oxygen uptake.

The Pvo_2 measurement is an alternative to Svo_2 in assessing oxygenation. Both are obtained from mixed venous blood. Of the two, the Svo_2 should be more reliable since it is solely a function of arterial oxygen delivery and oxygen uptake. In contrast, Pvo_2 depends on the Svo_2 *and* on the position of the oxygen dissociation curve. Venous blood is more acidotic than arterial blood; hence the venous oxygen dissociation curve is shifted to the right of the arterial curve. For a given Svo_2, the more the rightward shift of the curve, the higher the Pvo_2. Other factors besides pH will also influence the curve, such as the concentration of 2,3-diphosphoglycerate; thus the exact relationship of Svo_2 to Pvo_2 cannot be predicted in sick patients. If the Pvo_2 is used to assess oxygenation, it must be measured and not simply estimated from the Svo_2. An Svo_2 measurement of 75% could represent a range of Pvo_2 values depending on the position of the oxygen dissociation curve.

Clinical problem 9

What are the Svo_2 and Pvo_2 in each of the following situations? In each, the lungs and acid-base state are normal in a 30-year-old patient; the barometric pressure is 760 mm Hg, and the alveolar-arterial partial pressure of oxygen difference is normal.

 a. Cardiac output, 5 L/min; FIo_2, 0.21; hemoglobin, 15 gm%; oxygen uptake 250 ml/min
 b. Same as in *a*, except cardiac output is 2.5 L/min
 c. Same as in *a*, except FIo_2 is 1.00
 d. Same as in *a*, except hemoglobin content is 8 gm%

Clinical problem 10

A 69-year-old woman with progressive congestive heart failure is being treated in the intensive care unit. Because of a decreasing urinary output, a Swan-Ganz catheter is inserted in her pulmonary artery. The patient's cardiac output and her mixed venous oxygen measurements are obtained along with her arterial blood gas measurements: cardiac output, 2.9 L/min; Pao_2, 74 mm Hg; Sao_2, 92%; Cao_2, 14.5 vol%; Svo_2, 54%; and Pvo_2, 26 mm Hg.

The patient is treated with intravenous dobutamine, a drug that stimulates the myocardium to augment cardiac output. Three hours later the following measurements are obtained: cardiac output, 3.8 L/min; Pao_2, 76 mm Hg; Sao_2, 93%; Cao_2, 14.5 vol%; Svo_2, 65%; Pvo_2, and 34 mm Hg.

Do her mixed venous oxygen measurements (Svo_2, Pvo_2) reflect the arterial oxygen measurements (Pao_2, Sao_2)? How is the change in mixed venous oxygen measurements explained?

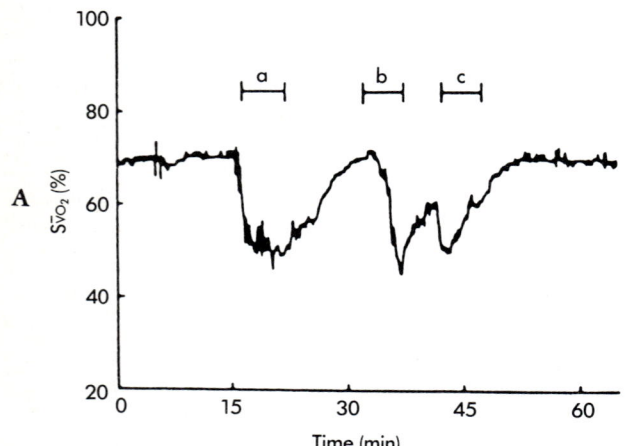
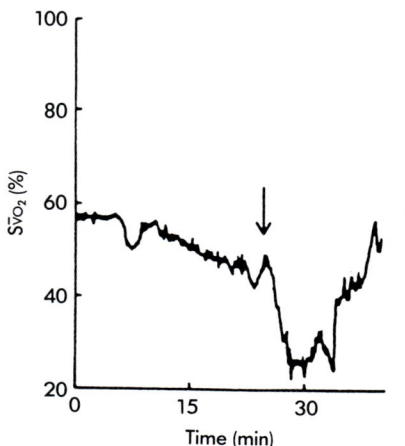

Fig. 6-5. Changes in Svo_2 when monitored continuously. **A**, Effect on Svo_2 of *a*, suctioning the patient's tracheal tube, *b*, bathing and weighing the patient, and *c*, turning the patient and changing his bed linen. Note the prolonged duration of the Svo_2 of less than 60%. **B**, Gradual decline in Svo_2 over the first 20 minutes heralded onset of cardiac arrest *(arrow)* for which resuscitation was successful. (From Baele, P.L., McMichan, J.C., Marsh, H.M., et al.: Anesth. Analg. **61:**513-517, 1982.)

Obviously, a mixed venous oxygen measurement is done only on very sick patients in whom there is reason to suspect inadequate oxygen delivery. There may also be technical problems in obtaining a proper sample—it is not a simple test to be performed repeatedly (see Chapter 8). A fiberoptic sensor in some models of the Swan-Ganz catheter allows for continuous measurement of Svo_2. This modification greatly improves the monitoring of mixed venous oxygenation and also demonstrates how clinical changes can affect mixed venous oxygenation (Fig. 6-5). Fig. 6-5, *A*, demonstrates that routine nursing procedures (tracheal suctioning and weighing) can *lower* Svo_2. Fig. 6-5, *B*, shows the Svo_2 tracing from a patient who developed cardiac arrest. Before the arrest, the Svo_2 declined precipitously and, in fact, heralded the problem.*

Mixed venous oxygen measurement represents a sophisticated attempt to answer the sometimes difficult question about the adequacy of overall oxygenation. However, for the vast majority of patients, measurement of arterial oxygen content will be sufficient to assess oxygenation.

SUMMARY

The second clinical question concerning oxygenation asks if oxygenation is adequate for the patient. This is sometimes a difficult question to answer. Unlike the first question posed in Chapter 5 (Are the lungs transferring oxygen properly?), the answer to this question must always include information from the patient's history and physical examination. The most important laboratory measurement to help answer this question is the arterial oxygen content (Cao_2). Cao_2 is the amount of oxygen in the blood measured in ml O_2/100 ml blood and is determined by mutliplying the hemoglobin oxygen saturation (Sao_2) times the hemoglobin content (in gm/100 ml blood) times 1.34 ml O_2/gm hemoglobin (hemoglobin's oxygen binding capacity).

---

*In neither condition would an intermittent sampling technique, such as arterial blood gas analysis, be expected to diagnose the rapid change in oxygenation.

Carbon monoxide affects oxygenation in two ways. First, it prevents oxygen from binding to hemoglobin, thus reducing the Sao_2; for every percent carboxyhemoglobin, Sao_2 is reduced 1%. Second, when carbon monoxide binds to hemoglobin, it causes a leftward shift of the oxygen dissociation curve, thus causing hemoglobin to hold onto oxygen more tightly than when carboxyhemoglobin is not present.

In critical illnesses such as shock or sepsis, the Cao_2 alone may be insufficient to determine the adequacy of oxygenation. In such situations, cardiac output, arterial oxygen transport, oxygen uptake, and mixed venous oxygen saturation may be measured. Unfortunately, such information can only be obtained with the aid of right heart catheterization, an invasive technique.

Mixed venous oxygen saturation (Svo_2) can be measured continuously by using a pulmonary artery catheter that is equipped with a special fiberoptic sensor. Continuous Svo_2 measurement has proved useful in monitoring the adequacy of oxygenation in critically ill patients. A low Svo_2 indicates inadequate oxygen delivery for the body's needs. If the Svo_2 is normal, overall oxygenation is probably adequate, provided that there is not significant regional hypoperfusion, left-to-right shunting, or interference with mitochondrial oxygen uptake.

REVIEW QUESTIONS

State whether each of the following is true or false.
1. Units for oxygen content are ml O_2/gm hemoglobin.
2. When Pao_2 is 100 mm Hg, Sao_2 is 98%, and hemoglobin content is 15 gm%, 86% of the available oxygen is carried on hemoglobin.
3. Mixed venous Po_2 increases one mm Hg with each mm Hg increase in Pao_2.
4. In a critically ill patient at rest, reduced Svo_2 indicates inadequate oxygen delivery to the tissues.
5. A P_{50} of 33 mm Hg indicates a reduced Sao_2 for a given Pao_2.

6. Arterial oxygen delivery is the product of cardiac output times arterial oxygen content.
7. Anemia can lower arterial Po_2 in the face of venous admixture.
8. To maintain oxygen uptake in the presence of a falling cardiac output, there must be a concomitant increase in the arterial-venous oxygen content difference.
9. Carbon monoxide shifts the oxygen dissociation curve to the left.
10. Methemoglobin shifts the oxygen dissociation curve to the right.

References

Baele, P.L., McMichan, J.C., Marsh, H.M., et al.: Continuous monitoring of mixed venous oxygen saturation in critically ill patients, Anesth. Analg. **61**:513, 1982.

Comroe, J.H., Jr., and Botelho, S.: The unreliability of cyanosis in the recognition of arterial hypoxemia, Am. J. Med. Sci. **214**:1, 1947.

Winter, P.M., and Miller, J.N.: Carbon monoxide poisoning, JAMA **236**:1502, 1976.

Suggested readings

Filley, G., Beckwith, H., Reeves, J., et al.: Chronic obstructive pulmonary disease: oxygen transport in two clinical types, Am. J. Med. **44**:26, 1968.

Kandel, G., and Aberman, A.: Mixed venous oxygen saturation: its role in the assessment of the critically ill patient, Arch. Intern. Med. **143**:1400, 1983.

Kasnitz, P., Drurger, G.L., Yorra, F., et al.: Mixed venous oxygen tension and hyperlactatemia, JAMA **236**:570, 1976.

Miller, M.J.: Tissue oxygenation in clinical medicine: an historical review, Anesth. Analg. **61**:527, 1982.

Mithoefer, J., Holfand, F., and Keighley, J.: The effect of oxygen administration on mixed venous oxygenation in chronic obstructive pulmonary disease, Chest **66**:122, 1974.

See also General References in Appendix G.

chapter 7
Acid-base balance

OUTLINE

Hydrogen ion homeostasis
Concept of pH
Buffer systems
Henderson-Hasselbalch equation
Does the patient have an acid-base disorder?
Calculated vs. measured HCO_3^-
Acid-base nomogram
Acidemia and alkalemia
Acidosis and alkalosis
Anion gap
Primary vs. compensatory processes
Acid-base map
In vivo titration curve for carbon dioxide
Base excess
Acute vs. chronic respiratory disorders
Acute vs. chronic metabolic disorders
Mixed acid-base disorders
Clinical approach to acid-base diagnosis

HYDROGEN ION HOMEOSTASIS

"Life is a struggle, not against sin, not against the Money Power, not against malicious animal magnetism, but against hydrogen ions."

H.L. MENCKEN

Mencken was neither a physician nor physiologist, but he knew the importance of hydrogen ions. Enzyme systems operate at an optimal hydrogen ion concentration ($[H^+]$), and variation from this optimal can markedly affect enzyme activity. For the blood plasma, optimal $[H^+]$ is 40 nanomoles/L. As shown in Table 7-1, the importance of H^+ is out of proportion to its miniscule concentration.

Strictly speaking, hydrogen ions are protons and do not exist in the naked state in body fluids; instead

Table 7-1. Plasma ion concentrations

Ion*	nmoles/L	mEq/L
H^+	40	4×10^{-5}
K^+	4,000,000	4
Ca^{++}	2,500,000	5
Mg^{++}	1,000,000	2
Na^+	140,000,000	140

*K^+, Potassium ion; Ca^{++}, calcium ion; Mg^{++}, magnesium ion; Na^+, sodium ion.

they react with water (H_2O) to form hydronium ions, such as H_3O^+ and $H_5O_2^+$. For clinical purposes H^+ can be used to represent these hydrated protons.

Because $[H^+]$ is so critical to enzyme function yet the absolute concentration is small and difficult to manipulate, the concept of pH was developed and is now universally used to represent $[H^+]$.*

CONCEPT OF pH

The pH is the negative logarithm of the hydrogen ion concentration ($[H^+]$):

$$pH = -\log [H^+] \quad (1)$$

A pH of 7.4 represents a $[H^+]$ of 40 nmoles/L, or 4×10^{-8} moles/L (for univalent ions, mmoles/L equal mEq/L). By definition pH does not have units.

Since pH is the negative log of $[H^+]$, the lower the pH, the greater the $[H^+]$ and hence the greater the acidity; the higher the pH, the lower the $[H^+]$ and the greater the alkalinity (or the less the acidity). Use of a logarithmic expression also means that a pH change of one whole unit, e.g., from 7.0 to 8.0, represents a *tenfold* change in $[H^+]$.

Table 7-2 shows the relationship between pH and the relative acidity of the blood. A pH change from 7.40 to 7.30 represents a 25% *increase* in blood $[H^+]$. A similar numerical change of conventional measurement, such as an increase in serum uric acid from 7.3 mg% to 7.4 mg%, represents only a 1.4% increase.

The range of normal arterial pH (7.36 to 7.44) encompasses approximately two standard deviations of the normal population; anything outside this range is considered abnormal. Clinically, the "safe" range for pH is approximately 7.30 to 7.52;

---

*Strictly speaking, pH reflects, but does not exactly equal, $[H^+]$. The pH is a measure of relative acidity and therefore is useful for clinical purposes. Reasons for using pH as opposed to $[H^+]$ have been debated; it would probably be less confusing to use $[H^+]$ when discussing blood acidity, but pH is a firmly entrenched concept and is used throughout this chapter.

Table 7-2. pH and hydrogen ion concentration

Blood pH	$[H^+]$ (nmoles/L)
Acidemia	
7.00	100
7.10	80
7.30	50
Normal	
7.40	40
Alkalemia	
7.52	30
7.70	20
8.00	10

within this range, pH *per se* is not usually life-threatening. A pH outside this range is potentially life-threatening because of altered enzymatic activity and enhanced myocardial irritability, and direct steps should be taken to return the pH to normal. Although 7.30 to 7.52 may at first seem a narrow range, it represents a $[H^+]$ ranging from 50 to 30 nmoles/L or a change from the normal 40 nmoles/L of plus or minus 25%. A similar range for serum sodium is 175 to 105 mEq/L!

BUFFER SYSTEMS

A buffer system counteracts the effects of adding acid or alkali to the blood. The resulting pH change is less than if the buffer were not present. Blood contains two basic buffer systems: bicarbonate and nonbicarbonate. Each consists of a weak acid or acids and their conjugate base or bases.

The bicarbonate system buffers the effects of fixed acids and alkalies that are added to the blood; the acid component is H_2CO_3 and the base is HCO_3^-. The nonbicarbonate system consists mainly of proteins and phosphates and serves to buffer changes in carbon dioxide. These two systems are represented by the equations in Fig. 7-1. Since the nonbicarbonate system is a heterogeneous group of compounds, the acid component is represented by HBuf and the base by Buf^-. Note that

Acid-base balance

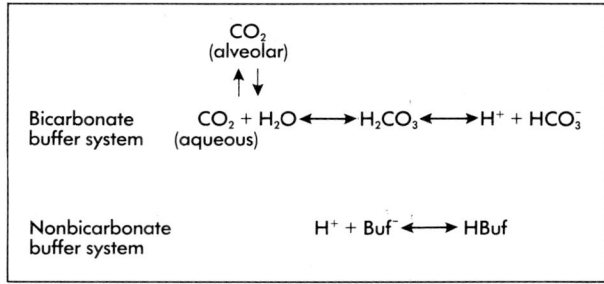

Fig. 7-1. Bicarbonate and nonbicarbonate buffer system. The two systems are in equilibrium with each other.

carbon dioxide is part of an open system, since any buildup in plasma (aqueous or dissolved CO_2) can be excreted by healthy lungs.

The bicarbonate and nonbicarbonate buffer systems are in equilibrium with each other. Measuring the components of either system will give the hydrogen ion concentration ($[H^+]$) or the pH of the blood. However, since the nonbicarbonate system is a heterogeneous group of molecules, it is easier to measure the bicarbonate buffer components in order to determine pH.

An extremely small quantity of H_2CO_3 is present in the blood compared with dissolved CO_2 (approximately 1 to 400). Since H_2CO_3 is in equilibrium with dissolved CO_2, the latter (measured as $Paco_2$) can be used as the acid component in calculating pH. Therefore measurement of HCO_3^- and $Paco_2$ will provide the pH.

HENDERSON-HASSELBALCH EQUATION

The Henderson-Hasselbalch equation relates blood pH to the components of the bicarbonate buffer system, as shown in Equation 2.

$$pH = pK + \log \frac{HCO_3^-}{0.03 \, (Paco_2)} \quad (2)$$

where pK is the negative log of the dissociation constant of carbonic acid and has the value 6.1. The pH of the blood is equal to the pK of the bicarbonate buffer system *plus* the logarithm of the following ratio—bicarbonate concentration ($[HCO_3^-]$) over 0.03 times the arterial partial pressure of carbon dioxide ($Paco_2$). The constant 0.03 converts $Paco_2$ from mm Hg to mmoles/L. Inserting normal values gives 7.4, the normal blood pH.

$$pH = 6.1 + \log \frac{24 \text{ mmoles/L}}{0.03 \, (40 \text{ mm Hg})} \quad (3)$$

$$pH = 6.1 + \log \frac{24}{1.2} \quad (4)$$

$$pH = 6.1 + \log 20 = 6.1 + 1.3 = 7.4 \quad (5)$$

It is not necessary to memorize the full Henderson-Hasselbalch equation to intelligently manage acid-base disorders. It *is* important to understand that pH reflects a ratio of HCO_3^- to $Paco_2$.

The bicarbonate buffer system is the most important of the body's buffer systems for several reasons. This system provides the major way to buffer the additions of fixed acid and alkali to the blood. Since one of its components is carbon dioxide, the system is open, i.e., the respiratory system allows for excretion of huge amounts of carbon dioxide. Also, since carbon dioxide is readily diffusible across all cell membranes, the results of buffering can be reflected quickly in intracellular compartments.

Since there are three variables in the bicarbonate buffer system (Equation 2), measurement of any two will define the third. The body preferentially wants to maintain normal pH and does so by altering the numerator (HCO_3^-) or denominator (Pa_{CO_2}) of the Henderson-Hasselbalch equation as necessary.

DOES THE PATIENT HAVE AN ACID-BASE DISORDER?

It is important to recognize when a patient has an acid-base disorder since that recognition is the first step toward diagnosis and therapy. If any of the three variables in the Henderson-Hasselbalch equation are abnormal, the answer to this question is *yes*. Any acid-base derangement will be reflected in one or more components of the bicarbonate system: pH, Pa_{CO_2}, HCO_3^- (see the box on p. 20 for the range of normal values).

A single abnormal component, even without knowledge of the other two, always indicates an acid-base disorder. This is particularly important since an abnormal HCO_3^- is often found in venous blood (as part of the serum electrolytes measurement) without a concomitant blood gas measurement. An abnormal HCO_3^- value alone cannot define or diagnose an acid-base disorder but nonetheless points to its presence. For example, an elevated HCO_3^- suggests either metabolic alkalosis or respiratory acidosis.

Clinical problem 1

A 79-year-old woman was hospitalized for dehydration and for cellulitis in her left leg. She received meperidine (Demerol) for pain and diazepam (Valium) for agitation. On the third hospital day she was found to be lethargic and unarousable. Review of her serum electrolytes measurements over the 3 days revealed the following information:

Day	Serum HCO_3^-
1	35 mEq/L
2	36 mEq/L
3	36 mEq/L

No blood gas analysis was obtained until Day 3. What probably happened to this woman?

CALCULATED VS. MEASURED HCO_3^-

Incorrect therapeutic decisions can occur if blood gas values are accepted at face value. They should always be examined for physiologic correctness, particularly when considering acid-base disorders, which seem prone to misdiagnosis. For example, a Pa_{CO_2} of 49 mm Hg, pH of 7.35, and HCO_3^- of 16 mEq/L may be interpreted as a *metabolic acidosis* (low pH and low HCO_3^-) when in fact there is a transcription error: the HCO_3^- should be 26 and cannot possibly be 16 if the pH is 7.35 and the Pa_{CO_2} is 49 mm Hg.

Such errors can be avoided if it is remembered that HCO_3^-, Pa_{CO_2}, and pH must satisfy the Henderson-Hasselbalch equation. If Pa_{CO_2} and pH have been measured, arterial HCO_3^- can be calculated and does not have to be measured. The HCO_3^- *is* routinely measured as one of the serum electrolytes (on venous blood), and this measurement can pose a problem when a comparison is made with the blood gas HCO_3^-. Often, the measured venous HCO_3^- does not agree with the arterial HCO_3^- that has been *calculated* from the Henderson-Hasselbalch equation. When this happens there are several possible reasons as shown in the box on p. 133.

Note that the pK of 6.1, on which the calculated HCO_3^- is based, may vary among patients. The significance of such variation is somewhat controversial (Hood and Campbell, 1981). At most, the variation is slight (± 0.012 for extreme conditions) and would not account for the wide discrepancy often found between measured venous HCO_3^- and calculated arterial HCO_3^-.

Clinical problem 2

A 54-year-old-man is hospitalized with congestive heart failure. His arterial blood pH is 7.52, P_{CO_2} is 44 mm Hg, and HCO_3^- is 34 mEq/L. Measured venous HCO_3^- is 24 mEq/L. What is his acid-base status?

ACID-BASE NOMOGRAM

Since the Henderson-Hasselbalch equation deals with the log of two variables in a ratio (Equation

> **POSSIBLE REASONS FOR MEASURED VENOUS HCO_3^- NOT AGREEING WITH CALCULATED ARTERIAL HCO_3^-**
>
> **PHYSIOLOGIC REASONS**
>
> 1. The venous HCO_3^- measurement is actually the total CO_2 content and is not identical to the plasma HCO_3^- calculated from the Henderson-Hasselbalch equation. Total CO_2 content includes *all* the acid-labile forms of carbon dioxide, of which plasma HCO_3^- constitutes approximately 95%. Hence the normal value for measured venous HCO_3^- (total CO_2 content) is approximately 2 to 3 mEq/L higher than calculated arterial HCO_3^-.
> 2. In critically ill or unstable patients, the pK of the bicarbonate buffer system may not be 6.1, thus rendering calculation of HCO_3^- inaccurate (Hood and Campbell, 1981).
> 3. The venous sample may be drawn at a time different from that of the arterial sample used for blood gas analysis, and thus reflect a true change in acid-base status.
>
> **TECHNICAL REASONS**
>
> 1. The blood-drawing technique may alter venous HCO_3^-, e.g., tourniquet placement may create a transient lactic acidosis, lowering the HCO_3^-.
> 2. The blood gases are usually measured within minutes after the arterial sample is obtained, whereas the serum electrolytes may not be measured for an hour or more after the venous sample is drawn. The venous sample's HCO_3^- may change if the blood is not stored anaerobically or if its measurement is delayed.
> 3. If pH and Pa_{CO_2} are inaccurately measured, the calculation of HCO_3^- will be inaccurate as well.
> 4. The venous HCO_3^- or the arterial HCO_3^- may be transcribed incorrectly.

2), knowing the pH and the Pa_{CO_2} does not lend itself to easy mental calculation of the HCO_3^-. Several nomograms have been developed that graphically solve the Henderson-Hasselbalch equation; they provide a solution to the equation as well as an introduction to diagnosing clinical acid-base problems.

The nomogram in Fig. 7-2 plots the P_{CO_2} on the abscissa against the pH on one ordinate and hydrogen ion concentration ($[H^+]$) on the other. The HCO_3^- isopleths (lines of equal HCO_3^-) radiate out from the left lower corner of the graph. (There are other ways of graphing the Henderson-Hasselbalch equation; for example, some nomograms plot Pa_{CO_2} against HCO_3^-, with pH lines radiating out in a fan-shape. All are equally valid, but I prefer the nomogram in Fig. 7-2 because it emphasizes what is actually measured: pH and Pa_{CO_2}.)

The following are two examples using the Henderson-Hasselbalch nomogram:

1. Given a pH of 7.1 and a Pa_{CO_2} of 70 mm Hg, what is the HCO_3^-? Drawing a line horizontally from a pH of 7.1 to where it intersects a vertical line up from a Pa_{CO_2} of 70 mm Hg, the HCO_3^- is 21 mEq/L.
2. Given a pH of 7.4 and a Pa_{CO_2} of 10 mm Hg, what is the HCO_3^-? Doing the same procedure shown in the first example, the lines intersect the HCO_3^- isopleth at 6 mEq/L.

The same HCO_3^- values may be obtained by solving the Henderson-Hasselbalch equation; this nomogram merely does the calculation for you.

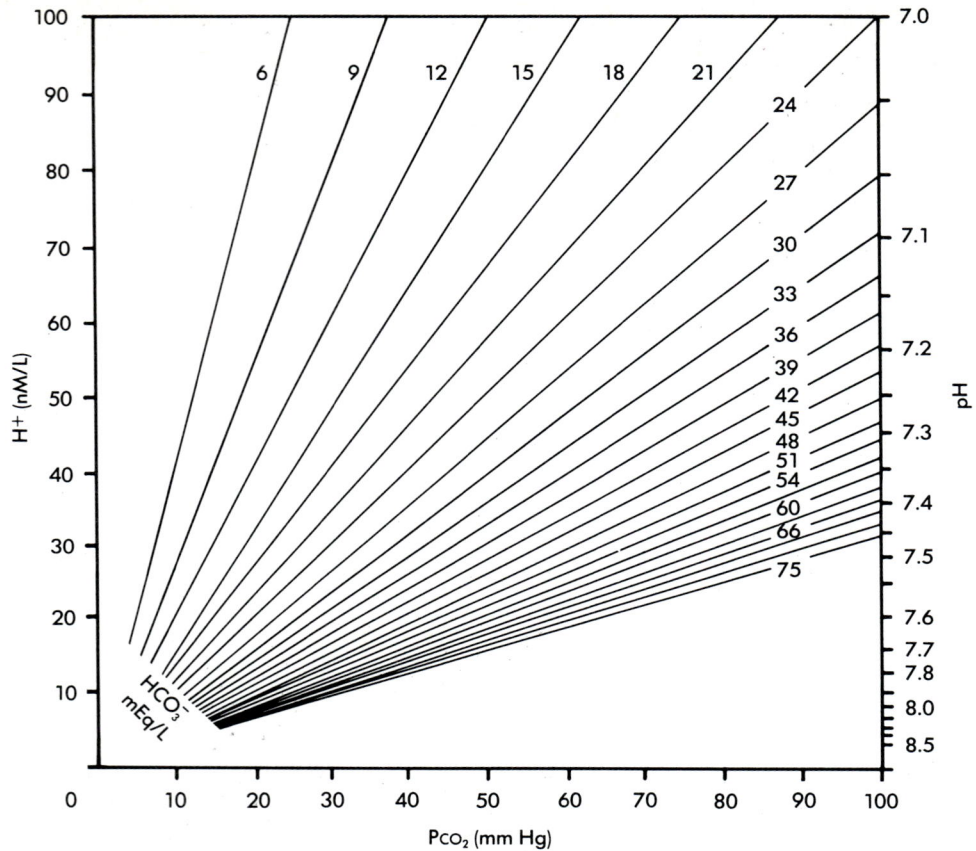

Fig. 7-2. Graphic solution of the Henderson-Hasselbalch equation.

ACIDEMIA AND ALKALEMIA

In the past there was much confusion over the terminology of acid-base disorders. This confusion arose mainly because some workers looked at acid-base disorders in terms of blood changes only, whereas others viewed the same disorders as in vivo, physiologic processes. Both the "laboratory" and "clinical" proponents were often saying the same thing but were using different terms. Agreement was reached in the 1960's, and there is now an internationally accepted terminology, one that adopts a clinical approach.

In terms of pH, the blood can reflect either *ac-idemia* or *alkalemia*. Acidemia indicates an acid pH (less than 7.36), and alkalemia indicates an alkaline pH (greater than 7.44). The terms acidemia and alkalemia provide no specific information about acidosis vs. alkalosis, metabolic disorder vs. respiratory disorder, or the underlying clinical causes. To characterize a patient's blood as having acidemia or alkalemia, only one value is needed: pH.

ACIDOSIS AND ALKALOSIS

Since pH is determined by a ratio of HCO_3^- to $PaCO_2$, the Henderson-Hasselbalch equation may be conveniently reduced for clinical use to

$$\text{pH} \simeq \frac{\text{HCO}_3^-}{\text{Paco}_2}$$

The kidneys are responsible for maintaining HCO_3^-, and the lungs are responsible for maintaining Paco_2 (see Chapter 4). Thus

$$\text{pH} \simeq \frac{\text{Kidneys (slow)}}{\text{Lungs (fast)}}$$

Since the kidneys affect HCO_3^- changes slowly (from hours to days) and since the lungs may affect changes in Paco_2 quickly (within minutes), the ratio determining pH is viewed as *slow* over *fast;* this concept is important when considering the compensatory changes for acid-base disturbances.

For example, a compensation that involves altering the HCO_3^- occurs relatively slowly.

Understanding acid-base disorders depends on knowing how the kidneys and the lungs act and react to the acid-base disorder. This knowledge leads to the concept of acidosis and alkalosis.

In contrast to acidemia and alkalemia, which refer to the *in vitro* determination of blood pH, acidosis and alkalosis refer to the *physiologic processes occurring in the patient.* Acidosis and alkalosis cannot be fully characterized without reference to the patient's history, physical examination, serum electrolyte values, and other relevant laboratory data. Acidosis and alkalosis cannot be defined by reference to blood changes only.

The numerator of the Henderson-Hasselbalch

DEFINITIONS OF ACID-BASE TERMS

DISORDERS IN THE BLOOD

Acidemia. A low blood pH (less than 7.36)
Alkalemia. A high blood pH (greater than 7.44)
Hypocapnia. A low Paco_2 (less than 36 mm Hg)
Hypercapnia. A high Paco_2 (greater than 44 mm Hg)

DISORDERS IN THE PATIENT

Metabolic acidosis. A primary physiologic process that causes a decrease in the serum bicarbonate and, when not complicated by other acid-base disorders, lowers the blood pH.
Metabolic alkalosis. A primary physiologic process that causes an increase in the serum bicarbonate and, when not complicated by other acid-base disorders, raises the blood pH.
Respiratory acidosis. A primary physiologic process that leads to an increased Paco_2 and, when not complicated by other acid-base disorders, lowers the blood pH.
Respiratory alkalosis. A primary physiologic process that leads to a decreased Paco_2 and, when not complicated by other acid-base disorders, raises the blood pH.
Compensatory process. Not a primary acid-base disorder, but a change that follows a primary disorder. A compensatory process attempts to restore the blood pH to normal and is not appropriately termed acidosis or alkalosis. The compensatory process for each primary disorder is given below.

Primary disorder	*Compensatory process*
Metabolic acidosis	Hyperventilation (lower Paco_2)
Metabolic alkalosis	Hypoventilation (raise Paco_2)
Respiratory acidosis	Renal HCO_3^- retention
Respiratory alkalosis	Renal HCO_3^- excretion

equation, HCO_3^-, is called the *metabolic component*, and the denominator, Pa_{CO_2}, is called the *nonmetabolic* or *respiratory component* (the term respiratory is used henceforth instead of nonmetabolic). There may be both metabolic and respiratory causes of acid-base disorders. The primary change determines the type of disorder; these disorders are defined in the box on p. 135.

Compensatory processes are secondary changes; as such, they occur *after* the primary process has begun and occur solely as an attempt to correct the pH change brought about by the primary disorder. Compensatory changes are not termed acidosis or alkalosis.

Acidosis and alkalosis refer to what is happening in the patient, not necessarily to what is manifested in the blood. For example, a low pH may reflect an acidosis alone or may indicate an acidosis *plus* an alkalosis. If the physiologic process causing the disorder is uncomplicated by other acid-base disorders, then the blood is appropriately acidemic (low pH) from an acidosis or alkalemic (high pH) from an alkalosis. However, if another acid-base disorder is present, the resulting pH may be high or low. So-called mixed acid-base disorders are common in patients with respiratory disease and are discussed in a later section.

The box below lists some clinical conditions responsible for the primary acid-base disorders. Keep in mind that acidosis and alkalosis are *physiologic processes* caused by a clinical disturbance that result in a tendency to reduce or elevate HCO_3^- or

---

CLINICAL CAUSES OF THE PRIMARY ACID-BASE DISORDERS

METABOLIC ALKALOSIS

Potassium loss
Corticosteroids
Diuretics
Vomiting or nasogastric suction

RESPIRATORY ACIDOSIS

Depression of central nervous system respiratory center
Severe impairment of chest bellows
Severe lung and/or airways disease

RESPIRATORY ALKALOSIS

Anxiety
Sepsis
Central nervous system lesions
Aspirin overdose
Liver failure
Hypoxemia
Interstitial lung disease
Acute lung and airways disease

METABOLIC ACIDOSIS

Increased anion gap	No increased anion gap (hyperchloremic acidosis)
Uremia	Renal HCO_3^- loss
Ketoacidosis	Renal tubular acidosis
Lactic acidosis	Interstitial nephritis
Intoxicants	Early renal failure
Aspirin overdose	Gastrointestinal HCO_3^- loss
Methanol	Diarrhea
Ethylene glycol	Ureteral diversion procedures
Paraldehyde	Carbonic anhydrase inhibitors
	Acids containing chloride (e.g., HCl, NH_4Cl)
	Hyperalimentation

Paco₂. The list is not exhaustive, but it does include many clinical causes of acid-base disorders.

ANION GAP

A useful aid in diagnosing both simple and mixed acid-base disorders is the anion gap (AG). The AG is the difference between the principal measured cations and anions. The measured cations are sodium (Na^+) and potassium (K^+), and the measured anions are chloride (Cl^-) and bicarbonate (HCO_3^-). Since potassium is of relatively low concentration, it is usually ignored when calculating the AG.

$$AG = Na^+ - (Cl^- + HCO_3^-) \qquad (6)$$

The normal AG is 12 ± 4 mEq/L and is a result of the presence of anion proteins, sulfates, and other molecules that are not routinely measured with the serum electrolytes. An elevated AG is almost always caused by *metabolic acidosis*. However, not all cases of metabolic acidosis manifest an elevated AG. The AG is elevated when the metabolic acid added to the blood contains an "unmeasured" anion, such as lactate or ketones. States of metabolic acidosis that add no unmeasured anion to the blood do not elevate the AG and are called *hyperchloremic metabolic acidosis*. In hyperchloremic metabolic acidosis the reduced HCO_3^- is replaced by chloride, which is measured as part of the serum electrolytes.

Clinical problem 3

A patient with a Paco₂ of 50 mm Hg and an anion gap of 20 mEq/L has the following electrolyte values: Na^+, 145 mEq/L; Cl^-, 104 mEq/L. What is the patient's pH?

PRIMARY VS. COMPENSATORY PROCESSES

A metabolic acidosis or metabolic alkalosis is a physiologic acid-base disorder in which the primary change is in the HCO_3^-. A respiratory acidosis or respiratory alkalosis is one in which the primary change is in the Paco₂. The key word is *primary*, meaning *first* change. If HCO_3^- changes first and then Paco₂ changes as a compensatory event, the basic process is metabolic, not respiratory, and the patient has a metabolic acidosis or metabolic alkalosis with respiratory compensation. Similarly, if the primary event is a change in Paco₂ and HCO_3^- changes as compensation, the basic process is either respiratory acidosis or respiratory alkalosis with metabolic compensation.

From the basic relationship expressed by the Henderson-Hasselbalch equation, what is the primary change and the compensatory response for metabolic acidosis? The body wants to keep pH in the normal range so that, given a primary event, the compensatory response should be predictable.

In *metabolic acidosis*, the primary event leads to reduction of HCO_3^-. This reduction may arise from an actual loss of HCO_3^- (renal or gastrointestinal) or from the buffering of fixed acid (e.g., lactic acid). Initially,

Primary event

$$\downarrow pH \simeq \frac{\downarrow HCO_3^-}{Paco_2}$$

As HCO_3^- decreases, pH falls. The body responds by decreasing the denominator (i.e., by hyperventilating) as much as possible. (The amount of hyperventilation is discussed in the section on confidence bands.)

This decrease in the denominator alters pH back toward normal:

Primary event plus compensatory response

$$\downarrow pH \simeq \frac{\downarrow HCO_3^-}{\downarrow Paco_2}$$

A smaller arrow than that shown for HCO_3^- is shown for the decrease in Paco₂ because the compensatory Paco₂ change is not of the same magnitude as the primary HCO_3^- change. As a result pH does not return completely to normal but remains somewhat decreased.

A common clinical cause of metabolic acidosis is lactic acidosis. For example, suppose a patient in shock produces enough lactic acid to lower his

Table 7-3. Primary event and compensatory response for acid-base disorders

Acid-base disorder	Primary event	Compensatory response
Metabolic acidosis	$\downarrow pH \simeq \dfrac{\downarrow HCO_3^-}{Paco_2}$	$\downarrow pH \simeq \dfrac{\downarrow HCO_3^-}{\downarrow Paco_2}$
Metabolic alkalosis	$\uparrow pH \simeq \dfrac{\uparrow HCO_3^-}{Paco_2}$	$\uparrow pH \simeq \dfrac{\uparrow HCO_3^-}{\uparrow Paco_2}$
Respiratory acidosis	$\downarrow pH \simeq \dfrac{HCO_3^-}{\uparrow Paco_2}$	$\downarrow pH \simeq \dfrac{\uparrow HCO_3^-}{\uparrow Paco_2}$
Respiratory alkalosis	$\uparrow pH \simeq \dfrac{HCO_3^-}{\downarrow Paco_2}$	$\uparrow pH \simeq \dfrac{\downarrow HCO_3^-}{\downarrow Paco_2}$

HCO_3^- to 12 mEq/L or half of normal. Before any compensatory response occurs, i.e., when the $Paco_2$ is still normal, the pH will be 7.10.

Primary event

$$\downarrow pH \simeq \dfrac{\downarrow HCO_3^-}{Paco_2} \qquad pH = pK + \log \dfrac{12}{40} = 7.10$$

The compensatory response of hyperventilation, e.g., lowering the $Paco_2$ to 30 mm Hg results in a ratio of HCO_3^- to $Paco_2$ that elevates pH to 7.30.

Primary event plus compensatory response

$$\downarrow pH \simeq \dfrac{\downarrow HCO_3^-}{\downarrow Paco_2} \qquad pH = pK + \log \dfrac{12}{30} = 7.30$$

A pH of 7.30 is not normal, but it is a lot safer than 7.10. The compensatory response in this example is hyperventilation and the response should not be termed respiratory alkalosis. Alkalosis implies a primary physiologic process; hyperventilation is only a secondary or compensatory phenomenon. This differentiation is not just an exercise in semantics; the terminology helps to distinguish between single acid-base disorders and mixed acid-base disorders, an area that is often confusing.

Table 7-3 shows the basic relationship of the Henderson-Hasselbalch equation for each of the primary acid-base disorders and their compensatory responses. The arrows represent relative changes in the components of the bicarbonate buffer system.

ACID-BASE MAP

To know how much compensation to expect for each acid-base disorder, the arrows in Table 7-3 must be replaced with real numbers. Studies of some primary acid-base disorders have defined the actual human compensation when the disorder is uncomplicated by another primary acid-base disturbance.

A summary of this work appears in Fig. 7-3. This figure is the same nomogram as in Fig. 7-2, with the addition of superimposed radiating *confidence bands* for the primary acid-base disorders. When confidence bands are placed on the nomogram, the entire arrangement is called an *acid-base map*.

The confidence bands are areas in which 95% of the studied population fell when their blood gas results were plotted. For example, to generate the band for metabolic acidosis, blood gas results from patients with uncomplicated diabetic ketoacidosis were obtained before they received treatment. The blood gas data were analyzed statistically, and a narrow band was drawn that included 95% of the values for pH and $Paco_2$.

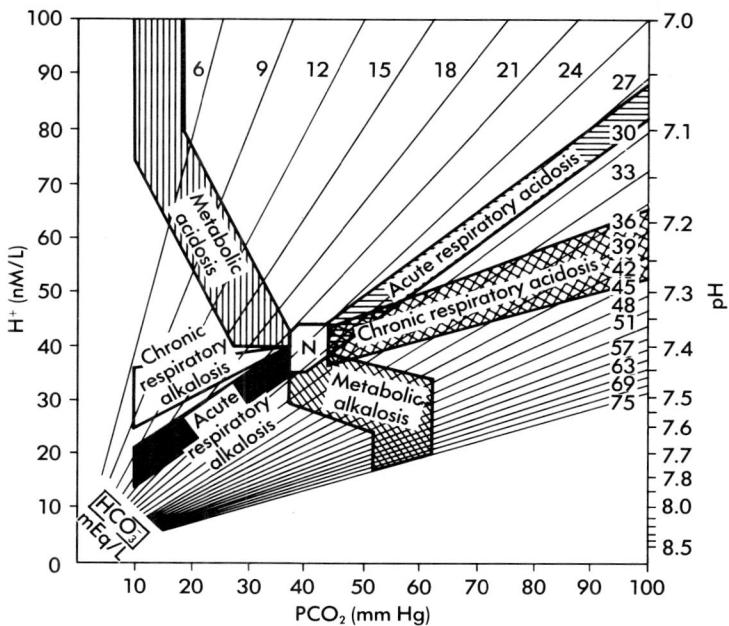

Fig. 7-3. Acid-base map. (From Goldberg, M., Green, S.B., Moss, M.L., et al.: JAMA **223**:269-275, 1973, Copyright 1973, American Medical Association.)

IN VIVO TITRATION CURVE FOR CARBON DIOXIDE

The long, diagonal band in Fig. 7-3 defines the in vivo titration curve for carbon dioxide (including its confidence limits). This curve was developed from two separate studies. To determine the band for respiratory alkalosis, patients undergoing elective surgery (e.g., routine hysterectomy) were acutely hyperventilated while under the effects of general anesthesia, and arterial samples were collected. A steady state was reached in 10 minutes, and blood gas results from this group defined the band for acute respiratory alkalosis.

To generate the band for acute carbon dioxide retention, healthy human volunteers breathed 5% and 7% carbon dioxide in an environmental chamber, and blood gas samples were collected from an indwelling arterial line. A steady state was also reached in 10 minutes, and blood gas results from these subjects defined the band for acute respiratory acidosis. These two bands, when connected, represent the in vivo titration curve for carbon dioxide and show how the healthy person titrates acute changes in carbon dioxide.

Note that a sudden change in the Pa_{CO_2} of 20 mm Hg alters the HCO_3^- approximately 2 to 3 mEq/L. Since this change occurs within 10 minutes, it reflects a biochemical reaction only and has nothing to do with renal compensation, which occurs much later. The direction of change is predicted by the hydration equation for carbon dioxide (Equation 7). As carbon dioxide is acutely retained, it combines with water and the equation is driven to the right, forming more HCO_3^-. As carbon dioxide is acutely excreted, the equation is driven to the left and HCO_3^- falls.

(Alveolar)
$$CO_2$$
$$\updownarrow$$
$$CO_2 + H_2O \leftrightarrow H_2CO_3 \leftrightarrow H^+ + HCO_3^- \quad (7)$$
(Dissolved)

The amount of change in HCO_3^-, and hence the resulting pH, cannot be predicted from the mere addition of carbon dioxide to blood. Carbon dioxide is buffered in the interstitium and intracellular compartments, and only in vivo human studies can show the actual result of buffering an acute change in carbon dioxide.

From the in vivo band, it can be noted that for every 10 mm Hg acute increase in the $Paco_2$, the pH decreases approximately 0.07 units; every 10 mm Hg decrease in the $Paco_2$ raises the pH approximately 0.08 units. This is a shorthand way of memorizing the carbon dioxide titration curve. Knowing the expected changes in both pH and HCO_3^- sharpens diagnostic ability.

Clinical problem 4

A patient initially has a pH of 7.14, a $Paco_2$ of 70 mm Hg, and a HCO_3^- of 23 mEq/L. How would you describe the likely acid-base disorder(s)?

BASE EXCESS

Base excess is an in vitro measurement that was introduced to characterize the metabolic component of acid-base disorders. Base excess was widely used before studies showed the human response to primary acid-base disorders (the in vivo confidence bands). Although the confidence bands are more accurate than base excess in diagnosing the metabolic component, base excess is still calculated and reported in many blood gas laboratories. However, for the novice base excess is a confusing concept and probably impedes understanding of acid-base problems.

To calculate base excess, the blood sample is equilibrated at two CO_2 tensions different from the patient's $Paco_2$, the pH is measured at both CO_2 levels, and the interpolated pH at $Paco_2$ of 40 mm Hg is used to calculate a *standard* bicarbonate (normal 24 mEq/L). Any change from this standard bicarbonate represents the metabolic component of the acid-base problem. The actual base excess (reported in mEq/L) is a derived value; the deviation from the standard bicarbonate is multiplied by a factor that takes into account hemoglobin content. If the patient's bicarbonate (calculated from blood gas measurements) is above the derived value, a positive base excess is present (i.e., a component of metabolic alkalosis); if the patient's bicarbonate is below the derived value, a negative base excess is present (i.e., a metabolic acidosis component).

A scientific critique of the base excess concept is provided in the article by Schwartz and Relman (1963).

ACUTE VS. CHRONIC RESPIRATORY DISORDERS

The acid-base map introduces the terms *acute* and *chronic*. In acid-base terminology these terms are synonymous with *compensated* and *uncompensated;* on the acid-base map, these terms apply only to respiratory acidosis and respiratory alkalosis.

- *Acute respiratory acidosis* occurs when carbon dioxide is retained acutely; it is the state of affairs *before* the kidneys have had a chance to compensate by retaining any HCO_3^-.
- *Chronic respiratory acidosis* occurs when the retained carbon dioxide has been, to some degree, buffered by the kidney's retention of HCO_3^-. The pH is higher than in acute respiratory acidosis, but it is still below 7.4. The HCO_3^- retention does not begin for at least a few hours and may take up to 3 days for maximal compensation.
- *Acute respiratory alkalosis* occurs when carbon dioxide is blown off acutely, before the kidneys have had a chance to compensate by excreting HCO_3^-. As with acute CO_2 retention, this change can occur quickly (within minutes) and may last for hours before there is any compensation.
- *Chronic respiratory alkalosis* occurs when the

reduction of carbon dioxide is compensated for by the renal excretion of HCO_3^-. The pH is lower than in acute respiratory alkalosis, but it is still above 7.4. The HCO_3^- excretion does not begin for at least a few hours and takes up to 3 days for maximal compensation.

The terms *chronic* and *compensation* do not imply "normal pH" (Fig. 7-3). Maximal compensation simply means that the body has done everything it can to return the pH toward normal. Rarely does compensation return pH *to* normal. A normal pH in the face of an acid-base disorder strongly suggests a mixed picture, with two or more primary disorders balancing each other. Occasionally patients can have a pH in the normal range when they have chronic respiratory acidosis or metabolic alkalosis, but the pH still does not return to the patient's true normal pH. For example, if a patient's normal pH is 7.40, compensation for respiratory acidosis might return it to 7.37 or 7.38 but not to 7.40.

ACUTE VS. CHRONIC METABOLIC DISORDERS

Why are there no acute bands for metabolic acidosis and metabolic alkalosis? The confidence bands shown for the metabolic disorders are in fact chronic. Patients whose blood gas values defined these bands had their condition long enough to reach their maximal physiologic compensation.

The compensation for metabolic acidosis occurs much more quickly than the compensation for respiratory disorders; in response to an acute reduction of HCO_3^-, the maximal reduction of $PaCO_2$ occurs within 12 to 24 hours.

Not much is known about how long it takes for the maximal compensation of metabolic alkalosis. Except when massive amounts of HCO_3^- are given to a patient, acute metabolic alkalosis is practically unknown in clinical practice. Also, not all patients seem to compensate for metabolic alkalosis with hypoventilation, making the band for metabolic alkalosis the least well characterized. Otherwise healthy people do not usually retain carbon dioxide to compensate for metabolic alkalosis, whereas patients suffering from severe lung disease or dehydration commonly retain carbon dioxide to compensate for this disorder.

Although acute and chronic changes are fairly well-defined for metabolic acidosis, acid-base maps generally omit the acute change. Fig. 7-4 shows the time course for acute metabolic acidosis based on the results from one human study (Pierce, Fedson, Brigham, et al., 1970); in this study patients who had cholera developed severe metabolic acidosis and took 11 to 24 hours to achieve maximal compensation. Their blood gas values moved along the pathway shown. Thus it should be kept in mind that a patient with early, uncomplicated metabolic acidosis may manifest blood gas values that do not fall into the commonly presented band for this disorder.

If the patient has had metabolic acidosis for at least 12 hours, his blood gas values can reasonably be expected to fall into the chronic metabolic acidosis confidence band (Fig. 7-3). After this period, gas values that fall above the band suggest a problem with compensation, e.g., a concomitant respiratory acidosis; gas values that fall below the band suggest a concomitant respiratory alkalosis.

Clinical problem 5

A patient initially has a $PaCO_2$ of 36 mm Hg, a pH of 7.10, and HCO_3^- of 13 mEq/L. He is in shock. How do you explain the patient's acid-base state?

The pitfall in diagnosing metabolic acidosis discussed above is one of several caveats regarding the acid-base map. Acid-base maps have probably been more abused than properly used. Although this map is used in figuring out acid-base problems, especially mixed disorders, it is important to point out pitfalls from the beginning. Most pitfalls can be avoided by practicing the author's First Law of Acid-Base Maps: *The acid-base map does not diagnose any acid-base disorder. Reliable diag-*

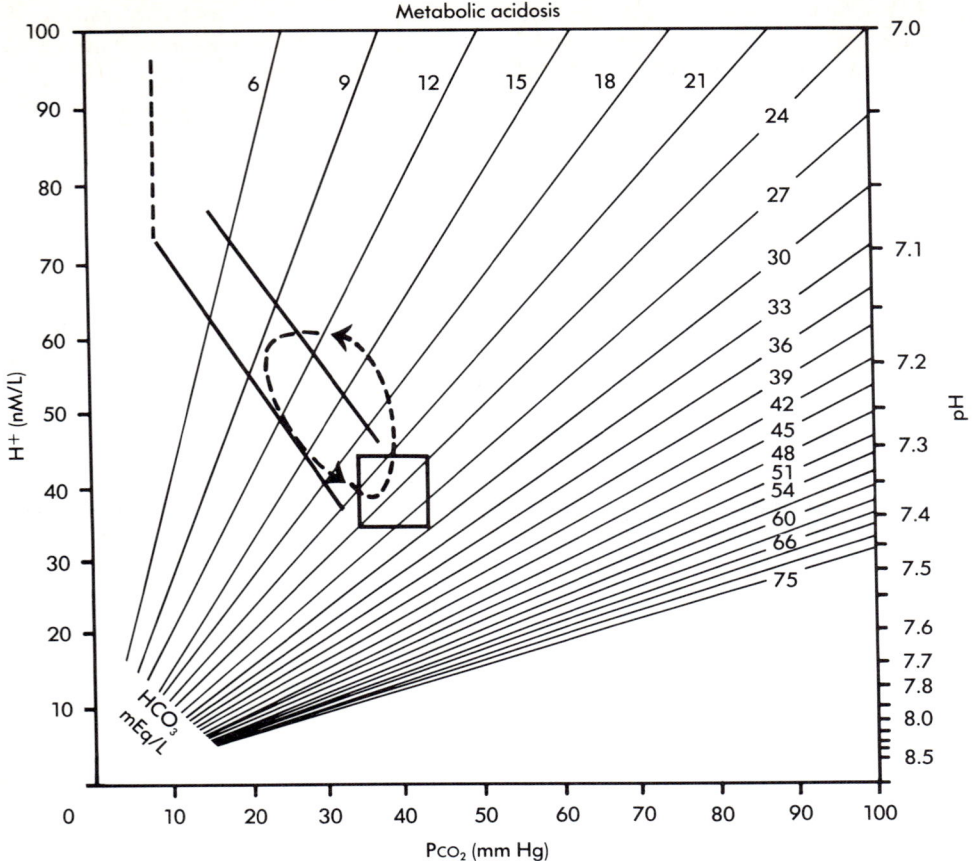

Fig. 7-4. Time course for compensation of metabolic acidosis. (Based on data from Pierce, N.F., Fedson, D.S., Brigham, K.L., et al.: Ann. Intern. Med. **72:**633, 1970.)

nosis can only be made clinically, in conjunction with the blood gas values and the other laboratory data.

With this caveat firmly emblazoned, the following are realistic uses of the acid-base map:
1. To help confirm the presence of a primary acid-base disorder
2. To help rule out a primary disorder as the sole cause of a patient's acid-base disturbance
3. To help follow a patient's hour-to-hour or day-to-day course

Clinical problem 6

A 45-year-old man comes to the emergency room complaining of shortness of breath that he says began a few days ago. A blood gas analysis shows a pH of 7.35, a Pa_{CO_2} of 60 mm Hg, and a Pa_{O_2} of 37 mm Hg. How would you characterize the patient's acid-base status?

Clinical problem 7

A comatose young woman is brought to the hospital. Blood gas analysis shows a pH of 7.1 and a Pa_{CO_2} of 90 mm Hg. What is her acid-base status?

MIXED ACID-BASE DISORDERS

So far simple or uncomplicated acid-base disorders have been emphasized. Patients with pulmonary disease often have two or more acid-base disorders occurring at the same time (see the box below); they are called mixed, or complicated, acid-base disorders. As a general rule, the more severe an acid-base disorder, the more likely it will be accompanied by *another* primary acid-base disturbance. For example, patients with severe respiratory acidosis (e.g., a Pa_{CO_2} of 80 mm Hg) are more likely to manifest accompanying metabolic acidosis than when the respiratory acidosis is mild to moderate (e.g., a Pa_{CO_2} of 50 mm Hg). This is simply because they are more likely to be severely hypoxemic or have cardiovascular impairment. The acid-base map is especially useful in sorting out these mixed disorders.

Theoretically, since the physiologic processes and not the blood pH define acid-base disorders, any possible combination of disorders, even three or more, may occur in one patient. Unusual but explainable combinations are listed in the box on this page.

Mixed acid-base problems are illustrated by the remaining cases. Detailed treatment of acid-base disorders, although outside the scope of this book, is discussed to some extent in these cases. The real key to treatment is understanding acid-base physiology in the clinical setting. This understanding, more than anything, assures rational management, whatever the underlying disturbance.

MIXED ACID-BASE DISORDERS

Common

Respiratory acidosis plus metabolic acidosis
Respiratory acidosis plus metabolic alkalosis
Respiratory alkalosis plus metabolic acidosis
Respiratory alkalosis plus metabolic alkalosis

Uncommon

Metabolic acidosis plus metabolic alkalosis
Respiratory acidosis plus respiratory alkalosis
Respiratory acidosis plus metabolic acidosis plus metabolic alkalosis
Respiratory alkalosis plus metabolic acidosis plus metabolic alkalosis
Metabolic acidosis plus respiratory acidosis plus respiratory alkalosis
Metabolic alkalosis plus respiratory acidosis plus respiratory alkalosis

---

Clinical problem 8

Part A. A 53-year-old man initially presented to the emergency room where he was found to have the following blood gas values while breathing room air: pH, 7.51; Pa_{CO_2}, 50 mm Hg; Pa_{O_2}, 40 mm Hg; and HCO_3^-, 39 mEq/L. His acid-base disorder is best characterized as which of the following?
 a. Metabolic alkalosis
 b. Metabolic alkalosis and respiratory acidosis
 c. Respiratory acidosis with metabolic compensation
 d. Indeterminable without more information

Part B. This patient was found to have congestive heart failure. (His initial blood gas values are given in Part A.) He was treated with low FI_{O_2} and diuretics. Three days later his pH was 7.38, Pa_{CO_2} was 60 mm Hg, HCO_3^- was 34 mEq/L, and Pa_{O_2} was 73 mm Hg while he was breathing 24% inspired oxygen, and he was clinically improved. How would his acid-base status be characterized at this point?

Clinical problem 9

A patient with several days duration of protracted vomiting is admitted to the hospital in a dehydrated state.

The following laboratory values are obtained:

Arterial blood gas values
pH, 7.51
$Paco_2$, 50 mm Hg
HCO_3^-, 39 mEq/L

Electrolytes
Na^+ 155 mEq/L
K^+, 5.5 mEq/L
Cl^-, 90 mEq/L
HCO_3^-, 40 mEq/L

Miscellaneous
Blood urea nitrogen, 121 mg%
Fasting glucose, 77 mg%

Which of the following most closely describes his acid-base status?
  a. Severe metabolic alkalosis
  b. Severe respiratory acidosis
  c. Respiratory acidosis plus metabolic alkalosis
  d. Metabolic alkalosis plus metabolic acidosis
  e. Respiratory acidosis plus respiratory alkalosis

Clinical problem 10

A 52-year-old woman has been artificially ventilated for 2 days following a drug overdose. Her blood gas values have been stable for the past 12 hours at pH, 7.45 and $Paco_2$, 25 mm Hg. Serum electrolytes studies reveal Na^+, 142 mEq/L; HCO_3^-, 18 mEq/L; Cl^- 100 mEq/L; and K^+, 4 mEq/L. How would you access her acid-base status?

Clinical problem 11

An 18-year-old girl is admitted to the intensive care unit because of an acute asthma attack that is unresponsive to treatment received in the emergency room. Her blood gas values while breathing room air show pH, 7.45; $Paco_2$, 25 mm Hg; Pao_2, 55 mm Hg; and Sao_2, 87%. Her peak expiratory flow rate is 95 L/min (predicted normal, 520 L/min). She continues to receive asthma medication (intravenous aminophylline and corticosteroids).

Two hours later she seems more tired, and her peak flow is less than 60 L/min. Blood gas values while breathing 40% inspired oxygen show pH, 7.20; $Paco_2$, 52 mm Hg; Pao_2, 65 mm Hg. At this point intubation and assisted ventilation are considered. What is her acid-base status?

Clinical problem 12

A 72-year-old man is admitted in shock with a blood pressure of 70 mm Hg measured by palpation. He has a history of chronic obstructive pulmonary disease and is also receiving treatment for a heart condition. An initial arterial blood gas analysis while he was breathing 40% oxygen shows $Paco_2$, 70 mm Hg; pH, 7.1; Pao_2, 35 mm Hg; and Sao_2, 58%. He is intubated, and a subsequent blood gas analysis also while breathing 40% oxygen reveals pH, 7.3; $Paco_2$, 40 mm Hg; and Pao_2, 87 mm Hg. The anion gap is elevated at 22 mEq/L. What is the patient's acid-base status?

CLINICAL APPROACH TO ACID-BASE DIAGNOSIS

The means to diagnose acid-base disorders, both simple and complicated, have been explained. Acid-base disorders refer to what is happening in the patient and represent physiologic processes, not just blood gas values. This concept allows diagnosis and management of difficult acid-base disorders. A rational approach to acid-base diagnosis and management is suggested below:

1. Find the acid-base disorder—serum HCO_3^- or arterial blood gas measurement.
2. Based on a full clinical assessment (history, physical examination, detailed laboratory review), explain the blood gas values in terms of physiologic processes and underlying clinical conditions.
3. Correct the pH if it is outside the range of 7.30-7.52.
4. Treat the underlying clinical condition.

SUMMARY

To maintain homeostasis, the body tries to keep the hydrogen ion concentration ($[H^+]$) at approximately 40 nmoles/L or the pH close to 7.40. Deviation from this $[H^+]$ is minimized by buffering systems, all of which are in equilibrium with one another; the largest is the bicarbonate buffer system. Any change in acid-base status is reflected in the components of the bicarbonate buffer system—

the bicarbonate ion (HCO_3^-) and the arterial partial pressure of carbon dioxide (Pa_{CO_2}). The Henderson-Hasselbalch equation relates pH to HCO_3^- and Pa_{CO_2}.

There are four primary acid-base disorders, each with a compensatory response that minimizes the change in pH. Compensatory responses are not named alkalosis or acidosis. Metabolic acidosis tends to lower the pH and the HCO_3^- (compensatory response is hyperventilation). Metabolic alkalosis tends to raise the pH and the HCO_3^- (compensatory response is hypoventilation). Respiratory acidosis tends to raise the Pa_{CO_2} and lower the pH (compensatory response is renal retention of HCO_3^-). Respiratory alkalosis tends to lower the Pa_{CO_2} and raise the pH (compensatory response is renal excretion of HCO_3^-). Compensatory processes do not return the pH to normal; a truly normal pH in the presence of an acid-base disorder (e.g., pH of 7.40 and Pa_{CO_2} of 25 mm Hg) indicates the presence of at least two primary acid-base disorders.

Each primary acid-base disorder should be viewed as a physiologic process caused by a specific clinical problem or disease and not simply as changes in blood gas values. This approach allows for unraveling complex or mixed acid-base disorders, which are particularly common in patients with severe respiratory disease.

REVIEW QUESTIONS

State whether each of the following is true or false.
1. Metabolic acidosis is present whenever the arterial pH is less than 7.35 and Pa_{CO_2} is less than 35 mm Hg.
2. In acute respiratory acidosis, bicarbonate initially rises because of the reaction of carbon dioxide with water and the formation of H_2CO_3.
3. If every cation and every anion were measured in the serum, there would be no "anion gap."
4. By definition, a patient cannot have a state of metabolic acidosis and a state of metabolic alkalosis at the same time.
5. If pH and Pa_{CO_2} are both above normal, bicarbonate must also be above normal.
6. The denominator of the Henderson-Hasselbalch equation equals 1.2 mEq/L when Pa_{CO_2} equals 40 mm Hg.
7. One reason the measured serum bicarbonate may not agree with the value calculated from the pH and the Pa_{CO_2} is the variation of the bicarbonate buffer system's pK value.
8. Diarrhea leads to metabolic alkalosis through the loss of gastrointestinal hydrogen ions.
9. A serum bicarbonate above normal, if accurate, always indicates an acid-base disorder.
10. The compensation for chronic respiratory acidosis is renal excretion of bicarbonate.

References

Goldberg, M., Green, S.B., Moss, M.L., et al.: Computer-based instruction and diagnosis of acid-base disorders, JAMA **223**:269, 1973.

Hood, I., and Campbell, E.J.M.: Is pK OK? (editorial), N. Engl. J. Med. **306**:864, 1982.

Mencken, H.L.: Exeunt Omnes, The Smart Set, p. 139, Dec. 1919.

Pierce, N.F., Fedson, D.S., Brigham, K.L., et al.: The ventilatory response to acute base deficit in humans, Ann. Intern. Med. **72**:633, 1970.

Schwartz, W.B., and Relman, A.S.: A critique of the parameters used in the evaluation of acid-base disorders, N. Engl. J. Med. **268**:1382, 1963.

Suggested readings

General

Brackett, N.C.: An approach to clinical disorders of acid-base balance, South. Med. J. **67**:1084, 1974.

Cohen, J.J., and Kassiner, J.P.: Acid/base, Boston, 1982, Little, Brown & Co.

Elkington, J.R.: Acid-base disorders and the clinician, Ann. Intern. Med. **63**:893, 1965.

Masoro, E.J., and Siegel, P.D.: Acid-base regulation: its physiology, pathophysiology and the interpretation of blood gas analysis, Philadelphia, 1977, W.B. Saunders Co.

McCurdy, D.K.: Mixed metabolic and respiratory acid-base disturbances: diagnosis and treatment, Chest Suppl. **62**:35, 1972.

Winters, R.W.: Terminology of acid-base disorders, Ann. Intern. Med. **63**:837, 1965.

See also General References in Appendix G.

Respiratory disorders

Arbus, G.S., Hebert, L.A., Levesque, P.R., et al.: Characterization and clinical application of the "significance band" for acute respiratory alkalosis, N. Engl. J. Med. **280**:117, 1969.

Brackett, N.C., Cohen, J.J., and Schwartz, W.B.: Carbon dioxide titration curve of normal man, N. Engl. J. Med. **272**:6, 1965.

Brackett, N.C., Wingo, F., Muren, O., et al.: Acid-base response to chronic hypercapnia in man, N. Engl. J. Med. **280**:124, 1969.

Gennari, F.J., Goldstein, M.B., and Schwartz, W.B.: The nature of the renal adaption to chronic hypocapnia, J. Clin. Invest. **51**:1722, 1972.

Ingram, R.H., Jr., Miller, R.B., and Tate, L.A.: Acid-base response to acute carbon dioxide changes in chronic obstructive pulmonary disease, Am. Rev. Respir. Dis. **108**:225, 1973.

Robin, E.D., Bromberg, P.A., and Tushan, F.S.: Carbon dioxide in body fluids, N. Engl. J. Med. **280**:162, 1969.

Schwartz, W.B., Brackett, N.C., and Cohen, J.J.: The response of extracellular hydrogen ion concentration to graded degrees of chronic hypercapnia: the physiologic limits of the defense of pH, J. Clin. Invest. **44**:281, 1965.

van Ypersele de Strihou, C., Brasseur, L., and DeConnick, J.: The carbon dioxide response curve for chronic hypercapnia in man, N. Engl. J. Med. **275**:117, 1966.

Metabolic disorders

Albert, M.S., Dell, R.B., and Winters, R.W.: Quantitative displacement of acid-base equilibrium in metabolic acidosis, Ann. Intern. Med. **66**:312, 1967.

Emmet, M., and Narins, R.G.: Clinical use of the anion gap, Medicine (Baltimore) **56**:38, 1977.

Fulop, M.: The ventilatory response in severe metabolic acidosis, Clin. Sci. Mol. Med. **50**:367, 1976.

Fulop, M.: Hypercapnia in metabolic alkalosis, N. Y. State J. Med. **76**:19, 1976.

Goldring, R.M., Cannon, P.J., Heinemann, H.O., et al.: Respiratory adjustment to chronic metabolic alkalosis in man, J. Clin. Invest. **47**:188, 1968.

Jarboe, T.M., Penman, R.W., and Luke, R.G.: Ventilatory failure due to metabolic alkalosis, Chest Suppl. **61**:61, 1972.

Lifschitz, M.D., Brasch, R., and Buomo, A.J.: Marked hypercapnia secondary to severe metabolic alkalosis, Ann. Intern. Med. **77**:405, 1972.

Madias, N.E., Ayus, J.C., and Adrogue, H.J.: Increased anion gap in metabolic alkalosis, N. Engl. J. Med. **300**:1421, 1979.

Oh, M.S., and Carroll, H.J.: The anion gap, N. Engl. J. Med. **297**:814, 1977.

Oliva, P.B.: Severe alveolar hypoventilation in a patient with metabolic alkalosis, Am. J. Med. **52**:817, 1972.

Perez-Guerra, F.: Hypercapnia during iatrogenically induced metabolic alkalosis, Chest **65**:108, 1974.

Tuller, M.A., and Mehdi, F.: Compensatory hypoventilation and hypocapnia in primary metabolic alkalosis, Am. J. Med. **50**:281, 1971.

van Ypersele de Strihou, C., and Frans, A.: The respiratory response to chronic metabolic alkalosis and acidosis in disease, Clin. Sci. Mol. Med. **45**:439, 1973.

Webb, J.: Severe hypercapnia associated with a nonrespiratory alkalosis, Br. J. Dis. Chest **72**:62, 1978.

chapter 8
Pulmonary circulation

OUTLINE

Pulmonary vs. systemic circulation
Pulmonary hypertension and right heart failure
Causes of pulmonary hypertension
Assessment of hemodynamic status
Swan-Ganz catheterization
Insertion of Swan-Ganz catheter—pressure tracings
Hemodynamic measurements and calculations
Pulmonary artery wedge pressure—measurement
Pulmonary artery wedge pressure—what does it represent?
Pitfalls and complications in hemodynamic monitoring
Hemodynamic monitoring in clinical practice

PULMONARY VS. SYSTEMIC CIRCULATION

Historically, physiologic assessment of the pulmonary circulation has lagged behind the measurement of lung mechanics and gas exchange. Although the systemic circulation is easily accessible for evaluation (e.g., routine blood pressure measurement), the pulmonary circulation was, until recently, hidden from view. This situation changed significantly with the introduction of cardiac catheterization in the 1950's. Even so, catheterization was a highly specialized test for years and was not routinely used in pulmonary patients. With the introduction of *bedside* right-sided heart catheterization in 1970, the clinical study of pulmonary hemodynamics entered a new era. The bedside catheter has allowed the study of pulmonary circulation in critically ill patients and has permitted the continuous monitoring of a patient's disease and its response to therapy. The result has both enhanced the knowledge of cardiopulmonary disease and contributed directly to patient care.

A review of the normal pulmonary circulation is helpful before discussing bedside catheterization. Fig. 2-12 diagrams the systemic and pulmonary circulations; Table 8-1 outlines the paths of blood flow for each circulation and lists the major physiologic differences between the two.

Table 8-1. Systemic and pulmonary circulations

	Systemic circulation	Pulmonary circulation
Path of blood	Left atrium → Left ventricle → Systemic arteries → Systemic capillaries → Systemic veins → Right atrium → Right ventricle	Right atrium → Right ventricle → Pulmonary arteries → Pulmonary capillaries → Pulmonary veins → Left atrium → Left ventricle
Function	Carries oxygenated blood from the left side of the heart through the systemic arteries to all the organs and tissues After delivering oxygen and receiving carbon dioxide in the systemic capillaries, returns deoxygenated blood through the systemic veins to the right atrium where the pulmonary circulation begins	Carries deoxygenated blood from the right side of the heart and through the pulmonary arteries to the lungs After receiving oxygen and delivering carbon dioxide in the pulmonary capillaries, returns oxygenated blood through the pulmonary veins to the left atrium where the systemic circulation begins
Pressure	Relatively high-pressure system; range of normal mean systemic arterial pressure is 70 to 105 mm Hg; easily measured with blood pressure cuff	Relatively low-pressure system; range of normal mean pulmonary artery pressure is 10 to 22 mm Hg; can only be measured with pulmonary artery catheter
Cause of elevated pressure	Unknown in majority of cases; renal disease in some patients; hypoxemia not a cause	Usually can be determined from full clinical picture; hypoxemia, left-sided heart failure, and destruction of pulmonary vascular bed among known causes
Treatment of elevated pressure	Low-salt diet; weight reduction if overweight; if necessary, many different types of antihypertensive drugs are available, including diuretics	Depends on cause; for heart failure, digoxin and diuretics often effective; for hypoxemia-induced pulmonary hypertension, continuous oxygen therapy is treatment of choice; in some cases, e.g., primary pulmonary hypertension, there is no effective treatment

PULMONARY HYPERTENSION AND RIGHT HEART FAILURE

Pulmonary hypertension is defined as a mean pulmonary artery pressure greater than 22 mm Hg. Pulmonary hypertension can occur from several physiologic causes and disease processes (Table 8-2); the hypertension may be transient, as in reversible conditions such as an asthma attack, or chronic, as in emphysema. In some patients, two or more causes may contribute to pulmonary hypertension (e.g., left ventricular heart failure and pulmonary emboli).

Right heart failure is a decompensated state of the right ventricle and can result from sustained or severe pulmonary hypertension of any origin. When the right ventricle is unable to pump its full cardiac output against the elevated pulmonary pressure, systemic venous pressure increases and fluid "backs up" in the systemic veins. Untreated, the patient will manifest leg edema, ascites, liver engorgement, and weight gain. In the absence of left ventricular failure, there is no excess fluid in the alveoli, and the lungs will remain clear on chest x-ray. A chest x-ray from a patient with right-side heart failure is shown in Fig. 8-1; note the cardiomegaly and the absence of pulmonary infiltrates. Treatment of right heart failure attempts to relieve the pulmonary hypertension and uses low sodium intake and diuretic therapy to help mobilize excess body fluid.

Table 8-2. Causes of pulmonary hypertension

Disease or condition	Underlying mechanism(s)
Lung diseases, including all forms of restrictive and obstructive lung conditions	Hypoxemia; loss of pulmonary blood vessels; acidosis
Heart disease, including left ventricular heart failure, mitral valve disease, congenital heart disease	Increased pulmonary capillary hydrostatic pressure
Pulmonary thromboembolic disease	Pulmonary artery narrowing; loss of pulmonary blood vessels
Pulmonary arteritis	Pulmonary artery narrowing; loss of pulmonary blood vessels
High altitude	Hypoxemia
Hypoventilation	Hypoxemia; acidosis
Chest wall deformity	Hypoxemia, acidosis; pulmonary artery narrowing
Idiopathic	Loss of pulmonary blood vessels; pulmonary artery narrowing

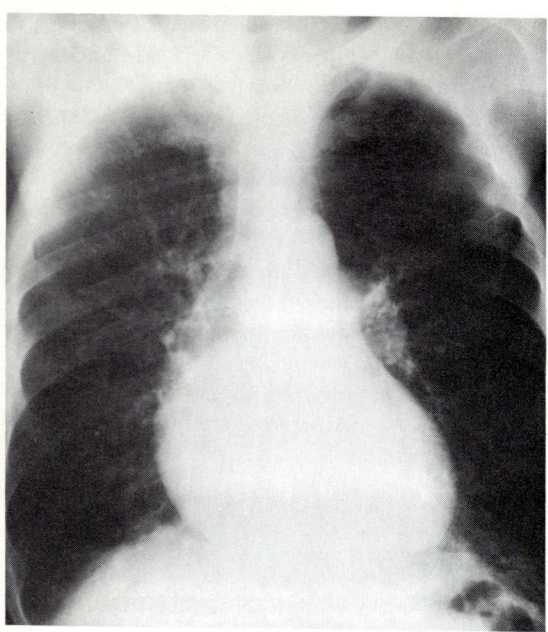

Fig. 8-1. Chest x-ray of a patient with pulmonary hypertension and right-sided heart failure. Note the enlarged heart (caused by an enlarged right ventricle), the enlarged pulmonary arteries, and the absence of lung infiltrates.

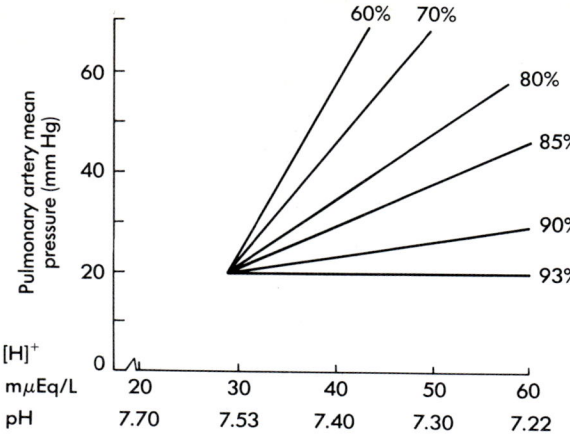

Fig. 8-2. Effect of hypoxemia (reduced SaO_2) and acidosis on mean pulmonary artery pressure. Percentages refer to SaO_2. See text for discussion. (From Mathay, R.A., and Berger, H.J.: Cardiovascular performances in chronic obstructive pulmonary diseases, Med. Clin. North Am. **65**(3):489-524, 1981; reprinted with permission from W.B. Saunders Co. Reproduced from J. Clin. Invest. **43**:1146-1162, 1964, by copyright permission of the American Society for Clinical Investigation.)

CAUSES OF PULMONARY HYPERTENSION

Lung disease, a common cause of pulmonary hypertension, usually operates through one of the mechanisms listed in Table 8-2. *Hypoxemia,* a frequent manifestation of lung disease, is one of the most common physiologic mechanisms causing pulmonary hypertension. Fig. 8-2 demonstrates the effect of hypoxemia on mean pulmonary artery pressure, as well as demonstrating the interrelationship with *acidosis*. At normal pH, the arterial percent saturation of hemoglobin with oxygen (SaO_2) must decline to approximately 75% to achieve a doubling of mean pulmonary artery pressure. When pH is 7.3, the same doubling of pulmonary artery pressure occurs when the SaO_2 is approximately 82%.

Both hypoxemia and acidosis cause pulmonary hypertension by constricting the small, muscular pulmonary arteries (those less than 0.2 mm in diameter). The exact mechanism for the vasoconstriction is unknown. The vasoconstriction may be caused by hypoxia- or acidosis-mediated release of vasoactive substances or by a direct effect on pulmonary artery smooth muscle.

Hypoxemia is a clinically important cause of pulmonary hypertension because it is potentially reversible. Continuous oxygen therapy does reduce mortality from hypoxemic chronic obstructive pulmonary disease (see Chapter 9).

Another cause of pulmonary hypertension is the loss of pulmonary vasculature. Patients with severe emphysema can actually have near normal PaO_2 yet

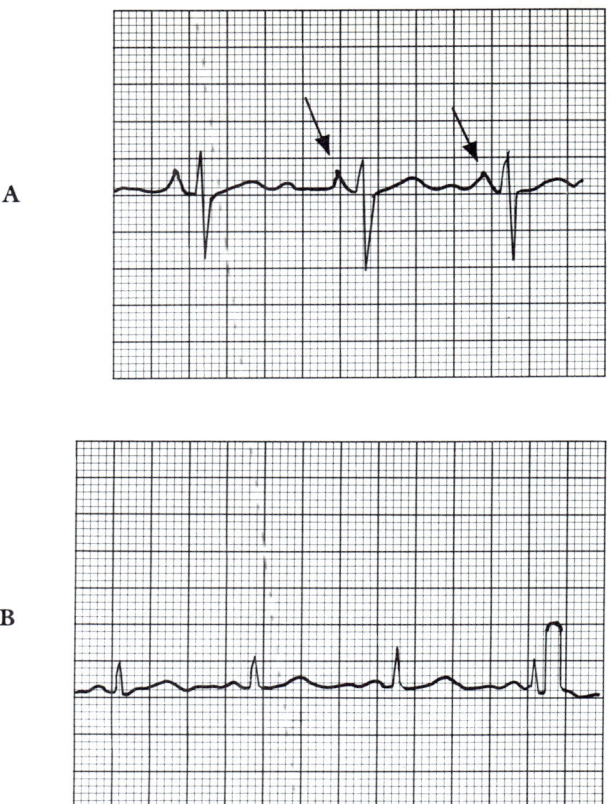

Fig. 8-3. ECG readings. **A,** An example of P-pulmonale (large, peaked P waves in lead II [*arrows*]), which represents right artrial dilation that results from increased pulmonary artery and right ventricular pressures. **B,** A normal ECG.

manifest severe pulmonary hypertension because the destruction of lung tissue in emphysema may remove *both* alveoli and pulmonary capillaries. The remaining lung has mostly high-ventilation–perfusion ratios that lead to increased dead space but not to significant hypoxemia (see Chapter 5). However, since there is a less vascular bed through which the right ventricle can pump its cardiac output, the pulmonary artery pressure is increased.

Cor pulmonale refers to any right ventricular manifestation of pulmonary hypertension caused by lung disease. Cor pulmonale usually manifests as one or more signs of right-sided heart strain—the effects of pulmonary hypertension on the right ventricle or right atrium (see the box on p. 152). Cor pulmonale is not synonymous with right heart failure. Of course, the basic cause of cor pulmonale, pulmonary hypertension, may also lead to right-sided heart failure.

Perhaps the most common cause of pulmonary hypertension is *left heart failure*. (The most common causes of left heart failure are arteriosclerosis and systemic hypertension.) In left heart failure fluid backs up in the left atrium and in the pul-

> **SIGNS OF COR PULMONALE**
>
> **Physical examination**—increased intensity of second (pulmonic) heart sound; right ventricular heave when palpating anterior chest wall
> **Chest x-ray film**—enlargement of pulmonary arteries and right ventricular dilation
> **Electrocardiogram**—evidence of right-sided heart strain, such as tall R wave in precordial leads or tall, peaked P wave in lead II (Fig. 8-3)

monary circulation, resulting in increased pulmonary artery pressures. Treatment is usually with digoxin and diuretics and is directed at the left ventricle. Unless the patient is hypoxemic, supplemental oxygen can be expected to have little benefit.

Mitral valve disease can cause profound heart failure and pulmonary hypertension by interfering with the flow of blood from the left atrium to the left ventricle; this interference can occur either through mitral stenosis (narrowing of the mitral orifice) or mitral regurgitation (ejection of blood back into the atrium during systole). Both conditions are easily diagnosed using noninvasive cardiac methods and are potentially correctable with mitral valve surgery. Years ago rheumatic fever was the principal cause of severe mitral valve disease. Rheumatic heart disease is now relatively uncommon in the United States, and as a consequence, the prevalence of severe mitral valve disease has decreased over the years. Nonetheless, mitral valve disease should always be considered when pulmonary hypertension is present without an obvious cause.

Pulmonary emboli are clots that usually arise in the deep veins of the thigh and pelvis, break off, and travel to lodge in one or more of the pulmonary arteries. If not fatal to the patient, these clots will usually dissolve with time; on occasion they organize and thrombose in situ. Both acute pulmonary emboli and pulmonary thrombi (emboli that organize and do not dissolve) are potential causes of pulmonary hypertension. Pulmonary embolism is a relatively common clinical condition and should always be considered as a cause of otherwise unexplained pulmonary hypertension.

Other, rarer causes of pulmonary hypertension are congenital heart disease, pulmonary arteritis (inflammation of the pulmonary arteries), and chest wall deformity. Within each category listed in Table 8-2 are many different disease entities, far too numerous to mention.

Pulmonary hypertension may also be of completely unknown origin (idiopathic). *Idiopathic pulmonary hypertension* has a predilection for young and middle-aged women and usually presents with the insidious onset of dyspnea. Diagnosis is made by catheterization of the right side of the heart, measurement of pulmonary artery pressures, and by ruling out all other possible causes (e.g., heart and lung disease). There is no effective treatment for this disorder, although several vasodilators have been tried on an experimental basis. Idiopathic pulmonary hypertension is usually fatal within 5 years from the time of diagnosis.

ASSESSMENT OF HEMODYNAMIC STATUS

Hemodynamic status refers to the status of the pressure and the flow within the pulmonary and systemic circulation. Patients manifesting shock, heart failure, pulmonary hypertension, fluid overload, and many other problems have altered hemodynamic status. In clinical practice, there are two levels of hemodynamic assessment. The first level is noninvasive, meaning without cardiac catheterization or arterial pressure monitoring. Noninvasive hemodynamic assessment includes the history, physical examination, chest x-ray studies, pulmonary function tests, arterial blood gas measurement, observation of the patient's response to treatment and, occasionally, noninvasive heart studies such as the echocardiogram. In the vast majority of respiratory patients, hemodynamic status can be assessed noninvasively.

Clinical problem 1

A 64-year-old man is admitted to the hospital because of dyspnea and leg edema. He has a long history of cigarette smoking. Previous pulmonary function studies showed severe, chronic airways obstruction.

When examined, the patient has decreased breath sounds in both lung bases. The intensity of his second heart sound is increased; his pulse is 120/min, and his blood pressure is 135/72 mm Hg. The patient's abdomen is enlarged, suggesting ascites, and he has bilateral leg edema. A chest x-ray film shows an enlarged heart without lung infiltrates (see Fig. 8-1). While breathing room air, his Pa_{O_2} is 45 mm Hg, Pa_{CO_2} is 47 mm Hg, and pH is 7.35.

Based on this information, how would you assess this patient's hemodynamic status?

Clinical problem 2

A 65-year-old man is brought to the hospital after being found unresponsive on the floor of his apartment. On evaluation, he is alert but confused; his skin and mucous membranes are very dry. Vital signs are as follows: systolic blood pressure, 90 mm Hg in the supine position (by palpation over the brachial artery); pulse, 96 and regular; respiratory rate, 20/min; and body temperature, 97.4° F. In the sitting position the patient's blood pressure falls to 60 mm Hg systolic, and his pulse increases to 110/min. A chest x-ray film shows a normal-sized heart with no pulmonary infiltrates, and an ECG shows only sinus tachycardia. Routine blood tests are ordered, including serum electrolytes.

His hemodynamic status most likely reflects which of the following:
  a. Cardiogenic shock
  b. Pulmonary hypertension
  c. Adult respiratory distress syndrome (ARDS)
  d. Severe dehydration
  e. Labile blood pressure
Is invasive hemodynamic monitoring indicated?

The second level of hemodynamic assessment is invasive and requires cardiac catheterization and arterial pressure monitoring. Until the early 1970's, catheterization was only possible in a special laboratory, and studies were usually limited to noncritically ill patients with valvular or coronary disease. The advent of the Swan-Ganz catheter, first introduced in 1970, made bedside catheterization feasible and revolutionized hemodynamic evaluation. In practice, most patients requiring bedside catheterization also have a small cannula inserted in a peripheral artery (usually radial) for continuous blood pressure monitoring. In addition, cardiac rate and rhythm are continuously monitored in all catheterized patients.

Clinical problem 3

A 43-year-old man has surgery for a gunshot wound to his abdomen. During surgery he receives 6 units of whole blood, plus several liters of normal saline. After surgery the patient is sent to the intensive care unit in stable condition. Four hours later his blood pressure falls to 80/50 mm Hg, and he becomes very tachypneic. Chest x-ray shows infiltrates in both lung fields; the heart size is indeterminant. An electrocardiogram shows sinus tachycardia at 120/min.

The most likely diagnosis is which of the following:
  a. Adult respiratory distress syndrome (ARDS)
  b. Cardiogenic shock
  c. Pulmonary hypertension
  d. Pulmonary embolism
  e. Pneumonia
Is invasive hemodynamic monitoring indicated?

SWAN-GANZ CATHETERIZATION

The first cardiac catheterization is now legendary. Working alone in 1929, a German physician named Werner Forssmann threaded a urologic catheter through a vein in his arm and into his heart. This procedure was done clandestinely since he did not have official approval for such a daring experiment. Dr. Forssmann took a chest x-ray, which demonstrated the catheter's position, and he published the procedure as a brief report. Cardiac catheterization did not become a clinically useful test, however, until the late 1940's, following the work of Dr. Dickinson W. Richards and Dr. Andre Cournand. For cardiac catheterization's revolutionary effect on cardiac diagnosis, all three physicians shared the 1956 Nobel Prize for Medicine.

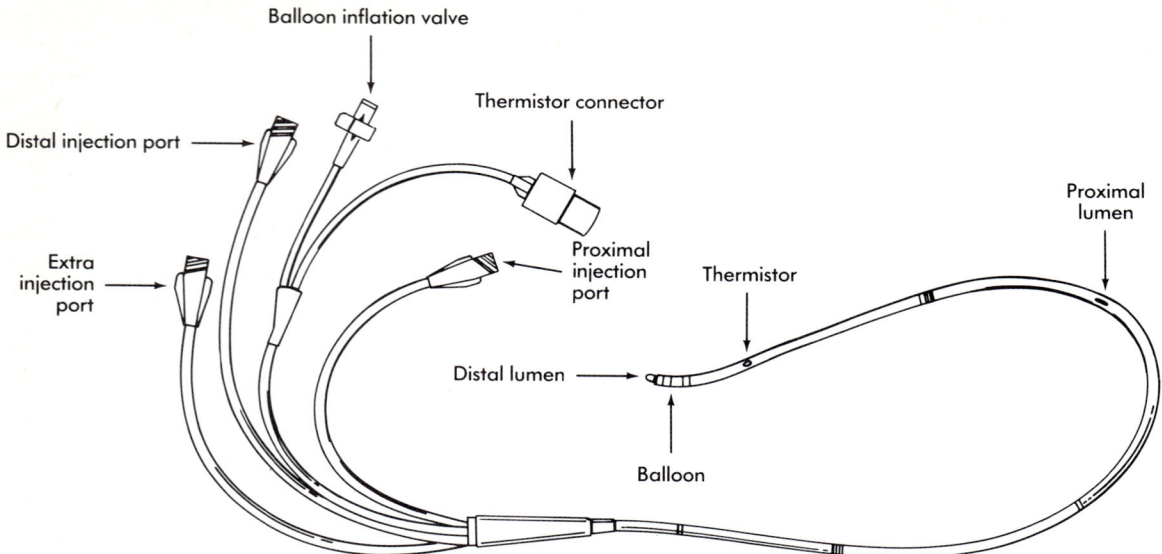

Fig. 8-4. The quadruple channel Swan-Ganz catheter. The most distal channel *(distal injection port)* is for pulmonary artery pressure measurement; blood can also be aspirated from this channel for mixed venous oxygen measurements. A second channel *(balloon inflation valve)* is used to inflate/deflate the distal balloon. A third channel *(proximal injection port),* which exits 30 cm from the catheter tip, is used for central venous (right atrial) pressure monitoring and fluid infusion. The fourth channel *(extra injection port),* which is not present on all catheters, can be used for continuous infusion of hyperalimentation fluids. The thermistor connector plugs into a bedside cardiac output computer.

In 1970 Swan, Ganz, Forrester, et al. published their now famous study of a special flow-directed, balloon-tipped catheter. The Swan-Ganz catheter made bedside catheterization of the right side of the heart a feasible procedure.* The catheter was originally introduced to assess patients suffering from acute myocardial infarction. Subsequently it has been used to assess patients who have a wide variety of hemodynamic and fluid problems. A general approach is to use the catheter in unstable patients when, by noninvasive means, the hemodynamic or fluid status is uncertain. The catheter provides measurements of right-sided heart pressure, pulmonary artery pressure, pulmonary artery wedge pressure, and cardiac output. An unstable patient's hemodynamic status cannot be reliably assessed clinically, so bedside catheterization is an important procedure in critical care units.

The Swan-Ganz catheter is shown in Fig. 8-4. The catheter is basically a thin, flexible tube with an inflatable rubber balloon surrounding the distal end. The balloon is inflated by injecting a maximum of 1.5 cc air through a part on the proximal end. The catheter's position within the pulmonary artery, with the balloon inflated, is shown in Fig. 8-5. In the center of the catheter runs a channel

---

*Swan-Ganz is a brand name for the catheter marketed by Edwards Laboratories of California and is named for Dr. Swan and Dr. Ganz, the senior authors of the original paper. Although other companies produce right-sided heart catheters for bedside use, the term "Swan-Ganz" has now become synonymous with this technique.

Pulmonary circulation

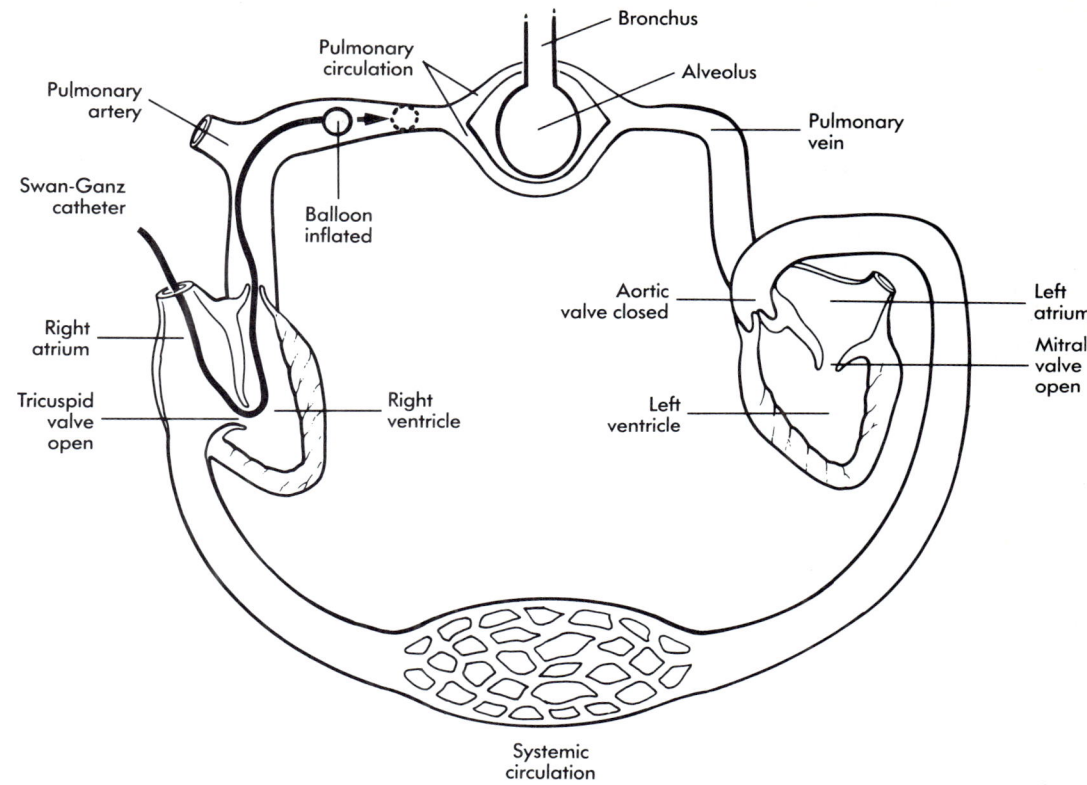

Fig. 8-5. Swan-Ganz catheter in wedge position. The heart, shown here separated into its right and left chambers, is in diastole. The Swan-Ganz catheter, with its balloon inflated, is gradually floated into the wedge position (dotted circle), occluding a pulmonary artery.

through which fluids can be infused or blood aspirated. One or more additional channels in the catheter can be used to administer fluids.*

In the preceding chapters, interaction between the heart and the lungs has not been a point of emphasis. However, anyone managing patients with the aid of the Swan-Ganz catheter can appreciate the heart-lung interaction. Often, changing one parameter to provide improved cardiac function has a profound effect on gas exchange, for better or worse.

Swan-Ganz catheterization is a sophisticated technique that requires an experienced person to insert the catheter and to wisely interpret and use the hemodynamic data obtained. A brief summary follows of the indications for use of the Swan-Ganz catheter, the catheter's route of insertion, and the measurements obtained from the catheterization.

Indications

In general terms, Swan-Ganz catheterization should be used when a reasonably accurate he-

---

*Some right-sided heart catheters incorporate a fiberoptic bundle that can continuously measure oxygen saturation (see Chapter 6).

modynamic assessment cannot be made noninvasively. Specifically, the catheter should be used when knowing any of the following values may affect therapy and benefit the patient: cardiac output; pulmonary artery pressures; pulmonary artery wedge pressure; mixed venous partial pressure of oxygen (Pvo_2), or mixed venous oxygen saturation (Svo_2). These measurements may be obtained one time only or, as is more common, over a period of hours to days (hemodynamic monitoring). Catheters equipped with a special fiberoptic bundle can continuously monitor pulmonary artery oxygen saturation.

Route of insertion

Any large vein can be used for insertion of the Swan-Ganz catheter. The most commonly used veins are the internal jugular, the subclavian, the external jugular, and the brachial. Catheterization is performed under sterile conditions (the physician wears a sterile gown and sterile gloves) at the patient's bedside.

Measurements

To obtain *pressure* measurements, the catheter is connected to a transducer, which is calibrated by using a mercury manometer. The transducer electronically converts the vascular pressure readings so that they can be displayed digitally or graphically on chart paper. All pressures are recorded in mm Hg.

Cardiac output is measured by using the thermodilution technique. Ten milliliters of saline are rapidly injected through the catheter's central venous pressure port, which exits in the right atrium. The saline, which can be either room temperature or iced to 0° C, changes the temperature of the blood in the pulmonary artery. The change in temperature is sensed by a thermistor at the distal end of the catheter (Fig. 8-4), which is located in the pulmonary artery. This thermistor is connected, through a port on the proximal end, to a small computer that sits at the patient's bedside. Almost immediately after the saline is injected, the computer calculates cardiac output based on the rapidity of the temperature change in the pulmonary artery.

Mixed venous oxygen measurement is performed on a pulmonary artery blood sample that is obtained from the most distal port of the catheter; this sample should be obtained only when the catheter is in the nonwedged position. If the catheter is equipped with a special fiberoptic sensor, the Svo_2 can be continuously monitored.

INSERTION OF SWAN-GANZ CATHETER—PRESSURE TRACINGS

The flow-directed catheter requires careful bedside monitoring of vascular pressure tracings during its insertion. The pressure tracings are used to determine the catheter's position. In practice, these pressure tracings are continuously monitored on an oscilloscope as the catheter is advanced; in addition, the ECG is continuously observed for any disturbance of cardiac rhythm.

A guide to catheter insertion follows, with reference to the pressure tracings at each point of insertion as shown in Fig. 8-6. This is *not* meant to be a specific guide to catheter insertion. The catheter manufacturer's instructions should always be observed, and the catheter should only be inserted, or the insertion should be directly supervised, by an experienced physician. Distances refer to the position of the catheter as shown in Fig. 8-6. Each distance is from the point of insertion, assuming that the internal jugular vein is the portal of entry and that the patient is an average-sized adult. The use of other venous access routes results in different catheter distances to the right atrium, the right ventricle, and the wedge position.

Superior vena cava. The first pressure reading obtained, approximately 5 to 10 cm from the point of insertion, is the central venous pressure (CVP). Normal CVP is less than 10 mm Hg. The operator continues to advance the catheter into the right atrium.

Right atrium. The right atrium is approximately 15 cm from the point of insertion. Right atrial pressure is normally less than 10 mm Hg,

Pulmonary circulation

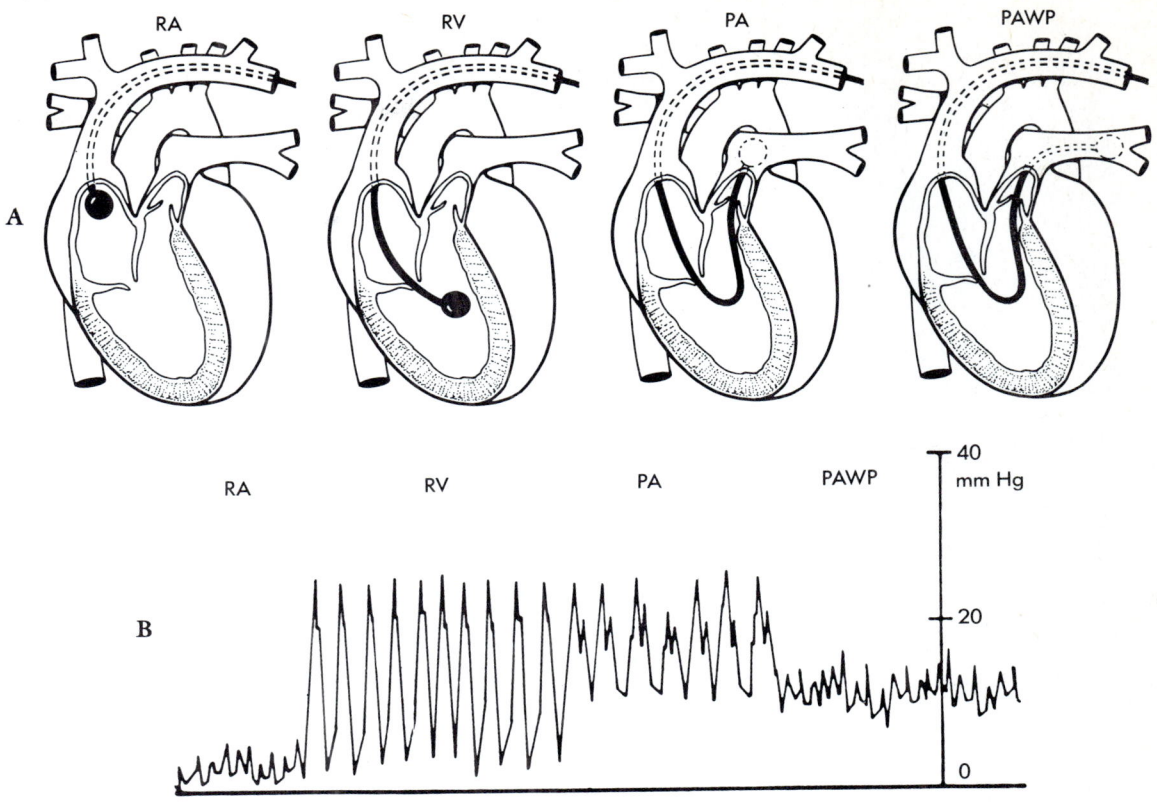

Fig. 8-6. **A**, Swan-Ganz catheter position in heart. **B**, As monitored by pressure tracings. (*RA*, pressure tracing from right atrium; *RV*, pressure tracing from right ventricle; *PA*, pressure tracing from pulmonary artery; *PAWP*, pulmonary artery wedge pressure tracing.)

and the pressure tracing also represents the CVP. At this point the balloon tip is safely inflated with 1.5 cc of air. As the catheter is gently advanced, the balloon tip "floats" across the tricuspid valve into the right ventricle.

Right ventricle. The right ventricle is approximately 25 cm from the point of insertion. The RV pressure tracing is distinctive, marked by a systolic pressure of approximately 25 mm Hg and an end-diastolic pressure close to zero. From this point the catheter is continually advanced. (If more than 15 cm of catheter is advanced and if it remains within the right ventricle, the catheter is coiling or knotting upon itself; the balloon should be deflated, and the catheter should be pulled back to the right atrium and advanced again.) As the catheter crosses the pulmonic valve, another distinctive pressure tracing heralds its entry into the main pulmonary artery.

Main pulmonary artery. The main pulmonary artery (PA) is approximately 35 cm from the point of insertion. Normal PA pressure is approximately 24/10 mm Hg, with a PA diastolic pressure distinctly higher than the right ventricular end-

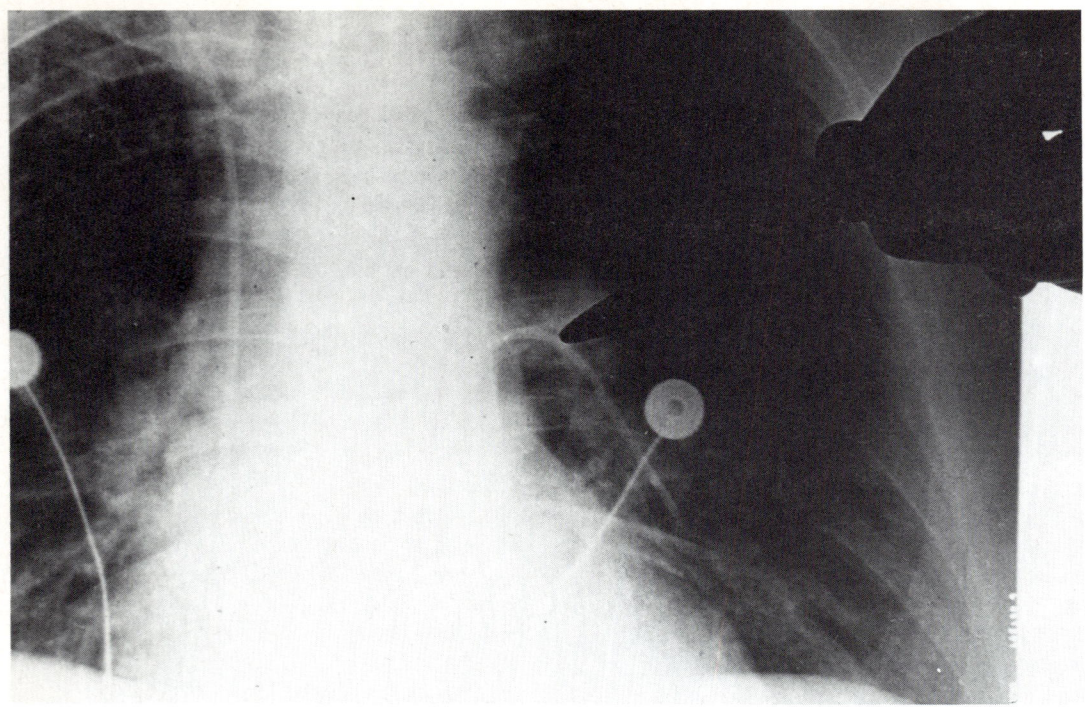

Fig. 8-7. Chest x-ray showing Swan-Ganz catheter in the patient's left pulmonary artery. A ballpoint pen is pointing to the catheter.

diastolic pressure. From this point the catheter is continually advanced until it *wedges* in one of the pulmonary artery branches.

Pulmonary artery branches. The pulmonary artery branches are approximately 40 cm from the point of insertion. The wedge pressure tracing is also distinctive and is marked by an overall flattening when compared to the pulmonary artery tracing. The "hills" and "valleys" of the normal wedge pressure tracing reflect left atrial diastole and systole. The actual wedge pressure reading is usually taken as the *mean* of this pressure curve and ranges from 6 to 12 mm Hg.

At this point a chest x-ray is obtained to check for catheter position and to make sure no complication occurred during the insertion, such as knotting of the catheter or pneumothorax. Fig. 8-7 shows a chest x-ray with the Swan-Ganz catheter in proper position.

HEMODYNAMIC MEASUREMENTS AND CALCULATIONS

The various measurements that are obtained from Swan-Ganz catheterization are used to calculate several derived values. Table 8-3 lists the usual measurements obtained by this technique, plus those measurements available from peripheral arterial cannulation. Table 8-4 lists the most common values that are calculated from the basic measurements.

Table 8-3. Basic measurements from Swan-Ganz catheterization and arterial cannulation

Measurement	Normal range
From Swan-Ganz catheter	
Central venous pressure	<10 mm Hg
Right arterial pressure	<10 mm Hg
Right ventricular pressure	15 to 30 mm Hg
Right ventricular pressure, diastolic	0 to 8 mm Hg
Pulmonary artery pressure, systolic	15 to 28 mm Hg
Pulmonary artery pressure, diastolic	5 to 16 mm Hg
Pulmonary artery pressure, mean	10 to 22 mm Hg
Pulmonary artery wedge pressure, mean	6 to 12 mm Hg
Cardiac output	4 to 7 L/min
Heart rate	60 to 80 beats/min
Oxygen saturation of mixed venous blood	70% to 75%
Partial pressure of oxygen in mixed venous blood	35 to 40 mm Hg
From peripheral arterial line	
Systemic arterial pressure, systolic	100 to 140 mm Hg
Systemic arterial pressure, diastolic	60 to 90 mm Hg
Systemic arterial pressure, mean	70 to 105 mm Hg
Arterial blood gases	See box on p. 20

Clinical problem 4

A critically ill patient is being managed in the intensive care unit with the aid of a Swan-Ganz catheter and a peripheral arterial cannula. The patient's initial measurements are shown below. (All pressures are in mm Hg.)

From Swan-Ganz catheter		*From peripheral arterial line*	
Central venous pressure	5	Systemic arterial pressure, systolic	89
Pulmonary artery pressure, systolic	38	Systemic arterial pressure, diastolic	54
Pulmonary artery pressure, diastolic	26	Systemic arterial pressure, mean	66
Pulmonary artery pressure, mean	31		
Pulmonary artery wedge pressure, mean	24		
Heart rate	120/min		
Cardiac output	3.1 L/min		

Based on the patient's weight and height, his body surface area is 1.8 m^2 (obtained from a standard body surface area nomogram). Calculate cardiac index, stroke volume, stroke index, systemic vascular resistance, and pulmonary vascular resistance (see the formulas in Table 8-4). What is wrong with the patient?

Table 8-4. Common values calculated from hemodynamic measurements

Value	Formula*	Normal range
Cardiac index	$\dfrac{Q_T \text{ (L/min)}}{\text{Body surface area (m}^2\text{)}}$	2.8 to 4.2 L/min/m^2
Stroke volume	$\dfrac{Q_T \text{ (ml/min)}}{\text{Heart rate (beats/min)}}$	50 to 80 ml/beat
Stroke index (SI)	$\dfrac{\text{Stroke volume (ml/beat)}}{\text{m}^2}$	30 to 65 ml/beat/m^2
Left ventricular stroke work index	SI × (MSAP − PAWP) × 0.0136	43 to 61 gm-meters/m^2
Right ventricular stroke work index	SI × (MPAP − CVP) × 0.0136	7 to 12 gm-meters/m^2
Systemic vascular resistance†	$\dfrac{\text{MSAP} - \text{CVP (mm Hg)}}{Q_T \text{ (L/min)}}$	11 to 18 mm Hg/L/min
Pulmonary vascular resistance†	$\dfrac{\text{MPAP} - \text{PAWP (mm Hg)}}{Q_T \text{ (L/min)}}$	1.5 to 3.0 mm Hg/L/min
% Shunt	$\dfrac{C_{CO_2} - C_{aO_2}}{C_{CO_2} - C_{vO_2}}$	<5%
Oxygen uptake	$Q_T \times (C_{aO_2} - C_{vO_2})$	150 to 300 ml O$_2$/min

*MSAP, mean systemic arterial pressure; CVP, central venous pressure; MPAP, mean pulmonary artery pressure; PAWP, pulmonary artery wedge pressure (mean); m^2, square meters of body surface area; Q_T, cardiac output; C_{CO_2}, C_{aO_2}, and C_{vO_2}, oxygen content in end-capillary blood, arterial blood, and mixed venous blood, respectively.

†In many textbooks, the resistance formula is multiplied by a conversion factor of 80 to obtain resistance units of dynes × sec × cm^{-5}. Either formula is correct. When dynes × sec × cm^{-5} is used, the normal range for systemic vascular resistance (SVR) is approximately 880 to 1440 and for pulmonary vascular resistance (PVR) is approximately 150 to 240.

PULMONARY ARTERY WEDGE PRESSURE—MEASUREMENT

Although the Swan-Ganz catheter is used for several measurements (see Table 8-3), the most useful measurement is the pulmonary artery wedge pressure (PAWP). Many factors can influence this measurement, and its proper interpretation in critically ill patients is not a simple matter. At the very least, correctly using PAWP requires knowledge of the full clinical situation, plus some familiarity with how respiration can affect pulmonary blood flow. Before discussing clinical use of the PAWP, its actual measurement is discussed in greater detail.

To measure PAWP, the catheter tip with the balloon inflated is "wedged" into a branch of the pulmonary artery (see Figs. 8-5 and 8-6). When the flow of the column of blood is interrupted by the inflated balloon, the tip of the catheter measures *downstream pressure*. Since it is the pulmonary artery branch that is occluded, downstream pressure is the pulmonary *venous* pressure. Pulmonary venous pressure reflects left atrial pressure and, under certain conditions, left ventricular end-diastolic pressure. Changes in these three pressures can profoundly affect gas exchange, and since left-sided pressures are not directly measurable at the bedside, PAWP is the "window" through which these important pressures are viewed.

PAWP cannot accurately reflect left-side pressures unless it is measured accurately; an incorrectly recorded PAWP is worse than none at all. There are two principal ways to check that an accurate PAWP is being measured.

1. The pressure waveform obtained with the wedged catheter should be characteristic of left atrial pressure (Fig. 8-6) and should represent a distinct change from the pulmonary artery pressure tracing. The PAWP pressure tracing should appear only with the balloon inflated; as soon as the balloon is deflated, the pulmonary artery waveform should reappear.
2. The mean wedge pressure should be lower than or equal to the diastolic pulmonary artery pressure. A mean wedge pressure higher than the diastolic pulmonary artery pressure suggests that something other than true wedge pressure is being measured; this incorrect measurement may occur when the balloon is inflated in a very small arterial branch ("overwedging" the catheter).

Another method used to check for true wedge position, but one not widely practiced, is to aspirate blood from the catheter when the balloon is inflated. If the catheter is occluding the pulmonary artery, the blood aspirated from the distal tip comes from the downstream pulmonary capillaries and should be fully oxygenated (i.e., close to 100% saturated). By contrast, mixed venous blood (obtained from a nonwedged pulmonary artery position) should be relatively desaturated. However, the pressure generated during aspiration may draw blood from a pulmonary shunt, or the catheter tip may reside in a low ventilation/perfusion region; for these reasons a partially oxygenated blood sample does not rule out a true wedged position.

For technical reasons it is often difficult to obtain repeated measurements of PAWP; among reasons for this difficulty are catheter migration within the pulmonary artery and balloon rupture. When PAWP is within a few mm Hg of diastolic pulmonary artery pressure, the latter can usually substitute for PAWP. When diastolic pulmonary artery pressure is much higher than PAWP, pulmonary hypertension is present, and diastolic pulmonary artery pressure cannot substitute for wedge pressure.

Clinical problem 5

How would you interpret the following pressures (in mm Hg) obtained from Swan-Ganz catheterization? In which patients could diastolic pulmonary artery pressure substitute for PAWP?

    Patient A. PAP, 24/12; PAWP, 12
    Patient B. PAP, 35/23; PAWP, 11
    Patient C. PAP, 43/23; PAWP, 22

A major problem in hemodynamic monitoring

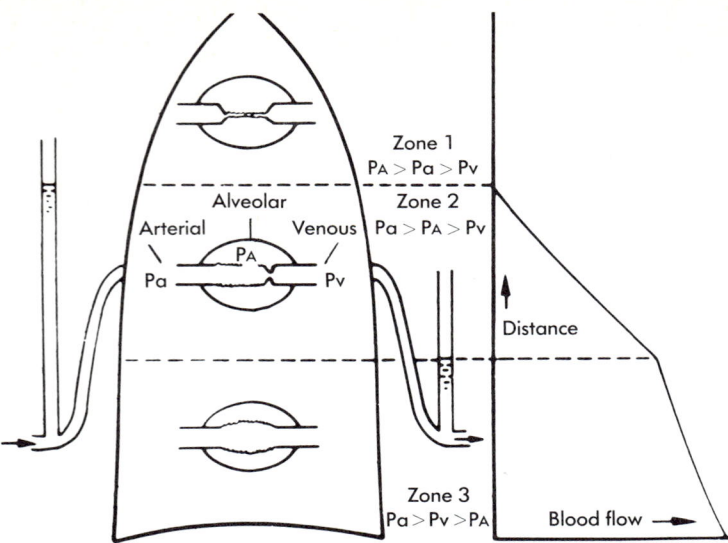

Fig. 8-8. Three zones of the lung in the upright position. See text for discussion. (From West, J.B., Dollery, C.T., and Naimark, A.: J. Appl. Physiol. **19**:713, 1964.)

is how to measure PAWP in a patient whose breathing is assisted by a ventilator, particularly if the patient is receiving positive end expiratory pressure (PEEP).* Do the increased airway pressures alter PAWP measurement?

The answer to this question depends on three main factors: (1) fluid status of the patient; (2) level of airway pressure; and (3) position of the Swan-Ganz catheter tip within the patient's thorax.

The relationship of pulmonary vascular pressures to alveolar pressures can be used to divide the lung into three zones (Fig. 8-8). Since gravity has a profound effect on blood flow within the lungs, in the upright lung there is relatively less blood flow per unit long volume at the apices than at the bases (see also Fig. 5-7). As a result, pulmonary artery pressure and blood flow are lowest at the top of the upright lung and highest at the bottom. By contrast, alveolar pressure is constant throughout the lung.

In Zone 1, near the top, the alveolar pressure (P_A) is greater than both the pulmonary artery (Pa) pressure and the pulmonary venous (Pv) pressure. As a result, there is no blood flow in Zone 1. Zone 1 is not normally present in healthy lungs, but in respiratory patients (particularly those receiving artificial ventilation) there may be a Zone 1 of varying size.

Much larger is Zone 2, where Pa is greater than P_A and where P_A is greater than Pv, at least during much of the respiratory cycle. Zone 2 blood vessels behave like collapsible tubes surrounded by a pressure chamber (so-called "Starling resistors"), so that blood flow is determined by the difference between the arterial pressure and the alveolar pressure. This pressure difference is perhaps best appreciated during positive pressure ventilation; when alveolar pressure rises in Zone 2 units, pulmonary capillary blood flow may cease and resume only when alveolar pressure falls. In any situation,

---

*PEEP is a ventilator maneuver that keeps airway pressure above atmospheric pressure throughout the breathing cycle and is discussed further in Chapters 9 and 10.

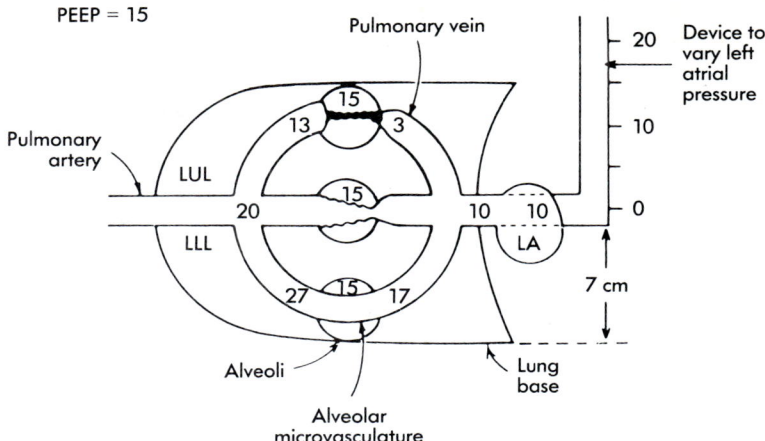

Fig. 8-9. Three zones of the lung in the supine position. This model assumes that a PEEP of 15 cm H_2O is transmitted to the alveoli and remains constant in all the alveoli. Vascular pressures vary depending on the vertical height of the blood column (and are given in cm H_2O for comparison with alveolar pressures). Pulmonary artery pressure is 13 cm H_2O at the top of the lung, 20 cm H_2O in the middle of the lung, and 27 cm H_2O at the bottom of the lung. This difference in vascular pressure, in relation to the constant alveolar pressure, creates the three zones. At the top of the lung *(Zone 1)*, there is no blood flow since alveolar pressure *(PA)* exceeds both pulmonary arterial pressure *(Pa)* and pulmonary venous pressure *(Pv)*. A small Zone 2 exists in the middle where Pa is greater than PA, but where PA is greater than, or close to, Pv. Finally, in Zone 3, both Pa and Pv exceed PA, and there is continuous blood flow. (*LUL,* left upper lung; *LLL,* lower left lung; *LA,* left atrium.) (From Tooker, J., Huseby, J., and Butler, J.: Am. Rev. Respir. Dis. **117:**721-725, 1978.)

as blood flow increases toward the bottom of the lung because of gravity, Pv approaches PA, and there is a decreasing tendency of blood vessels to collapse.

Finally, in Zone 3 Pv is always greater than PA (and still less than Pa), so pulmonary blood flow is uninterrupted, even during expiration.

The three-zone lung model's pressure relationships also hold true in the supine patient (Fig. 8-9). The left atrium serves to demarcate the three zones. Zone 2 is at or close to the level of the atrium. Zone 1 lies above the atrium because the blood flow there is reduced by gravity; below the atrium, where blood flow is increased because of gravity, is Zone 3. These zones are *not* fixed in size, but instead are affected by *both artificial ven-tilation and the patient's hemodynamic (fluid) status.*

Artificial ventilation, by increasing alveolar pressures, can convert areas of Zone 2 into Zone 1 and areas of Zone 3 into Zone 2. For example, when a ventilator pushes air into the lungs, alveolar pressure may increase to the point of cutting off all blood flow; during exhalation, when alveolar pressure decreases, blood flow may then resume; such alternation of blood flow would define a Zone 2 region. Where alveolar pressures are such that no blood flows during the breathing cycle, a Zone 1 area exists; conversely, Zone 3 is the area where alveolar pressures never cut off blood flow.

During artificial ventilation airway pressures are much greater than they are during normal breathing, and PA can increase so that it exceeds either Pv (creating a Zone 2) or Pa (creating a Zone 1). The higher the airway pressure that is generated by the ventilator (peak inspiratory pressure *or* end expiratory pressure), the higher the alveolar pressure, and the greater the effect on pulmonary blood flow. Although an increase in the size of Zones 1 and 2 is a predictable result of artificial ventilation, *neither the magnitude nor the clinical effect of the increases can be accurately predicted.* Arterial blood gas measurements must be monitored to assess the effects of artificial ventilation on gas exchange.

Hypovolemia, by lowering pulmonary vascular pressure, can also convert areas of Zone 3 into Zone 2 or areas of Zone 2 into Zone 1. Generally, the more dehydrated the patient, the smaller is Zone 3 and the larger are Zones 1 and 2. A combination of artificial ventilation and dehydration can create relatively large Zones 1 and 2 and a correspondingly smaller Zone 3.

Many studies have attempted to clarify how artificial ventilation and intravascular fluid status affect pulmonary artery wedge pressure (PAWP). If the Swan-Ganz catheter tip is in Zone 1 or in Zone 2, the positive alveolar pressure can give a falsely high reading of PAWP; in fact, alveolar pressure may be measured and not PAWP. If the patient is not receiving PEEP, this problem can usually be circumvented by measuring PAWP only at the end of exhalation (Fig. 8-10). Without PEEP, end-exhalation alveolar pressure will be atmospheric (0), and a true wedge pressure measurement should be obtained.

PAWP measurement is more complex when the patient is receiving PEEP because end-exhalation pressure is always above atmospheric pressure. Some authors have recommended that patients be taken off PEEP when PAWP is measured, but this is not a good idea if for no other reason than the patient needs the PEEP and removing it could worsen oxygenation. Furthermore, the patient will remain on PEEP at all other times, so PAWP should be known while PEEP is being used. There is no easy solution to this dilemma, but several studies provide some reassurance. In general, PEEP of 10 cm H_2O or less in a euvolemic patient does not influence PAWP to a significant degree. If there is concern that the patient is dehydrated, a fluid bolus (100 to 200 cc of intravenous saline) should be given before accepting a PAWP measurement as accurate.

More importantly, since the Swan-Ganz catheter is flow-directed, the catheter tip usually ends in

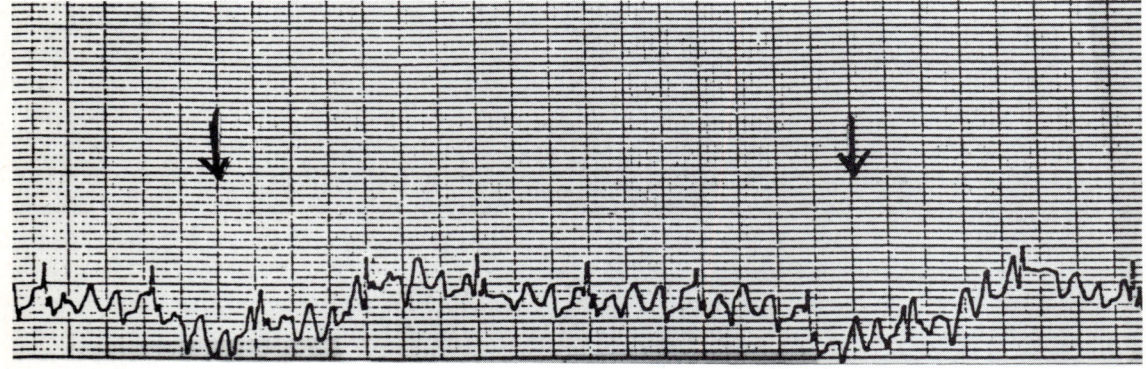

Fig. 8-10. Measurement of pulmonary artery wedge pressure (PAWP) during artificial ventilation. PAWP should be measured at the end of exhalation *(arrows),* where the influence from positive airway pressure is minimal.

Zone 3 where the influence of PEEP is minimal. (Since the vertical catheter position cannot be gauged with the routine anteroposterior chest x-ray film, some authors recommend obtaining a lateral film to check for catheter placement.) The important thing is to appreciate the potential influence of airway pressures and of PEEP on PAWP measurement and not to accept any measurement as valid without considering these influences.

PULMONARY ARTERY WEDGE PRESSURE—WHAT DOES IT REPRESENT?

The previous discussion deals mainly with artifact of measurement. Assuming an accurate, artifact-free pulmonary artery wedge pressure (PAWP) is measured, just what does it represent?

PAWP measurement is used to obtain information about the status of the left side of the heart and the pulmonary circulation distal to the catheter tip. There are thus two fundamental reasons for measuring PAWP: (1) as a guide to pulmonary capillary hydrostatic pressure, and (2) as a guide to filling pressures of the left atrium and ventricle.

Before the advent of Swan-Ganz catheterization in 1970, this hemodynamic information could be obtained only (at the bedside) by measurement of the central venous pressure (CVP). For CVP measurement a long catheter (approximately one third the length of a Swan-Ganz catheter) was placed in a large vein and then was connected to a vertical column of water. If there were no obstruction between the venous end of the catheter and the water column, the CVP was accurately recorded by observing the water level. Using this method, CVP in a healthy person is under 12 cm H_2O (under 10 mm Hg).

Before the ability to measure PAWP, the CVP was used to indicate the left atrial and pulmonary venous pressures on the assumption that these pressures were transmitted unchanged to the pulmonary arteries, the right side of the heart, and the central venous system. Experience with the Swan-Ganz catheter has shown this transmission of pressures

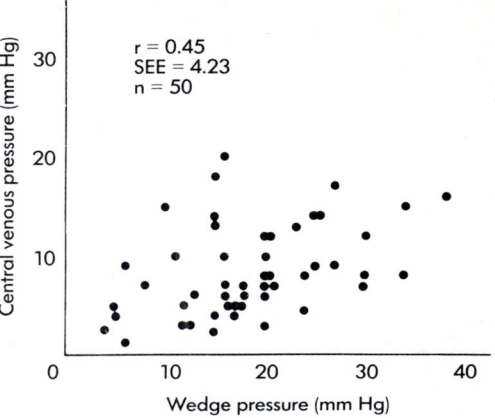

Fig. 8-11. Poor correlation between central venous pressure and pulmonary artery wedge pressure measurement. (*r*, Correlation of coefficient; *SEE*, standard error of estimate; *n*, number of patients studied.) (From Forrester, J.S., Diamond, G., McHugh, T.L., et al.: Reprinted by permission of N. Engl. J. Med. **285**:190-193, 1971.)

does *not* occur in many situations (Fig. 8-11). There is often a lack of correlation between CVP and PAWP, and it is now accepted that CVP is no substitute for PAWP in critically ill patients or in a patient with an acute myocardial infarction.

PAWP as a guide to pulmonary capillary hydrostatic pressure. Except when PAWP is elevated by artifact (as from artificial ventilation), PAWP is a measure of the capillary hydrostatic component that tends to force plasma fluid into the pulmonary interstitium. This force, usually between 6 and 12 mm Hg, is opposed by the capillary oncotic pressure (normal value, 20 to 25 mm Hg) so that fluid does not accumulate in the lungs. The higher the PAWP or the lower the capillary oncotic pressure, the greater is the leaking tendency.

Although oncotic pressure can be directly measured on a pulmonary artery blood sample with an oncometer, it can also be assessed by the serum total protein or albumin concentration (normal values, 6 to 8 gm% and 3.8 to 5.0 gm%, respectively). The serum protein concentration correlates with the measured oncotic pressure; if the proteins are low, oncotic pressure is also reduced. A low oncotic pressure per se should not lead to pulmonary edema, but it can definitely contribute to pulmonary edema arising from increased hydrostatic pressure.

In any event, when an imbalance in oncotic and hydrostatic forces results in pulmonary edema, measurement of PAWP can provide important therapeutic information. (The physiologic mechanisms in pulmonary edema are discussed further in Chapter 11.)

When the only contributor to pulmonary edema is increased hydrostatic pressure, there is a useful correlation between PAWP and the chest x-ray. If PAWP is less than 18 mm Hg the x-ray should not show any signs of pulmonary edema. The minimal to moderate changes caused by pulmonary edema (beginning with a slight vascular redistribution to the upper lobes) may be found when PAWP is between 18 to 25 mm Hg. Above 25 mm Hg, frank changes of pulmonary edema may be seen, and the higher the PAWP is the more severe the x-ray appearance. To make these correlations it is important that the chest x-ray be obtained close to the time that the PAWP is measured.

For example, if the chest x-ray shows definite pulmonary edema and if an accurate PAWP measurement is 10 mm Hg before the patient has received any treatment, the cause definitely is not left-sided heart failure. Conversely, if the PAWP measurement is 35 mm Hg and the chest x-ray film is perfectly clear, either the PAWP is in error or the chest x-ray belongs to someone else!

Clinical problem 6

Following is the initial wedge pressure in three different patients, along with their blood pressure readings and serum albumin levels (pressures are in mm Hg; serum albumin is in gm%). On the basis of physical examination and chest x-ray films, each patient is suffering from pulmonary edema.

Patient A. Blood pressure, 70/50; PAWP, 7; serum albumin, 4.1

Patient B. Blood pressure; 135/83; PAWP, 27; serum albumin, 3.4

Patient C. Blood pressure, 125/75; PAWP, 16; serum albumin, 2.6

In regard to capillary hydrostatic pressure as a cause of pulmonary edema, how do you interpret each wedge pressure measurement?

PAWP as a guide to left heart filling pressures. The relationship of PAWP to left heart hemodynamics is a complex one. This relationship can be simplified somewhat by examining the relationship between PAWP and left atrial pressure (LAP), left ventricular end-diastolic pressure (LVEDP), and left ventricular end-diastolic volume (LVEDV), which is a critical determinant of left ventricular function.

PAWP measurement would be most useful if the following were always true: (1) PAWP equals LAP equals LVEDP; and (2) LVEDP accurately reflects LVEDV so that an increase or a decrease in LVEDV proportionately changes LVEDP.

These ideal conditions are often assumed to be present during hemodynamic measurement, but in unhealthy patients they may not hold. Chronologic review of the Swan-Ganz literature reveals increasing sophistication in the understanding of this fact plus a better appreciation of the possible pitfalls in interpreting PAWP measurement.

Generally there is good correlation between PAWP and LAP, even in patients with heart disease, including those who have mitral stenosis. The difficulty arises in the correlation between PAWP and LVEDP. Before discussing this correlation, we will examine why it is important to know the LVEDP.

During diastole, blood from the left atrium flows past the mitral valve to fill the left ventricle. The more the myocardium is stretched, the more the blood volume that is ejected during systole increases. The degree of myocardial stretch at the end of diastole is often referred to as *preload*; with increasing preload, up to a point, the work produced by the myocardium (left ventricular stroke work) increases. This relationship is the essence of Starling's law of the heart (Fig. 8-12).

The degree of myocardial stretch is usually measured in vitro on isolated muscle preparations. In vivo, the degree of stretch correlates with the left ventricular end-diastolic volume (LVEDV). According to Starling's law, LVEDV is the left ventricular preload and bears the same relationship to left ventricular stroke work as does the degree of myocardial muscle stretch.

Stroke volume can also be substituted for left ventricular stroke work. Thus in vivo, Starling's law of the heart relates LVEDV to stroke volume (Fig. 8-13)—*the higher the LVEDV (up to a point), the higher the stroke volume*. Since cardiac output is the stroke volume times the heart rate, at a constant heart rate the same Starling relationship exists for LVEDV vs. cardiac output.

Shifts of the Starling curve can occur as a result of anything that alters myocardial contractility; the curve can be shifted to the left (increased contractility, as may occur from inotropic drugs) or to the right (decreased contractility, as may occur from myocardial infarction). A Starling curve shifted to the left will have an increased cardiac output for a given LVEDV; a curve shifted to the right will have a decreased cardiac output for a given LVEDV (Fig. 8-13).

Starling's law is often reinterpreted to relate left ventricular end-diastolic *pressure* (LVEDP) to cardiac output (Fig. 8-13). LVEDP is the "filling pressure" of the left ventricle, i.e., the left ventricular pressure at the end of diastole. As the filling pressure increases (presumably reflecting filling volume), cardiac output increases, again up to a point. *If* this relationship is true and *if* PAWP accurately reflects LVEDP, PAWP can then be used as a measure of left ventricular preload. As a measure of

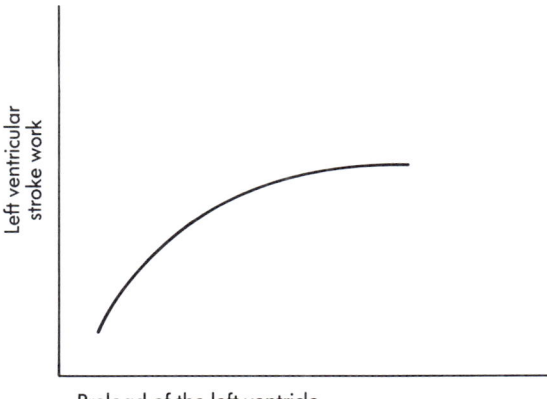

Fig. 8-12. The Starling curve relates the degree of myocardial stretch (measured as end-diastolic fiber length) to the degree of muscle work *(left ventricular stroke work)*. The former is the preload of the left ventricle and, in vivo, correlates with the left ventricular end-diastolic volume.

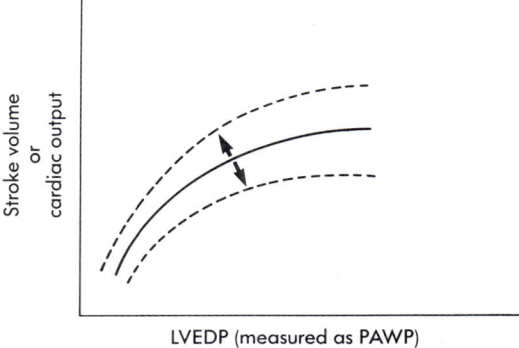

Fig. 8-13. The Starling curve in clinical practice. In clinical practice the stroke volume (or cardiac output) is used in place of left ventricular stroke work, and the left ventricular end-diastolic pressure (LVEDP) is used in place of left ventricular end-diastolic volume (LVEDV). This reinterpretation of the Starling curve allows pulmonary artery wedge pressure (PAWP) to serve as the basic measurement of left ventricular preload on the assumption that PAWP equals LVEDP and that LVEDP accurately reflects LVEDV. Changes in myocardial contractility affect the quantitative relationship between preload and stroke volume. The middle curve represents the normal relationship. Changes in contractility of the myocardium can displace the Starling curve to the left (increased contractility) or to the right (decreased contractility).

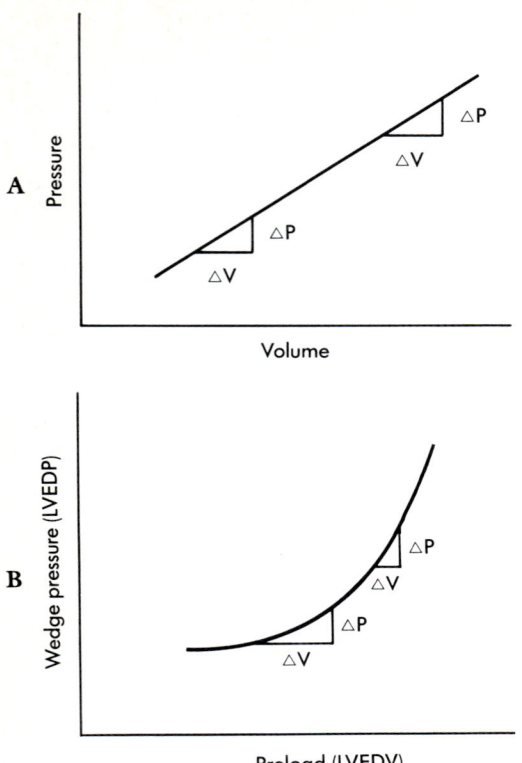

Fig. 8-14. Left ventricular compliance curve—LVEDV vs. LVEDP. **A,** Idealized ventricular compliance curve, a linear function. The same change in pressure at any part of the straight line reflects the same change in volume. **B,** Actual ventricular compliance curve, a curvilinear function. The same change in pressure at different parts of the curve reflects a different change in volume.

preload, PAWP can serve as a valuable guide to therapy.

Clinical problem 7

Two patients have reduced urine output and systemic hypotension. Assuming their problem is caused by hemodynamic instability, how would you manage each patient based on the following information?

        Patient A. PAWP, 4 mm Hg
        Patient B. PAWP, 28 mm Hg

In many cases PAWP accurately reflects left ventricular filling pressure (LVEDP) and can be used as a guide to patient management. However, the relation between LVEDP and LVEDV is not a straight line (Fig. 8-14, *A*) but instead is curvilinear (Fig. 8-14, *B*). Ventricular compliance is the change in volume (LVEDV) per the change in distending pressure (LVEDP). Because this relationship is not linear, a change in LVEDP (and hence PAWP) cannot be assumed to reflect accurately a change in ventricular preload; in Fig. 8-14, *B*, a small pressure change in the ascending limb of the curve reflects the same volume change as does a large pressure change near the top of the curve. Furthermore, ventricular compliance curves are greatly altered with heart disease so that relationships between pressure and volume can be even more distorted; in the low-compliant, stiff left ventricle, a high LVEDP may actually reflect a relatively small LVEDV.

Positive end expiratory pressure (PEEP) can also affect ventricular compliance by increasing the intrathoracic pressure so that the pressure surrounding the left ventricle is increased. This effect is similar to the one PEEP has on elevating PAWP. Normally, at end-exhalation, the thoracic pressure surrounding the left ventricle is at, or close to, atmospheric pressure (zero). With PEEP this surrounding pressure may be positive (above atmospheric). As a result, a higher than normal LVEDP will be required to achieve a given ventricular volume, and the ventricle's compliance will be reduced. Fig. 8-15 shows how changes in left ventricular preload may not be reflected in the LVEDP.

In summary, there are several situations where PAWP may *not* reflect the true preload (LVEDV) of the left ventricle. These situations are summarized in the box on p. 170. Obviously, the true relationship of PAWP (as measured with the Swan-Ganz catheter) and the left ventricular preload is a complex one, especially when the patient is receiving artificial ventilation or when there is altered left ventricular compliance. There is no easy way to account for the multitude of factors listed in the

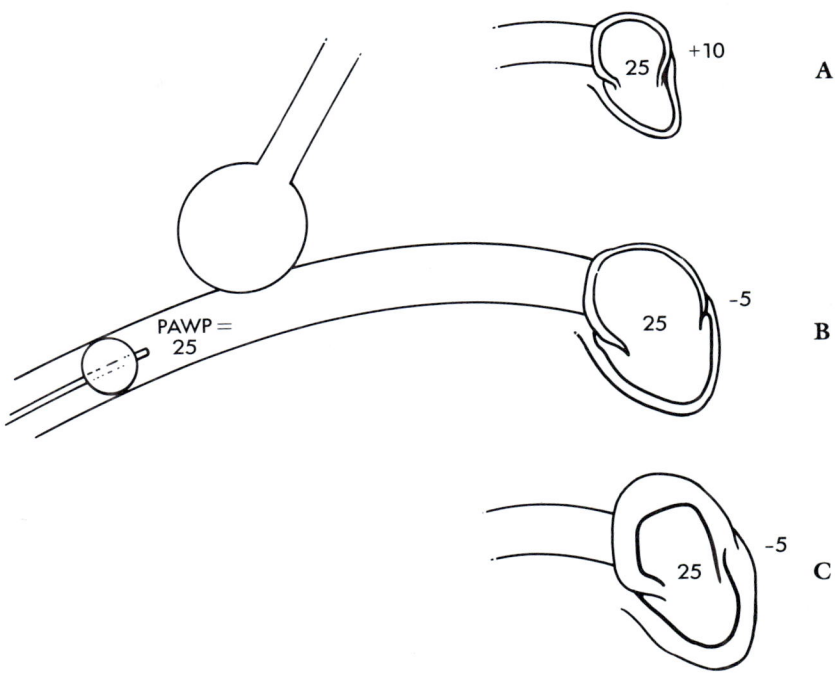

Fig. 8-15. The pulmonary artery wedge pressure (PAWP) reflects left ventricular end-diastolic pressure (LVEDP), but LVEDP may not accurately reflect left ventricular preload. The relationship is shown of the PAWP to the left ventricular preload (left ventricular volume) in three situations. In each situation PAWP is elevated to 25 mm Hg and accurately reflects an LVEDP of 25 mm Hg. **A,** The cause of the PAWP elevation is increased pleural pressure (+10 mm Hg), which might occur from positive end-expiratory pressure (PEEP) therapy. The increased pleural pressure adds to the LVEDP and is therefore reflected in the PAWP. However, the true left ventricular preload (left ventricular volume) is normal. **B,** The cause of PAWP elevation is an elevated left ventricular volume; pleural pressure is normal at −5 mm Hg. Thus PAWP accurately reflects an elevated left ventricular preload. **C,** The cause of PAWP elevation is a stiff left ventricle, which might occur from myocardial ischemia. PAWP and pleural pressure are the same as in **B,** and left ventricular preload (left ventricular volume) is normal. (Modified from O'Quin, R., and Marini, J.J.: Am. Rev. Respir. Dis. **128:**320, 1983.)

> **SITUATIONS WHERE PAWP MAY NOT ACCURATELY REFLECT LEFT VENTRICULAR PRELOAD***
>
> 1. **PAWP is less than LVEDP.**
>
>   Aortic regurgitation
>   Reduced left ventricular compliance (see number 3)
>
> 2. **PAWP is greater than LVEDP.**
>
>   When catheter tip is in Zone 1 or 2; may occur from artificial ventilation, with or without PEEP or from volume depletion
>   Atrial myxoma
>   Thoracic tumors pressing on pulmonary veins
>   Mitral stenosis or regurgitation
>   Increased left ventricular compliance (see number 3)
>
> 3. **PAWP equals LVEDP, but LVEDP does not correlate with LVEDV.**
>
> | *Decreased left ventricular compliance* | *Increased left ventricular compliance* |
> |---|---|
> | Increased right ventricular volume | Decreased right ventricular volume |
> | Pericardial tamponade | Removal of pericardium |
> | Some drugs, e.g., isoproterenol | Some drugs, e.g., nitroglycerin |
> | High LVEDV | Low LVEDV |
> | Tachycardia | Bradycardia |
> | PEEP | |
> | Myocardial ischemia and infarction | |
> | Myocardial hypertrophy | |
>
> *Ideal Situation—PAWP equals LAP equals LVEDP, and LVEDP is proportional to LVEDV. When this is true, PAWP can be used as a measure of left ventricular preload.

box except to follow the patient closely, gauging changes in cardiac output, oxygenation, and urine output with changes in wedge pressure. PAWP is another, albeit important, measurement, that should never substitute for intelligent clinical assessment of the patient.

PITFALLS AND COMPLICATIONS IN HEMODYNAMIC MONITORING

There are probably more pitfalls and complications from use of Swan-Ganz catheterization than from any other technique mentioned in this book. Some of the potential pitfalls were discussed in the previous section on pulmonary artery wedge pressure. Pitfalls are errors in judgment or management; complications refer to problems with the technique itself. The box on p. 171 lists the common pitfalls and complications of this technique.

This list is by no means complete, but it does represent most of the problems likely to be encountered. Despite the potential for problems, one should not hesitate to use hemodynamic monitoring in the right situation. Properly used, hemodynamic monitoring (including arterial cannulation and blood gas analysis) can provide an accurate physiologic picture of critically ill patients.

PITFALLS AND COMPLICATIONS IN HEMODYNAMIC MONITORING

Pitfalls (errors in judgment or management)

1. Inappropriate indications (when less invasive methods are just as good and when data will not change therapy)
2. Obtaining data incorrectly (inaccurate machine calibration and incorrect transducer placement)
3. Misusing data (improper interpretation of data obtained)
4. Not checking all relevant or related data before making therapeutic decisions (data such as chest x-ray, serum albumin, and urine output)
5. Not removing catheter when hemodynamic data are no longer used or are no longer useful in patient management

Complications from the technique

1. Ruptured or torn pulmonary or tricuspid valve
2. Pneumothorax (usually from subclavian insertion)
3. Pulmonary thrombosis and hemorrhage, including rupture of pulmonary artery
4. Right-sided endocardial damage (including hemorrhage, thrombus, and infection)
5. Knotting or kinking of catheter
6. Thrombosis in venous site of insertion
7. Cardiac arrhythmias, including heart block
8. Infection at site of insertion or at catheter tip
9. Balloon rupture
10. Loss of guide wire or portion of catheter within the venous system

HEMODYNAMIC MONITORING IN CLINICAL PRACTICE

Table 8-5 shows typical hemodynamic changes in some common clinical conditions; these changes represent the "pure" cases. Many patients have more than one problem, e.g., adult respiratory distress syndrome (discussed in Chapter 11) and left-sided heart failure. To make things even more complicated, pulmonary edema can be aggravated by low oncotic pressure.

Clinical problem 8

A 60-year-old diabetic woman is admitted to the hospital because of dehydration and a urinary tract infection. When admitted, her temperature is 100.7° F. Treatment is begun using antibiotics and intravenous fluids. On the morning of her third hospital day, she develops respiratory distress manifested by tachypnea, and her temperature rises to 102° F. Her blood pressure, normal on admission, falls to 88 mm Hg systolic. A chest x-ray film, also normal on admission, now shows bilateral infiltrates. She is transferred to the intensive care unit and a Swan-Ganz catheter is inserted through her right internal jugular vein. Initial measurements and calculations are as follows:

Pulmonary artery pressure	27 mm Hg systolic
	12 mm Hg diastolic
	21 mm Hg mean
Pulmonary artery wedge pressure	7 mm Hg
Cardiac output	6.3 L/min
Cardiac index	4.1 L/min/m^2
Systemic vascular resistance	8.3 mm Hg/L/min

How do you interpret these hemodynamic data?

Table 8-5. Some hemodynamic changes in common clinical conditions*

Condition	Chest x-ray infiltrates	SAP	SVR	QT	PAP	PAWP
Adult respiratory distress syndrome	Both sides	Variable	Variable	Variable	Variable	Normal to decreased
Left-sided heart failure	One or both sides	Normal to decreased	Increased	Decreased	Increased	Increased
Septic shock	None, one, or both sides	Decreased	Decreased	Increased	Normal to decreased	Normal to decreased
Dehydration	None	Decreased	Increased	Normal to decreased	Normal to decreased	Decreased
Pulmonary hypertension	None	Normal	Normal	Normal	Increased	Normal

*Many conditions overlap so that the typical hemodynamic changes may not manifest in an individual patient. For example, a patient with sepsis and heart failure may have decreased cardiac output; a patient with adult respiratory distress syndrome and heart failure may have an increased PAWP. SAP, systemic arterial pressure; SVR, systemic vascular resistance; QT, cardiac output; PAP, pulmonary arterial pressure; PAWP, pulmonary artery wedge pressure.

Clinical problem 9

A 68-year-old man is hospitalized following a cerebrovascular accident that has left him unable to speak or eat. The patient is alert and understands directions. His recovery is slowed by development of right lower lobe aspiration pneumonia; blood gas measurement shows a PaO_2 of 65 mm Hg while the patient is breathing nasal oxygen at 2 L/min. He is treated with intravenous fluids, antibiotics, and nasogastric feedings, but by the fourth hospital day his condition has deteriorated; his PaO_2 is now 55 mm Hg while breathing 50% oxygen through a face mask, and he is unresponsive. Portable chest x-ray shows bilateral infiltrates compatible with pneumonia. The patient is intubated and provided artificial ventilation.

At this point differential diagnosis includes bilateral pneumonia, adult respiratory distress syndrome, and congestive heart failure. A Swan-Ganz catheter and arterial line are placed and the following information is obtained:

Pulmonary artery pressures	35 mm Hg systolic
	23 mm Hg diastolic
	29 mm Hg mean
Systemic artery pressures	140 mm Hg systolic
	72 mm Hg diastolic
	100 mm Hg mean
Pulmonary artery wedge pressure	22 mm Hg mean
Central venous pressure	10 mm Hg
Cardiac output	5.4 L/min
Cardiac index	3.1 L/min/m^2
Systemic vascular resistance	19 mm Hg/L/min

How do you interpret these data?

Clinical problem 10

A comatose 65-year-old man is brought to the emergency room. Initial blood gas analysis reveals marked respiratory acidosis, with pH of 7.05, $Paco_2$ of 86 mm Hg, and Pao_2 of 36 mm Hg (FIo_2 of 0.21). The patient is intubated and is transferred to the intensive care unit. His chest x-ray shows clear lung fields and a slightly enlarged heart. Because of his very small urine output and systemic hypotension, a Swan-Ganz catheter and an arterial cannula are placed in the patient.

Initial and subsequent hemodynamic data are shown below. During a 10-hr period, the patient received intravenous dextrose and saline at a rate of approximately 200 ml/hr. How do you interpret these data?

	1 PM	3 PM	11 PM
Pulmonary arterial pressure (mm Hg)	53/26	50/25	48/24
Pulmonary artery wedge pressure (mm Hg)	9	14	16
Systemic arterial pressure (mm Hg)	95/65	110/73	115/75
Cardiac output, L/min	4.5	4.8	5.1
Cardiac index, L/min/m²	2.7	2.8	2.9
Tidal volume (cc)	800	800	800
Respiratory rate/min	12	12	12
FIo_2	0.50	0.40	0.40
pH	7.23	7.35	7.38
$Paco_2$ (mm Hg)	65	58	51
Pao_2 (mm Hg)	123	90	94

SUMMARY

In contrast to the systemic circulation, the pulmonary circulation is a low pressure, high capacitance system. Pulmonary hypertension, a common physiologic problem, can be found in many different diseases, including virtually all chronic heart and lung conditions. Mechanisms of pulmonary hypertension include hypoxemia, loss of pulmonary vasculature, increased pulmonary capillary hydrostatic pressure, and pulmonary artery narrowing.

Bedside measurement of pulmonary artery pressures and resistances and measurement of right ventricular cardiac output can be obtained with the balloon-tipped, flow-directed (Swan-Ganz) right heart catheter. In selected patients, Swan-Ganz catheterization can provide useful information about hemodynamic status. The most frequently obtained Swan-Ganz measurement is pulmonary artery wedge pressure (PAWP). Under ideal conditions PAWP reflects the left atrial and the left ventricular filling pressures and the left ventricular preload (left ventricular volume); at such times PAWP is a valid guide to fluid therapy. In some situations, however, such as when positive end-expiratory pressure is being delivered or when left ventricular compliance is reduced, PAWP may not accurately reflect left ventricular preload and may give a false impression of the patient's fluid status. PAWP measurement must be interpreted cautiously and must always be evaluated in conjunction with the full clinical, radiologic, laboratory, and hemodynamic picture.

Apart from the improper interpretation of Swan-Ganz data, another potential pitfall involves leaving the catheter in place beyond its period of clinical usefulness. In addition, many complications can occur with Swan-Ganz catheterization, including venous thrombosis, pulmonary hemorrhage, and cardiac arrhythmias.

REVIEW QUESTIONS

State whether each of the following is true or false.

1. Normal pulmonary artery pressure is one half the systemic artery pressure.
2. Pulmonary artery pressure will increase in the presence of arterial hypoxemia and decrease in the presence of arterial acidosis.
3. Swan-Ganz catheterization allows for direct measurement of left ventricular pressures.
4. Hallmarks of septic shock are elevated cardiac output and reduced systemic vascular resistance.
5. If available, hemodynamic monitoring is indicated for all cases of severe dehydration.
6. The Swan-Ganz catheter can be used to obtain a sample of mixed venous blood from the pulmonary artery.
7. Cor pulmonale is right-sided heart failure caused by pulmonary hypertension.
8. The pulmonary artery wedge pressure is used to calculate pulmonary vascular resistance.
9. In primary pulmonary hypertension, the pulmonary artery diastolic pressure is higher than the pulmonary artery wedge pressure.
10. Pulmonary edema may occur without an elevation of pulmonary artery wedge pressure.

References

Enson, Y., Giuntini, C., Lewis, M.L., et al.: The influence of hydrogen ion concentration and hypoxia on the pulmonary circulation, J. Clin. Invest. **43**:1146, 1964.

Forrester, J.S., Diamond, G., McHugh, T.J., et al.: Filling pressures in the right and left sides of the heart in acute myocardial infarction, N. Engl. J. Med. **285**:190, 1971.

Grossman, W.G., editor: Cardiac catheterization and angiography; Philadelphia, 1980, Lea & Febiger.

Matthay, R.A., and Berger, H.J.: Cardiovascular performance in chronic obstructive pulmonary diseases, Med. Clin. North Am. **65**(3):489, 1981.

O'Quin, R., and Marini, J.J.: Pulmonary artery occlusion pressure: clinical physiology, measurement, and interpretation, Am. Rev. Respir. Dis. **128**:319, 1983.

Swan, H.J.C., Ganz, W., Forrester, J.S., et al.: Catheterization of the heart in man with use of a flow-directed balloon-tipped catheter, N. Engl. J. Med. **283**:447, 1970.

Tooker, J., Huseby, J., and Butler, J.: The effect of Swan-Ganz catheter height on the wedge pressure-left atrial pressure relationship in edema during positive-pressure ventilation, Am. Rev. Respir. Dis. **117**:721, 1978.

West, J.B., Dollery, C.T., and Naimark, A.: Distribution of blood flow in isolated lung: relation to vascular and alveolar pressures, J. Appl. Physiol. **19**:713, 1964.

Suggested readings

Connors, A.F., Castele, R.J., Farhat, N.Z., et al.: Complications of right heart catheterization: a prospective autopsy study, Chest **88**:567, 1985.

Connors, A.F., McCaffree, D.R., and Gray, B.A.: Evaluation of right-heart catheterization in the critically ill patient acute myocardial infarction, N. Engl. J. Med. **308**:263, 1983.

Eaton, R.J., Taxman, R.M., and Avioli, L.V.: Cardiovascular evaluation of patients treated with PEEP, Arch. Intern. Med. **143**:1958, 1983.

Elliott, C.G., Zimmerman, G.A., and Clemmer, T.P.: Complications of pulmonary artery catheterization in the care of critically ill patients: a prospective study, Chest **76**:647, 1979.

Forrester, J.S., Diamond, G., Chatterjee, K., et al.: Medical therapy of acute myocardial infarction by application of hemodynamic subsets, N. Engl. J. Med. **295**:1356, 1976.

Jardin, E., Farcot, J.C., Boisante, I., et al.: Influence of positive endexpiratory pressure on left ventricular performance, N. Engl. J. Med. **304**:387, 1981.

Raper, R., and Sibbald, W.J.: Misled by the wedge? The Swan-Ganz catheter and left ventricular preload, Chest **89**:427, 1986.

Rowley, K.M., Clubb, K.S., Smith, G.J., el. al.: Right-sided infective endocarditis as a consequence of flow-directed pulmonary-artery catheterization, N. Engl. J. Med. **311**:1152, 1984.

Shaver, J.A.: Hemodynamic monitoring in the critically ill patient, N. Engl. J. Med. **308**:277, 1983.

Sprung, C.L., editor: The pulmonary artery catheter: methodology and clinical applications, Baltimore, 1983, University Park Press.

Swan, H.J.C.: The role of hemodynamic monitoring in the management of the critically ill, Crit. Care Med. **3**:83, 1975.

Timms, R.M., Khaja, F.U., and Williams, G.W.: Hemodynamic response to oxygen therapy in chronic obstructive pulmonary disease, Ann. Intern. Med. **102**:29, 1985.

Weil, M.H. and Rackow, E.C.: Critical care medicine: caveat emptor, Arch. Intern. Med. **143**:1391, 1983.

Wiedemann, H.P., Matthay, M.A., and Matthay, R.A.: I. Cardiovascular-pulmonary monitoring in the intensive care unit, Chest **85**:537, 1984.

Wiedemann, H.P., Matthay, M.A., and Matthay, R.A.: II. Cardiovascular-pulmonary monitoring in the intensive care unit, Chest **85**:656, 1984.

See also General References in Appendix G.

chapter 9

Oxygen therapy

OUTLINE

Oxygen as a drug
Terminology in oxygen therapy
When to institute oxygen therapy
Classification of oxygen therapy
Low-supplemental FIO_2 therapy
High-supplemental FIO_2 therapy
Potential harm from oxygen therapy
Positive airway pressure and oxygen therapy
Hyperbaric oxygen
Monitoring oxygen therapy—clinical signs and PaO_2
Blood transfusion—effect on PaO_2 and oxygen content
Artificial blood
Methods of home oxygen therapy
Indications for home oxygen therapy

OXYGEN AS A DRUG

When used in medical therapy, oxygen is a drug. Like any drug, it has certain indications, contraindications, and harmful effects (see the box on p. 176). Oxygen is also one of the oldest drugs, having been used for therapeutic intent since shortly after its discovery in 1774 (see Introduction). In the entire nineteenth century, oxygen therapy, when given at all, was apt to be accompanied by totally unfounded claims and consequently dismal results (Fig. 9-1). In fact, only in the last two decades has the medical profession learned to use oxygen wisely; this use has been made possible by the widespread availability of blood gas measurement and the broader understanding of pulmonary physiology.

The partial pressure of oxygen in arterial blood (PaO_2) can be thought of as the drug level; unlike most drug levels, the PaO_2 measurement is usually available within minutes from an arterial blood sample. This measurement allows the effects of oxygen therapy to be followed closely, and to avoid both underoxygenating and overoxygenating the patient.

Virtually every hospital now has liquid oxygen piped from a central source into the patient rooms. Liquid systems have largely replaced the individual green tanks or cylinders that contain dry oxygen gas under high pressure, which were commonplace in all hospitals. Oxygen is 100% pure and dry when it leaves the wall outlet. By the time the oxygen reaches the patient, it usually has been humidified and diluted with room air (Fig. 9-2).

In years past, oxygen was occasionally combined with carbon dioxide and administered as "carbogen," a mixture no longer used. A helium-oxygen mixture is also sometimes used in patients with severe obstructive lung disease; the rationale is that low-density helium, which replaces the higher-density nitrogen, allows oxygen to enter obstructed airways more easily (Spearman, Sheldon, and Egan, 1982). Although the helium-oxygen mixture has its advocates, the mixture is not widely

> **OXYGEN AS A DRUG**
>
> **Indications**
>
> Low arterial partial pressure of oxygen (PaO_2) and/or low percent saturation of oxygen in arterial blood (SaO_2)
>
> **Contraindications**
>
> In premature infants unless hypoxemia is life-threatening; in adults when PaO_2 or SaO_2 is adequate and there is no clinically significant stress on the cardiopulmonary system
>
> **Dose**
>
> Fraction of inspired oxygen (FIO_2) above 0.21, up to 1.00
>
> **Method of administration**
>
> As inhaled gas, either at ambient barometric pressure or under positive (above atmospheric) pressure
>
> **Blood level**
>
> Measured as PaO_2; normal PaO_2 is age-dependent and ranges from 70 to 100 mm Hg while patient is breathing ambient air at sea level
>
> **Harmful effects**
>
> Time- and FIO_2-dependent; may manifest as (1) pulmonary toxicity, (2) blunting of hypoxic drive (in hypercapnic patients), (3) absorption atelectasis, or (4) retrolental fibroplasia in premature infants

Regardless of the fraction of inspired oxygen (FIO_2), supplemental oxygen must be humidified by bubbling the gas through a sterile water supply that is attached at the source of the oxygen (e.g., near the wall outlet, as in Fig. 9-2). Medical oxygen is a dry gas; the humidity added to the gas should at least match the humidity present in the room air to prevent drying and crusting of the patient's secretions. If the upper airway is bypassed by a tracheostomy or an endotracheal tube, the inspired oxygen must be both thoroughly humidified and warmed (usually to approximately 30° C).

As with any drug, both a dose and a route of delivery must be designated when prescribing oxygen. The dose of solid or liquid drugs is given in milligrams or in some other unit of weight and is usually administered orally or parenterally (intravenous or intramuscular). Oxygen dosage, on the other hand, is expressed as FIO_2 and is administered by inhalation only.* Even though inhalation is the only route for oxygen therapy, the apparatus to deliver the gas must still be chosen—e.g., nasal cannula, face mask, or artificial ventilator.

Another difference in prescribing oxygen, compared with most medications, is it is needed continuously. Oxygen lack cannot be corrected by a "twice a day" dosage or a "prn" (as needed) order.† To be of benefit, supplemental oxygen must be inhaled continuously. The body does not store any significant amount of oxygen; once the patient is removed from supplemental oxygen, his blood level (PaO_2) will fall within minutes to room air value.

---

*In the nineteenth century oxygen was also given by enema, intraperitoneally, and subcutaneously; all methods were ineffective. Today supplemental oxygen is occasionally applied directly to gangrenous or pregangrenous limbs to promote healing and prevent further tissue destruction. Except for local application purposes, the only noninhalation method used today is extracorporeal membrane oxygenation during cardiac bypass.

†Intermittent dosage was the *only* way supplemental oxygen was prescribed in the nineteenth century. Despite its clear lack of benefit from a physiologic perspective, oxygen therapy was nonetheless claimed as a panacea for a wide variety of respiratory and nonrespiratory conditions (see Fig. 9-1).

used in medical practice and is not discussed further here.

Oxygen is routinely mixed with anesthetic gases, but this mixture is confined mainly to the operating room. Apart from this use and the occasional use of the helium-oxygen mixture mentioned above, oxygen is always administered either pure (100%) or diluted with ordinary air.

Oxygen, or Vital Air,

IN THE
CURE OF DISEASES:

TO WHICH ARE ADDED,
A FEW EXPERIMENTS

ON THE
VEGETATION OF PLANTS,

ILLUSTRATED WITH FIVE ENGRAVINGS.

By DANIEL HILL, M.D. SURGEON,
HONORARY MEMBER OF THE MEDICAL SOCIETY AT GUY'S HOSPITAL,
AND FELLOW OF THE HORTICULTURAL SOCIETY.

Sed ne verba dare nos discat quispiam, et assertiones speciosas tantum facere sine fundamento, et non justa de causa innovare: **tria confirmanda veniunt**: quibus positis, necessario hanc sequi veritatem, et rem palam esse arbitror.—Harvey, Exercitatio Anatomica de Motu Cordis, caput nonum.

THE SECOND EDITION, WITH AN APPENDIX.

London:
PRINTED FOR F. C. & J. RIVINGTON,
ST. PAUL'S CHURCH-YARD, AND WATERLOO-PLACE, PALL-MALL;
T. CADELL, STRAND; J. HATCHARD, PICCADILLY; AND
J. CALLOW, PRINCE'S STREET, SOHO.

1820.

Fig. 9-1. Cover from an 1820 monograph on oxygen therapy. Another century would elapse before oxygen would be used in a scientific manner. (Translation of Latin quote: "But lest anyone say that we cheat and merely make plausible assertions without a basis and advance new views without a just cause, there are three suppositions which come up for confirmation. If these are stated, then I think the truth which I advocate automatically follows and the fact is plain to all." [From Harvey, W.: Movement of the heart and blood, an anatomic essay, 1957. Courtesy of Charles C Thomas, Publisher, Springfield, Ill. Translated by K.J. Franklin.])

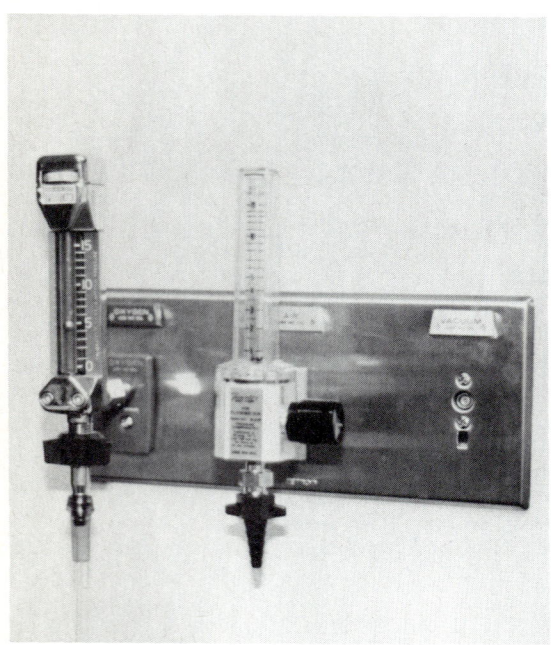
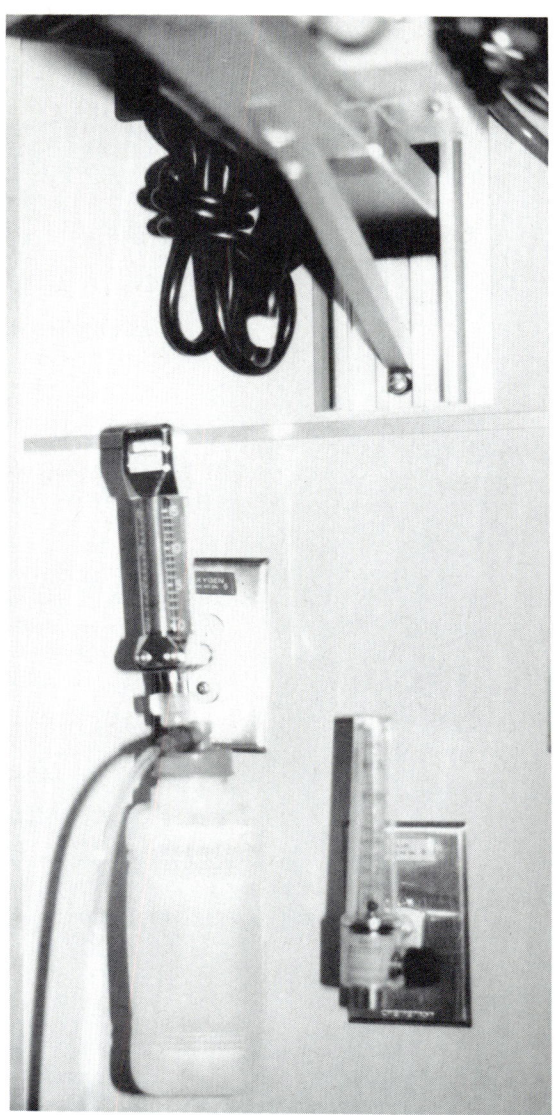

Fig. 9-2. One hundred percent oxygen is delivered from the wall source (piped in from a central supply of liquid oxygen) to the patient. **A,** An oxygen gauge *(left)* without a source of humidification attached; oxygen may be used in this manner for short periods of time, e.g., a few hours. For continuous therapy (as in virtually all hospitalized patients), it is necessary to provide humidification. **B,** An oxygen gauge with a bottle of sterile water attached; oxygen bubbled through this apparatus is thus humidified. The tubing leading from the bottle can be connected to any type of oxygen appliance (see Figs. 9-3 and 9-4).

Clinical problem 1

Given the following information, calculate how long it would take an apneic individual to use half his oxygen supply. Assume that before the patient's apnea the FIO_2 was 0.21.

Functional residual capacity, 3 L; total blood volume, 5 L; arterial oxygen content, 20 ml O_2/100 ml; metabolic oxygen uptake, 250 ml O_2/min.

TERMINOLOGY IN OXYGEN THERAPY

FIO_2 vs. percent. The FIO_2 is the fraction of inspired oxygen, which is written as a decimal, e.g., 0.21 or 0.40. Oxygen is also referred to as a percentage, e.g., 21% or 40%. When prescribing oxygen therapy, either term (FIO_2 or percentage) is appropriate, and these terms are often used interchangeably. In this book, FIO_2, meaning a decimal fraction, is frequently used. At other times oxygen may be referred to as a percentage.

Low- vs. high-oxygen therapy. An FIO_2 between 0.21 and 0.40 is usually called *low*, which is sometimes confusing since low ought to imply an FIO_2 of *less than* 0.21. To avoid confusion, either the FIO_2 should be specified or the wording qualified, e.g., low-supplemental FIO_2.

More confusing perhaps is that the terms "low flow" and "high flow" are sometimes used instead of specifying an FIO_2. *Flow* is another of those overworked terms, like ventilation and shunt, that often lack precise meaning. Flow may refer to the L/min at which oxygen exits from the wall outlet or to the L/min at which the enriched air flows past the patient's face. Flow or flow rate does not equate with the FIO_2, and such terms should not be used in lieu of a specific FIO_2.

Technically, a *low-flow oxygen system* is one in which some of the patient's inspired air comes from the room air; the oxygen system is not able to deliver all the air the patient inspires. Oxygen delivery through a nasal cannula or nasal prongs is a good example—some of the inspired air is pure oxygen, and the rest is from unenriched (room) air.

A *high-flow oxygen system* delivers all the inspired air, so that the patient inhales no room air. A Venturi face mask is an example of this system.

With any flow system, the supplemental FIO_2 may be high or low. When prescribing oxygen, one should first decide what FIO_2 the patient needs. Only then does it make sense to decide on the method of oxygen delivery.

WHEN TO INSTITUTE OXYGEN THERAPY

Ambient air has an FIO_2 of 0.21, regardless of the altitude. *Oxygen therapy* means to prescribe some enrichment of the inspired air so that the FIO_2 is above 0.21; this enrichment is also called *supplemental oxygen*. There is no specific blood gas value that calls for instituting oxygen therapy. Generally, symptomatic patients with SaO_2 less than 90% or PaO_2 less than 60 mm Hg should receive supplemental oxygen; this recommendaton includes patients whose work of breathing has increased in order to maintain an adequate SaO_2.

Even accepting these guidelines for oxygen therapy, clinical application is variable. A patient's symptoms may not always be clearly caused by oxygen lack. Conversely, many patients with an SaO_2 less than 90% have no symptoms. In practice, some patients are also prescribed oxygen without their necessarily manifesting hypoxemia. Examples include suspected heart attack patients and asthmatic patients who are receiving treatment for bronchospasm. An FIO_2 between 0.21 and 0.40 is usually harmless unless the patient has carbon dioxide retention.

Clinical problem 2

Which of the following patients would likely benefit from supplemental oxygen? All blood gas values are measured with the patient breathing room air (FIO_2, 0.21); RR is the respiratory rate.
a. A 54-year-old man with chronic obstructive pulmonary disease who is comfortable at rest; his baseline blood gas values show a PaO_2 of 44 mm Hg, a $PaCO_2$ of 53, an SaO_2 of 83%, and an RR of 20.

b. A 33-year-old patient with chronic renal insufficiency and a hemoglobin of 5 gm%; blood gas values show a PaO_2 at rest of 67 mm Hg, a $PaCO_2$ of 29 mm Hg, an SaO_2 of 91%, and an RR of 22.
c. A 27-year-old man with pneumonia; blood gas values while breathing room air show a PaO_2 of 67 mm Hg, a $PaCO_2$ of 28 mm Hg, an SaO_2 of 93%, and an RR of 32.
d. A 78-year-old woman suffering from chronic dementia; blood gas values show a PaO_2 of 72 mm Hg, a $PaCO_2$ of 38 mm Hg, an SaO_2 of 93%, a pH of 7.41, and an RR of 18.
e. A 52-year-old woman with chronic congestive heart failure; blood gas values are a PaO_2 of 54 mm Hg, a $PaCO_2$ of 31 mm Hg, an SaO_2 of 90%, a pH of 7.51, and an RR of 26.

CLASSIFICATION OF OXYGEN THERAPY

The box below presents a simple physiologic classification of oxygen therapy as used in clinical practice. Although the devices and the techniques used to deliver oxygen change over the years, the basic physiology of oxygen therapy does not. This classification takes into account the two major decisions made whenever oxygen therapy is prescribed—the amount of supplemental oxygen (FIO_2) to use and the method or device used to deliver the FIO_2.

LOW-SUPPLEMENTAL FIO_2 THERAPY

In severely hypoxemic patients, low-supplemental FIO_2 therapy can be effective because of the shape of the oxygen dissociation curve in the region of low PaO_2, i.e., less than 60 mm Hg (see Chapter 6). A small increase in PaO_2, from 45 to 55 mm Hg, will increase the SaO_2 and the oxygen content appreciably without significantly reducing the hypoxic breathing stimulus. Ideally, an FIO_2 as close to 0.21 as possible should be administered that will (1) improve the patient's oxygenation and (2) not raise arterial partial pressure of carbon dioxide ($PaCO_2$) more than a few mm Hg.

Any patient in need of supplemental oxygen who is retaining carbon dioxide but who does not require artificial ventilation should receive low-supplemental FIO_2. There are two widely used devices, the nasal cannula and the Venturi face mask, that allow 100% oxygen from the source to mix with

---

CLASSIFICATION OF OXYGEN THERAPY

AMOUNT OF SUPPLEMENTAL FIO_2

1. Low—more than 0.21, less than 0.40
2. High—0.40 or greater

DEVICE OR METHOD OF DELIVERY (any of the following may be used to deliver either low- or high-supplemental FIO_2)

1. Ambient air pressure
   A. Low-flow system, e.g., nasal cannula, some face masks
   B. High-flow system, e.g., Venturi face masks
2. Positive airway pressure
   A. Continuous positive airway pressure (no machine ventilation)
   B. Intermittent positive pressure ventilation (artificial or machine ventilation)
   C. Hyperbaric chamber

room air so that the FIO_2 reaching the patient is less than 40%.

Nasal cannula

A nasal cannula (also called nasal prongs) fits comfortably inside a patient's nostrils (Fig. 9-3). Oxygen delivered through the cannula at 1 to 3 L/min is usually considered low-supplemental FIO_2, although the actual FIO_2 may be above 0.40. A given liter flow cannot be precisely correlated with an FIO_2 because the final FIO_2 is a mixture of 100% oxygen inhaled from the nasal cannula plus a varying amount of room air (FIO_2, 0.21). The amount of room air depends on the patient's pattern of breathing, including the tidal volume and the time taken for each inspiration. There is no widely accepted method for calculating or estimating nasal cannula FIO_2 even when all these factors are considered.

Shapiro, Harrison, Kacmarek, et al. (1985) propose the following method for calculating FIO_2. (This method is presented here for didactic purposes to illustrate the influence of the breathing pattern on FIO_2.) An "anatomic reservoir" is in the patient's upper airways and is assumed to be approximately 50 cc in size (one third of anatomic dead space); this area includes the nasal passages and the throat area behind the mouth and nose. The anatomic reservoir is generally filled with 100% oxygen from the nasal cannula; this oxygen is inhaled at the beginning of each tidal volume breath. Assume the following: tidal volume, 600 ml; inspiratory time, 1 sec; and nasal oxygen flow rate, 3 L/min or 50 ml/second.

Each tidal volume breath then consists of 50 ml reservoir oxygen (100% oxygen) plus 50 ml nasal flow oxygen (100% oxygen) plus 500 ml room air (21% oxygen). Calculating the final FIO_2 (0.XX):

Reservoir + Nasal + Room air = Final
oxygen   oxygen   oxygen   oxygen.

50 (1.00) + 50 (1.00) + 500 (0.21) = 600 (0.XX)

$$0.XX = \frac{205}{600} = 0.34 \text{ or } 34\% \text{ oxygen}$$

The final FIO_2 depends heavily on the patient's tidal volume and respiratory rate, with the latter a determinant of the inspiratory time. For this reason, a specific FIO_2 cannot be assumed from a nasal cannula flow rate.

Clinical problem 3

Calculate the FIO_2 for the following situations. Assume that the anatomic reservoir is 50 ml and that it stays filled with 100% oxygen.

a. A patient with severe chronic obstructive pulmonary disease is prescribed nasal oxygen at 2 L/min; tidal volume is 300 ml and inspiratory time is 1 second.

b. A patient with pneumonia is given nasal oxygen at 2 L/min; tidal volume is 500 ml and inspiratory time is 1 second.

c. A patient with chest pain is given nasal oxygen at 2 L/min; tidal volume is 600 ml and inspiratory time is 1.5 seconds.

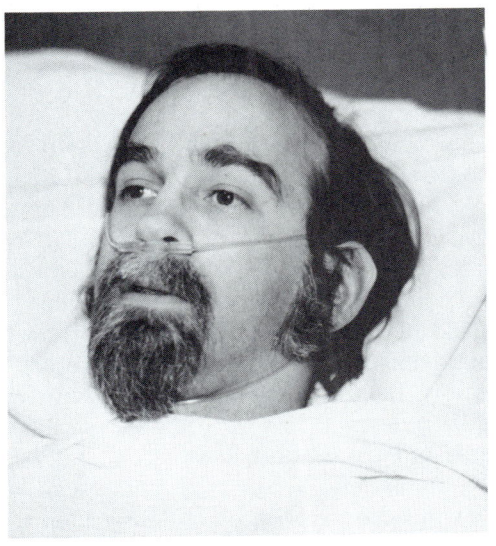

Fig. 9-3. Nasal cannula used for oxygen therapy.

Venturi face mask

Patients with unstable respiratory failure and hypercapnia often breathe as a result of an hypoxic stimulus; a high FIO_2 can remove this stimulus and can result in a decreased drive to breathe. At the time this effect was discovered, available face masks delivered too high an FIO_2. In the quest for better control, a new type of mask was introduced in the 1960's—the Venturi face mask (Fig. 9-4).

The Venturi face mask works on the Bernoulli principle—when a stream of gas is pushed through a narrow orifice, the pressure on the outside of the stream *falls* as a result of the increased velocity of gas passing through the restricted orifice. Any other gas in the vicinity of this reduced pressure will be entrained by the speeding gas stream. In the Venturi mask, a specified liter flow of pure oxygen enters the base of the mask through a narrowed orifice; just past this orifice are openings for room air to enter (entrained by the Bernoulli effect) and to mix with the oxygen (Fig. 9-5). The critical feature of the mask is the size of the opening through which oxygen enters the base of the mask.

The liter flow of oxygen is not critical in the Venturi mask, although it must be in a specified range. For example, the 0.24 Venturi mask is designed to deliver an FIO_2 of 0.24 to the patient's face if the flow rate of oxygen entering the base of the mask is 3 to 5 L/min. A flow rate in this range with the 0.24 Venturi mask will entrain 25 L of room air for every liter flow of oxygen. In the following calculation, the figures in parentheses represent FIO_2; 0.XX is the new FIO_2 achieved with the Venturi face mask.

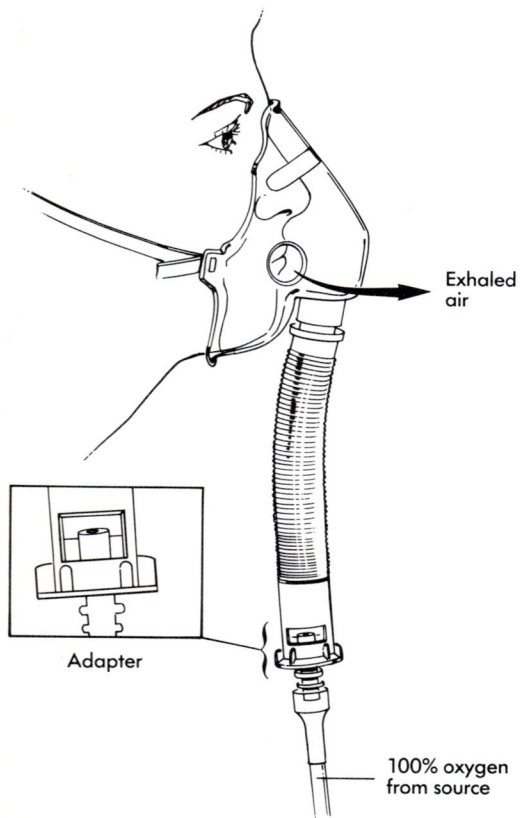

Fig. 9-4. Venturi face mask. Adapters for the mask are shown in Fig. 9-5. Changing the adapter *(inset)* and the oxygen flow rate will change the fraction of inspired oxygen received by the patient (see Table 9-1).

4 L/min	+	100 L/min	=	104 L/min
(1.00)		(0.21)		(0.XX)
(From oxygen source)		(Entrained air)		(Final oxygen flow)

$$0.XX = \frac{25 \text{ L/min}}{104 \text{ L/min}} = 0.24$$

The ability to deliver fairly precise FIO_2 is but one advantage of this mask. The other is high airflow, i.e., a high liter flow of enriched air past the patient's mouth and nose. For the 0.24 Venturi mask, airflow is 104 L/min. This high flow effectively prevents the patient from rebreathing any exhaled air and carbon dioxide since his own minute ventilation is only a small fraction of the total air flow. Table 9-1 lists the popular sizes of Venturi masks along with the manufacturer's recommendations for oxygen liter flow.

Unfortunately, Venturi masks have drawbacks. Many patients experience facial discomfort after a few hours' use, and the masks cannot be worn while the patient is eating. The result is that Venturi

Oxygen therapy

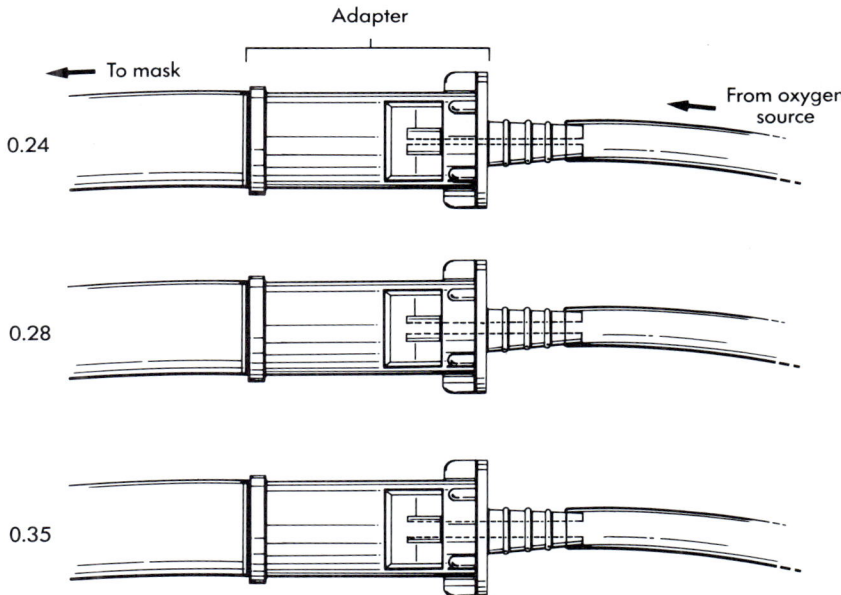

Fig. 9-5. A cross section of three separate adapters for the Venturi face mask for delivery of 0.24, 0.28, and 0.35 fraction of inspired oxygen (FIO_2). The only difference among the three adapters is the size of the orifice *(dotted lines)* through which pure (100%) oxygen enters the mask. The larger the orifice is, the higher the resulting FIO_2 will be.

Table 9-1. Venturi masks—recommendations for oxygen flow

Mask size ($FIO)_2$	Ratio air/O_2	Recommended flow of oxygen into mask (L/min)	Airflow past patient's mouth and nose (L/min)
0.24	25/1	4	104
0.28	10/1	4 to 6	44 to 66
0.31	7/1	6 to 8	48 to 64
0.35	5/1	8 to 10	48 to 60
0.40	3/1	8 to 12	32 to 48
0.50	1.75/1	12	33

masks are not practical for long-term oxygen therapy. Nasal cannulas, despite their inability to deliver precise FIO_2, are much better tolerated; except in the unstable carbon dioxide-retaining patient, nasal cannulas are preferred over face masks.

HIGH-SUPPLEMENTAL FIO_2 THERAPY

High-concentration oxygen can safely be used if the patient if not retaining carbon dioxide and should be employed for any hyperventilating, hypoxemic patient. It is a mistake to give low-supplemental FIO_2 to such a patient. Consider a man with pneumonia who has a $PaCO_2$ of 30 mm Hg and a PaO_2 of 40 mm Hg; he needs his hypoxemia corrected quickly and is in no danger of hypoventilating from a high FIO_2. An FIO_2 above 0.40 can be achieved by the use of a variety of face masks and, if necessary, by intubation and artificial ventilation. Although a high FIO_2 can also be achieved with a nasal cannula, face masks are generally used for this purpose (except for the intubated patient).

There are three main types of masks used to provide high FIO_2—the Venturi, discussed previously; the simple face mask; and the nonrebreathing or partial rebreathing face mask. The simple face mask is nothing more than a plastic mask connected to an oxygen hose. Oxygen flow rates of 5 to 8 L/min into the base of the simple face mask generally provide an FIO_2 between 0.40 and 0.70; however, as is true when using the nasal cannula, the final FIO_2 depends on the patient's own breathing pattern.

The nonrebreathing face mask can be used to give an FIO_2 above 60%. A plastic bag hangs down from the base of this mask and serves as an oxygen reservoir; this bag stays filled with 100% oxygen, which is fed in from the wall outlet (Fig. 9-6, A). The patient's inspired oxygen comes from the reservoir bag, and a one-way valve prevents expired air from entering this bag. The reservoir bag must always be filled; otherwise, excess ventilation will occur from the entry of room air, and the intended high FIO_2 will be diluted.

Nonrebreathing face masks are capable of delivering over 90% oxygen; the final FIO_2 depends on the liter flow fed into the mask, how tightly the mask fits the patient's face, and how well the one-way valve prevents rebreathing of exhaled air. If the valve between the bag and mask is removed, some exhaled air will be inhaled and the FIO_2 will be lower; a mask configured this way is sometimes referred to as a "partial rebreathing" face mask (Fig. 9-6, B).

A nonrebreathing face mask (or any other type of high FIO_2 mask) is used for the nonintubated patient who is very hypoxemic but not at risk for carbon dioxide retention, such as the patient with early adult respiratory distress syndrome or mild pulmonary edema (see Chapter 11). Treatment of carbon monoxide poisoning is another instance where a high FIO_2 is indicated (see the section on hyperbaric oxygenation).

Finally, high FIO_2 can be delivered under positive airway pressure, a technique that includes both continuous positive airway pressure and artificial ventilation. These subjects are discussed later in this chapter and more thoroughly in Chapter 10.

POTENTIAL HARM FROM OXYGEN THERAPY

The cutoff between low- and high-supplemental FIO_2 at 0.40 is in part arbitrary (why not 0.39 or 0.41) but is also in part based on clinical and experimental evidence of potential harm resulting from a high FIO_2. In clinical practice, the most important problems resulting from oxygen therapy are pulmonary toxicity, absorption atelectasis, and reduction of hypoxic ventilatory drive.

Pulmonary toxicity. Oxygen in high concentration can cause lung damage. At ambient air pressure, this damage is time- and FIO_2-dependent and correlates with high alveolar oxygen pressure (PAO_2) rather than arterial oxygen pressure (PaO_2). Thus 100% oxygen at ½ atmosphere is approximately the same (in terms of PAO_2 and oxygen toxicity) as 50% oxygen at 1 atmosphere.

Although much research remains to be done on

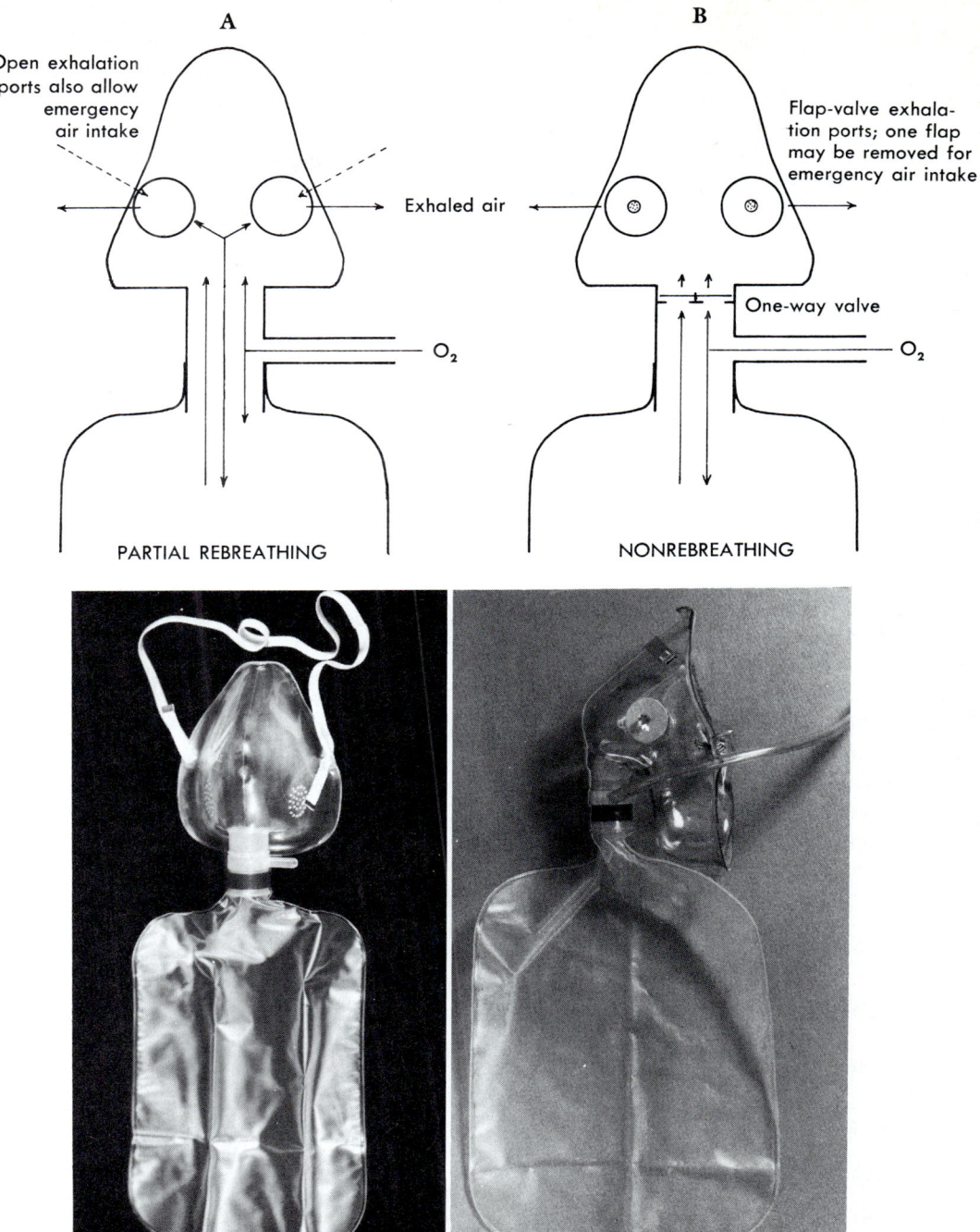

Fig. 9-6. Partial rebreathing and nonrebreathing oxygen face masks used to deliver high concentrations of oxygen. **A,** Mask lacks one-way valve between bag reservoir and mask, permitting some rebreathing of exhaled air. **B,** With one-way valve in place, the fraction of inspired oxygen can go above 0.90. (From Spearman, C.B., Sheldon, R.L., and Egan, D.F.: Egan's fundamentals of respiratory therapy, St. Louis, The C.V. Mosby Co.)

pulmonary oxygen toxicity, two points are certain: (1) an FIO_2 of 0.21 is safe; and (2) an FIO_2 of 1.00 is highly toxic in animals when administered for more than a day and is very irritating when inspired for a few hours by healthy humans. Limited studies on ventilated patients suggest that an FIO_2 above 0.80 is also toxic when administered for more than a few days. The pulmonary toxicity shows up as an exudative reaction in the alveoli; the lung pathology is similar to that seen in the adult respiratory distress syndrome (see Chapter 11). Thus an FIO_2 close to 1.00 can cause the very disease it is often employed to treat.

By extrapolation from experimental data, an FIO_2 less than 0.40 at atmospheric pressure is probably safe indefinitely; higher FIO_2s run a correspondingly higher risk of causing oxygen toxicity, and the risk increases the longer the oxygen is inhaled (Fig. 9-7).

Absorption atelectasis. When high concentrations of oxygen are administered, particularly FIO_2s close to 1.00, nitrogen is washed out of the alveoli and the blood, leaving only oxygen and carbon dioxide in the alveoli. Alveoli that are part of lung units with a low ventilation-perfusion ratio (see Chapter 5) tend to shrink because inert nitrogen is washed out by the high-oxygen concentration. As the remaining oxygen is absorbed into the pulmonary capillaries, the alveoli collapse, increasing the amount of venous admixture since blood perfusing the collapsed alveoli is no longer oxygenated. The net effect is that a patient's hypoxemia can actually worsen when on a high FIO_2.

Reduction of hypoxic ventilatory drive. Another possible harm from high FIO_2 is seen in hypercapnic patients. Until the widespread availability of arterial blood gas measurement, which came about in the 1960's, oxygen therapy was given empirically without objective measurement of need or benefit. Also before blood gas measurement, relatively crude methods of oxygen delivery, such as oxygen tents, usually meant the administration of a high FIO_2. Beginning in the late 1940's, astute physicians in England noticed that many patients with chronic obstructive pulmonary disease did worse when breathing a high FIO_2 than when inhaling room air or a low-supplemental FIO_2. Thus was born the concept of low-supplemental oxygen for some patients.

After much study, it was learned that carbon dioxide-retaining patients have a blunted carbon dioxide response and that elevated carbon dioxide does not stimulate their breathing as it does in normal subjects. For this reason, the main breathing stimulus in carbon dioxide-retaining patients is usually hypoxemia.

Consider the following blood gas values from a patient with chronic obstructive pulmonary disease: pH, 7.31; PaO_2, 45 mm Hg; $PaCO_2$, 67 mm Hg (FIO_2, 0.21). If this patient, who may appear confused, cyanotic, and dyspneic, receives high FIO_2, his PaO_2 could rise to over 100 mm Hg, blunting the hypoxic drive to breathe. Since he has already lost the carbon dioxide drive, he could decrease his minute ventilation to a dangerously low level.

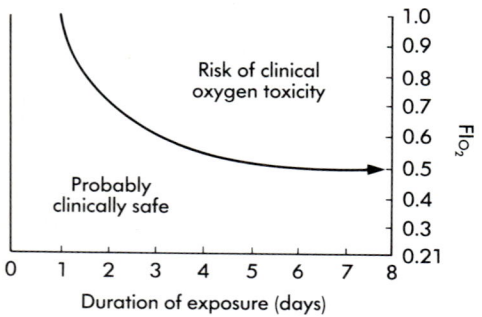

Fig. 9-7. Pulmonary oxygen toxicity is time- and FIO_2-dependent. (Modified from Luce, J.M., Tyler, M.L., and Pierson, D.J.: Intensive respiratory care, Philadelphia, 1984, W.B. Saunders Co.)

Clinical problem 4

A man with chronic obstructive pulmonary disease has the following blood gas values while breathing room air: pH, 7.35; $PaCO_2$, 50 mm Hg; and PaO_2, 38 mm Hg. Which set of blood gas values would most likely appear when this patient is breathing 28% oxygen?

Oxygen therapy

a. pH, 7.38; Pa_{CO_2}, 55; Pa_{O_2}, 45
b. pH, 7.32; Pa_{CO_2}, 62; Pa_{O_2}, 41
c. pH, 7.45; Pa_{CO_2}, 45; Pa_{O_2}, 73
d. pH, 7.31; Pa_{CO_2}, 57; Pa_{O_2}, 57
e. pH, 7.40; Pa_{CO_2}, 40; Pa_{O_2}, 88

Clinical problem 5

A patient with chronic obstructive pulmonary disease has the following blood gas values, which were obtained 3 hours apart.

1. pH, 7.37; Pa_{CO_2}, 53; Pa_{O_2}, 48; FI_{O_2}, 0.21
2. pH, 7.35; Pa_{CO_2}, 65; Pa_{O_2}, 68; FI_{O_2}, 0.31
   (through a face mask)

If the patient takes off his face mask, assuming there is no change in the Pa_{CO_2}, what will happen to his Pa_{O_2}?

There are other potential hazards of oxygen therapy. Retrolental fibroplasia (retinopathy of prematurity [ROP]) can occur in premature infants who receive high FI_{O_2}. Since this problem was widely publicized in the 1950's, oxygen is no longer routinely used in premature infants, but ROP has not disappeared (Campbell, Ball, Ellis, et al. 1983; Flynn, 1984). Many premature infants are in need of supplemental oxygen, so ROP is still a major clinical concern.

Several complications of oxygen therapy relate more to its administration than to the drug itself, e.g., drying of mucous membranes from inadequate humidification, nasal sores from the plastic tubing, and nasal stuffiness.

POSITIVE AIRWAY PRESSURE AND OXYGEN THERAPY

Either low- or high-supplemental FI_{O_2} may be given under positive airway pressure. Switching from ambient to positive airway pressure without a change in FI_{O_2} or the patient's Pa_{CO_2} often results in a higher Pa_{O_2}; this increase is best explained by the improvement in the ventilation-perfusion relationships that results from the increased airway pressure.

There are basically three ways to deliver oxygen under increased airway pressure—continuous positive airway pressure (CPAP), machine or artificial ventilation, or a hyperbaric chamber. Of the three, CPAP is the newest to be used in clinical medicine. With CPAP there is no machine pushing air in under positive pressure. Instead, the patient does all the breathing on his own against a resistance that creates a positive airway pressure. CPAP can be set up using either a tight fitting face mask or an endotracheal tube inserted into the trachea. In either case CPAP tends to be uncomfortable for the patient. (CPAP and artificial ventilation are discussed further in Chapter 10.)

HYPERBARIC OXYGEN

The oldest method of delivering oxygen under positive airway pressure is through a hyperbaric chamber. This method was thoroughly investigated by the Frenchman Paul Bert in the 1870's. He even devised a traveling hyperbaric chamber that could be moved from hospital to hospital! Hyperbaric chambers have long been used for decompression sickness and a host of other medical problems ranging from gangrene to senility.

The hyperbaric chamber is rarely used in pulmonary medicine today mainly because it is of no proven benefit for pulmonary diseases. However, one occasional use is for the victims of severe carbon monoxide poisoning. High-oxygen pressures allow oxygen to compete better with carbon monoxide for the Fe^{++} binding site of hemoglobin, thus speeding the dissociation of carboxyhemoglobin (HbCO) and the excretion of carbon monoxide. In addition to speeding the dissociation of HbCO, hyperbaric oxygen can dissolve enough oxygen in plasma (6 ml/100 ml plasma when the patient is breathing 100% oxygen at 3 atmospheres) to sustain life, even if HbCO is 100%. In less severe cases (or if a hyperbaric chamber is unavailable, which is the case in most hospitals), high concentration oxygen (as close to 100% as feasible) at atmospheric pressure is used; this oxygen can be delivered with a nonrebreathing face mask or, if necessary, with intubation and artificial ventilation.

The half-life of HbCO at atmospheric pressure (when breathing air and 100% oxygen) and at 2.5

Table 9-2. Hyperbaric oxygenation

Atmospheres*	FIO$_2$	Po$_2$ atm†	PAO$_2$‡	Pao$_2$§	Sao$_2$‖	Cao$_2$¶
1	0.21	160	102	100	0.97	19.80
2	0.21	319	261	250	1.00	20.85
3	0.21	479	421	400	1.00	21.30
4	0.21	638	581	550	1.00	21.75
1	1.00	760	673	640	1.00	22.02
2	1.00	1520	1433	1390	1.00	24.27
3	1.00	2280	2193	2140	1.00	26.52
4	1.00	3040	2953	2890	1.00	28.77

*For example, one atmosphere equals sea level barometric pressure (PB) of 760 mm Hg; 2 atmospheres equal PB of 1520 mm Hg.
†Po$_2$ atm = Po$_2$ in the atmosphere = FIO$_2$ × PB.
‡PAO$_2$ = (FIO$_2$ × (PB − 47)) − (1.2 × Pco$_2$), when FIO$_2$ = 0.21 and Pco$_2$ = 40 mm Hg. PAO$_2$ = (FIO$_2$ × (PB − (PB − 47)) − Pco$_2$, when FIO$_2$ = 1.00 and Pco$_2$ = 40 mm Hg.
§Pao$_2$ is an estimated value assuming healthy lungs and a normal slight increase in P(A-a)o$_2$ with increasing PAO$_2$.
‖Sao$_2$, percent saturation of hemoglobin with oxygen
¶Cao$_2$, arterial oxygen content in ml O$_2$/100 ml blood, assuming hemoglobin content equals 15 gm%; includes dissolved fraction

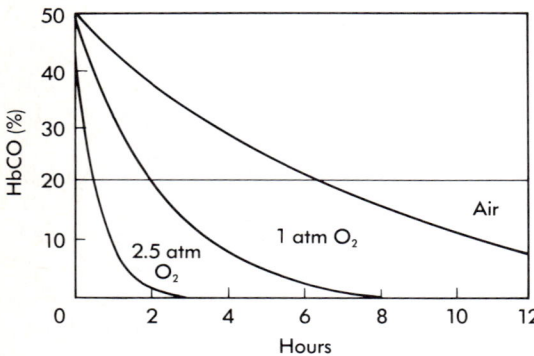

Fig. 9-8. Half-life of carboxyhemoglobin (HbCO) at atmospheric and hyperbaric pressures. The patient has a 50% HbCO level, a potentially lethal amount. If the patient were breathing room air, 12 hours would be needed to reach a HbCO level below 10%. If the patient were breathing 100% oxygen at atmospheric pressure *(1 atm O$_2$)*, all carbon monoxide would be eliminated in approximately 8 hours. If the patient were in a hyperbaric chamber and breathing 100% oxygen at 2.5 atm, the carbon monoxide would be eliminated in less than 3 hours. (From Winter, P.M., and Miller, J.N.: JAMA **236:**1502-1504, Copyright 1976, American Medical Association.)

atmospheres (when breathing 100% oxygen) is shown in Fig. 9-8. The changes in blood oxygenation with the use of a hyperbaric chamber are listed in Table 9-2.

Clinical problem 6

A patient with carbon monoxide poisoning has the following blood gas values: Pao$_2$, 80 mm Hg; Paco$_2$, 37 mm Hg; Sao$_2$, 47%; HbCO, 46%. After the patient has breathed 100% oxygen for 2 hours at 2.5 atmospheres, his HbCO level is 4%. Assuming there is no significant ventilation-perfusion imbalance, what are the Po$_2$ atm, PAO$_2$, Pao$_2$, and Sao$_2$ at this point?

MONITORING OXYGEN THERAPY— CLINICAL SIGNS AND Pao$_2$

The goal of oxygen therapy is to improve organ and tissue oxygenation. There is no practical way to monitor tissue oxygenation, so in practice patients are monitored both for clinical improvement and for an increase in Pao$_2$. Clinical improvement is usually manifested by improvement in the signs of hypoxemia—e.g., altered mental status, tachycardia, tachypnea, dyspnea, and cyanosis. How-

Oxygen therapy

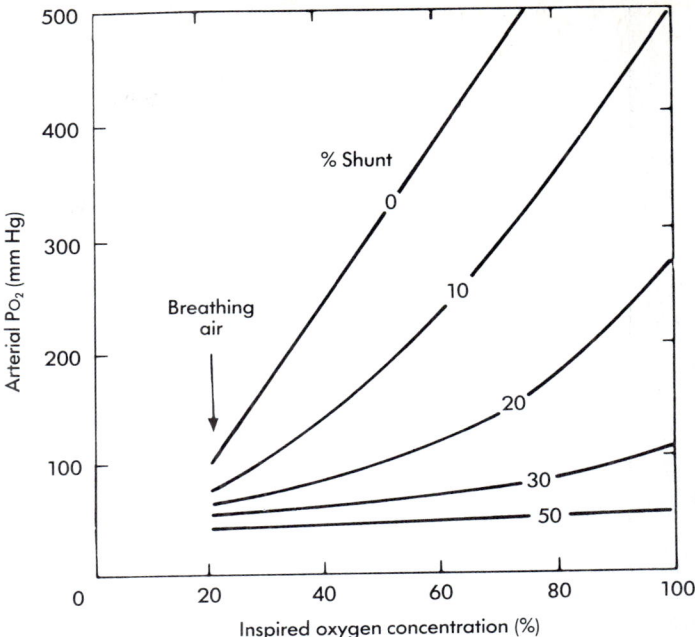

Fig. 9-9. Effect of shunt on arterial partial pressure of oxygen (Pa_{O_2}) as inspired oxygen concentration is increased. The higher the % shunt, the less the increase will be with a given increase in oxygen concentration. Only representative values are shown; other parameters, such as cardiac output and hemoglobin concentration, also affect the resulting Pa_{O_2}. (From West, J.B.: Pulmonary pathophysiology, Baltimore, © 1982, The Williams & Wilkins Co.)

ever, many hypoxemic patients do not manifest these signs. Also, signs suggesting hypoxemia may be present but may be unrelated to oxygen lack (e.g., dyspnea caused by asthma).

Improvement in Pa_{O_2} (or Sa_{O_2}) is the single best measurement to show benefit from supplemental oxygen therapy. If the Pa_{O_2} does not improve, the use of supplemental oxygen is probably not working.* Before blaming the disease for the lack of improvement, the patient must be examined to determine if he is, in fact, receiving the supplemental oxygen; many a face mask is found on the floor instead of the patient's face! A Pa_{O_2} that does not improve while the patient is breathing supplemental oxygen implies either a physiologic or anatomic right-to-left shunt (see Chapter 5).

How much should Pa_{O_2} improve? With healthy lungs, an increase in alveolar P_{O_2} ($P_{A_{O_2}}$) can be predicted from the abbreviated alveolar air equation ($P_{A_{O_2}} = P_{I_{O_2}} - P_{CO_2}$). When the barometric pressure is 760 mm Hg, every increase in $F_{I_{O_2}}$ of 0.10 (e.g., $F_{I_{O_2}}$ change from 0.21 to 0.31 or from 0.40 to 0.50) should improve $P_{A_{O_2}}$ approximately 70 mm Hg.

However, as $F_{I_{O_2}}$ is increased, the Pa_{O_2}, even in healthy subjects, does not go up by the same amount as the $P_{A_{O_2}}$. As a result, the normal alveolar-arterial oxygen pressure difference

---

*In some instances Pa_{O_2} may stay the same while the patient's work of breathing, as manifested by hyperventilation, improves. In such instances the $P(A-a)_{O_2}$ should improve.

$(P(A-a)O_2)$ widens as FIO_2 is increased (see Fig. 5-4). In lung disease the degree of PaO_2 improvement is invariably *less* than that predicted for healthy lungs because some areas have low V/Q ratios and shunting. Fig. 9-9 shows how various degrees of shunting can affect PaO_2 when FIO_2 is increased.

There are two implications for oxygen therapy demonstrated by Fig. 9-9. First, a patient with a large shunt may do almost as well (in terms of PaO_2) while breathing 60% or 70% oxygen as when breathing 100% oxygen. One should never leave a patient on 100% oxygen without first trying lower FIO_2s. Second, given a patient who has a shunt or a significant venous admixture, the $P(A-a)O_2$ cannot be used as a reliable guide to gas exchange when the FIO_2 is changed. The ratio of PaO_2 to PAO_2 is a more reliable parameter (see Fig. 5-5).

When should an arterial blood gas analysis be obtained after changing the FIO_2? With healthy lungs, only a few minutes are needed for the PaO_2 to reach equilibrium with a new FIO_2. In diseased lungs, reaching equilibrium takes longer, depending on the disease and the amount of "slow space," or poorly filling alveoli, in the lungs. In severe chronic obstructive pulmonary disease, as long as 15 to 20 minutes can be needed to achieve a new equilibrium. A safe interval for checking a blood gas-value after an FIO_2 change is 30 minutes, by which time virtually all patients should reach a new equilibrium.

BLOOD TRANSFUSION—EFFECT ON PaO_2 AND OXYGEN CONTENT

It is easy to understand how blood transfusion can improve the blood's oxygen content since the latter is a direct function of the hemoglobin content. Less understood is that blood transfusion can improve PaO_2, at least in conditions where there is increased venous admixture (right-to-left shunt or areas of low ventilation/perfusion). The explanation for this improvement lies in the effect of mixed venous oxygen content (CvO_2) on PaO_2 (see Table 5-3). The lower the CvO_2, the more the venous blood will depress the PaO_2 as it is shunted past the lungs. Transfusion, by providing more oxygen content to the tissues, raises the mixed venous oxygen content; if the amount of venous admixture is unchanged after transfusion, the resulting PaO_2 should be higher.

ARTIFICIAL BLOOD

For years attempts have been made to find some blood substitute that could safely be transfused and that could carry extra oxygen. Such a product, called Fluosol-DA, is now available. Fluosol-DA is an emulsion of perfluorochemicals that carries oxygen in dissolved form; there is no hemoglobin or other compound to chemically bind oxygen. The solubility of oxygen in Fluosol-DA is approximately three times that of oxygen in plasma; with a fraction of inspired oxygen of 1.00 (a PaO_2 over 600 mm Hg), approximately 6 ml O_2/100 ml Fluosol-DA can be carried in solution (i.e., dissolved). Although this oxygen content is well below the normal oxygen content of blood (20 ml O_2/100 ml), in acute operative or traumatic situations 6 ml O_2/100 ml can significantly improve oxygen delivery. In one study, benefit was found only when 100% oxygen was inhaled but not on lower FIO_2 (Tremper, Friedman, Levine, et al. 1982; Geyer, 1982). Thus some risk of oxygen toxicity is present when Fluosol-DA is used in this manner.

METHODS OF HOME OXYGEN THERAPY

Home oxygen therapy is now widely used for many patients, particularly those suffering chronic obstructive pulmonary disease (COPD). The increased use of home oxygen therapy has been spurred by three concurrent developments: (1) improvement in the technology and the methods for delivering home oxygen; (2) scientific studies proving the efficacy of continuous oxygen in COPD; and (3) the assumption of payment by Medicare and other insurance plans.

The physiologic principles underlying home oxygen therapy are the same as those that apply to oxygen therapy in the hospital. The major differ-

Oxygen therapy

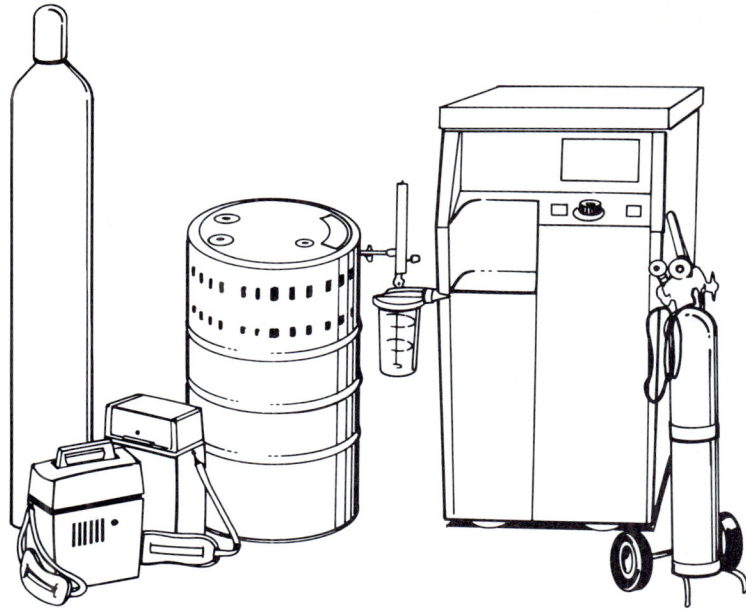

Fig. 9-10. Equipment used to deliver supplemental oxygen in the home. *Left,* the large cylinder, once commonplace, has been generally replaced either by liquid oxygen systems, the wide cylinder in the middle of the picture, or by oxygen concentrators, the large boxlike structure. With the liquid oxygen system, smaller containers (left of liquid oxygen cylinder) can be filled, allowing patients to leave home for a few hours. The oxygen concentrator is powered by electricity and is not portable, although patients may still leave home with the aid of small pressurized oxygen tanks (shown on wheels).

ences are in the types of apparatus used, and in the indications for instituting oxygen therapy.

For home use there are three types of systems (Fig. 9-9). The oldest system uses oxygen tanks or cylinders; these tanks are always colored green and contain oxygen gas in compressed form. Oxygen in the tank, under pressure of 1500 pounds per square inch (psi), is converted to lower pressure by a series of valves. The tanks are exchanged by the oxygen supply company, with delivery frequency determined by the patient's liter flow rate and length of use. For limited portability, smaller tanks are provided on wheels (Fig. 9-10).

A second method is the liquid oxygen system; it is, in principle, the same system used in hospitals but on a smaller scale and designed specifically for home use. A liquid oxygen container (represented by the two large canisters in Fig. 9-10; see also Fig. 9-11) is placed in the patient's home and is filled periodically from a source in a truck brought to the residence. Liquid oxygen has the advantage of allowing more oxygen to be stored at one time (compared to tanks of compressed oxygen). An additional advantage is that portable containers can be filled from the liquid oxygen systems in the patients' homes, something not possible with the other two systems (Figs. 9-11 and 9-12).

The third method of delivering home oxygen is through an oxygen extractor or concentrator. This ingenious device uses normal house current (see Fig. 9-10). The machine uses a molecular sieve to increase oxygen concentration by trapping nitrogen

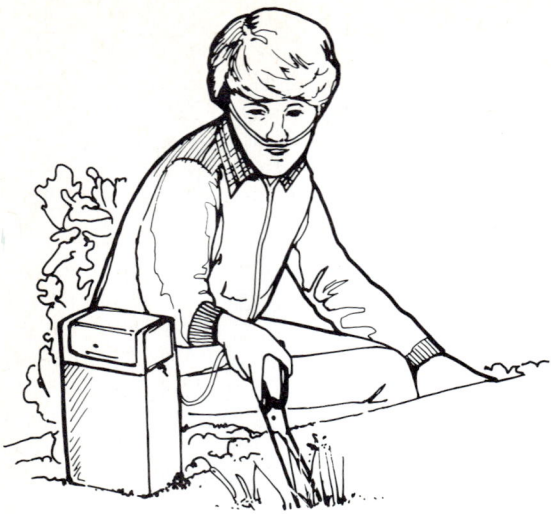

Fig. 9-11. A woman who is gardening while using a portable liquid oxygen container. This container, filled from a cylinder like the one in Fig. 9-10, allows the use of continuous oxygen for hours outside the home.

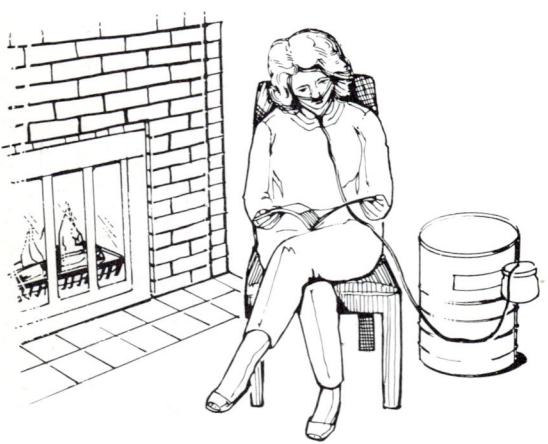

Fig. 9-12. A woman sitting by a fireplace while using a liquid oxygen system. This position is safe as long as there is no direct contact between the flames and the oxygen system. Note the oxygen tubing from the canister to her nose.

and separating it from the oxygen; this procedure effectively converts the oxygen concentration from 21% to over 90%. As is true with the other two systems, the actual amount of oxygen received by the patient is determined by the liter flow rate. The three systems are compared in Table 9-3.

Unfortunately, despite the undoubted benefit of supplemental oxygen for many patients, there are several obstacles to effective home use. These obstacles are summarized in the following discussion.

Continuous administration. Given the need for supplemental oxygen, continuous delivery is necessary since the body does not store oxygen to any appreciable extent. Only a few minutes' supply is available in the circulating blood; once that supply is exhausted, death ensues. This oxygen supply is in marked contrast to the food-supply, which is stored as protein and fat and which can keep a fasting person alive for many days. Hypoxemic patients would logically benefit from receiving supplemental oxygen all the time, but this is imprac-

Table 9-3. Three oxygen systems for home use

Compressed air (tanks)	Liquid oxygen	Oxygen concentrator
High pressure, 2200 psi*	Low Pressure, 50 psi	Low Pressure, 7 to 10 psi
Size for H cylinder, 9 in by 56 in high	13 in diameter by 24 in high	Variable, e.g., 2 ft by 1 ft by 1 ft
High center of gravity, narrow base	Low center of gravity, broad base	Low center of gravity, broad base
6900 gaseous L	13,800 gaseous L	Continuous oxygen supply
155 lbs full	30 lbs empty, 70 lbs full	Approximately 95 lbs
No increase in electric bill	No increase in electric bill	Variable increase in electric bill

*psi, pounds per square inch

tical because of inconvenience and cost.

Inconvenience. Supplemental oxygen must come from either heavy tanks or from cumbersome electrical apparatus and hence is confining. To receive continuous oxygen, patients must be sedentary or carry bulky equipment if they wish to leave home (Fig. 9-11). Unfortunately, portable oxygen equipment does not allow excursions for more than a few hours.

Because of the inconvenience of oxygen use, most patients compromise. They use oxygen mainly at night and during the day only when they feel a need for it or when it is otherwise convenient to use. Many people suffer the symptoms of hypoxemia rather than be confined, carry bulky equipment, or be seen in public with a tube in their nose. Certainly both the inconvenience and the stigma some patients feel are obstacles to continuous oxygen use. Conversely, the patient's continuous need is an obstacle to truly effective oxygen therapy.

Cost. The cost of the oxygen varies depending on the amount and the duration of its use. Oxygen used at 2 L/min for 12 hours a day can cost up to several hundred dollars a month. For some patients a large percentage of the total cost is subsidized by insurance carriers or Medicare.

Discomfort. Continuous home oxygen is almost always delivered through a nasal cannula. Prolonged use of the cannula tends to cause irritation and erythema in the area of nasal contact. Some patients also complain of headache and find no relief unless they remove the cannula.

Toxicity. The potential harm from oxygen toxicity was discussed earlier. Pulmonary toxicity is not usually a problem since the fraction of inspired oxygen for home use is usually less than 0.40. However, carbon dioxide–retaining patients must be cautioned not to turn up the liter flow rate without clear medical guidance.

INDICATIONS FOR HOME OXYGEN THERAPY

Until the last few years, there was little proof that home oxygen therapy actually benefited patients. One study published in 1975 (Stewart, Hood, and Block) showed that 12 patients with severe chronic obstructive pulmonary disease (COPD) demonstrated an improvement in quality of life and a decrease in the number of hospital admissions; however, after follow-up for an average of 2 years, half the patients had died.

A large scale, multicenter study (known as the nocturnal oxygen therapy trial [NOTT]) provided evidence that continuous oxygen therapy is indeed beneficial in a select group (Ann. Intern. Med., 1980). Treatment with either 12 or 24 hours of continuous oxygen therapy was given to 203 patients with hypoxemic COPD. Criteria for entry into the study included a resting PaO_2 of 55 mm Hg or less or a PaO_2 of 59 mm Hg or less in the presence of edema, polycythemia, or cor pulmonale. The flow rate ranged from 1 to 4 L/min, depending on the degree of improvement as demonstrated by arterial blood gas analysis. The two groups (12- and 24-hour oxygen therapy groups) were well-matched for disease severity, and the compliance with the oxygen therapy was judged good. Overall mortality in the 12-hour oxygen therapy group was 1.94 times that in the continuous oxygen group (Fig. 9-13). Although there was no specific physiologic parameter to explain the difference in mortality, the end result was proof enough of the ultimate benefit.

Another large scale study from England (Lancet, 1981) compared the use of 15-hour oxygen therapy with no oxygen therapy. The oxygen-treated patients had significant improvement in survival. This study and the NOTT study lead to the following conclusion: for treatment of severe hypoxemia, especially when the resting PaO_2 is 55 mm Hg or less, the longer the patient uses oxygen the better is survival; 24 hours per day of continuous oxygen is better than 12 hours per day, and 12 hours per day is better than none.

Because of the expense and other problems inherent in home oxygen therapy, patients should be optimized before committing them to this therapy. Many patients with acute exacerbation of their un-

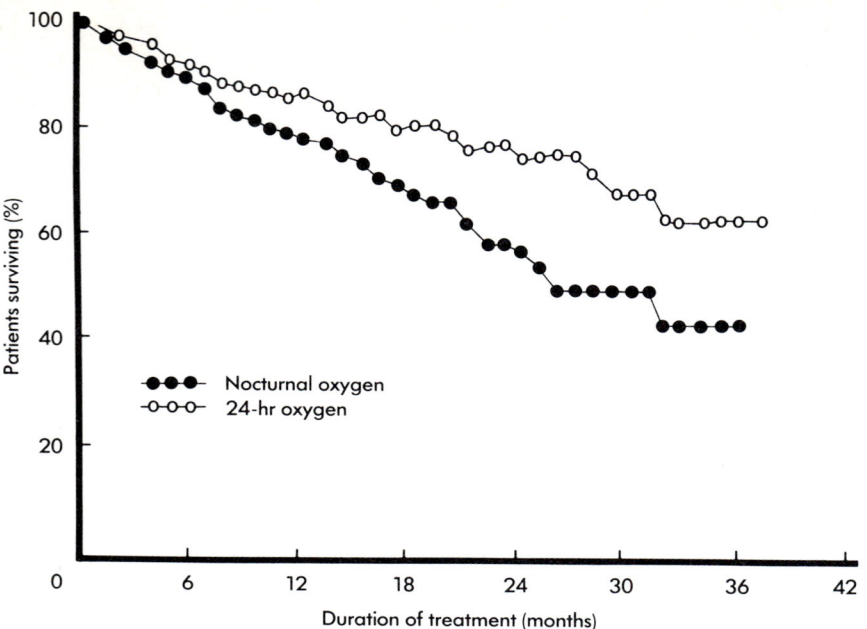

Fig. 9-13. Survival curves in nocturnal oxygen therapy trial (NOTT) study. Upper curve *(open circles)* shows survival rates for patients receiving 24 hours of continuous oxygen; lower curve *(solid circles)* shows survival rates for patients receiving only nocturnal (12 hours) oxygen. Survival differences at 12, 24, and 36 months are statistically significant. (From Petty, T.L.: Ambulatory oxygen, New York, 1983, Thieme-Stratton, Inc., redrawn from Ann. Intern. Med. **93**:391-398, 1980.)

derlying lung disease will initially manifest severe hypoxemia; after appropriate treatment, the PaO_2 will often improve to a point where home oxygen therapy will not be of significant benefit. For this reason the NOTT study did not admit any patient until after he had received 3 weeks of treatment with bronchodilators and antibiotics; only then were blood gas samples drawn and determinations made about who qualified for oxygen therapy.

In summary, determining who will benefit from home oxygen therapy requires a thorough evaluation, which includes arterial blood gas analysis after optimal medical treatment of the patient's pulmonary problem. Home oxygen therapy should not be ordered without such an evaluation.

SUMMARY

The use of supplemental oxygen is a common medical therapy in many cardiopulmonary conditions. Like any other drug, supplemental oxygen has proper indications, contraindications, and dosage levels. The dose, the fraction of inspired oxygen (FIO_2), can range from above 0.21 to 1.00. Any FIO_2 can be delivered at atmospheric pressure (via a nasal cannula or a face mask) or under positive airway pressure (e.g., artificial ventilation).

For medical therapy FIO_2 is arbitrarily divided into *low* vs. *high,* with the cutoff between the two at 0.40. Low-supplemental oxygen (between 0.21 and 0.40) is indicated for patients who are chronic carbon dioxide retainers or for patients with a mild degree of hypoxemia. High-supplemental oxygen (0.40 or above) is indicated for severely hypoxemic patients who do not retain carbon dioxide.

The terms *low flow* and *high flow* refer to the amount of oxygen-enriched air that the delivery system provides the patient. Low-flow systems, such as nasal cannulas and some face masks, deliver only part of the patient's inspired air; the rest is inhaled from the surrounding room air. For this reason a specific FIO_2 cannot be inferred when a patient is using a nasal cannula; the amount of room air inhaled through the patient's mouth is unknown. High-flow systems, such as Venturi face masks and artificial ventilators, provide enough oxygen-enriched air to meet the patient's total ventilatory needs. A Venturi mask can be used when a precise FIO_2 must be delivered.

Oxygen toxicity is time- and FIO_2-dependent. Oxygen toxicity can manifest in several ways, including direct lung damage leading to pulmonary fibrosis, absorption atelectasis, and reduction of hypoxic ventilatory drive. Retinopathy in premature infants is also a risk from a high FIO_2.

Oxygen therapy is now commonly prescribed for chronically ill, nonhospitalized patients. Studies have demonstrated that home oxygen therapy for patients with chronic obstructive pulmonary disease can reduce long-term mortality.

REVIEW QUESTIONS

State whether each of the following is true or false.

1. Low-supplemental oxygen therapy is defined as a fraction of inspired oxygen (FIO_2) above 0.21 (room air) but less than 0.40.
2. The only recognized complication of oxygen therapy in adults is pulmonary fibrosis.
3. The Venturi mask is part of a high-flow system that is used to deliver supplemental oxygen.
4. Two L/min nasal oxygen is equivalent to 28% inspired oxygen.
5. Home oxygen therapy can be safely delivered from a machine that extracts oxygen from the atmosphere.
6. Chronic oxygen therapy has been found to reduce the mortality rate from hypoxemic chronic obstructive pulmonary disease.
7. Artificial blood is a protein substance that binds oxygen at roughly one half the capacity of human hemoglobin.
8. Twenty-one percent oxygen delivered at 3 atmospheres carries the same risk for oxygen toxicity as 63% oxygen delivered at 1 atmosphere.
9. In treating carbon monoxide poisoning, the higher the FIO_2 the more rapidly carbon monoxide is removed from the blood.
10. The critical determinant of FIO_2 in the Venturi system is the liter flow rate of oxygen into the mask.

REFERENCES

Campbell, P.B., Ball, M.V., Ellis, F.D., et al.: Incidence of retinopathy of prematurity in a tertiary newborn intensive care unit, Arch. Ophthalmol. **101:**1686, 1983.

Continuous or nocturnal oxygen therapy in hypoxemic chronic obstructive lung disease: a clinical trial, Ann. Intern. Med. **93:**391, 1980.

Flynn, J.T.: Oxygen and retrolental fibroplasia: update and challenge, Anesthesiology **60:**397, 1984.

Geyer, P.P.: Oxygen transport in vivo by means of perfluorochemical preparations (editorial), N. Engl. J. Med. **307:**304, 1982.

Long-term domiciliary oxygen therapy in chronic hypoxic cor pulmonale complicating chronic bronchitis and emphysema: report of the Medical Research Council Working Party, Lancet **1:**681, 1981.

Petty T.L.: *Ambulatory oxygen,* New York, 1983, Thieme-Stratton, Inc.

Shapiro, B.A., Harrison, R.A., Kacmarek, R.M., et al.: *Clinical application of respiratory care,* ed. 3, Chicago, 1985, Year Book Medical Publishers, Inc.

Spearman, C.B., Sheldon, R.L., and Egan, D.F.: *Egan's fundamentals of respiratory therapy.* St. Louis, 1982, The C.V. Mosby Co.

Stewart, B.N., Hood, C.I., and Block, A.J.: Long-term results of continuous oxygen therapy at sea level, Chest **68:**486, 1975.

Tremper, K.K., Friedman, A.E., Levine, E.M., et al.: The preoperative treatment of severely anemic patients with a perfluorochemical oxygen-transport fluid, Fluosol-DA, N. Engl. J. Med. **307:**277, 1982.

Suggested readings

Barach, A.L.: Hypercapnia in chronic obstructive lung disease—an adaptive response to low flow oxygen therapy (editorial), Chest **66:**112, 1974.

Friedman, S.A., Weber, B., Briscoe, W.A., et al.: Oxygen therapy: evaluation of various air-entraining masks, JAMA **228:**474, 1974.

Fulmer, J.D., and Snider, G.L.: ACCP-NHLBI National conference on oxygen therapy, Chest **86:**234, 1984.

Myers, R.A.M., Snyder, S.K., Linberg, S., et al.: Value of hyperbaric oxygen in suspected carbon monoxide poisoning, JAMA **246:**2478, 1981.

Nishimura, N., and Sugi, T.: Changes of hemodynamics and O_2 transport associated with the perfluorochemical blood substitute, Fluosol-DA, Crit. Care Med. **12:**36, 1984.

Petty, T.L., and Neff, L.M.: The history of long-term oxygen therapy, Respir. Care **28:**859, 1983.

Schacter, E.N., Littner, M.R., Luddy, P., et al.: Monitoring of oxygen delivery systems in clinical practice, Crit. Care Med. **8:**405, 1980.

Timms, R.M., Kvale, P.A., Anthonisen, N.R., et al.: Selection of patients with chronic obstructive pulmonary disease for long-term oxygen therapy, JAMA **245:**2514, 1981.

See also General References in Appendix G and references in Chapter 6.

chapter 10
Artificial ventilation

OUTLINE

Intubation and artificial ventilation
Indications for artificial ventilation
Mode of artificial ventilation and FI_{O_2}
Normal breathing vs. ventilator breathing
Controlled ventilation
Assist-control ventilation
Intermittent mandatory ventilation
Ventilator settings
Ventilator compliance
High-frequency ventilation
Positive end-expiratory pressure
Continuous positive airway pressure
Complications of artificial ventilation
Ventilator weaning

INTUBATION AND ARTIFICIAL VENTILATION

When the patient's respiratory system can no longer provide adequate oxygenation and/or ventilation, artificial ventilation with supplemental oxygen is available. To receive artificial ventilation, the patient must first be intubated; intubation involves the insertion of a large-bore endotracheal tube into the trachea (Fig. 10-1).* The route of insertion can be through the nose or mouth or directly into the trachea through a surgical incision

---

*Occasionally a patient can be artificially ventilated without intubation, but this is not practical in most clinical situations.

(tracheostomy). One end of the endotracheal tube is surrounded by an inflatable rubber balloon; when filled with air, the balloon creates an airtight seal in the trachea. The other end of the tube is connected to two flexible, wide-bore hoses, through a Y connector; one hose is for inspiration and the other, for expiration. The expiratory hose can be connected to a spirometer or to a bellows to measure expiratory volume (Fig. 10-2).

The endotracheal tube, with its balloon inflated, allows the machine (artificial ventilator) to push air into the patient's lungs under positive (above atmospheric) pressure. Since air cannot escape around the tube, it enters the lungs and takes part in gas exchange. The machine then allows air to be passively exhaled through the endotracheal tube; after exhalation the patient is ready to receive the next ventilatory cycle. In practice, a variety of machines and types of endotracheal tubes is used, but the principle for their use is the same.

Sometimes patients are intubated when, although there is no need for artificial ventilation, there is a need to assure a patent airway (see the box on p. 198). The two broad indications for *intubation only* are (1) threatened airways obstruction and (2) definite airways obstruction. Either indication must be based solely on the clinical examination, although arterial blood gas measurement is often helpful to assure that artificial ventilation is not necessary.

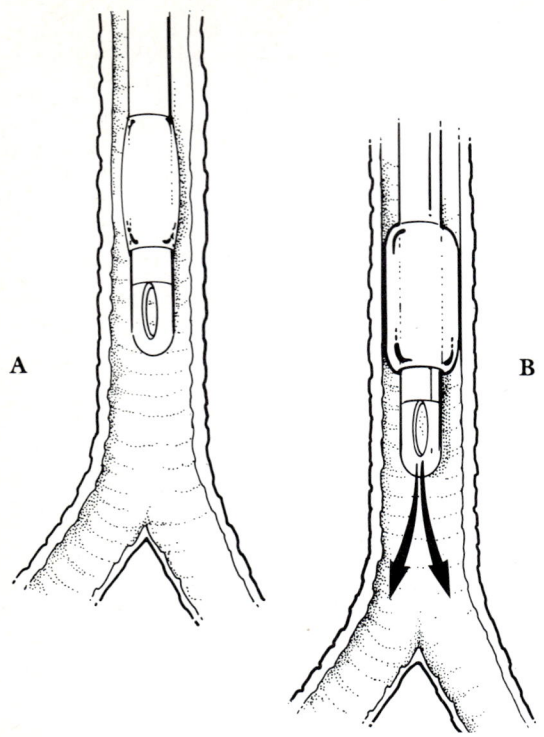

Fig. 10-1. Endotracheal tube in the trachea. **A,** Balloon deflated. **B,** Balloon inflated. Air that is pushed through the tube enters the lungs since it cannot escape around the tube when the balloon is inflated.

CRITERIA FOR INTUBATION AND ARTIFICIAL VENTILATION

Intubation only (oxygenation and ventilation are adequate)

1. Threatened airways obstruction—e.g., deep coma
2. Definite airways obstruction—e.g., laryngeal edema, tracheal tumor

Intubation and artificial ventilation (oxygenation and/or ventilation are not adequate)

1. Apnea
2. Impaired alveolar ventilation (as assessed by Pa_{CO_2}) when accompanied by *one or more* of the following:
    a. Depressed mental status
    b. Increasing fatigue
    c. Reduced Pa_{O_2} that cannot otherwise be corrected
    d. Severely deranged pH that cannot otherwise be corrected
    e. Compromise of upper airways (e.g., by secretions)
3. Low Pa_{O_2} (e.g., less than 60 mm Hg):
    a. That cannot be improved with an FI_{O_2} less than 0.50, and
    b. That is causing symptoms or seriously impairing bodily function

Artificial ventilation 199

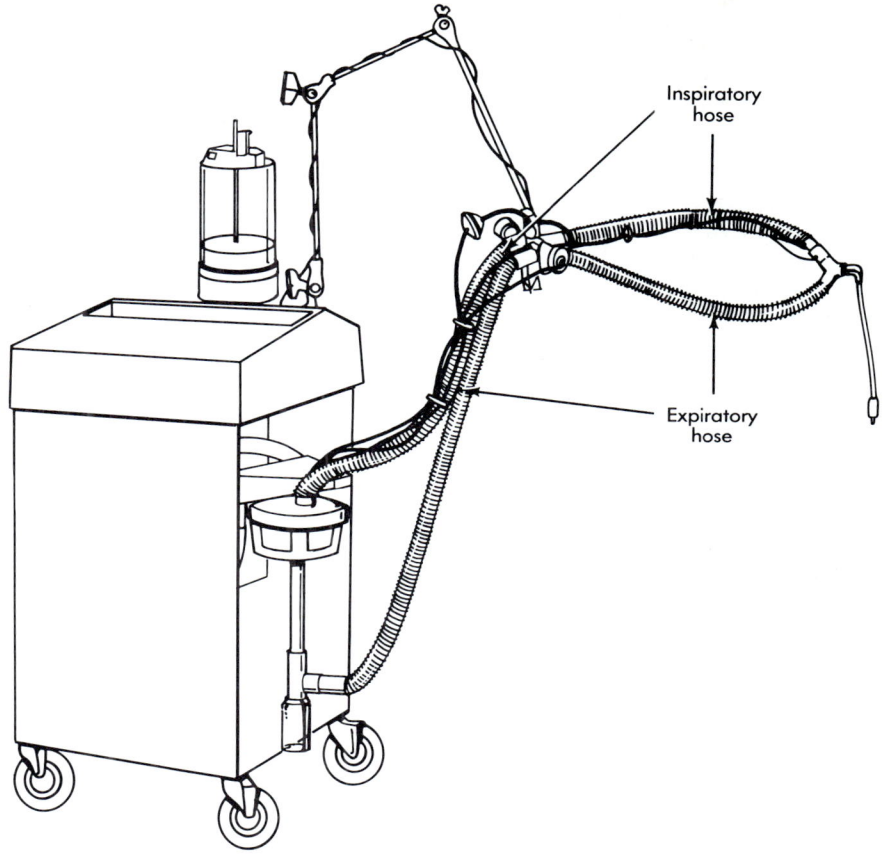

Fig. 10-2. Ventilator connected to endotracheal tube. One hose is part of the inspiratory circuit that delivers air to the patient; the other is part of the expiratory circuit. This ventilator is an example of a conventional volume ventilator. See text for discussion.

Probably the most common reason for intubation only is deep coma—the patient is totally unresponsive, except perhaps to deep pain, but has adequate oxygenation and ventilation. An endotracheal tube is placed in such a patient to assure a patent airway since airways occlusion is always possible from the patient's tongue receding into the oropharynx or from inspissated secretions in the upper airways. An endotracheal tube is not placed in the patient (as is sometimes thought) to prevent aspiration. There is no evidence that using a soft-cuffed tube prevents aspiration; indeed, clinical experience suggests that the act of intubation itself can lead to aspiration pneumonia. Therefore the assessment of deep coma should be based on the entire physical examination. Absence of the gag reflex, per se, is not a reliable guide for the need for intubation.

The other common indication for intubation only is definite airways obstruction. Patients with laryngeal edema, tracheal tumor, macroglossia, and other upper airway problems may initially be seen with stridor. When such obstruction is assessed as life-threatening (e.g., based on arterial blood gas analysis, or presence of cyanosis, extreme degree of muscular effort to breath, or shock) a secure airway is mandatory. Of course it may be difficult to pass an endotracheal tube, in which case an emergency tracheostomy or cricothyroidotomy may be necessary.

INDICATIONS FOR ARTIFICIAL VENTILATION

Earlier artificial ventilation was discussed in relation to alveolar ventilation (Chapter 4) and to oxygenation (Chapter 6). Impairment of alveolar ventilation (assessed by Pa_{CO_2}) and/or oxygenation (assessed by Pa_{O_2}) are the only physiologic reasons for instituting artificial ventilation. Although artificial ventilation can lead to better cardiac, renal, or cerebral function, the basic goal for its use must be to improve the Pa_{O_2} and/or the Pa_{CO_2} or to reduce the FI_{O_2} or the amount of work needed to maintain blood gas values at an acceptable level. Criteria for instituting artificial ventilation, listed in the box on p. 198, can be applied in all cases. For example:

- Patients undergoing cardiopulmonary resuscitation are intubated and artificially ventilated to reverse the inevitable hypercapnia and hypoxemia.
- During general anesthesia patients are routinely ventilated to prevent the hypercapnia and hypoxemia that would otherwise result.
- Patients are sometimes intubated even though their Pa_{CO_2} is in the normal range. This may be justified if the work of breathing is at the patient's limit and if decompensation is feared. In such cases the goal of artificial ventilation is to relieve the patient of some or all of the work of breathing and to maintain Pa_{CO_2} at an acceptable level.
- Patients are occasionally intubated to improve oxygenation even though the Pa_{O_2} may be above 50 mm Hg. This is justified if the FI_{O_2} is dangerously high *and* if the patient is in respiratory distress and not improving. Again the goal is to maintain an adequate Pa_{O_2}.
- Intubation may be warranted if excessive, uncontrolled *hyper*ventilation results in a dangerously high pH. For example, a patient with central neurogenic hyperventilation (e.g., from a brainstem tumor) may have a Pa_{CO_2} of 6 mm Hg, a pH of 7.67, and a Pa_{O_2} of 120 mm Hg while breathing room air. Artificial ventilation with the addition of drug-induced muscle paralysis may be the only way to control the severe alkalemia.

The last example is an unusual situation, but it does reinforce the main point—artificial ventilation is indicated only when there is a need to improve or control the Pa_{O_2} and/or Pa_{CO_2}. Obviously, good clinical judgment is necessary when deciding about intubation, especially when the Pa_{CO_2} is in the normal range or the Pa_{O_2} is above 50 mm Hg.

Clinical problem 1

Based on criteria presented in the box on p. 198, which of the following cases would warrant immediate intubation and artificial ventilation?

a. A 50-year-old man is comatose from drug overdose. Pa_{CO_2} is 51 mm Hg, Pa_{O_2} is 76 mm Hg, and pH is 7.31 while breathing room air.
b. A 29-year-old man is alert but in respiratory distress and is breathing 42 times/min. Pa_{CO_2} is 38 mm Hg, pH is 7.42, and Pa_{O_2} is 47 mm Hg while breathing 60% oxygen through a face mask.
c. A 61-year-old woman who has severe emphysema is alert but is in moderate respiratory distress; her respiratory rate is 24/min. Pa_{O_2} is 75 mm Hg while breathing nasal oxygen at 2 L/min, Pa_{CO_2} is 59 mm Hg, and the pH is 7.37. Her chest x-ray is clear.
d. A 29-year-old woman is suffering from diabetic ketoacidosis. Her pH is 7.10, Pa_{CO_2} is 26 mm Hg, and Pa_{O_2} is 110 mm Hg while breathing room air.
e. A 31-year-old drug addict responds briefly to the administration of Narcan (a narcotic antagonist) by opening her eyes and crying out and then lapses back into a state of semnistupor. Pa_{CO_2} is 31 mm Hg, pH is 7.38, and Pa_{O_2} is 89 mm Hg while breathing 3 L/min nasal oxygen.

MODE OF ARTIFICIAL VENTILATION AND FIO₂

Once the decision is made to institute artificial ventilation, the fraction of inspired oxygen (FIo$_2$) and the mode of ventilation must be chosen. Choosing an FIo$_2$ is no more difficult than picking a number, albeit one based on the patient's clinical problem and the reason for intubation. For example, a patient who is intubated mainly for hypercapnia will usually be adequately oxygenated with an FIo$_2$ under 0.40. A patient intubated because of severe hypoxemia or during cardiopulmonary resuscitation may need an initial FIo$_2$ of 1.00. In all cases, a blood gas analysis should be repeated in the first half hour after treatment, and adjustments should be made to keep the Pao$_2$ between 60 and 90 mm Hg at the lowest FIo$_2$ possible.

Choosing the mode of ventilation is often more difficult for several reasons. First, confusion often exists over ventilator terminology, with many of the commonly used terms no more than abbreviations (e.g., PEEP and IMV). Second, no widely accepted *best mode* of artificial ventilation is available; intensivists frequently debate in the literature about which mode is best for which patients. Third, with the exception of respiratory therapists, most hospital personnel, including all but a handful of physicians and nurses, do not understand the altered physiology of artificially ventilated patients.

NORMAL BREATHING VS. VENTILATOR BREATHING

Learning ventilator physiology should not be attempted without first understanding the changes in airway pressure during normal breathing. Fig. 10-3, *A,* shows the changes in airway pressure in the mouth during spontaneous, quiet breathing. Airway pressure during inspiration is negative (allowing air to enter the lungs) and is positive during expiration. Also, there is normally a brief expiratory pause, when airway pressure remains at atmospheric pressure.

The basic difference between normal breathing and artificial ventilation can be seen in the changes

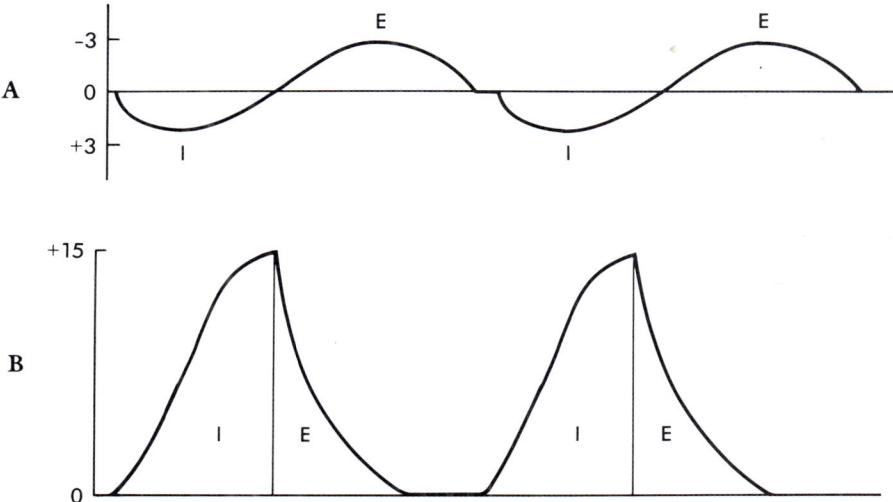

Fig. 10-3. Airway pressures during normal quiet breathing, **A,** and controlled positive pressure ventilation, **B.** Pressures are in cm H$_2$O; *O* represents atmospheric pressure. Pressures above the line are positive (higher than atmospheric); pressures below the line are negative (subatmospheric). (*I,* inspiration; *E,* expiration)

in airway pressure with each breath (Fig. 10-3, *B*). As used today, artificial ventilation is almost always positive (above atmospheric) and *intermittent*. Generically, most artificial ventilation is therefore intermittent positive pressure ventilation (IPPV).* It is important to remember that IPPV fundamentally alters the normal airway pressures; this fact accounts for most of its benefits and complications. The three main modes of IPPV are discussed in the next section.

CONTROLLED VENTILATION

The earliest mode of intermittent positive pressure ventilation (IPPV) was controlled ventilation.† Note the pressure relationships during controlled ventilation (Fig. 10-3, *B*); there is no negative pressure because all ventilation is accomplished by the machine with no patient effort required. In contrast to normal breathing, airway pressure during controlled ventilation is positive during inspiration and also positive during expiration. To achieve an adequate tidal volume, the ventilator "pushes" air into the lungs, resulting in a peak airway pressure higher than that reached during any part of normal breathing. Peak pressure marks the end of inspiration and the beginning of expiration; as in normal breathing, expiration during controlled ventilation is passive. As the lungs' elastic recoil brings them toward functional residual capacity, air is exhaled. Airway pressure at the end of expiration is again atmospheric (zero) until the next machine breath begins.

As a result of the higher peak pressure and the fact that airway pressure is positive throughout the breathing cycle, *mean* airway pressure during IPPV is higher than in normal breathing. The higher mean airway pressure improves gas exchange *and* accounts for some of the complications of artificial ventilation.

Controlled ventilation is the mode of ventilation used when the patient is completely paralyzed or otherwise unable either to breathe on his own or to initiate ventilator breaths. Controlled ventilation becomes unnecessarily limiting when the patient can contribute to his own minute ventilation.

ASSIST-CONTROL VENTILATION

Assist-control ventilation was the next mode to evolve after controlled ventilation (Fig. 10-4, *A*). Assist-control ventilation allows the patient to initiate ventilator breaths, providing the advantage of cycling the ventilator when the patient is ready and of lessening the need to suppress the patient's own drive to breathe. The transient negative pressure shown in Fig. 10-4, *A*, represents the patient's inspiratory effort; the machine senses the negative pressure and obliges by pushing in the next ventilator breath.

With the assist-control mode, both a tidal volume and a minimal respiratory rate must be selected in case the patient stops breathing. For example, if the ventilator is set for 12 breaths/min with a tidal volume of 700 cc, the patient will receive this as a *minimum*. If the patient chooses to breathe 20 time a minute, 20 will be the respiratory rate, and the volume of each breath will be 700 cc. Assist-control ventilation thus has the advantage of allowing the patient to choose his own respiratory rate, with each initiated breath guaranteeing an adequate tidal volume. If the respiratory rate of the patient is controlled by properly functioning chemoreceptors, the assist-control mode should result in optimal alveolar ventilation.

Of course each breath is only initiated by the patient but is completed by the machine. Respiratory muscles are not fully used during assist-control breathing, so muscle atrophy resulting from

---

*IPPV should not be confused with IPPB, intermittent positive pressure *breathing*. IPPB is used only to deliver medication or to provide "inhalation treatments" and not for support of alveolar ventilation.

†Although controlled ventilation was the earliest positive pressure mode, negative pressure ventilation actually preceded it as a means of artificial ventilation. Negative pressure was used by the old iron lungs, or "tank respirators," that contained the patient's entire body except for his head. Negative pressure ventilation is rarely employed today and, when used at all, is usually administered through machines (Cuirass respirators) that fit around the thorax only (see Introduction).

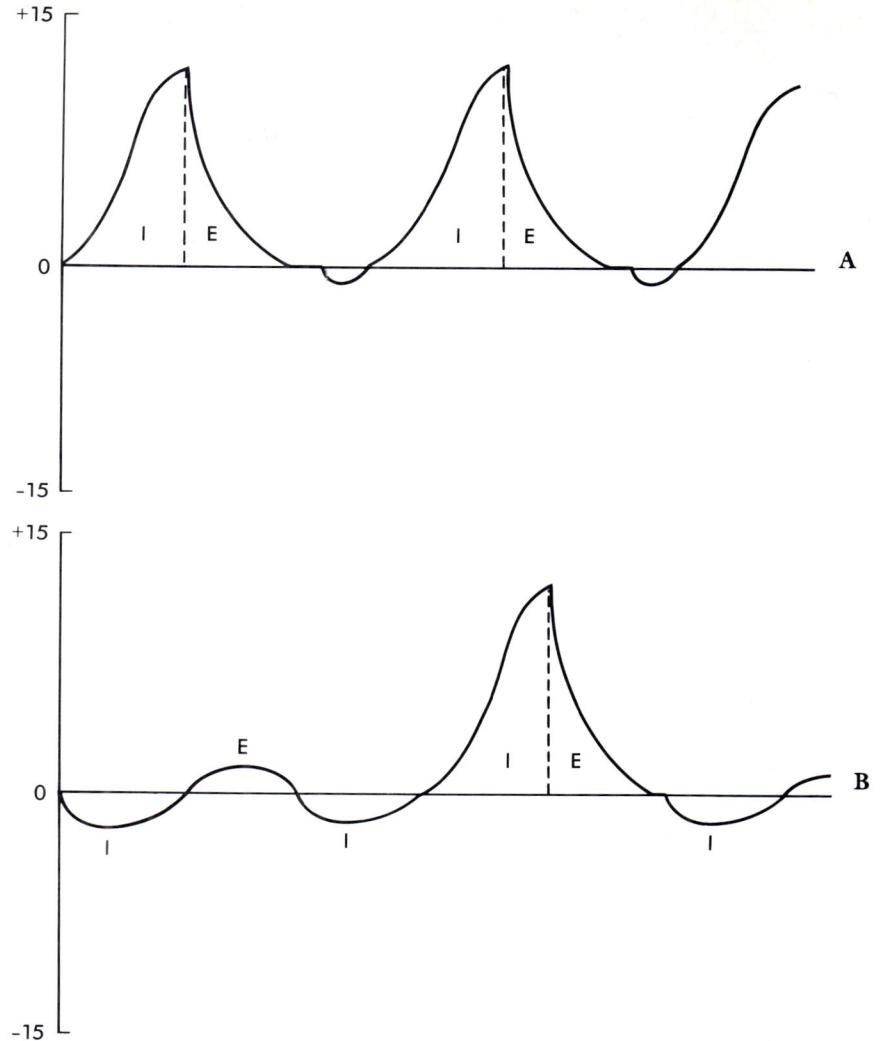

Fig. 10-4. Airway pressures during assist-control ventilation, **A**, and intermittent mandatory ventilation, **B**. Pressures are in cm H_2O.

disuse could develop if assist-control ventilation is used for long periods. Another potential problem arises if the patient breathes too fast, which may occur, for example, with central nervous system disorders, toxic or febrile states, and sepsis. In these conditions, tachypnea occurring without the patient breathing through a ventilator might be accompanied by shallow tidal volumes. Because the ventilator delivers a full tidal volume for each patient-initiated breath, the minute ventilation is much higher than needed and can lead to severe respiratory alkalosis.

Another problem that results from a rapid respiratory rate is a shortened time interval for expiration. When the patient is tachypneic, there is less time for exhalation of the full tidal volume; each patient-initiated ventilator breath occurs too soon, and the patient often appears to be "fighting the ventilator." Partly for these reasons, assist-control ventilation is no longer used as often as the next mode of ventilation, intermittent mandatory ventilation.

INTERMITTENT MANDATORY VENTILATION

Intermittent mandatory ventilation (IMV) allows the patient to interact with the ventilator in a more physiologic manner than with the control or assist-control modes. In the IMV mode, both the tidal volume and the number of machine breaths are also set, but they are only delivered *intermittently,* alternating with the patient's own breathing efforts. Between the ventilator's intermittent *mandatory* breaths, the patient breathes spontaneously, setting his own tidal volume and respiratory rate (Fig. 10-4, *B*). IMV is made possible by a valve that can alternate the inspiratory circuit between the ventilator and room air. To maintain a constant fraction of inspired oxygen (FIO_2), the room air is enriched with the same FIO_2 as is delivered from the ventilator (Fig. 10-5).

Many machines are designed so that the ventilator breath is delivered in synchrony with the patient's own inspiratory effort; this is called synchronous IMV or SIMV. IMV is only for the patient who has an intact respiratory center and who can accomplish the work of breathing. IMV is popular for weaning chronically ventilated patients from the ventilator; the number of IMV (machine) breaths can be gradually decreased, over a period of weeks if necessary, all the way down to 1/min or less.

Although IMV was introduced as a weaning technique, it is also a common ventilatory mode in patients not being weaned. The difference between the two uses of IMV (weaning vs. full-ventilatory maintenance) is in the number of IMV breaths/minute (assuming the patient is spontaneously breathing). Arbitrarily, seven or less IMV breaths/minute is considered a weaning mode, with the patient's spontaneous breathing constituting a major part of the total ventilation. Eight or more IMV breaths/minute is tantamount to full-ventilatory support in most people, even though the patient is breathing spontaneously between ventilator breaths. Although eight breaths/min is an arbitrary dividing line, this division serves to emphasize that IMV can be used for two different purposes.

Since its introduction in 1973, there has been a minor controversy over whether IMV is really better than assist-control ventilation as a full-ventilatory mode or is better than the old "trial and error" technique as a weaning technique. In the trial and error method, the patient is judged ready to be weaned and then simply is disconnected from the ventilator; close observation of the patient after disconnection is obviously important (see the section on Ventilator Weaning later in this chapter).

Drs. Shapiro and Cane (1984) have addressed the issue of IMV vs. assist-control-ventilation by calling attention to the fact that IMV is the only clinically available technique for providing *partial-ventilatory support,* i.e., for ventilator weaning. They define partial-ventilatory support as a ventilator rate of 7/min or less with the patient "providing a physiologically significant degree of spontaneous ventilation." Anything more than this rate is "full-ventilatory support" and can be provided by controlled ventilation, assist-control ventilation *or* IMV.

For full-ventilatory support, there is no proof that IMV or assist-control ventilation is a better technique. From a practical standpoint, IMV is now the most common technique for full-ventilatory support, replacing both control and assist-control modes in popularity. For partial-ventilatory support, debating IMV vs. assist-control ventilation is pointless since the latter is not a weaning mode.

In summary, the three choices for full support are control ventilation, assist-control ventilation, and IMV. If only partial-ventilatory support is to be provided, IMV is the only available mode. When using IMV, the number of ventilator breaths/minute determines if the patient is receiving partial- (7 or less) or full- (8 or more) ventilatory support.

Artificial ventilation

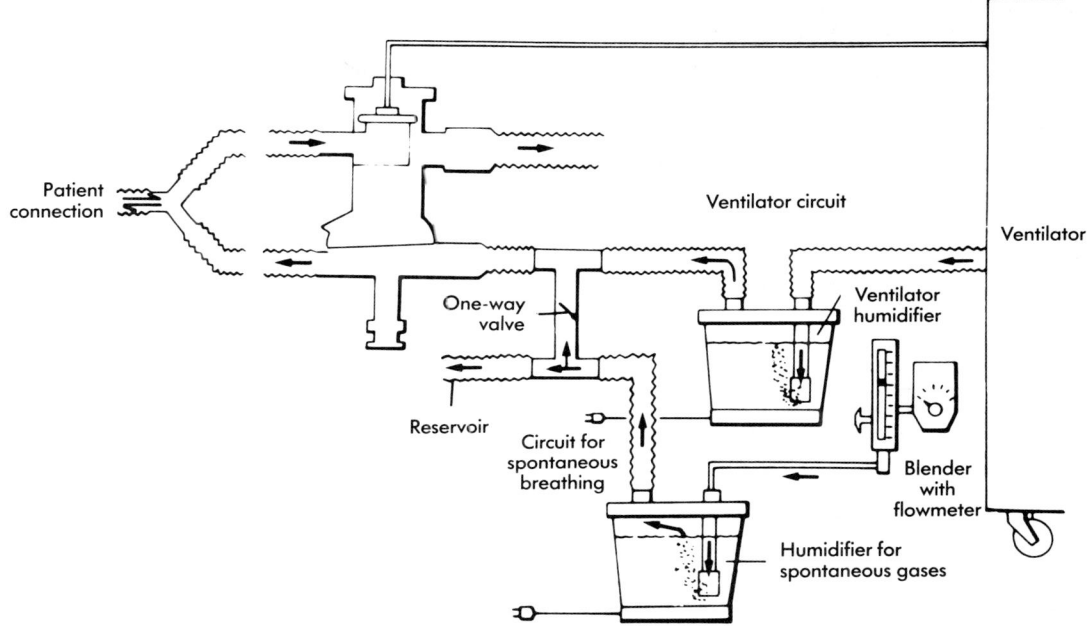

Fig. 10-5. Example of an intermittent mandatory ventilation (IMV) circuit. IMV is made possible by a one-way valve that closes when the ventilator delivers air but that can be opened by the patient's spontaneous breathing between ventilator-delivered breaths. In this figure the one-way valve separates the primary ventilator circuit from a parallel, nonventilator circuit that delivers the same FIO_2 as the ventilator. When the ventilator cycles, positive pressure is delivered to the patient and the one-way valve closes. Between mechanical breaths, the patient's spontaneous breathing can open the valve so that the patient can inhale air of the same FIO_2 and humidification as the air from the ventilator, but under ambient pressure. If desired, positive airway pressure can also be delivered through the IMV circuit; because the patient is breathing spontaneously, positive pressure through an IMV circuit represents continuous positive airway pressure alternating with ventilator breaths. (From McPherson, S.P., and Spearman, C.B.: Respiratory therapy equipment, ed. 3, St. Louis, 1985, The C.V. Mosby Co.)

Clinical problem 2

A decision is made to wean a 67-year-old man from the ventilator. Before weaning is begun, the machine is in the assist-control mode. The patient is initiating 16 breaths/min and is receiving 700 cc/breath. He is switched to IMV at a rate of 12/min and within a half hour is noted to be in respiratory distress with a total respiratory rate (machine-initiated plus spontaneous) of 20/min. Blood gas measurements obtained before and after the change to IMV are shown below. How would you explain the changes?

Ventilatory mode	Machine breaths (and tidal volume)	Spontaneous breaths	pH	$Paco_2$	Pao_2	FIO_2
Assist-control	16 (700 cc)	0	7.45	38	78	0.40
IMV	12 (700 cc)	8	7.39	47	65	0.40

VENTILATOR SETTINGS

Table 10-1 lists the principal ventilator settings for intermittent positive pressure ventilation when using conventional volume ventilators. These machines are by far the most commonly used for adult artificial ventilation and are called volume ventilators because they will generate whatever pressure is necessary (up to a limit) to provide the preset tidal volume. Pressure-cycled ventilators, which have the pressure preset, are rarely used for artificial ventilation today.

Each ventilator setting is adjusted by using a knob or a dial on the ventilator console (see Fig. 10-2). These settings determine whether the patient is receiving full- or partial-ventilatory support and, if full-ventilatory support, whether it is the control or assist-control mode. Also, the amount of positive end-expiratory pressure can be set for any of the ventilatory modes.

Fraction of inspired oxygen. A precise FIO_2 can be dialed on most volume ventilators. In addition, alarms can be set to sound if the delivered FIO_2 falls outside a certain range. For example, if the FIO_2 is set at 0.40, the limits can be set between 0.30 and 0.60; any delivered FIO_2 outside this range will sound an alarm.

Tidal volume and inspiratory pressure limit. A volume ventilator delivers a preset tidal volume regardless of the condition in the airways; presetting assures that the volume needed will be received by the patient. However, a potential danger exists if a major airway becomes unexpectedly obstructed or if something impedes air entry. In such cases delivery of the preset volume can result in a dangerously high airway pressure; to guard against this, an inspiratory pressure limit is always set along with the tidal volume. For example, setting the tidal volume for delivery of 700 cc might achieve a peak airway pressure of 30 cm H_2O; a *pressure limit* of 50 cm H_2O can be set at the same time. If, for example, the endotracheal tube slips into the patient's right main stem bronchus, the machine will attempt to deliver 700 cc to just one lung (half the previous lung volume), and the peak inspiratory pressure will acutely rise. Conceivably the elevated airway pressure could rupture the right lung or cause other damage. Instead, however, when 50 cm H_2O airway pressure is reached, the

Table 10-1. Principal ventilator settings for intermittent positive pressure ventilation while using conventional volume ventilators*

Setting	Typical range
Fraction of inspired oxygen	0.21-1.00
Tidal volume	400-1000 cc
Inspiratory pressure limit	Up to 80 cm H_2O
Respiratory rate	FVS, 8-30 or more breaths/min
	PVS, 7 or less breaths/min
	PVS can be accomplished only in the IMV mode, which allows the patient to breathe spontaneously between ventilator breaths
Peak inspiratory flow rate	20-100 L/min (to achieve inspiratory flow time of 0.5-1.5 sec)
Inspiratory sensitivity	Control mode, no sensitivity
	Assist-control mode, sensitivity dialed in (a variable control)
Positive end-expiratory pressure	1-30 or more cm H_2O
Inspiratory plateau or hold	0-2.0 seconds

*FVS, full-ventilatory support; PVS, partial-ventilatory support; IMV, intermittent mandatory ventilation

machine stops inspiration and an alarm sounds, perhaps after delivering only 400 cc. With this warning, the therapist or nurse can quickly investigate the problem. The alarm will sound each time airway pressure reaches the preset inspiratory pressure limit.

Respiratory rate. The respiratory rate is set by using a dial on the machine. For controlled ventilation, the rate equals the total number of ventilator breaths the patient will receive. For assist-control ventilation, the rate represents the *minimal* number of breaths; depending on the inspiratory sensitivity (also set by the machine), the patient may initiate more than the minimal amount. For intermittent mandatory ventilation, the respiratory rate is also the total number of ventilator breaths per minute; however, between the machine breaths, the patient may breathe spontaneously (Fig. 10-4 and 10-5).

Peak inspiratory flow rate. The peak inspiratory flow rate determines how fast each breath will be delivered to the patient and is therefore a determinant of inspiratory time. The faster the flow rate, the shorter the inspiratory time, and the more breaths that can be delivered per minute. Optimal inspiratory flow time is between 0.5 and 1.5 seconds and is usually achieved with a peak inspiratory flow rate between 40 and 70 L/min.

Sensitivity. Many volume ventilators include a dial labeled "sensitivity" or "inspiratory effort"; this setting determines how easily a patient can initiate a machine-delivered breath. When the sensitivity dial is turned all the way to the *off* position, no amount of patient effort will initiate a machine breath, and the machine is in the controlled ventilatory mode. As sensitivity is "dialed in," the ventilator changes to the assist-control mode, and it becomes much easier for the patient to initiate a machine breath. The sensitivity dial is not calibrated in units, but rather is adjusted by trial and error to the patient's own inspiratory efforts. However, the patient's inspiratory effort will show up as a negative (subatmospheric) deflection on the ventilator's pressure dial, usually between -0.5 and -2.5 cm H_2O.

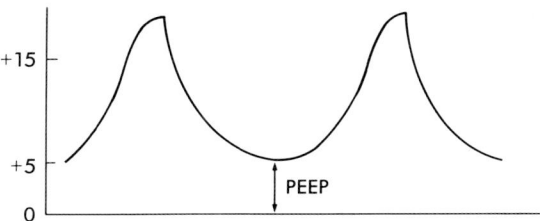

Fig. 10-6. Pressure tracing with positive end-expiratory pressure (PEEP). In this example a PEEP of 5 cm H_2O has been applied.

Positive end-expiratory pressure. On most ventilators manufactured today, PEEP can be simply set by dialing to a desired setting. The dial regulates an expiratory resistance valve that effectively keeps airway pressure above atmospheric pressure at end-expiration. PEEP may be used in the control, assist-control, or IMV modes. A PEEP pressure tracing is shown in Fig. 10-6; the use and complications of PEEP will be discussed in later sections.

Inspiratory plateau or hold. The inspiratory plateau or hold dial adds resistance to the expiratory circuit; the effect is to prolong inspiration and create a transient plateau pressure. Airway pressure is still zero at end-expiration (Fig. 10-7) in contrast to PEEP, which maintains a positive airway pressure at the end of expiration (see Fig. 10-6). Inspiratory plateau was originally used to improve oxygenation by providing a longer time for gas exchange, but PEEP is now used instead. Today, the principal use of inspiratory plateau is in measuring static compliance (see the section on Ventilator Compliance).

These ventilator settings (Table 10-1) represent the principal ones on volume ventilators. A glance at any modern ventilator may reveal several more knobs, alarms, and circuits than can be discussed here. Generally, other settings are determined by the respiratory therapy personnel whose knowledge of ventilators exceeds that of most physicians because the therapists work with ventilators daily. More detail on artificial ventilators is available in the texts listed in the references.

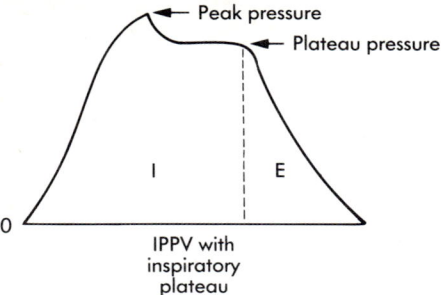

Fig. 10-7. Effect of inspiratory plateau. The principal effect is to prolong inspiration. In contrast to PEEP, inspiratory plateau allows the end-expiratory pressure to return to zero. The difference between peak pressure and plateau pressure is caused by airways resistance. The difference between plateau pressure and end-expiratory pressure is that amount of pressure needed to distend the system (tubing, lungs, chest wall), and the difference can be used to calculate system compliance. See text for further discussion.

The ranges for most ventilator settings are large (Table 10-1). Patients vary widely in their ventilatory requirements, and it is virtually impossible to predict settings that will provide a given patient with optimal blood gases. What settings should be chosen when initiating artificial ventilation? Generally, the initial tidal volume is set at approximately 10 to 15 cc/kg body weight, the respiratory rate is set between 10 to 16 per minute (control, assist-control, or IMV mode, depending on the clinical state), and the inspiratory flow rate is set at 40 to 60 L/min. PEEP is usually added later, depending on the patient's clinical course and the results of arterial blood gas analysis. Whatever settings are chosen, it is important to check the blood gas measurements within 30 minutes and to repeat the measurements within a few hours to assure a ventilatory steady state. Any time a ventilator setting that might affect Pao_2 or $Paco_2$ is changed, the blood gas analysis should be repeated within 30 to 60 min.

Clinical problem 3

A 60-year-old patient is in the hospital for treatment of a myocardial infarction. During the night she suffers acute pulmonary edema and requires cardiopulmonary resuscitation. Before the patient is intubated and artificial ventilation is begun, her blood gas measurements show pH of 7.06, $Paco_2$ of 61 mm Hg, and Pao_2 of 50 mm Hg while breathing 100% oxygen delivered by manual ventilation with an Ambu bag. The patient's estimated body weight is 50 kg (110 lbs). What initial ventilator settings would you choose for the following:
a. Fio_2
b. Tidal volume
c. Inspiratory pressure limit
d. Respiratory rate
e. Peak inspiratory flow rate
f. Inspiratory sensitivity
Would you provide PEEP?

Clinical problem 4

A 72-year-old man with severe chronic obstructive pulmonary disease is in the intensive care unit. His pH is 7.24, $Paco_2$ is 84 mm Hg, and Pao_2 is 58 mm Hg while breathing 28% oxygen through a Venturi mask. His chest x-ray suggests severe emphysema. Despite optimal drug therapy, his blood gas measurements cannot be improved, and he is almost unarousable. To prevent respiratory arrest, he is intubated and given artificial ventilation. His estimated body weight is 70 kg (150 lbs). What initial ventilator settings would you choose for the following:
a. Fio_2
b. Tidal volume
c. Inspiratory pressure limit
d. Respiratory rate
e. Peak inspiratory flow rate
f. Inspiratory sensitivity
Would you provide PEEP?

Clinical problem 5

A comatose 20-year-old patient is brought to the emergency room following an overdose of sleeping pills. Because of very shallow respirations and cyanosis, the patient is intubated before his blood gas results are known. Initial ventilator settings include a tidal volume (V_T) of 700 cc, a respiratory rate (RR) of 12/min, and an FIO_2 of 0.50. The patient has no spontaneous breathing. Blood gas results obtained (1) before intubation and (2) 20 minutes later show the following:

	pH	$Paco_2$	Pao_2	FIO_2	V_T	RR
(1)	7.10	79	38	Room air	0	0
(2)	7.25	56	117	50% oxygen	700	12

Following the second blood gas analysis, would you change the FIO_2, the tidal volume, or the respiratory rate? If so, what settings would you choose?

VENTILATOR COMPLIANCE

The concept of compliance was introduced in Chapter 3. Since compliance represents a change in volume/change in pressure, it is relatively easy to measure in ventilated patients. Ventilator compliance is a measure of the distensibility of the entire system, which includes the ventilator tubing, the chest wall, and the lungs. Compliance is often a valuable parameter to follow since any significant change may represent a change in the patient's respiratory condition.

In measuring system compliance, the volume is the amount of air delivered by the ventilator per breath, i.e., the tidal volume, which is easily measured by collecting the expired air from each breath. Determining the correct pressure to use in compliance measurement is a little more difficult.

If the patient is not receiving positive end expiratory pressure, the pressure at the beginning of inspiration is zero (atmospheric); the final pressure is the peak airway pressure. For purposes of discussion, assume a patient's tidal volume is 500 cc and his peak pressure is 20 cm H_2O. The net change is the pressure at end-inspiration (20 cm H_2O) minus the pressure at end-expiration (0 cm H_2O) or 20 cm H_2O. Is the compliance then 500 cc/20 cm H_2O or 25 cc/cm H_2O? Not exactly.

As discussed in Chapter 3, compliance is a static measurement. If the pressure change is measured during ventilator breathing, the amount of pressure being measured is that required to not only distend the lungs, but also to overcome airways resistance. If two patients with equally distensible lungs have different airways resistance, their compliance, measured during breathing, will be different.

To eliminate the pressure caused by airways resistance, the inspiratory plateau dial is quickly turned to the maximum at the end of inspiration; this setting creates a plateau of pressure. The plateau lasts for only a fraction of a second, but is long enough to be observed on the ventilator's pressure gauge. The difference between the peak airway pressure and plateau pressure reflects the amount of pressure needed to overcome airways resistance. The difference between plateau pressure and end-expiratory pressure is that amount of pressure needed to distend the lungs and is therefore used in the compliance measurement (Fig. 10-7).

Clinical problem 6

A 29-year-old man is intubated following an overdose of sleeping pills. He is receiving controlled ventilation at a tidal volume of 800 cc. The patient's peak airway pressure is 30 cm H_2O, his plateau pressure is 20 cm H_2O, and his end-expiratory pressure is 0. What is the static system compliance?

Clinical problem 7

a. A 35-year-old patient is receiving artificial ventilation for severe pneumonia. The ventilator settings are as follows: FIO_2, 0.60; tidal volume, 900 cc; and respiratory rate, 12/min. The peak pressure is 45 cm H_2O, the plateau pressure is 40 cm H_2O, and the PEEP pressure is 5 cm H_2O. What is the compliance of this system?

b. The peak pressure limit for the above patient is set at 60 cm H_2O. One hour later the machine alarm indicates that the pressure limit has been exceeded. The respiratory therapist increases the limit to 80 cm H_2O and takes new readings. The tidal volume is still 900 cc, but the peak pressure is now 68 cm H_2O, the plateau pressure is 64 cm H_2O, and the PEEP pressure is 5 cm H_2O. What is the system compliance at this point? How do you explain the change?

HIGH-FREQUENCY VENTILATION

Conventional intermittent positive pressure ventilation (IPPV) rarely exceeds 30 breaths/min, at

Table 10-2. Modes of high-frequency ventilation

Mode	Respiratory rate per minute	Tidal volume	Peak inspiratory pressure	Comment
High-frequency positive-pressure ventilation	50 to 150	3 to 5 cc/kg body weight	Low	Can be accomplished with some conventional volume ventilators
High-frequency jet ventilation	100 to 300	3 to 5 cc/kg body weight	Low	Short bursts delivered into upper airways; requires a special "jet" ventilator
High-frequency oscillation	900 to 3600	50 to 100 cc	Low	Uses piston pump or radio loudspeaker to oscillate column of gases in airway

least in adults. High-frequency ventilation (HFV) starts where conventional IPPV leaves off. Because HFV may provide tidal volume breaths *equal to or less than* the patient's dead space volume, it is a radically new mode of ventilation. (Conventional volume ventilation attempts always to provide a tidal volume greater than the patient's dead space.) Although originally introduced in the late 1960's in animal experiments, clinical experience with HFV is still very limited. Except in special situations, such as during laryngoscopy or bronchoscopy, HFV is not routinely used in clinical medicine.

Much confusion has centered around HFV, partly because it is new and partly because HFV includes several different modes (Table 10-2)—high-frequency positive-pressure ventilation, high-frequency jet ventilation, and high-frequency oscillation.

High-frequency positive-pressure ventilation (HFPPV) is simply a faster method of delivering conventional IPPV. Each breath is pushed into the patient's lungs through a pneumatic valve instead of through a mechanical on-off valve. The patient is intubated with a wide-bore endotracheal tube in the conventional manner (Fig. 10-1). Usual rates for HFPPV are 50 to 150 breaths per minute. HFPPV is commonly used during laryngoscopy and bronchoscopy.

High-frequency jet ventilation (HFJV) accounts for over 90% of the HFV used clinically. HFJV pushes "jets" of air into the airways through a small bore cannula, such as a 14-gauge or 16-gauge catheter. HFJV requires a different type of ventilator (a "jet" ventilator) from the conventional volume ventilator discussed so far. A pressure tracing from HFJV is shown in Fig. 10-8; below this tracing is one from conventional IPPV.

High-frequency oscillation (HFO) is the most radical technique of HFV and is also the most experimental. Air in the upper airways is merely oscillated or vibrated at 900 to 3600 vibrations/min! This vibration is accomplished by either a piston or a radio loudspeaker.

At present there is no clear advantage of HFV over conventional ventilation in treating respiratory failure. So far, the most important impact of HFV on respiratory therapy is the way the concept of artificial ventilation has been altered. It is now known that adequate alveolar ventilation can be achieved with tidal volumes equal to or smaller than the patient's dead space volume.

The mechanism or mechanisms by which HFV accomplishes alveolar ventilation are not well understood. One theory is that molecules on the periphery of the airways move more slowly than molecules in the center, allowing for a continuous circular movement of gas—fresh air travels down the center of the airway while stale air is exiting around the periphery. Whatever the mechanism, HFV works. Its main indications now are for ventilating patients with bronchopleural fistulas and for use

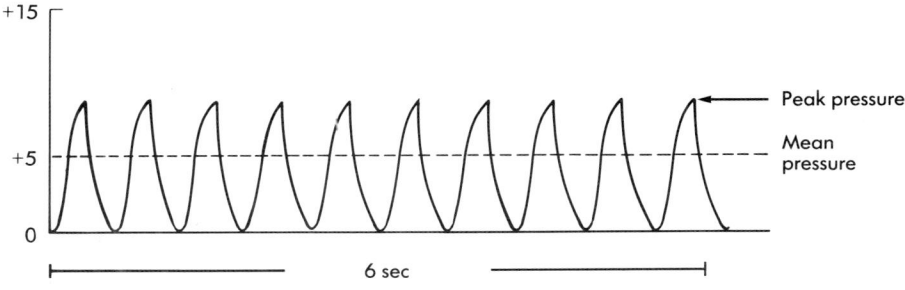

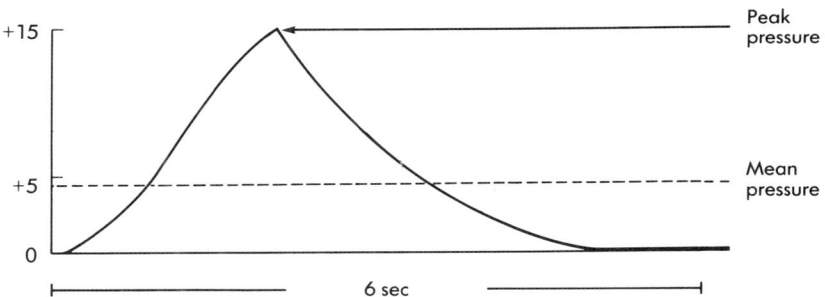

Fig. 10-8. Airway pressure during high-frequency jet ventilation (HFJV). **A,** HFJV. **B,** Conventional, intermittent positive pressure ventilation (IPPV). In the time it takes to deliver one IPPV breath, HFJV delivers approximately 10 breaths. In this example, HFJV delivers each breath at a lower peak pressure than is reached with IPPV, but the mean airway pressure is approximately the same. Pressures are in cm H_2O.

during bronchoscopy and laryngoscopy. In the management of adult respiratory distress syndrome and other forms of respiratory failure, HFV has not been shown to offer any significant advantage over conventional volume ventilation.

POSITIVE END-EXPIRATORY PRESSURE

For most ventilated patients, the machine-delivered fraction of inspired oxygen (FIO_2) will provide an adequate PaO_2. When this FIO_2 is above 0.60 and the PaO_2 remains inadequate, positive end-expiratory pressure (PEEP) is often employed. PEEP is used only to improve the PaO_2, not the $PaCO_2$. PEEP is an alteration of ventilator pressures so that airway pressure is positive (above atmospheric) *throughout* the breathing cycle. It may be used with any of the ventilatory modes discussed so far, including high-frequency ventilation (HFV).

PEEP was first introduced into clinical medicine in 1967 when physicians working in a Denver intensive care unit described their experience with adult respiratory distress syndrome (ARDS) patients (Ashbaugh, Bigelow, Petty, et al., 1967). Two of the patients received PEEP on an empiric basis, and their PaO_2 improved. PEEP has since been used routinely in the management of ARDS. A pressure curve for PEEP is shown in Fig. 10-6. Normally, airway pressure at end-expiration is atmospheric (measured at the mouth); with PEEP it

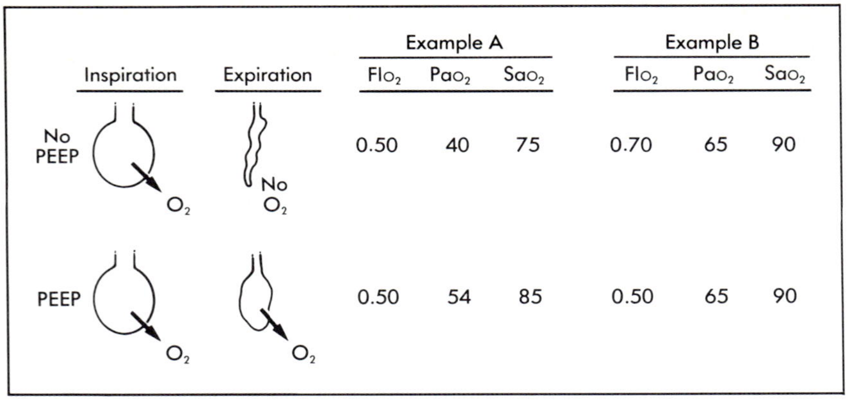

	Inspiration	Expiration	Example A			Example B		
			FIo$_2$	Pao$_2$	Sao$_2$	FIo$_2$	Pao$_2$	Sao$_2$
No PEEP			0.50	40	75	0.70	65	90
PEEP			0.50	54	85	0.50	65	90

Fig. 10-9. Effect of PEEP on oxygenation. During expiration with PEEP, airways that would otherwise collapse are kept open, allowing continued oxygen transfer. In Example A, the Pao$_2$ and Sao$_2$ improve while FIo$_2$ is unchanged. In Example B, the Pao$_2$ is maintained at an acceptable level while the FIo$_2$ is decreased from 0.70 to 0.50.

is above atmospheric. As commonly employed, PEEP pressures are usually between 5 and 20 cm H$_2$O above atmospheric pressure.

The mechanism by which PEEP improves oxygenation is not known for sure. Since PEEP increases functional residual capacity, it probably leads to better oxygenation by preventing end-expiratory collapse (Fig. 10-9). (Lung water studies have shown that PEEP does not diminish total lung water, but just redistributes it within the alveoli. Therefore PEEP cannot be considered a primary treatment for pulmonary edema.)

It is important to recognize that PEEP is measured in the upper airways and does not equal airway pressure in the alveolus. The PEEP is considerably dissipated by the time it reaches the alveoli. Yet it is the positive pressure at the alveolar level that both improves oxygenation and leads to complications. There is no practical way to know how much of the measured PEEP is present in the alveoli; the amount of dissipation depends on complex factors, including lung compliance and airways resistance. Nonetheless, as learned by experience and observation, a PEEP of less than 10 cm H$_2$O usually improves Pao$_2$ without significant complications; above this level, PEEP is more likely to be accompanied by complications, either barotrauma or a decrease in cardiac output (discussed later in this chapter).

CONTINUOUS POSITIVE AIRWAY PRESSURE

Another way of delivering positive airway pressure is through continuous positive airway pressure (CPAP). CPAP is positive end expiratory pressure (PEEP) without air being pushed in by a machine. With CPAP, inspiration is accomplished entirely by the patient's own muscular effort.* CPAP requires a tight seal to prevent escape of the positive air pressure, so it must be delivered through an endotracheal tube or a tightly sealed face mask. The changes in airway pressure with CPAP are similar to those in normal breathing except that both inspiratory and expiratory pressures are maintained above atmospheric pressure (Fig. 10-10).

Despite its theoretical advantages (no ventilator is necessary and mean airway pressure is less than with intermittent positive pressure ventilation

---

*The patient may be connected to a ventilator while receiving CPAP; in this situation the ventilator is not used to push air into the lungs but only serves as a source of oxygen-enriched air.

Artificial ventilation

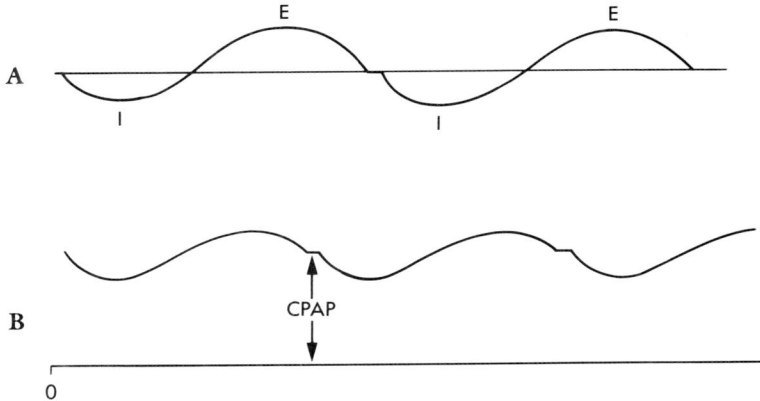

Fig. 10-10. Airway pressure during normal quiet breathing, **A**, and during continuous positive airway pressure (CPAP), **B**.

[IPPV]), CPAP is not widely used in adult medicine. CPAP is *not* a ventilatory mode (just as PEEP is not), and it is used only to augment oxygenation; machine-delivered ventilation is invariably more effective for this purpose. It is difficult to keep a tight-fitting face mask in place, and the mask is often uncomfortable for the patient. Despite its limitations, there are occasions when nonintubated patients can be aided by CPAP. The technique is always worth a try if a completely alert patient is suffering from oxygenation failure and avoiding artificial ventilation is desired.

CPAP is also sometimes used as a weaning technique during the interval between discontinuing a patient from IPPV and his extubation.

COMPLICATIONS OF ARTIFICIAL VENTILATION

Whenever machines take over a vital function, there is risk of complications; perhaps a complication does not occur every time in every patient, but one occurs often enough to cause a healthy wariness. Used appropriately, artificial ventilation can be life-saving and is well worth the risks; used inappropriately, the risks can outweigh the benefits. The box on p. 214 lists the more commonly observed complications of intubation and artificial ventilation. These complications may occur in any mode of intermittent positive pressure ventilation (IPPV). In addition, positive end expiratory pressure (PEEP) increases the likelihood of complications that arise from increased airway pressure.

Barotrauma manifests as subcutaneous emphysema, pneumothorax, or pneumomediastinum. A more serious problem is decreased cardiac output. The elevated intrathoracic pressure arising from IPPV can cause a decrease in venous return and hence a decrease in cardiac output. The problem is accentuated when PEEP is used. In fact patients may show a simultaneous *increase in arterial partial pressure of oxygen (PaO_2)* and *decrease in cardiac output*, with the net result of overall *decrease in oxygen transport* (Fig. 10-11). This decrease in oxygen transport is one reason why patients receiving PEEP are often monitored with a right-sided heart catheter (see Chapter 8).

The point at which PEEP maximally improves PaO_2 *and* oxygen transport is sometimes called "optimal" PEEP. However, this level of PEEP may not be optimal if accompanied by other problems, e.g., barotrauma. In truth, there is no consensus on what criteria constitute optimal PEEP. Determining optimal PEEP should probably *not* depend on sophisticated hemodynamic measure-

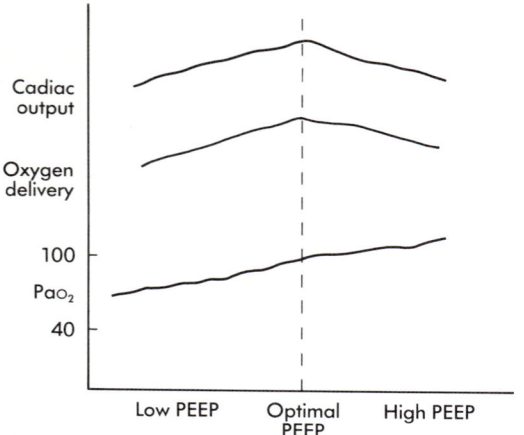

Fig. 10-11. Effect of PEEP on cardiac output and oxygen delivery. The Pa_{O_2} can increase while cardiac output and arterial oxygen delivery are decreasing. Optimal PEEP for a given patient can only be found by trial and error. See text for discussion.

ments, especially if the patient is receiving PEEP for a long period. In practice, optimal PEEP is usually the lowest level of PEEP that will give an adequate Pa_{O_2} on an FI_{O_2} of 0.6 or less.

Machine malfunction varies with the complexity and variety of machines in use. In practice, each machine is checked regularly (usually every hour) along protocols established by the manufacturer and each hospital's respiratory therapy department. Although today's volume ventilators are highly reliable, there is no substitute for constant surveillance by competent personnel. Quite literally, the patient's life depends on it.

The complications of PEEP are the same, qualitatively, as they are with any form of IPPV. Because mean airway pressure is higher with, than without, PEEP, barotrauma and decreased cardiac output tend to occur more commonly when PEEP is used. PEEP can be thought of as an exaggeration of conventional IPPV; it is not unique in causing complications of artificial ventilation.

POTENTIAL COMPLICATIONS OF INTUBATION AND ARTIFICIAL VENTILATION

From intubation
    Damage to teeth, mouth, and upper airways
    Intubation of esophagus
    Sedation-related complications (arrhythmia, further depression of ventilation, cardiac arrest)
From the tracheal tube
    Erosion of upper airways, e.g., pressure sores and tracheomalacia
    Accidental slippage of tube into a main stem bronchus
    Plugged tube, e.g., from mucus or secretions
From the increased airway pressure
    Barotrauma, e.g., pneumomediastinum and pneumothorax
    Decreased venous return and decreased cardiac output
    Increased physiologic dead space
Oxygen toxicity (only with high FI_{O_2})
Muscle atrophy from muscle disuse
Starvation from inadequate nutritional support
Gastric distention from air entering gastrointestinal tract
Accidents, e.g., disconnection from ventilator
Nosocomial infection, e.g., from machine or humidifier
Machine malfunction

Artificial ventilation

Clinical problem 8

A patient with severe emphysema is intubated because of progressive ventilatory failure. During his course of treatment the following blood gas values are obtained, all on an FIO_2 of 0.40 (V_T, tidal volume in cc; RR, respiratory rate; $\dot{V}_E$, minute ventilation in L/min; PP, peak ventilator pressure in cm H_2O; $Paco_2$ and Pao_2 are in mm Hg.):

Time	V_T	RR	$\dot{V}_E$	PP	pH	$Paco_2$	Pao_2
4:20 PM	500	12	6.0	30	7.35	48	76
5:30 PM	600	12	7.2	35	7.34	47	78
7:05 PM	700	12	8.4	38	7.31	54	75

Assuming no change has occurred in the clinical picture, how would you explain the rise in $Paco_2$?

VENTILATOR WEANING

If all patients undergoing general anesthesia are included, the vast majority of patients who receive artificial ventilation do not need to be weaned from the machine. When the underlying problem is rapidly corrected (as in recovery from anesthesia), the patient can simply be disconnected from the ventilator and extubated. For many chronically ill patients the procedure is not so simple. They often require prolonged artificial ventilation and a more gradual weaning from the machine.

Three steps are involved in weaning a patient from the ventilator (see box on p. 216). First, and most important, is to optimize the patient. The patient must be in as stable a condition as is feasible, which means improving or correcting conditions such as hypoxemia, anemia, fever, and metabolic alkalosis, as well as unstable cardiac conditions. Second, some assessment must be made showing that the patient can comfortably and adequately maintain oxygenation and ventilation without the machine. Third, the patient has to be removed (weaned) from the ventilator.

The physiologic parameters outlined in the box refer to the second step, assessing the patient's ability to oxygenate and ventilate without the machine. There has been an unfortunate tendency to view these parameters as rigid criteria for extubation. In fact these "weaning criteria" are merely physiologic guidelines and are not meant to predict who can or cannot be weaned. It is never necessary to perform all or even most of these measurements to wean a patient, and some measurements are totally inappropriate in certain situations. For example, measurement of the alveolar-arterial oxygen pressure difference ($P(A-a)O_2$) while the patient is breathing 100% oxygen would be ridiculous if the patient never required that fraction of inspired oxygen (FIO_2); this measurement and the shunt fraction measurement were at one time advocated for patients with severe adult respiratory distress syndrome, but they have no role in weaning a patient who was intubated primarily for ventilatory failure.

The other weaning measurements can give a useful index of the patient's ability to sustain ventilation. However, experienced physicians successfully extubate many patients without performing any of these tests. No good studies exist on the criteria for weaning chronically diseased patients. Indeed, some patients who are ambulatory and functioning at home would fail these tests.

Certainly a patient who exceeds these weaning criteria should have little trouble sustaining spontaneous ventilation. However, for the vast majority of patients, it is not necessary to measure anything more than arterial blood gases and the patient's respiratory rate; these measurements and simple observation are usually sufficient for ventilator weaning.

Clinical problem 9

A 59-year-old nonsmoking woman with no prior lung disease develops ARDS following a drug overdose. After

STEPS FOR WEANING PATIENT FROM THE VENTILATOR

1. **OPTIMIZE THE PATIENT.** Conditions requiring specific attention or correction before weaning is initiated include the following (in no particular order):

   Anemia
   Shock
   Starvation
   Thoracic pain
   Fever
   Infection

   Acid-base abnormalities, especially metabolic alkalosis and acidosis
   Electrolyte imbalance
   Sleep deprivation
   Reduced cardiac output
   Copious airway secretions

2. **ASSESS ABILITY OF PATIENT TO OXYGENATE AND TO VENTILATE WITHOUT THE MACHINE.** Physiologic criteria that have been used for this purpose include the following:

Tests of mechanics	Criterion
Tidal volume	At least 4 to 5 cc/kg
Vital capacity	At least 10 to 15 cc/kg
Peak inspiratory pressure	At least -20 to -30 cm H_2O*
Resting minute ventilation ($\dot{V}_E$)	Less than 10 L/min, with ability to at least double $\dot{V}_E$ voluntarily

Tests of oxygenation and ventilation	
FIO_2 that provides adequate PaO_2	0.40 or less, without PEEP
P (A-a)O_2 while breathing 100% oxygen	Less than 350 mm Hg
Shunt fraction while breathing 100% oxygen	Less than 20%
Dead space/tidal volume ratio	Less than 0.60

3. **WEAN THE PATIENT.** The two methods of weaning are:
   A. **Trial and error method.** Disconnect endotracheal tube from ventilator and connect to a T-piece containing humidified oxygen; repeat blood gas analysis in approximately 30 minutes and again before extubation. Carefully observe patient's respiratory rate and effort, blood pressure, and pulse.
   B. **Intermittent mandatory ventilation (IMV).** Gradually decrease number of IMV breaths per minute; monitor patient's respiratory rate and arterial blood gas values with each change in IMV.

*The more negative the number the better, i.e., -40 cm H_2O is more desirable than -30 cm H_2O

several weeks her oxygenation has improved, but she remains ventilator-dependent because of hypercapnia and severe restrictive impairment. She is alert and responsive. On an assist-control mode, the patient is initiating 24 breaths/min. The following measurements are obtained: PaO_2, 75 mm Hg; $PaCO_2$, 65 mm Hg; pH, 7.34; and mean expired PCO_2, 28 mm Hg.

What is the patient's ratio of dead space to tidal volume (V_D/V_T), and what does this ratio predict about weaning her from the ventilator?

Clinical problem 10

A 65-year-old man with a history of severe emphysema (FEV_1 of 900 cc, 40% of predicted; baseline arterial blood gas [ABG] analysis #1, below) is admitted to the intensive care unit because of acute pneumonia. Admission ABG analysis is #2. Despite the administration of appropriate antibiotics and low-supplemental oxygen therapy, the patient decompensates the night of admission (ABG analysis #3), and he is intubated. Over the next several days he gradually improves. On the fifth day he is receiving IMV at a rate of 8/min (ABG analysis #4) and appears alert and comfortable. He has a spontaneous (spont.) respiratory rate (in addition to the machine-delivered breaths) of 6/min. How would you proceed with ventilator weaning at this point?

ABG analysis	pH	$Paco_2$	Pao_2	Fio_2	Mode
#1 (baseline)	7.37	51	65	0.21	Spont.
#2 (admission)	7.35	54	45	0.28	Spont.
#3 (before intubation)	7.33	58	39	0.35	Spont.
#4 (5 days later)	7.37	47	78	0.30	IMV, 8/min; spont., 6 breaths/min

SUMMARY

Artificial ventilation is indicated for patients with life-threatening impairment of alveolar ventilation and/or oxygenation. Airway pressures with artificial ventilation differ fundamentally from normal breathing; in normal breathing airway pressure alternates between negative pressure (on inspiration) and positive pressure (on expiration). In the most common mode of artificial ventilation used today (intermittent positive pressure ventilation [IPPV]), airway pressure is positive on both inspiration and expiration.

For artificial ventilation a fraction of inspired oxygen (Fio_2) and a mode of ventilation must be chosen. The Fio_2 may range from 0.21 to 1.00. The most commonly employed modes of ventilation include control ventilation (machine initiates and delivers each breath), assist-control ventilation (patient initiates or triggers a machine-delivered breath), and intermittent mandatory ventilation (IMV, the patient can breathe spontaneously between mandatory ventilator breaths). Both control and assist-control modes are used for full-ventilatory support. IMV at 8 or more ventilator breaths/min is tantamount to full-ventilatory support; IMV at 7 or less breaths/min is considered partial-ventilatory support and is commonly used as a weaning mode.

Positive end-expiratory pressure (PEEP) is a method of improving oxygenation that can be used in any ventilatory mode. PEEP can be applied to an intubated, artificially ventilated patient or to a nonintubated patient through a tight-fitting face mask, in which case the technique is called CPAP. All forms of artificial ventilation have potential complications, which include barotrauma and reduction of cardiac output; these two problems are more commonly seen with the addition of high levels of PEEP.

Ventilator weaning includes three steps: (1) optimizing the patient, (2) assessing the patient's ability to oxygenate and ventilate without the machine, and (3) weaning the patient. There are two methods of weaning—removing the patient from the ventilator for short periods of time ("trial and error") and progressive reduction of IMV breaths/minute. Either method is adequate as long as the patient is carefully observed.

REVIEW QUESTIONS

State whether each of the following is true or false.
1. Artificial ventilation is indicated for any patient with a $Paco_2$ above 50 mm Hg and a pH less than 7.30.
2. Airway pressures found in normal breathing can be duplicated by artificial jet ventilation.

3. During controlled positive pressure ventilation, each breath is initiated by the patient.
4. During ventilation with positive end-expiratory pressure (PEEP), the pressure in the upper airways is always above atmospheric pressure.
5. A patient receiving intermittent mandatory ventilation (IMV) is able to alternate spontaneous breathing with machine breaths.
6. Continuous positive airway pressure (CPAP) is defined as a PEEP pressure maintained above 10 cm H_2O.
7. The appropriate FIO_2 during the initial stages of artificial ventilation is always 1.00 (100%).
8. With PEEP, a patient's PaO_2 may improve while the arterial oxygen delivery is decreasing.
9. Compared with conventional positive pressure ventilation, jet ventilation provides a lower peak airway pressure.
10. Successful ventilatory weaning requires the patient to have a V_D/V_T of less than 0.45.

References

Ashbaugh, D.B., Bigelow, D.B., Petty, T.L., et al.: Acute respiratory distress in adults, Lancet **2**:319, 1967.

Shapiro, B.A., and Cane, R.D.: IMV-AMV controversy: a plea for clarification and redirection, Crit. Care Med **12**:472, 1984.

Suggested readings

Cane, R.D., and Shapiro, B.A.: Mechanical ventilatory support, JAMA **254**:87, 1985.

Downs, J.B., Klein, E.F., Desautels, D., et al.: Intermittent mandatory ventilation: a new approach to weaning patients from mechanical ventilators, Chest **64**:331, 1973.

Feely, R.W., and Hedley-Whyte, J.: Weaning from controlled ventilation and oxygen, N. Engl. J. Med. **292**:903, 1975.

Hodgkin, J.E., Bowser, M.A., and Burton, G.G.: Respirator weaning, Crit. Care Med. **2**:96, 1974.

McPherson, S.P., and Spearman, D.B.: Respiratory therapy equipment, St. Louis, 1983, The C.V. Mosby Co.

Mushin, W.W., Rendell-Baker, L., Thompson, P.W., et al.: Automatic ventilation of the lungs, Oxford, 1980, Blackwell Scientific Publications, Ltd.

Pepe, P.E., Hudson, L.D., and Carrico, C.J.: Early application of positive end expiratory pressure in patients at risk for the adult respiratory distress syndrome, N. Engl. J. Med. **311**:281, 1984.

Rounds, S., and Brody, J.S.: Putting PEEP in perspective, N. Engl. J. Med. **311**:323, 1984.

Sahn, S.A., Lakshminarayan, S., and Petty, T.L.: Weaning from mechanical ventilation, JAMA **235**:2208, 1976.

Suter, P.M., Fairley, H.B., and Isenberg, M.D.: Optimum end-expiratory pressure in patients with acute pulmonary failure, N. Engl. J. Med. **292**:284, 1975.

See also General References in Appendix G.

chapter 11
Respiratory failure

OUTLINE

Definition of respiratory failure
Physiologic classification of respiratory failure
Clinical classification of respiratory failure
Acute vs. chronic respiratory failure
Pulmonary edema
Shunt equation
Adult respiratory distress syndrome
Physiologic manifestations of ARDS
Management of ARDS
A case of oxygenation respiratory failure
Respiratory failure in chronic obstructive pulmonary disease
A case of combined ventilatory and oxygenation failure in COPD

Previous chapters covered important aspects of gas exchange and lung mechanics. The subject of *respiratory failure* serves to "put it all together." No other clinical problem focuses so acutely the important aspects of respiratory physiology.

DEFINITION OF RESPIRATORY FAILURE

The respiratory system is the total integrative system dealing with respiration; this includes the brainstem medullary center, the chest bellows (including nerves, muscles, bones, and pleura), and the lungs (including the airways). Respiratory failure is defined in terms of the primary function of the respiratory system, which is to exchange oxygen and carbon dioxide with the atmosphere. This function is properly called external respiration to distinguish it from respiration (oxygen and carbon dioxide transfer) at the tissue level. Clinically, respiratory failure refers only to the external process and is defined as a state of *severely reduced arterial partial pressure of oxygen (Pa_{O_2}) and/or high arterial partial pressure of carbon dioxide (Pa_{CO_2}) when caused by a defect in the respiratory system*.

The clinical (i.e., bedside) estimation of Pa_{O_2} and Pa_{CO_2} is notoriously unreliable in sick patients. Hence respiratory failure must first be suspected, then blood must be drawn for blood gas analysis to confirm the diagnosis and begin management. Generally respiratory failure should be suspected in any patient who is comatose, obtunded, confused, or cyanotic or who has unexplained dyspnea, anxiety, restlessness, or aggressive behavior. These signs and symptoms may be manifestations of severe hypoxemia or hypercapnia. However, signs and symptoms are an unreliable guide to specific diagnosis and management; they are not invariably present and do not necessarily correlate with severity of blood gas abnormality (see Chapters 4 and 6). The only reliable clinical definition of respiratory failure is the absence of breathing.

There is no universal agreement on "cutoff" values for Pa_{CO_2} and Pa_{O_2} beyond which a patient is said to have respiratory failure. Commonly

Table 11-1. Oxygenation and ventilatory respiratory failure

Type of respiratory failure	Clinical examples	Blood gas changes		
		PaO_2*	$PaCO_2$	$P(A-a)O_2$
Oxygenation	Pneumonia, pulmonary edema	Low	Normal to low	High
Ventilatory	Drug overdose, poliomyelitis	Low	High	Normal
Oxygenation and ventilatory	Chronic obstructive pulmonary disease, severe asthma	Low	High	High

*In each case, PaO_2 is lower than predicted for the FIO_2. When breathing high FIO_2, PaO_2 can be adequate, e.g., 90 to 100 mm Hg, in the face of severe oxygenation failure.

quoted is a PaO_2 less than 60 mm Hg or a $PaCO_2$ above 50 mm Hg, while the patient is breathing room air at sea level. These criteria are arbitrary and leave out a large number of patients with profound respiratory failure under other circumstances, e.g., a patient with PaO_2 of 70 mm Hg while breathing 100% oxygen or a patient with $PaCO_2$ of 46 mm Hg and pH of 7.15 who is suffering a severe asthma attack. In both cases the lungs have failed to work properly, and the patient is in danger of dying from respiratory failure.

It is best to consider any elevation of $PaCO_2$ above 50 mm Hg as an indication of respiratory failure and to evaluate lower a $PaCO_2$ carefully in the clinical context. Similarly, any reduction of PaO_2 can be considered respiratory failure if (1) it is caused by a disorder in the respiratory system and (2) it cannot be maintained above 60 mm Hg without supplemental oxygen.

PHYSIOLOGIC CLASSIFICATION OF RESPIRATORY FAILURE

In terms of gas exchange, there are two physiologic types of respiratory failure. Table 11-1 lists common clinical examples of these physiologic types of respiratory failure and their accompanying gas exchange abnormalities.

Oxygenation failure. Oxygen failure is charaterized by low PaO_2, increased $P(A-a)O_2$, and normal or low $PaCO_2$. In oxygenation failure, the lungs have failed to transfer oxygen properly. Physiologically, it is always caused by venous admixture (ventilation/perfusion imbalance and/or right-to-left shunting) and is always manifested by elevated alveolar-arterial oxygen pressure difference ($P(A-a)O_2$). $PaCO_2$ may be normal but more commonly is reduced (alveolar hyperventilation). Oxygenation failure is always a manifestation of pulmonary parenchymal or airways disease.

Ventilatory failure. Ventilatory failure is characterized by low PaO_2, normal $P(A-a)O_2$, and high $PaCO_2$. The problem in ventilatory failure is that alveolar ventilation ($\dot{V}A$) is insufficient for the amount of carbon dioxide production. In "pure" ventilatory failure, PaO_2 is low *only because* $PaCO_2$ is high, and the $P(A-a)O_2$ is therefore normal. Ventilatory respiratory failure may occur from central nervous system depression or chest bellows impairment. The physiologic basis for pure ventilatory failure is decreased minute ventilation, increased dead space ventilation, or a combination of the two (see Chapter 4).

CLINICAL CLASSIFICATION OF RESPIRATORY FAILURE

The physiologic classification of respiratory failure (see Table 11-1) can be merged with a clinical classification based on the respiratory system's three main divisions—the respiratory control centers, the chest bellows, and the lungs and airways

Respiratory Failure

Table 11-2. Some clinical causes of respiratory failure

	Division of respiratory system (Type of respiratory failure)	
Respiratory control centers (Ventilatory)	**Chest bellows (Ventilatory)**	**Lungs/airways (Oxygenation alone or ventilatory plus oxygenation)**
Drug overdose	Kyphoscoliosis	Chronic obstructive pulmonary disease
Central nervous system medullary lesions	Flail Chest	Bronchitis
	Massive obesity	Emphysema
Pickwickian syndrome	Poliomyelitis	Asthma
Hypoventilation caused by metabolic alkalosis	Guillain-Barré syndrome	Pneumonia
	Myasthenia gravis	Pulmonary embolism
	Muscular dystrophy	Cystic fibrosis
	Paralyzing drugs	Interstitial fibrosis
		Pulmonary edema

(Table 11-2). Disease or dysfunction in any one of these areas can seriously impair gas exchange and lead to respiratory failure. Note that disease of either the medullary center or chest bellows alone (i.e., without lung involvement) can only result in pure ventilatory failure (increased arterial pressure of carbon dioxide [$PaCO_2$], and normal alveolar-arterial oxygen pressure difference [$P(A-a)O_2$]). This is because the only determinants of $P(A-a)O_2$ are V/Q imbalance, shunt, and diffusion barrier, and the lung is the only organ in which these physiologic problems can arise (see Chapter 5).

Note also that common lung diseases, such as asthma, bronchitis, and emphysema, are but a few of the many potential causes of respiratory failure. Respiratory failure can arise from a variety of clinical problems unrelated to primary lung disease.

ACUTE VS. CHRONIC RESPIRATORY FAILURE

Much of the literature refers to *acute* and *chronic* respiratory failure; however, use of these modifiers can obscure the overall picture. When applied to respiratory failure, acute and chronic do not generally indicate a specific disease or pathologic process. Acute has been applied to a variety of conditions causing respiratory failure, such as the adult respiratory distress syndrome (ARDS) and exacerbation of chronic obstructive pulmonary disease (COPD); in this context, acute usually means "requiring immediate medical attention" or refers to recent onset of symptoms.

Acute, as well as chronic, can apply to either oxygenation or ventilatory respiratory failure. The most common cause of respiratory failure is probably COPD, which can manifest as failure of oxygenation alone or as combined ventilatory and oxygenation failure. Such patients can be working and living relatively normal lives (chronic illness), or they can present in "acute" distress, as when beset by complications such as pulmonary infection. Conversely, ARDS, the most severe manifestation of oxygenation respiratory failure, is invariably acute in its presentation.

PULMONARY EDEMA

Pulmonary edema occurs when excess plasma enters the pulmonary interstitium and alveoli. Pulmonary edema is an acute clinical problem that is invariably accompanied by respiratory distress and tachypnea (unless the patient is obtunded) as well as reduced PaO_2 and increased $P(A-a)O_2$. The basic physiologic mechanism for the hypoxemia is ventilation-perfusion imbalance (see Chapter 5).

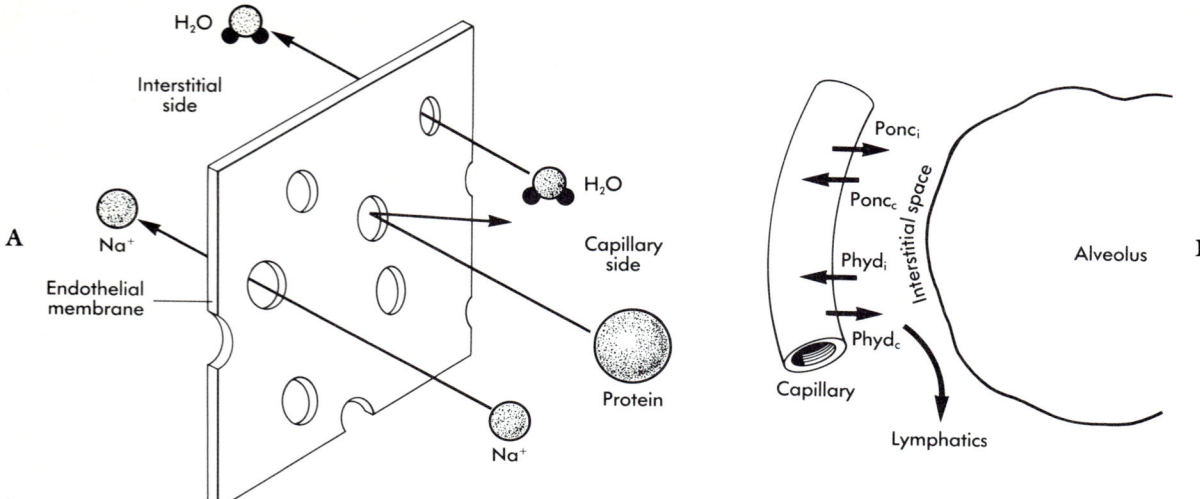

Fig. 11-1. **A,** Fluid transport from capillary to interstitial space. The intact endothelial membrane is permeable to water and to small solutes (e.g., Na⁺) but is impermeable to protein. In noncardiogenic pulmonary edema, proteins leak through the damaged membrane, flooding the interstitium and alveolar spaces. **B,** Balance of colloid and hydrostatic forces in pulmonary capillary. Colloid osmotic pressure is normally closely balanced against capillary hydrostatic pressure. Capillary hydrostatic pressure favors movement of fluid out of the capillary and is opposed by the hydrostatic pressure in the interstitial fluid. Colloid osmotic pressure of the plasma proteins tends to keep fluid in the capillary and is opposed by the osmotic pressure of proteins in interstitial fluid. The exact pressures (oncotic and hydrostatic) within the pulmonary capillary are not known for sure, but the net result is a slight and continuous leak of fluid out of the capillaries and into the pulmonary interstitium, where it is picked up by interstitial lymphatics. It is estimated that lymph flow from the lung is approximately 10 to 20 ml/min (Staub, 1978). When this balance of forces is upset so that fluid movement overwhelms lymphatic drainage, pulmonary edema results. ($Phyd_c$, hydrostatic pressure in pulmonary capillary; $Phyd_i$, hydrostatic pressure in pulmonary interstitium; $Ponc_c$, oncotic pressure in pulmonary capillary; $Ponc_i$, oncotic pressure in pulmonary interstitium.)

Normally, fluid in the pulmonary capillaries is balanced with fluid in the interstitium. A slight amount of capillary plasma (water and small solutes) continually enters the interstitium, where it is transported by the interstitial lymphatics to the systemic venous circulation (Fig. 11-1, *A* and *B*).

The forces that balance the capillary and interstitial fluid compartments are *hydrostatic* and *oncotic.* Hydrostatic pressure is the intravascular pressure tending to push fluid out of the pulmonary capillary; it reflects the filling pressure of the left side of the heart and is approximated by the pulmonary artery wedge pressure (PAWP; see Chapter 8).

Oncotic pressure is caused by large-molecular-weight molecules, mainly proteins. Oncotic pressure tends to keep fluid in the capillaries and thus opposes the capillary hydrostatic pressure. Although this pressure can be measured with an oncometer (normal value 20 to 25 mm Hg), it correlates with both the serum total protein and albumin concentration; if the total protein or albumin concentration is low, oncotic pressure is also reduced.

Table 11-3. Mechanisms in the pulmonary capillary that influence movement of fluid into the pulmonary interstitium

Mechanism	Normal	Factor favoring excess fluid movement	Common clinical cause	Type of pulmonary edema
Hydrostatic pressure	6 to 12 mm Hg*	Increased value	Left heart failure	Cardiac
Oncotic pressure	20 to 25 mm Hg†	Decreased value	Liver cirrhosis	Noncardiac
Membrane permeability	—	Increased permeability	Sepsis	Noncardiac

*Measured as pulmonary artery wedge pressure.
†Oncotic pressure can be qualitatively assessed by measurement of serum total protein or albumin, each of which correlates with the measured oncotic pressure. A low-oncotic pressure is rarely, if ever, a sole cause of pulmonary edema; however, it is definitely a contributory factor in presence of another mechanism.

Equation 1 (the Starling equation) relates the forces that account for net fluid filtration from the capillary to the interstitium (see also Fig. 11-1, *B*). Qf represents the fluid movement between the capillary (c) and the surrounding interstitium (i) and is the sum of the hydrostatic and oncotic forces in each space. K and K@ are coefficients for capillary membrane permeability for both fluid and protein, respectively.

$$Qf = Q \text{ hydrostatic} = Q \text{ oncotic}$$

$$Qf = K(Phyd_c - Phyd_i) - K@(Ponc_c - Ponc_i) \quad (1)$$

Thus fluid movement into the interstitium depends on three mechanisms—(1) pulmonary hydrostatic pressure, (2) serum oncotic pressure, and (3) permeability of the alveolar-capillary membrane (Table 11-3).

The physiologic mechanism in *cardiogenic* pulmonary edema is increased hydrostatic pressure. This results from failure of the left ventricle to pump blood normally; the result is a "backup" of blood in the pulmonary circulation and a flooding of the pulmonary interstitium and alveoli. Left-ventricular failure may occur from any disease that tends to weaken or damage the heart (e.g., myocardial infarction). In those cases where the hydrostatic pressure must be measured, a Swan-Ganz catheter is passed and measurement is taken of the pulmonary artery wedge pressure (see Chapter 8).

The physiologic mechanism in *noncardiogenic* pulmonary edema is increased membrane permeability, which is impossible to quantify clinically. In its most fulminant state, noncardiogenic pulmonary edema is called the adult (or infant) respiratory distress syndrome (ARDS or IRDS).

Low oncotic pressure is rarely, if ever, an isolated cause of pulmonary edema. Either type of pulmonary edema (cardiogenic from hydrostatic forces or noncardiogenic from increased permeability) may be aggravated by a low serum protein concentration.

SHUNT EQUATION

In Chapter 5 a distinction was made between right-to-left blood shunts and venous admixture. To review, venous admixture includes all pulmonary venous blood that returns to the left side of the heart unoxygenated. This lack of oxygenation may come about for several reasons: a right-to-left shunt, where the blood sees no alveolar air; low ventilation/perfusion (V/Q) ratios, where the amount of alveolar ventilation is less than capillary perfusion (see Chapter 5); and a diffusion barrier between the alveolar space and capillary blood.

In low V/Q and diffusion-impaired units, 100% oxygen will eventually fully oxygenate the capillary blood and eliminate the venous admixture (see

Chapter 5). When a patient is breathing 100% oxygen, the sole remaining cause of venous admixture will be right-to-left shunting; for this reason 100% oxygen is used when calculating the amount of shunt (discussed later in this chapter).

Inhaling 100% oxygen will not distinguish between *anatomic* and *physiologic* shunting. Anatomic shunting results from an abnormal connection between a pulmonary artery (or a right-sided heart chamber) and a pulmonary vein (or a left-sided heart chamber). Physiologic shunting occurs when blood in normally connected pulmonary vessels does not come into contact with alveolar air. Of the two types, physiolgoic shunting is much more common; it occurs in pulmonary edema and in most cases of oxygenation respiratory failure.

The amount of blood shunted from right to left, Qs, is usually calculated as a percentage of the cardiac output, QT and is symbolized Qs/QT. Normal Qs/QT, less than 3%, comes from bronchial circulation and blood serving the left-ventricular myocardium (thebesian vessels) that returns directly to the left side of the heart. In severe cases of oxygenation failure, as much as 40% of the cardiac output may be shunted. Generally, the higher the Qs/QT, the more severe the underlying pulmonary disease.

The actual calculation of Qs/QT is used more in research than in day-to-day intensive care practice. Studies that chart the effects of treatment modalities, such as positive end expiratory pressure (PEEP), often report changes in %shunt to show improvement or worsening of gas exchange. In clinical practice, there are simpler methods of showing improvement without resorting to the shunt calculation. In addition, as was discussed in Chapter 6, breathing 100% oxygen may cause absorption atelectasis and increase the Qs/QT.

Although I do not find routine shunt calculation a valuable clinical tool, the shunt equation is nonetheless useful for didactic purposes. It ties together many of the aspects of physiology so far discussed, such as venous admixture, oxygen content, and the alveolar air equation. For this reason, the shunt equation will be derived here and used in later clinical problems.

Fig. 11-2 shows a schematic of the lungs with a right-to-left shunt. Note that:

$$Q_T = \text{Total cardiac output}$$
$$Q_S = \text{Total shunted blood flow}$$
$$(Q_T - Q_S) = \text{Amount of cardiac output that is oxygenated}$$

It follows that:

$$Q_T = Q_S + (Q_T - Q_S). \quad (2)$$

Oxygen is added to the blood only through the lungs. In Fig. 11-2, that portion of Q_T that receives oxygen is $(Q_T - Q_S)$; by definition, Qs receives no oxygen. All oxygen in the arterial system must therefore come from the oxygen already in Qs (the mixed venous oxygen) and that delivered by $(Q_T - Q_S)$. Thus

$$\text{Oxygen transport in arterial blood} = \quad (3)$$
$$\text{Oxygen transport in shunted blood} +$$
$$\text{Oxygen transport in nonshunted blood}$$

Since oxygen transport is blood flow times oxygen content, the phrases in Equation 3 can be replaced with the respective blood flows and oxygen contents for arterial blood, shunted blood, and nonshunted blood.

$$(Q_T \times Ca_{O_2}) = (Q_S \times Cv_{O_2}) + \quad (3)$$
$$([Q_T - Q_S] \times Cc_{O_2})$$

where Ca_{O_2}, Cc_{O_2}, and Cv_{O_2} are, respectively, arterial, end-capillary, and mixed venous oxygen contents.

Rearranging Equation 3, the shunt equation is obtained.

$$\frac{Q_S}{Q_T} = \frac{Cc_{O_2} - Ca_{O_2}}{Cc_{O_2} - Cv_{O_2}} \quad (4)$$

Although Ca_{O_2} can be obtained from analysis of arterial blood gas, how are CcC_{O_2} and Cv_{O_2} obtained? Cv_{O_2} must come from measurement of mixed venous oxygen saturation, which requires a right-sided heart catheter (see Chapter 8). Cc_{O_2} is

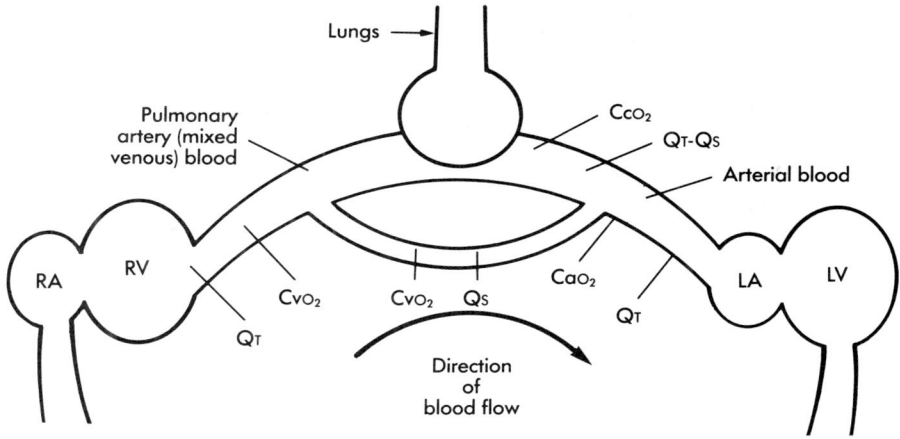

Fig. 11-2. Schematic of the lungs with a right-to-left blood shunt. (*RA*, right atrium; *RV*, right ventricle; *LA*, left atrium; *LV*, left ventricle.)

calculated by assuming that, while the patient is breathing 100% inspired oxygen, end-capillary P_{O_2} equals alveolar P_{O_2} and end-capillary hemoglobin is 100% saturated.

When a patient is inhaling 100% oxygen, the shunt equation calculates the actual right-to-left shunt. When the patient is breathing less than 100% oxygen, the equation provides the total venous admixture since it cannot be assumed that all low V/Q areas and diffusion barriers have been overcome.

Consider the following problem: A 54-year-old patient in the intensive care unit is being ventilated with 100% oxygen; barometric pressure is 747 mm Hg. His Pa_{O_2} is 123 mm Hg, Pa_{CO_2} is 35 mm Hg, Sa_{O_2} is 98%, Pv_{O_2} is 35 mm Hg, Sv_{O_2} is 68%, and hemoglobin content is 12 gm%. What is the Q_S/Q_T?

To calculate the shunt, first calculate the oxygen concentration in end-capillary blood (Cc_{O_2}), arterial blood (Ca_{O_2}), and mixed venous blood (Cv_{O_2}). Alveolar P_{O_2} is calculated using the alveolar air equation ($P_{A_{O_2}} = 665$ mm Hg). In calculating oxygen contents for the shunt equation, the dissolved fraction of oxygen must always be included, which is $0.003 \times P_{O_2}$.

$Cc_{O_2} = ([1.00 \times 1.34 \times 12] + [0.003 \times 665]) = 18.08$

$Ca_{O_2} = ([0.98 \times 1.34 \times 12] + [0.003 \times 123]) = 16.13$

$Cv_{O_2} = ([0.68 \times 1.34 \times 12] + [0.003 \times 35]) = 11.04$

Substituting in Equation 4,

$$\frac{Q_S}{Q_T} = \frac{1.95}{7.04} = 0.28 \text{ or } 28\% \text{ right-to-left shunt}$$

Some abbreviations of the shunt equation assume a value for ($Ca_{O_2} - Cv_{O_2}$) in their calculation, e.g., 5 vol%. Patients with oxygenation failure can manifest a wide range for ($Ca_{O_2} - Cv_{O_2}$), so accuracy of any shunt equation is questionable if a value for Cv_{O_2} is assumed. Without some measurement of mixed venous oxygen, one might just as well use $P(A-a)_{O_2}$ as an indicator of gas exchange impairment without bothering with shunt calculation.

ADULT RESPIRATORY DISTRESS SYNDROME

The adult respiratory distress syndrome (ARDS) is a type of fulminant, noncardiogenic pulmonary

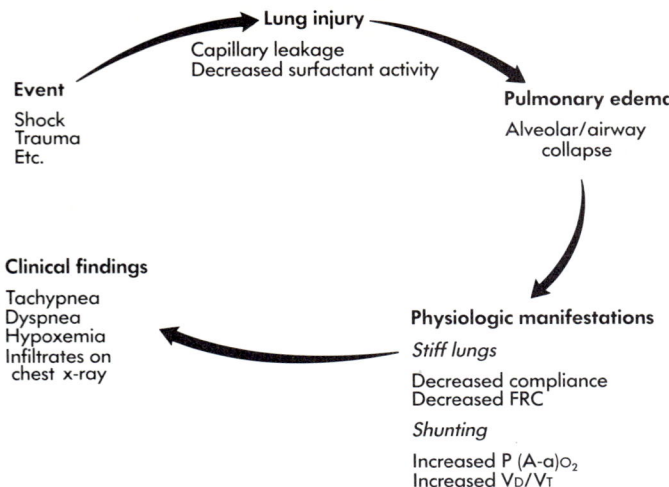

Fig. 11-3. Pathophysiology of adult respiratory distress syndrome.

edema. This syndrome has become widely recognized in the past 15 years, coincident with the spread of critical care units and arterial blood gas analysis. ARDS includes the following features:
1. Severe respiratory distress following an acute illness or injury
2. Pulmonary capillary leakage with normal pulmonary hydrostatic pressures (and therefore not caused by heart failure)
3. Chest x-ray showing bilateral "white-out" caused by extensive lung infiltration
4. Severe hypoxemia, usually not correctable with oxygen therapy at ambient air pressure (é.g., using nasal cannula, or conventional face mask)

Patients with underlying, chronic lung disease do not appear any more prone to develop ARDS than do previously healthy patients. In fact, the absence of any prior lung disease is typical of ARDS patients.

Since the first publication of the syndrome in 1967 (Ashbaugh, Bigelow, Petty, el al.), hundreds of cases have been reported in the literature. The estimated incidence of ARDS in the early 1970's was 150,000 new cases per year.

The most common causes or precipitating events of ARDS are listed in the box above. Patients suffering any of these medical problems may develop ARDS. The diversity of causes has prompted search for a unified pathophysiology. Various hy-

---

EVENTS THAT MAY PRECIPITATE ARDS

Hypotension ("shock lung")
Sepsis
Trauma (including nonthoracic)
Fat embolism
Transfusion reaction
Viral pneumonia
Aspiration pneumonia
Pancreatitis
Oxygen toxicity
Drug overdose

Table 11-4. Adult respiratory distress syndrome

Physiologic manifestations and their consequences	
Stiff lungs	**Consequences**
Decreased compliance	Requires more airway pressure for given volume of breath
Decreased functional residual capacity	Less lung volume for oxygen transfer
Shunting	
Increased $P(A-a)O_2$	High FIO_2 required for adequate oxygenation; also PEEP is often necessary
Increased V_D/V_T	More ventilation required for gas transfer because of large percentage of each breath going to dead space

potheses have tried to explain how these conditions lead to the capillary leakage characteristic of ARDS. Theories advocated include neurogenic causes, thromboembolic causes, circulating toxin, and fluid overload mechanisms. There are probably several underlying mechanisms, which are different for each clinical condition. Regardless, all cases of ARDS seem to share a common pathophysiology (Fig. 11-3 and Table 11-4).

PHYSIOLOGIC MANIFESTATIONS OF ARDS

The physiology of ARDS is characterized by *stiff lungs* and *shunting* (Table 11-4). Stiff lungs are manifested by their low-compliance, i.e., reduced change in lung volume per change in distending pressure. The lungs are stiff (low-compliance) because they are filled with a proteinaceous exudate that has leaked out of damaged pulmonary capillaries. For this reason it takes more airway pressure to achieve a given tidal volume in lungs of patients with ARDS than in healthy lungs.

Another manifestation of stiffness is reduced functional residual capacity (FRC). FRC is the volume of air in the lungs at the end of tidal volume. Reduced FRC occurs because the alveoli, filled with fluid, tend to collapse at the end of expiration. As a result, there is less lung volume to exchange oxygen throughout the breathing cycle. One of the major treatment modalities in ARDS, positive end-expiratory pressure, helps keep alveoli open at the end of expiration, thereby increasing FRC and facilitating oxygen transfer.

Shunting, the other major physiologic problem in ARDS, is manifested by both a blood shunt (venous admixture) and an "air shunt" (alveolar dead space). Blood is shunted past the collapsed alveoli, leading to venous admixture, which accounts for the profound hypoxemia of ARDS. At the same time *other* alveoli are relatively underperfused and overventilated, creating extra dead space or an increase in dead space/tidal volume (V_D/V_T). In a sense, air brought to these alveoli is "shunted" since it is met by decreased or absent perfusion.

The physiologic basis of both the blood shunt and the air shunt is profound V/Q imbalance (Fig. 11-4). ARDS exemplifies the most severe V/Q disturbance seen clinically. The early stage of ARDS is more related to the venous admixture than to the alveolar dead space since arterial blood gas measurements invariably show low PaO_2 *and* low $PaCO_2$. It is only in the late stages of unresolving ARDS that hypercapnia is manifested. (Blood gases are discussed in more detail later in this chapter in the case of oxygenation respiratory failure.)

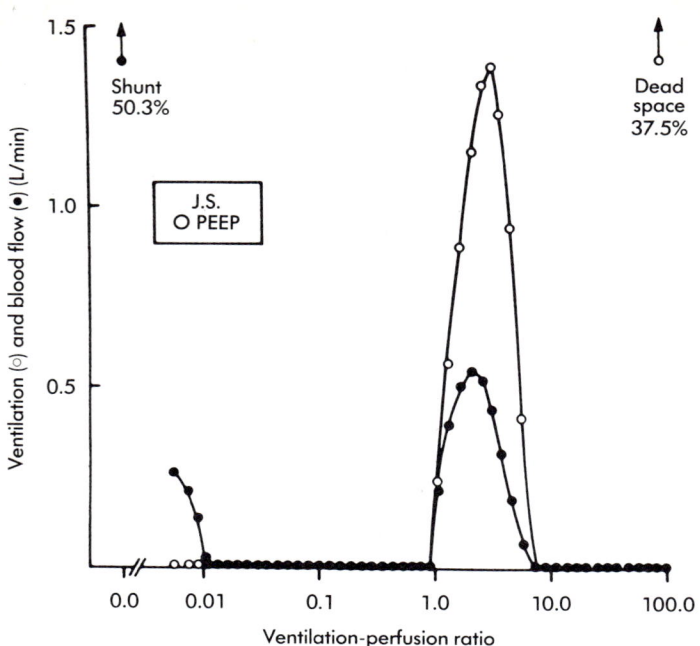

Fig. 11-4. Ventilation-perfusion curves from a young male patient with ARDS caused by viral pneumonia (compare with Fig. 5-9). Part of the pulmonary blood flow is well-ventilated, but a large proportion is also distributed to areas with either very little or no alveolar ventilation. In this example 50.3% of the blood flow "sees" no ventilation (i.e., is shunted). At the same time, 37.5% of the ventilation sees no perfusion (i.e., dead space). (From Dantzker, R.D., Brook, C.J., Dehart, P., et al.: Am. Rev. Respir. Dis. **120**:1042, 1979.)

MANAGEMENT OF ARDS

Management of ARDS is outlined in the box on p. 229. The major problem is severe hypoxemia, and the goal is to maintain adequate oxygenation in any way possible. Practically, this means maintaining PaO_2 above 60 mm Hg on a fraction of inspired oxygen (FIO_2) less than 0.50 to obviate the risk of oxygen toxicity (see Chapter 9).

To achieve this goal, in most cases the patient must be intubated and receive artificial ventilation along with a high FIO_2. Usually positive end expiratory pressure (PEEP) is also employed. PEEP is simply a ventilator maneuver that maintains airway pressure above atmospheric pressure at the end of expiration. PEEP causes an increase in functional residual capacity and a decrease in the amount of right-to-left shunting. PEEP can increase PaO_2 without an increase in FIO_2 or can allow for a lowering of FIO_2 without a reduction in PaO_2 (see also Chapter 10).

PEEP is not without its drawbacks, such as barotrauma and reduced cardiac output. Despite its potential disadvantages, many consider PEEP an important advance in the treatment of ARDS. Even so, overall mortality from ARDS is approximately 50% to 60%, unchanged since the first clinical description in 1967. Patients who recover from ARDS will usually have no major pulmonary problem. At most they seem to show only a slight restriction during pulmonary function testing or a small decrease in diffusing capacity. Thus ARDS seems to confer an "all or nothing" result on its

---

MANAGEMENT OF ARDS

1. Intubation and artificial ventilation
2. High supplemental FIO_2
3. Positive end expiratory pressure
4. Careful attention to fluid intake and output to keep patient on "dry side"; diuretic therapy is often employed for this purpose
5. Corticosteroids (variable indications)
6. Intensive nursing care, e.g., frequent turning of patient to prevent pressure sores and suctioning
7. Nutritional maintenance using nasogastric and/or intravenous feedings
8. Frequent monitoring and charting of:
   Blood gas measurements
   Chest x-ray studies
   Pulmonary wedge pressure and cardiac output (Swan-Ganz right-sided heart catheter)
   Ventilator pressures
   Patient's weight

---

victims, at least as regards pulmonary function.

The use of corticosteroids in ARDS is controversial; in practice their use depends on the precipitating clinical cause and the experience of the treating physician. Steroids are commonly used in treating septic shock and fat emboli, but their use in other conditions seems more variable. Diuretics are also frequently used to help keep the patient on the "dry side" and to prevent or treat overhydration that could worsen the pulmonary edema. Apart from attention to oxygenation (high FIO_2, PEEP), the most important principle of overall management is careful monitoring. Recovery from ARDS depends vitally on intensive care support; without it these patients would surely die.

A CASE OF OXYGENATION RESPIRATORY FAILURE

Included with this case is a series of multiple choice questions. For each question, select the one best answer. Unless otherwise stated, all values are at sea level, and barometric pressure is 760 mm Hg.

A 25-year-old man comes to the emergency room complaining of severe shortness of breath. He has had upper respiratory symptoms, mainly cough and fever, for the past 3 days. Dyspnea has been progressive. During examination he appears cyanotic and is in obvious distress. Inspiratory rales are heard at the left base, and a chest x-ray shows a left lower lobe pneumonia (Fig. 11-5). His temperature is 102° F, his WBC is 17,000/mm^3 with a slight leftward shift, and his hemoglobin is 14 gm%.

His ECG shows a sinus tachycardia with a rate of 110/min. Many white cells are seen in the patient's sputum, but no bacteria. Electrolytes are normal except for a serum HCO_3^- of 20 mEq/L. Arterial blood gas analysis, obtained with the patient breathing room air, shows the following:

pH	7.55
Pa_{CO_2}	25 mm Hg
Pa_{O_2}	38 mm Hg
Sa_{O_2}	78%
HCO_3^-	21 mEq/L
%HbCO	1.5%

1. The patient is severely hypoxemic as a result of:
   a. Hypoventilation and venous admixture
   b. Hyperventilation causing left shift of oxygen dissociation curve and reduced Sa_{O_2}
   c. Abnormal amounts of HbCO depressing Pa_{O_2}
   d. Ventilation-perfusion imbalance
   e. Decreased cardiac output leading to decreased oxygen transport
2. The patient's oxygen content, in ml O_2/100 ml, is approximately:
   a. 10 ml
   b. 12.5
   c. 14.6
   d. 16.0
   e. 18.0

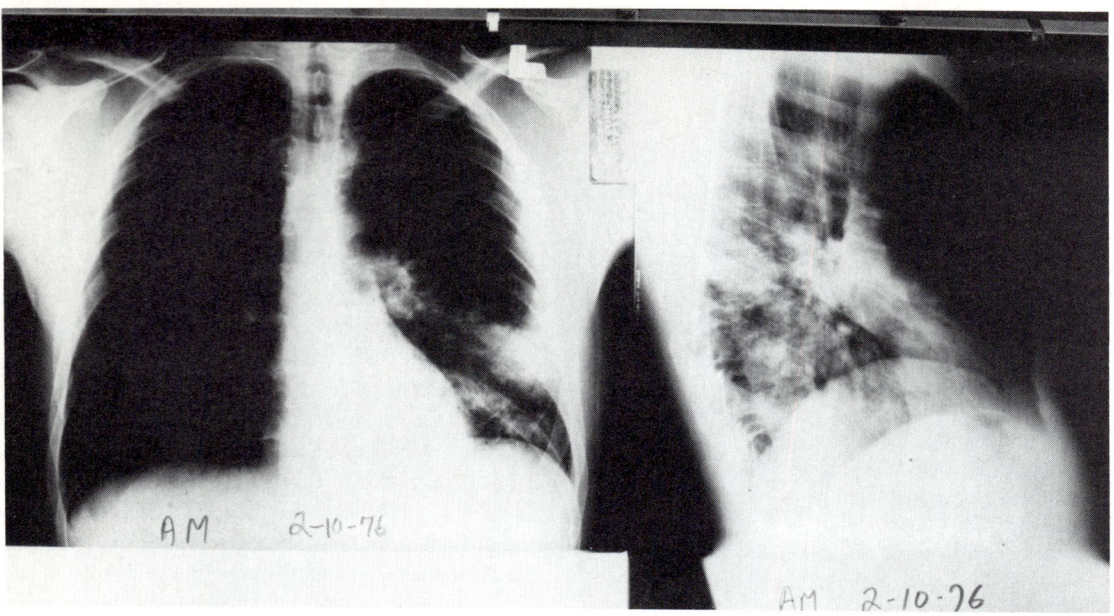

Fig. 11-5. Initial chest x-rays from a patient with oxygenation failure showing a left lower lobe pneumonia.

3. The patient's $P(A-a)O_2$, in mm Hg, is approximately:
   a. 15
   b. 108
   c. 82
   d. 115
   e. 662
4. The patient's acid-base status is best characterized as:
   a. Marked hyperventilation and metabolic acidosis
   b. Respiratory alkalosis and metabolic acidosis
   c. Chronic respiratory alkalosis
   d. Marked hyperventilation and acute respiratory alkalosis
   e. Respiratory alkalosis and metabolic alkalosis
5. At this point you would treat the patient with:
   a. Bicarbonate, low-supplemental FIO_2, and erythromycin
   b. 28% oxygen and erythromycin
   c. 40% oxygen by face mask and antibiotics
   d. A mixture of inhaled carbon dioxide and oxygen to lower pH and raise PaO_2
   e. 28% oxygen by face mask and blood transfusion to raise oxygen content

Twelve hours later the patient appears no better. By this time his FIO_2 has been changed several times, and he is receiving 90% oxygen from a nonrebreathing face mask. His PaO_2 is only 55 mm Hg. His chest x-ray now shows extensive *bilateral infiltrates* (Fig. 11-6), and his white count is up to 24,000/mm^3.

The patient now manifests the adult respiratory distress syndrome (ARDS)—acute onset of severe hypoxemia accompanied by bilateral "white-out"

Respiratory Failure

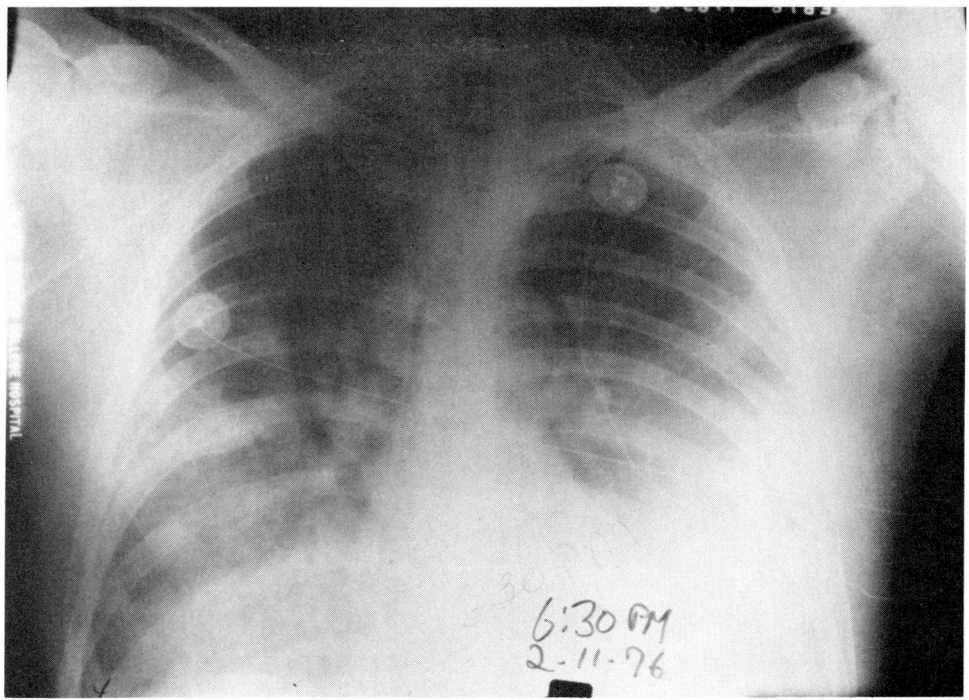

Fig. 11-6. Follow-up chest x-ray of the patient in Fig. 11-5. Note the extension of infiltrates throughout both lungs. What began as a left lower lobe "viral" pneumonia has rapidly progressed and, by the little understood mechanism of diffuse capillary leakage, has allowed proteinaceous fluid to leak into the interstitial and alveolar spaces throughout both lungs.

of the lungs. The cause is most likely viral or viral-like pneumonia.

At this point, because of oxygenation failure, the patient is intubated and given artificial ventilation. Ventilator settings include 100% inspired oxygen; controlled ventilation at 14 breaths/min; tidal volume of 700 cc; peak inspiratory pressure of 40 cm H_2O; and plateau pressure of 35 cm H_2O. Blood gas analysis shows the following:

pH	7.40
$Paco_2$	25 mm Hg
Pao_2	60 mm Hg
Sao_2	85%
Hemoglobin	13 gm%
HCO_3^-	15 mEq/L

6. Now the most likely cause of hypoxemia is:
   a. Hypoventilation
   b. A change in the position of his oxygen dissociation curve
   c. Areas of lung with perfusion but no ventilation
   d. Diffusion barrier caused by the pneumonia
   e. Not evident from above information

7. Arterial oxygen content, in ml O_2/100 ml blood, is:
   a. 12.2
   b. 14.8
   c. 16.4
   d. 17.4
   e. Indeterminant

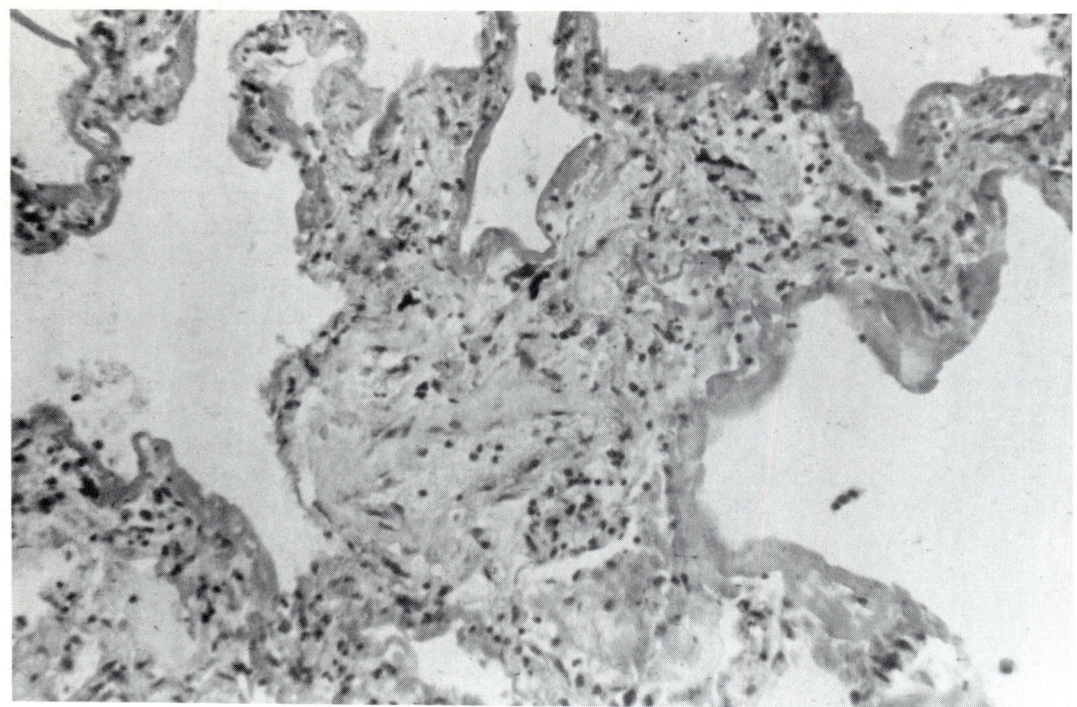

Fig. 11-7. Section of lung from a patient with ARDS. Note the thickening of the alveolar capillary membrane and the tremendous widening of the interstitium. Normally the interstitium is very thin and filamentous.

8. $P(A-a)O_2$, in mm Hg, is:
   a. 250
   b. 350
   c. 400
   d. 500
   e. Over 600

9. The static (system) compliance, in cc/cm H_2O, is:
   a. 17.5
   b. 20
   c. 35
   d. 40
   e. 50

A Swan-Ganz catheter is placed in the patient's pulmonary artery. Pulmonary capillary wedge pressure is 12 mm Hg, and cardiac output is 7 L/min; a mixed venous blood sample is obtained and found to have a PvO_2 of 34 mm Hg, and a SvO_2 of 65%.

10. The patient's tissue oxygen uptake, in ml O_2/min, is:
    a. 152
    b. 188
    c. 215
    d. 245
    e. 310

11. The patient's Q_S/Q_T is:
    a. 15%
    b. 29%
    c. 41%
    d. 56%
    e. Indeterminant without more information

12. The patient's acid-base status at this point is best characterized as:
    a. Chronic metabolic acidosis
    b. Chronic respiratory alkalosis
    c. Respiratory alkalosis plus metabolic acidosis
    d. Metabolic acidosis plus respiratory acidosis
    e. Indeterminate from the information given

The problem now is a marginal PaO_2 and oxygen content while breathing 100% inspired oxygen. There is a risk of oxygen toxicity (see Chapter 9). For this reason positive end expiratory pressure (PEEP) is instituted.

13. On a PEEP of 10 cm H_2O, the patient's PaO_2 rises to 110 mm Hg, and his $PaCO_2$ is still low at 31 mm Hg. The next step is to:
    a. Reduce PEEP to 5 cm H_2O and repeat the blood gas analysis
    b. Reduce FIO_2 to 0.80 and repeat the blood gas analysis
    c. Reduce PEEP to 5 cm H_2O and FIO_2 to 0.80 and repeat the blood gas analysis
    d. Continue on these FIO_2 and ventilator settings and repeat the blood gas analysis in a few hours
    e. Extubate the patient
14. A common complication of PEEP, particularly above 20 cm H_2O, is:
    a. Carbon dioxide retention
    b. Reduced PaO_2
    c. Reduced oxygen transport
    d. Oxygen toxicity
    e. Decreased oxygen uptake

This patient died. At autopsy his lungs were heavy and edematous. Microscopic sections revealed extensive hyalinization and fibrosis of the alveolar-capillary membrane and widening of the pulmonary interstitium (Fig. 11-7). The pathologic changes are typical of ARDS lungs that do not recover. No specific infecting organism was found.

RESPIRATORY FAILURE IN CHRONIC OBSTRUCTIVE PULMONARY DISEASE

A common cause of combined oxygenation and ventilatory failure is severe chronic obstructive pulmonary disease (COPD). COPD encompasses the conditions chronic bronchitis and emphysema and is almost always caused by long-term cigarette smoking. Fig. 11-8 contrasts a normal airway with one from a patient with chronic bronchitis and emphysema.

Classically, early symptomatic emphysema is manifested by dyspnea, yet blood gas measurements are not markedly abnormal. The pathologic abnormality is the destruction of the alveolar-capillary units, resulting in larger air spaces that are not adequately perfused. The major ventilation/perfusion (V/Q) problem is one of increased dead space, with relatively little venous admixture (Chapter 5). As long as the patient can maintain an increased minute ventilation to meet the need for adequate *alveolar* ventilation, arterial partial pressure of oxygen (PaO_2) and arterial partial pressure of carbon dioxide ($PaCO_2$) will stay near normal.

In contrast to emphysema, patients with severe chronic bronchitis often manifest a major blood gas abnormality: hypoxemia with or without hypercapnia. The hypoxemia is caused by narrowing of terminal bronchioles from bronchial wall thickening and excess mucus in the airway. This creates regions of low V/Q and consequently increased venous admixture (Chapter 5).

When the forced expiratory volume, 1 second (FEV_1) decreases to less than 30% of predicted, there is a definite risk of carbon dioxide retention (see Fig. 3-23). Why some patients with severe mechanical impairment retain carbon dioxide and others do not is an unsolved question. Patients who retain carbon dioxide tend to have lower tidal volumes, but measurements of forced vital capacity, FEV_1, minute ventilation, diffusing capacity, and volume of anatomic dead space show no significant differences between the two groups. The lower

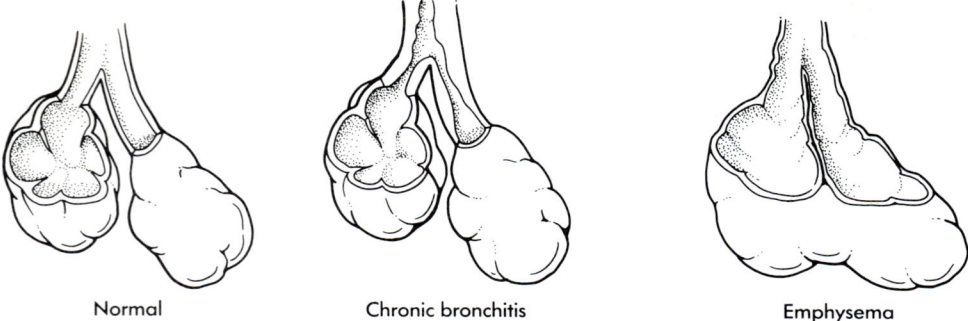

Fig. 11-8. Normal airway contrasted with chronic bronchitis and emphysema. Shown are representative sections of alveoli and airways, without their accompanying blood vessels. In chronic bronchitis the airways are narrowed but not destroyed. In emphysema the damage is extensive, and there is actual loss of alveolar walls and capillaries; note the coalescence of two alveoli into one larger dead space.

tidal volume leads to a reduction in alveolar ventilation, which accounts for the carbon dioxide retention, but why this pattern of breathing is chosen by some patients and not by others is unclear.

With progressive deterioration, either type of COPD will usually lead to severe hypoxemia, hypercapnia, cor pulmonale, overt heart failure, and death. Until the end, however, good medical management can often provide the patient some relief and perhaps halt if not reverse the course. The following case emphasizes the physiology presented in previous chapters.

A CASE OF COMBINED VENTILATORY AND OXYGENATION FAILURE IN COPD

Included with this case is a series of multiple choice questions. For each question, select the one best answer. Unless otherwise stated, all values are at sea level, and barometric pressure is 760 mm Hg.

A 65-year-old man comes to the emergency room in moderate respiratory distress. He has smoked an average of two packs of cigarettes daily for 45 years and has refused to quit smoking despite pleading by his family and physician. Pulmonary function tests during past visits showed marked airways obstruction consistent with severe COPD.

According to his history, the patient was "doing well" until a few days earlier when his cough and dyspnea worsened. As a consequence he cut down his smoking to approximately a half a pack a day.

During the examination the patient has obviously cyanotic fingers and lips, bilateral wheezing in both lung bases, and a few scattered rales. His respiratory rate is 30/min, and he is using accessory breathing muscles. Even so he is alert and oriented. His feet are edematous and there is a slight tremor in his hands.

His emergency room chest x-ray shows flattened diaphragms and some hyperinflation (Fig. 11-9). There is no radiologic evidence for congestive heart failure. The ECG shows evidence of right-sided heart strain but no ischemic changes.

His initial blood gas analysis, on a FIO_2 of 0.21, shows the following:

pH	7.36
$Paco_2$	60 mm Hg
Pao_2	35 mm Hg
Sao_2	51%
HCO_3^-	33 mEq/L
Hemoglobin	17 gm%

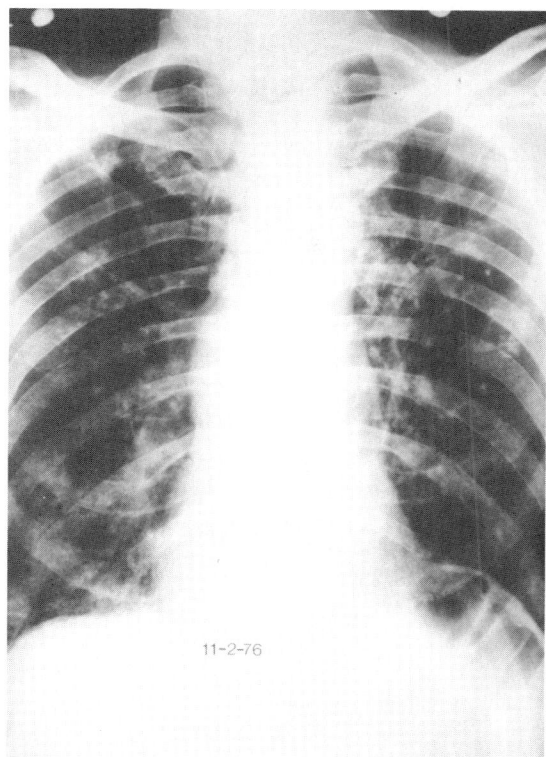

Fig. 11-9. Chest x-ray from a patient with chronic obstructive pulmonary disease (COPD). Both diaphragms are depressed consistent with hyperinflation from COPD. There is no definite infiltrate or evidence of pneumonia.

1. The most likely explanation for the patient's hypoxemia is:
   a. Right-to-left shunting alone
   b. V/Q imbalance alone
   c. Hypoventilation and V/Q imbalance
   d. Hypoventilation, V/Q imbalance, and increased level of carbon monoxide
   e. Diffusion barrier to oxygen transfer and V/Q imbalance
2. At this point you would prescribe:
   a. 50% inspired oxygen by face mask
   b. A nonrebreathing face mask to give high FIO_2
   c. Low supplemental FIO_2, e.g., 24% by face mask
   d. Artificial ventilation to bring down $PaCO_2$
   e. Phlebotomy of one unit of blood and 100% inspired oxygen
3. Your answer to the above is based on knowledge that:
   a. PaO_2 goes up as the $PaCO_2$ comes down.
   b. A small PaO_2 change in this part of the oxygen dissociation curve can lead to a relatively large change in SaO_2.
   c. In this region of the oxygen dissociation curve, high FIO_2 is needed to improve the SaO_2.
   d. Hypoxemia is life-threatening, and a patient's PaO_2 should be improved as quickly as possible.
   e. Removing hemoglobin while adding oxygen will improve overall oxygen transport.

The patient initially does well on your regimen. However, 6 hours later he is less alert, and he falls asleep when not aroused. A blood gas analysis reveals pH of 7.1, $PaCO_2$ of 80 mm Hg, and HCO_3^- of 24 mEq/L. You conclude he requires artificial ventilation because of *altered mental status, hypoventilation,* and *acidemia.*

4. His acid-base status before intubation is best characterized as:
   a. Acute respiratory acidosis
   b. Acute respiratory acidosis plus metabolic acidosis
   c. Chronic respiratory acidosis plus metabolic acidosis
   d. Metabolic acidosis and metabolic alkalosis
   e. Indeterminate from the information given

This patient is an example of the "blue-bloater," a term given to patients with severe chronic bronchitis who develop hypoxemia and right-sided heart failure. Despite these derangements, such patients can live for many years with good medical management. Treatment includes judicious use of oxygen, bronchodilators, an occasional course of steroids (if there is an asthmatic component), and of course smoking cessation. Potentially lethal are upper respiratory infections, pneumonia, and other acute pulmonary insults. Infection was the presumed cause of decompensation in this patient.

Ventilator settings are set at 16 breaths/min and tidal volume at 800 cc. Blood gas measurements obtained 1 hour after intubation on an FIO_2 of 0.40 show:

pH	7.30
$PaCO_2$	50 mm Hg
PaO_2	75 mm Hg
SaO_2	88%
HCO_3^-	24 mEq/L

5. At this point you would:
   a. Give one ampule (50 mEq) of bicarbonate and repeat the blood gas analysis
   b. Increase FIO_2 to 0.50
   c. Increase tidal volume to 1000 ml
   d. Increase breathing frequency to 20/min
   e. Not change the ventilator settings

Over the next few days the patient slowly improves with diuretics, steroids, antibiotics, and chest physiotherapy. By the third hospital day his wheezing has cleared, and he is alert and feeling better. He is now receiving intermittent mandatory ventilation, including 6 ventilator breaths/min, with tidal volume at 800 ml. His own respiratory rate is 10/min. On an FIO_2 of 0.28, he has the following blood gas measurements:

pH	7.56
$PaCO_2$	40 mm Hg
PaO_2	65 mm Hg
SaO_2	94%
HCO_3^-	35 mq/L
Hemoglobin	15 gm%

6. At this point you would:
   a. Extubate but maintain the same FIO_2
   b. Repeat the blood gas analysis in 6 hours and, if no worse, extubate, keeping the same FIO_2
   c. Use a T-piece at the same FIO_2 so that he can breathe entirely on his own through the endotracheal tube (i.e., disconnect from the respirator), repeat the blood gas analysis in a few hours, and, if the results are adequate, extubate (keeping the same FIO_2)
   d. Remove supplemental oxygen but keep the same ventilator settings and, if PaO_2 remains adequate, extubate
   e. Decrease the number of IMV breaths per minute while keeping the same FIO_2

7. Your answer to the above is based on the fact that:
   a. There are a number of complications of intubation, and the endotracheal tube should be removed as soon as possible.
   b. Blood gas measurements represent the status at a particular time, and that status may change rapidly; however, if the blood gas results are essentially the same over a period of time, the patient is more likely to remain stable.
   c. If a patient can breath on his own through an endotracheal tube, he will also be able to breathe without one.
   d. The patient will be breathing room air after discharge, so you must assure that his blood gas measurements are at least adequate on room air.
   e. The goal is to achieve his baseline state and not to extubate when his blood gas results are better than he can manage without ventilatory assistance.

8. Additional information that you would like at this time (choose the *one best* answer):
   a. Chest x-ray
   b. P_{50}
   c. % carboxyhemoglobin
   d. Serum electrolytes
   e. Serum calcium

9. Additional treatment that might be necessary at this point (choose the *one best* answer):
   a. Penicillin
   b. Blood transfusion
   c. Increasing FIO_2 to 0.40
   d. Potassium chloride
   e. Calcium gluconate

10. Following extubation and after discharge from the hospital, the patient does well, although he continues to smoke. When at his clinical best after discharge, the most likely set of arterial blood gas values he would have on room air is:

   a. PaO_2, 80; $PaCO_2$, 60; pH, 7.35; SaO_2, 90
   b. PaO_2, 58; $PaCO_2$, 55; pH, 7.37; SaO_2, 88
   c. PaO_2, 90; $PaCO_2$, 35; pH, 7.43; SaO_2, 90
   d. PaO_2, 38; $PaCO_2$, 67; pH, 7.38; SaO_2, 80
   e. PaO_2, 72; $PaCO_2$, 28; pH, 7.34; SaO_2, 93

SUMMARY

Respiratory failure is defined in terms of the primary function of the respiratory system—gas exchange. Respiratory failure is present whenever the arterial partial pressure of oxygen (PaO_2) is very low or the arterial partial pressure of carbon dioxide ($PaCO_2$) is elevated because of a problem in the respiratory system. Since the respiratory system includes the lungs and airways, the chest bellows apparatus, and the central nervous system (CNS) components that control ventilation, respiratory failure may be seen in a variety of clinical problems, not just primary lung disease. Except in the apneic patient, respiratory failure can only be diagnosed and managed with the aid of arterial blood gas measurements or their equivalent.

There are two broad physiologic types of respiratory failure: failure of oxygenation (oxygenation respiratory failure) and failure of ventilation (ventilatory respiratory failure). Oxygenation respiratory failure is always caused by a pulmonary problem, and its primary physiologic basis is usually ventilation-perfusion imbalance; it always manifests an elevation of $P(A-a)O_2$, the difference between alveolar and arterial PO_2. A severe form of oxygenation respiratory failure is the adult respiratory distress syndrome (ARDS). ARDS is a fulminant picture of noncardiac pulmonary edema and may arise from a variety of precipitating events, such as shock, trauma, and aspiration. As opposed to cardiac pulmonary edema, which is caused by an increase in pulmonary capillary hydrostatic pressure, ARDS results from damage to the capillary membrane so that plasma "leaks" into the interstitium and alveoli. In ARDS capillary hydrostatic pressure (measured as pulmonary artery wedge pressure) is within normal limits.

Ventilatory respiratory failure may be caused by disease of the lungs, the chest bellows, or the central nervous system (CNS); in pure ventilatory respiratory failure $P(A-a)O_2$ is not elevated. One common example of ventilatory respiratory failure is CNS depression from sedative overdose. Patients who present in respiratory failure from chronic obstructive pulmonary disease often manifest combined oxygenation and ventilatory respiratory failure, i.e., an elevation of both $PaCO_2$ and $P(A-a)O_2$.

REVIEW QUESTIONS

State whether each of the following is true or false.

1. All patients with respiratory failure have a PaO_2 lower than it would be without respiratory failure.
2. Oxygenation respiratory failure is always accompanied by increased alveolar-arterial PO_2 difference.
3. Patients with respiratory failure are invariably tachypneic.
4. Treatment of oxygenation respiratory failure always includes supplemental oxygen.
5. Ventilatory failure is always manifested by an increase in the alveolar-arterial PO_2 difference.
6. The definition of adult respiratory distress syndrome (ARDS) includes a pulmonary capillary wedge pressure above normal.
7. Pancreatitis is a recognized precipitating event of ARDS.
8. To calculate the percentage of cardiac output shunted past the lungs, one must measure or assume a value for the cardiac output.
9. Respiratory failure is present when the respiratory rate is less than 8 breaths/min in a comatose patient.
10. ARDS is one manifestation of end-stage emphysema.

References

Ashbaugh, D.G., Bigelow, D.B., Petty, T.L., et al.: Acute respiratory distress in adults, Lancet **2**:319, 1967.

Dantzker, R.D., Brook, C.J., Dehart, P., et al.: Ventilation-perfusion distributions in the adult respiratory distress syndrome, Am. Rev. Respir. Dis. **120**:1039, 1979.

Staub, N.C.: Pulmonary edema: physiologic approaches to management, Chest **74**:559, 1978.

Suggested readings

Bone, R.C., editor: Adult respiratory distress syndrome, Clin. Chest Med., **3**:1, 1982.

Bone, R.C.: Treatment of severe hypoxemia due to the adult respiratory distress syndrome, Arch. Intern. Med. **140**:85, 1980.

Campbell, E.J.M.: The management of acute respiratory failure in chronic bronchitis and emphysema, Am. Rev. Respir. Dis. **96**:626, 1967.

Fowler, A.A., Hamman, R.F., Zerbe, G.O., et al.: Adult respiratory distress syndrome: prognosis after onset, Am. Rev. Respir. Dis. **132**:472, 1985.

Martin, L.: Respiratory failure, Med. Clin. North Am. **61**:1369, 1977.

Matthay, M.A., editor: Symposium on pulmonary edema, Clin. Chest Med. **6**:3, 1985.

Montgomery, A.B., Stager, M.A., Carrico, C.J., et al.: Causes of mortality in patients with the adult respiratory distress syndrome, Am. Rev. Respir. Dis. **132**:485, 1985.

Petty, T.L.: Indicators of risk, course, and prognosis in adult respiratory distress syndrome (ARDS), Am. Rev. Respir. Dis. **132**:471, 1985.

Petty, T.L., and Ashbaugh, D.G.: The adult respiratory distress syndrome, Chest **60**:233, 1971.

Pontoppidan, H., Geffin, B., and Lowenstein, E.: Acute respiratory failure in the adult, N. Engl. J. Med. **287**:690, 1972.

Shapiro, B.A., Cane, R.D., and Harrion, R.A.: Positive end expiratory pressure therapy in adults with special reference to acute lung injury: a review of the literature and suggested clinical correlations, Crit. Care Med. **12**(2):127, 1984.

Sykes, M.K., McNicol, M.W., and Campbell, E.J.M.: Respiratory failure. ed. 2, Oxford, 1976, Blackwell Scientific Publications, Ltd.

See also General References in Appendix G.

chapter 12

Exercise physiology

OUTLINE

Exercise physiology
What happens during exercise?
Metabolism during exercise—aerobic vs. anaerobic
Pa_{CO_2} during exercise
The exercise test
Physiologic changes during exercise
Normal exercise parameters
Clinical use of physiologic exercise testing
Clinical interpretation of physiologic exercise testing

EXERCISE PHYSIOLOGY

The pulmonary physiology discussed so far deals largely with patients at rest. Many patients complain of dyspnea only during exercise or during minimal exertion, such as stair climbing. Their resting pulmonary function tests many be normal or, if abnormal, not reduced enough to explain the degree of exercise intolerance. Why does exercise either bring out or exacerbate dyspnea in some patients? How does exercise testing help diagnose the cause of dyspnea?

Exercise physiology, a relatively new field for clinical study, helps to answer these questions. Exercise physiology encompasses aspects of pulmonary, cardiac, and sports medicine, plus cellular metabolism and biochemistry. This chapter will concentrate on exercise physiology in the diagnosis of cardiopulmonary disease.

WHAT HAPPENS DURING EXERCISE?

During exercise much more oxygen and carbon dioxide are exchanged than at rest. This single metabolic fact accounts for the profound changes in cardiac, pulmonary, and circulatory physiology during exercise. Increased oxygen supply is provided by increases in both arterial oxygen delivery and tissue oxygen extraction; at the same time there is increased carbon dioxide transport on the venous side. The need for increased gas exchange by exercising muscles leads to the following general physiologic changes.

Metabolic changes. Increased oxygen consumption ($\dot{V}O_2$) and carbon dioxide production ($\dot{V}CO_2$) occur immediately with exercise. During aerobic metabolism, glucose and fats utilize oxygen to form adenosine triphosphate (ATP), the ultimate source of energy. There is very little oxygen stored in the body, so aerobic metabolism requires continuous delivery of oxygen from the atmosphere to the blood. Without oxygen, glucose is metabolized anaerobically, and the yield of ATP per glucose molecule is much less; in addition, lactic acid is generated as a by-product. Anaerobic metabolism is sufficient for short bursts of activity, but prolonged exercise requires oxygen as energy substrate.

Cardiac changes. Oxygen consumption ($\dot{V}O_2$)

is related to cardiac output by the Fick equation:

$$\dot{V}_{O_2} = Q_T \times (C_{aO_2} - C_{vO_2}) \quad (1)$$

where Q_T is cardiac output in ml/min, and $(C_{aO_2} - C_{vO_2})$ is the arterial-venous oxygen content difference in ml/100 ml blood. Since cardiac output is the product of stroke volume (SV) and heart rate (HR),

$$\dot{V}_{O_2} = SV \times HR \times (C_{aO_2} - C_{vO_2}) \quad (2)$$

Both SV and HR increase immediately with exercise, but stroke volume plateaus early. Further increases in cardiac output are largely due to increases in heart rate.

Systemic circulation changes. The extra cardiac output delivers more oxygen to exercising muscles. There is a redistribution of the systemic circulation, including vasodilation in the skin and working muscles and vasoconstriction in the visceral organs and nonworking muscles. The net effect of vascular redistribution is a decrease in systemic vascular resistance.

Oxygen extraction changes. Apart from increased cardiac output and vascular redistribution, a third mechanism to meet oxygen requirements is increased oxygen extraction from the arterial blood; this results in an increased arterial-venous oxygen content difference (Equation 1).

Pulmonary circulation changes. Pulmonary circulation also increases immediately with exercise. Unperfused alveoli become perfused (through recruitment of pulmonary capillaries), and underperfused units receive an increased blood supply. As a result, both pulmonary blood volume and the pulmonary diffusing capacity for oxygen increase.

Ventilation changes. As pulmonary blood flow increases, both minute ventilation ($\dot{V}_E$) and alveolar ventilation ($\dot{V}_A$) increase; in this way the lungs transfer more oxygen and carbon dioxide and keep pace with metabolic demands. Although both tidal volume (V_T) and respiratory rate increase with exercise, in the early stages an increase in V_T accounts for most of the rise in $\dot{V}_E$ and $\dot{V}_A$. At a point where V_T approaches approximately 60% of the vital capacity, further increases in ventilation come from increasing respiratory rate.

Hematologic changes. Although most of the increase in oxygen delivery is accounted for by increased cardiac output, in some individuals hemoglobin concentration may rise. This can occur by red cells entering the circulation from splenic and marrow reservoirs, as well as by reduction of plasma volume. The rise in hemoglobin does not occur in well-trained athletes, who tend to have higher resting blood volume than the general population. In any case the magnitude of hemoglobin increase is small, approximately 10%, and does not play a significant role in augmenting oxygen delivery during exercise.

METABOLISM DURING EXERCISE—AEROBIC VS. ANAEROBIC

Metabolically, there are two types of exercise, aerobic and anaerobic. Aerobic exercise uses oxygen as energy substrate to metabolize food to adenosine triphosphate (ATP) (see box on p. 241). When the supply of oxygen is no longer sufficient to meet the needs of exercising muscles, anaerobic metabolism begins. In anaerobic metabolism, glucose is converted to ATP without oxygen, and lactic acid is generated as a by-product. A healthy person can perform aerobic exercise for several hours; in contrast, pure anaerobic exercise can only be sustained for a few minutes before severe dyspnea and fatigue set in.

During short bursts of activity, such as sprinting, energy may be obtained only anaerobically. Otherwise, anaerobic metabolism occurs in addition to ongoing aerobic metabolism. Typically, anaerobic metabolism begins approximately midway between resting and maximal oxygen consumption. The point at which anaerobic metabolism begins is called the *anaerobic threshold* (AT). AT can be identified by a typical pattern of changes in the blood and in expired gases (see the next section).

Clinical problem 1

Concerning carbon dioxide production, what is the distinction between aerobic and anaerobic metabolism?

Exercise physiology

METABOLIC CHANGES DURING AEROBIC AND ANAEROBIC EXERCISE

During aerobic exercise, both glucose and fatty acids are metabolized. One molecule of glucose utilizes 6 molecules of oxygen and produces 6 molecules of carbon dioxide, for a metabolic respiratory quotient (RQ) of 1.0. For fatty acids, 23 molecules of oxygen are used for every 16 molecules of carbon dioxide produced, giving an RQ of 0.71. The average RQ during mild to moderate exercise (before anaerobic threshold) is approximately 0.85.

By contrast, anaerobic metabolism produces only 2 molecules of ATP per molecule of glucose; at the same time 2 molecules of lactic acid are produced, which, when buffered, generate carbon dioxide in excess of that from aerobic metabolism.

AEROBIC METABOLISM

$$C_6H_{12}O_6 + 6\ O_2 \rightarrow 6\ CO_2 + 6\ H_2O + 36\ ATP \quad (RQ = 1.0)$$
(Glucose)

$$C_{16}H_{32}O_2 + 23\ O_2 \rightarrow 16\ CO_2 + 16\ H_2O + 130\ ATP \quad (RQ = 0.71)$$
(Fatty acid)

ANAEROBIC METABOLISM

$$Glucose + 2\ ADP \rightarrow 2\ H^+\ lactate^- + 2\ ATP$$
(Lactic acid)

$$H^+\ lactate^- + Na^+HCO_3^- \rightarrow Na^+\ lactate^- + H_2CO_3$$
$$H_2CO_3 \rightarrow H_2O + CO_2$$

Pa_{CO_2} DURING EXERCISE

A common misconception is that respiratory effort during exercise indicates hyperventilation, i.e., low arterial partial pressure of carbon dioxide (Pa_{CO_2}). In fact, Pa_{CO_2} is kept remarkably constant during mild to moderate exercise before anaerobic threshold is reached. The constancy of Pa_{CO_2} can be explained by the Pa_{CO_2} equation (Chapter 4):

$$Pa_{CO_2} = \frac{\dot{V}_{CO_2} \times k}{\dot{V}_A} \quad (3)$$

During aerobic exercise, carbon dioxide production ($\dot{V}_{CO_2}$) and alveolar ventilation ($\dot{V}_A$) increase proportionately, resulting in an unchanged Pa_{CO_2} (Fig. 12-1). Only with anaerobic exercise does Pa_{CO_2} fall and then only as compensation for the lactic acidosis.

Take a jog around the block but do not push to your limit. After 5 to 10 minutes you will be huffing and puffing, but not hyperventilating.

Clinical problem 2

In the resting steady state, a well-trained jogger has an RQ of 0.8, end-tidal P_{CO_2} of 40 mm Hg, and a minute ventilation of 6 L/min. After 5 minutes on a treadmill at 2.5 mph, the following expired gas measurements are obtained: $\dot{V}_{CO_2}$ of 800 ml/min, $\dot{V}_{O_2}$ of 1000 ml/min, end-tidal P_{CO_2} of 39 mm Hg, and minute ventilation of 30 L/min. What are alveolar and arterial P_{CO_2} at this point?

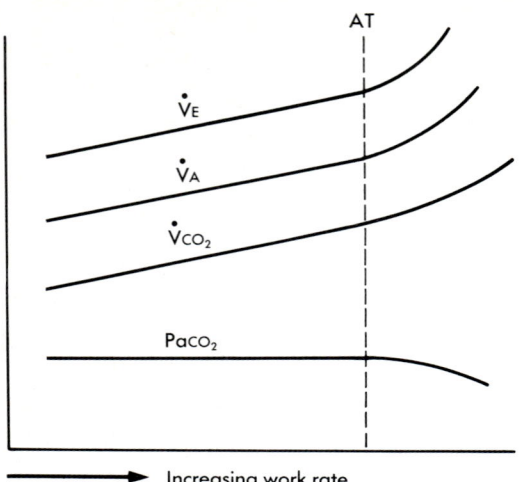

Fig. 12-1. Changes in minute ventilation ($\dot{V}_E$), alveolar ventilation ($\dot{V}_A$), metabolic carbon dioxide production ($\dot{V}_{CO_2}$), and arterial partial pressure of carbon dioxide (Pa_{CO_2}) during exercise. $\dot{V}_{CO_2}$ represents the total metabolic load of carbon dioxide presented to the lungs for excretion, including carbon dioxide produced from buffering lactic acid. $\dot{V}_E$, $\dot{V}_A$, and $\dot{V}_{CO_2}$ rise proportionately during submaximal exercise, so Pa_{CO_2} stays constant. After anaerobic threshold *(AT)* is reached, $\dot{V}_E$ and $\dot{V}_A$ rise proportionately more than $\dot{V}_{CO_2}$, so Pa_{CO_2} falls; this hyperventilation occurs as compensation for the lactic acidosis.

THE EXERCISE TEST

Exercise testing requires measuring one or more physiologic parameters during a supervised, graded exercise test. Typically these measurements are performed as the patient either walks on a treadmill or cycles on a bicycle ergometer. The test is usually "graded" in that the work necessary to continue exercising is progressively increased, either by making the treadmill go faster (and raising its angle from the floor) or by increasing the resistance of the bicycle wheel as the subject pedals.

Table 12-1 lists many of the measurements obtained during a physiologic exercise test, grouped according to the equipment required. The first group of measurements can be obtained without a mouthpiece but does require continuous monitoring of the patient's ECG. Included in this group is noninvasive measurement of arterial oxygen saturation (Sa_{O_2}), which can be accomplished with an ear or finger oximeter (Fig. 12-2).

Working down the list in Table 12-1, each group of measurements becomes progressively more "invasive." Measurements in the second group require the collection of expired gases, which means the subject must keep a mouthpiece in place while exercising. The mouthpiece is connected through hoses to instruments that sample and measure expired oxygen and carbon dioxide; a typical setup is shown in Fig. 12-3. The third group of measurements is obtained from arterial blood and re-

Table 12-1. Measurements during graded exercise testing

Level of test	Measurements
Group 1	No mouthpiece
	Patient response and symptoms
	Heart rate
	Blood pressure
	ECG
	Sa_{O_2} by oximetry
Group 2	Mouthpiece, oxygen, and carbon dioxide analyzer
	Respiratory rate
	Tidal volume
	Minute ventilation
	End-tidal gas measurements
	$\dot{V}_{O_2}$ and O_2-pulse
	$\dot{V}_{CO_2}$
	Respiratory quotient
Group 3	Arterial line
	Blood gas values—Pa_{O_2}, Pa_{CO_2}, and pH
	HCO_3^- and lactate
	V_D/V_T
Group 4	Right-sided heart catheter
	Pulmonary artery pressures
	Cardiac output
	Mixed venous P_{O_2} and S_{O_2}

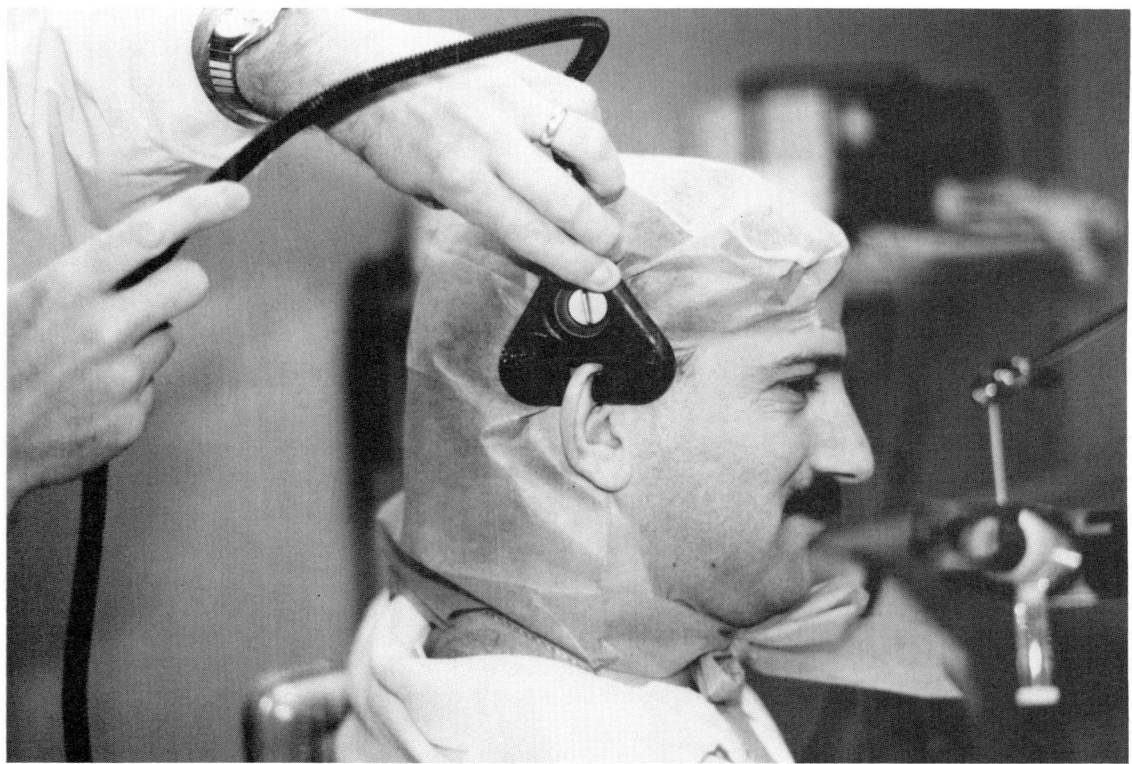

Fig. 12-2. A type of oximeter used in the exercise test. The oximeter fits over the upper part of the ear (Hewlett Packard Model No. 47201A). The patient exercises with the oximeter attached, allowing for continuous, noninvasive measurement of oxygen saturation (see also Fig. 12-3).

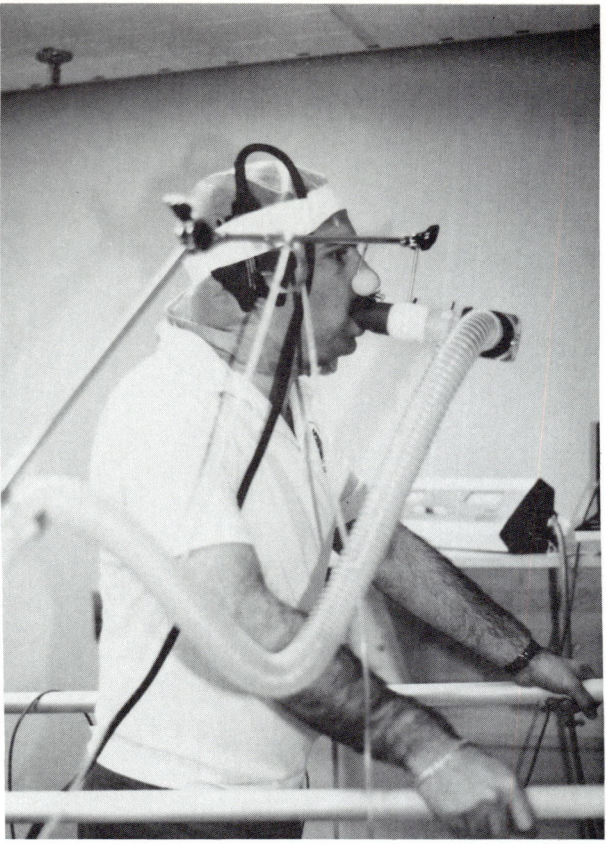

Fig. 12-3. The exercise test. The patient is prepared to exercise on a treadmill. In addition to the ear oximeter (kept in place by a headband), he has a mouthpiece in place that is connected to large-bore tubing. All expired air will go through the tubing to instruments that continuously measure the concentration of expired gases.

quires an indwelling arterial catheter. Finally, the test can be performed with a right heart catheter in place, a technique that is only rarely necessary.

Obviously, not all the measurements listed in Table 12-1 are recorded in every exercise test; measurements must be tailored to the problem being evaluated.

PHYSIOLOGIC CHANGES DURING EXERCISE

Fig. 12-4 graphs many of the parameters that can be measured during the graded exercise test (see groups presented in the box on p. 242). The abscissa for each group represents increasing work, i.e., a progressive increase in treadmill speed or in

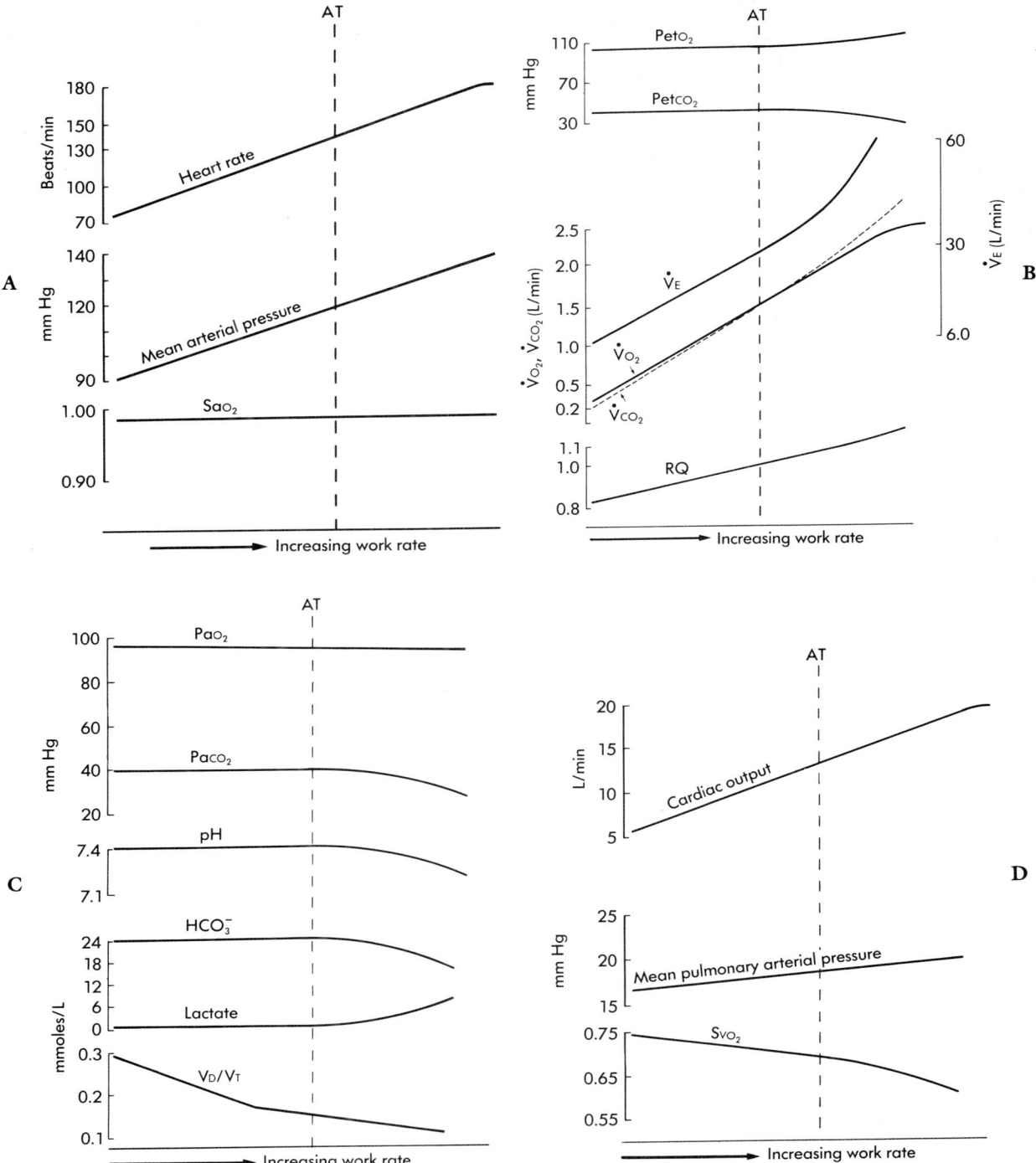

Fig. 12-4. Physiologic changes during exercise. **A,** Group 1 data, **B,** Group 2 data; **C,** Group 3 data; and **D,** Group 4 data. *AT* = anaerobic threshold.

PHYSIOLOGIC CHANGES AT ANAEROBIC THRESHOLD (AT)

Anaerobic threshold occurs at different work rates for different individuals. In practice it is not always easy to discern a subject's AT. Sometimes there is no sharp demarcation from either expired or arterial gas values to show a specific point where AT truly begins. Nonetheless, the concept of AT is a valid one, and the greater the number of measurements, the more likely the point of anaerobic threshold will be determined. (See also Fig. 12-4).

MEASURED IN EXPIRED GASES (From Group 2 measurements, Table 12-1)

- Respiratory quotient ($\dot{V}_{CO_2}/\dot{V}_{O_2}$) increases above 1.0 as relatively more carbon dioxide is blown off than oxygen is consumed.
- End-tidal P_{CO_2} (Pet_{CO_2}) falls.
- There is an increase in slope of both $\dot{V}_E$ and $\dot{V}_{CO_2}$, but $\dot{V}_E$ increases more than $\dot{V}_{CO_2}$, reflecting compensation for the metabolic acidosis.
- Slope of $\dot{V}_{O_2}$ remains unchanged; hence $\dot{V}_E/\dot{V}_{O_2}$ increases.
- There is an increase in $P(A-a)_{O_2}$, reflecting an increasing P_{AO_2} (measured as Pet_{O_2}) and a constant Pa_{O_2}.

MEASURED IN BLOOD (From Group 3 measurements, Table 12-1)

- Lactic acid, a product of anaerobic metabolism, increases.
- As HCO_3^- buffers lactic acid, HCO_3^- falls almost millimole for millimole with the rise in lactic acid.
- As exercise increases beyond AT, Pa_{CO_2} decreases to compensate for the developing metabolic acidosis.

---

bicycle wheel resistance. Work is usually measured in kilopond-meters (kpm); one kpm is the work required to move a one kilogram mass a vertical distance of one meter against gravity. Work per unit time is power or kpm/min, which is often converted into watts (600 kpm/min is roughly equal to 100 watts). For example, a 70-kg person walking on a treadmill at 3 mph, 5% grade, generates approximately 300 kpm/min or 50 watts of power.

In clinical practice, actual work rates are not usually stated. Instead, the exercise test is quantitated in terms of the patient's oxygen uptake ($\dot{V}_{O_2}$). Normal resting $\dot{V}_{O_2}$ is approximately 3.5 ml/min/kg. Multiples of resting $\dot{V}_{O_2}$ are called METS so that 10 METS equal 35 ml/min/kg. The intensity or severity of the exercise test is quantitated in terms of either the absolute oxygen consumption (ml O_2/min) or the number of METS.

The parameters listed in the box above and graphed in Fig. 12-4 are discussed in the next section. The values displayed represent typical changes for an adult of average physical fitness. The physiologic changes at anaerobic threshold are also summarized in this box.

Group 1 measurements

Patient response and symptoms can give valuable information about overall exercise capability. Sometimes the patient is so uncoordinated that the test is invalid. Treadmills and bicycles are foreign to many patients, so the examiner has to make sure the test is at least valid before collecting data.

Common reasons for exercise intolerance are dyspnea, fatigue, leg pain, and chest pain. Leg pain may be a clue to developing lactic acidosis but can also be caused by shoe discomfort or orthopedic problems. Careful questioning can reveal the reason. Any chest pain or discomfort should be correlated with the ECG. If a patient quits because of dyspnea or fatigue, the collected data should reveal whether the problem's origin is cardiac, respiratory, or poor fitness (see section Clinical Interpretation of Physiologic Exercise Testing).

Heart rate rises immediately during exercise and continues to increase linearly along with $\dot{V}O_2$. $\dot{V}O_2$ reaches a maximal limit and plateaus because heart rate does so. The predicted maximal heart rate declines with age:

Max heart rate = 210 − (0.65 × Age in years) (4)

Both diastolic and systolic *blood pressures* increase with increasing exercise, systolic proportionately much more than diastolic. Mean arterial pressure increases from approximately 90 mm Hg at rest to 140 mm Hg at maximal oxygen consumption.

The *electrocardiogram* normally shows sinus tachycardia without arrhythmia or abnormal ventricular beats.

Arterial oxygen saturation (SaO_2) is unchanged during exercise, reflecting the constant arterial partial pressure of oxygen (PaO_2).

Group 2 measurements

Minute ventilation ($\dot{V}E$) increases linearly along with $\dot{V}O_2$ until anaerobic threshold (AT) is reached. At AT, $\dot{V}E$ rises to compensate for the increase in carbon dioxide production. Normally ventilation does not limit exercise. Maximal ventilation achieved during exercise is usually approximately 65% to 75% of the maximal voluntary ventilation (MVV).* At low levels of work, increase in $\dot{V}E$ is caused mainly by an increase in *tidal volume;* at high work rates, increases in *respiratory rate* account for most of the rise in $\dot{V}E$.

Normally, *end-tidal gas measurements* ($PetO_2$ and $PetCO_2$) reflect alveolar gas values; end-tidal partial pressure of oxygen ($PetO_2$) and partial pressure of carbon dioxide ($PetCO_2$) are constant until anaerobic threshold, at which point $PetO_2$ rises and $PetCO_2$ falls.

---

*The MVV is measured at rest by having the patient breathe as rapidly and deeply as possible for 12 seconds and multiplying the 12-second ventilation by 5 to obtain a figure in L/min.

At rest, *oxygen uptake* ($\dot{V}O_2$) is approximately 250 to 300 ml/min or approximately 3.5 ml/min/kg. $\dot{V}O_2$ increases during aerobic exercise and is the single best measurement of the total exercise effort. The lower the $\dot{V}O_2$ for a given amount of work, the more aerobically fit is the person. Thus if two people are doing the same work, e.g., walking on a treadmill at 2 mph for 5 minutes, the one with the lowest oxygen uptake is considered more physically fit.

As work increases, $\dot{V}O_2$ increases in a linear fashion and eventually plateaus. This plateau, which for a healthy person occurs only after the onset of anaerobic threshold (very heavy exercise), is called the maximal $\dot{V}O_2$ ($\dot{V}O_2$ max). The level of exercise (work rate) can increase beyond $\dot{V}O_2$ max, but the rate of oxygen uptake will remain flat because cardiac output cannot increase further. For a given type of exercise (e.g., bicycle or treadmill), work intensity, and level of training, there is a constant $\dot{V}O_2$ max for each individual. $\dot{V}O_2$ max increases as fitness improves (Fig. 12-5). For most adults without cardiopulmonary disease, $\dot{V}O_2$ max is between 2 and 3 L/min, which is approximately 10 times the resting $\dot{V}O_2$. World class athletes can reach a $\dot{V}O_2$ max of over 4 L/min.

The following equations predict $\dot{V}O_2$ max, in

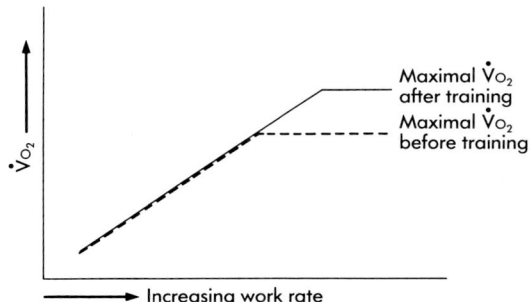

Fig. 12-5. Maximal $\dot{V}O_2$ ($\dot{V}O_2$ max) before and after training. The slope of the $\dot{V}O_2$ curve is unchanged with exercise training. Training produces a greater $\dot{V}O_2$ max and increases the work load at which anaerobic threshold begins.

L/min, for men and women (Jones and Campbell, 1982):

Men—
$$\dot{V}_{O_2} \text{ max} = 4.2 - (0.032 \times \text{Age}) \pm 0.4 \quad (5)$$

Women—
$$\dot{V}_{O_2} \text{ max} = 2.6 - (0.014 \times \text{Age}) \pm 0.4 \quad (6)$$

O_2-pulse is $\dot{V}_{O_2}$/heart rate and is another useful index of fitness. O_2-pulse increases with increasing exercise. In healthy patients O_2-pulse ranges from 2.5 to 4 ml O_2/heart beat at rest to 10 to 15 ml O_2/heart beat at maximal exercise. At any given work rate, O_2-pulse is higher in the fit person than in the unfit.

Clinical problem 3

A 40-year-old man is referred for an exercise test before undertaking a mountain climbing expedition. He exercises to his maximal endurance and quits because of dyspnea. At this point his oxygen uptake is 2.80 L/min and his heart rate 176/min. Is he physically fit?

Carbon dioxide production increases immediately during exercise. Below AT, the extra carbon dioxide presented to the lungs for excretion comes from food metabolism. Above AT, additional carbon dioxide enters the blood from buffering of lactic acid (see the box on p. 241).

Respiratory quotient (RQ), measured as carbon dioxide elimination over oxygen uptake by the lungs, increases as the AT is approached. On a regular diet, RQ during mild to moderate exercise is approximately 0.85. At AT, RQ goes above 1.0. The rise above 1.0 is caused by the increase in $\dot{V}_{CO_2}$ compared to $\dot{V}_{O_2}$, as extra carbon dioxide enters the blood from the buffering of lactic acid, (see box on p. 241). This RQ does not reflect the *metabolic* exchange of oxygen and carbon dioxide, which cannot go higher than 1.0 (1.0 is the value when only carbohydrates are metabolized).

Group 3 measurements

PaO_2 and $P(A-a)O_2$. The alveolar-arterial oxygen pressure difference ($P(A-a)O_2$) does not change at low work levels but increases at AT, caused mainly by an increase in alveolar partial pressure of oxygen (PAO_2); generally arterial partial pressure of oxygen (PaO_2) stays fairly constant throughout exercise. Part of the increase in PAO_2 is caused by hyperventilation after AT is reached. However, at rest an increase in PAO_2 would also increase PaO_2, and this does not occur during exercise; constant PaO_2 may be caused by a reduced mixed venous oxygen content counterbalancing the effect of an increased PAO_2.

Arterial partial pressure of carbon dioxide ($PaCO_2$) stays remarkably constant below AT. Above AT, $PaCO_2$ and end-tidal PCO_2 ($PetCO_2$) normally fall, largely as a result of compensation for the developing lactic acidosis.

Lactate, pH, and HCO_3^- are fairly constant until AT, at which point lactate increases from the anaerobic metabolism of glucose; also at this point, pH and HCO_3^- begin to fall as the lactic acid is buffered in the blood.

V_D/V_T. Calculation of V_D/V_T (ratio of dead space to tidal volume) requires measurement of both the expired and the arterial PCO_2 (see Equation 9, Chapter 4). V_D/V_T normally falls with exercise. Initially the decrease is rapid as a result of the large increase in tidal volume. As respiratory rate begins to account for most of the increase in the minute ventilation, the decline in V_D/V_T slows.

Group 4 measurements

Cardiac output may increase severalfold and is the single most important mechanism for satisfying the increased oxygen uptake during exercise. In early exercise the cardiac output increases as a result of both an increase in stroke volume and in the heart rate. Stroke volume plateaus early so that further increases are caused by the heart rate.

Pulmonary artery pressures rise only slightly during exercise despite the enormous increase in cardiac output sent through the pulmonary circulation.

Mixed venous PO_2 and oxygen saturation fall because of increased oxygen extraction by the exercising tissues.

In any state of impaired exercise tolerance, one or more of the previous physiologic parameters are abnormal, either its absolute value or its value relative to the work rate achieved. For example, a cardiac patient might produce lactic acid after walking only 2 minutes at 1 mph a work rate well below the normal anaerobic threshold.

NORMAL EXERCISE PARAMETERS

Like most effort-dependent tests, there is a wide range of normal values for exercise testing. Care should be taken to use the normal values appropriate to the patient being studied, particularly regarding age and sex. Table 12-2 shows normal values for a group of 77 healthy middle-aged men who were evaluated because of a history of asbestos exposure (Hansen, Sue, and Wasserman, 1984). These men had no evident cardiopulmonary disease (except for pleural thickening evidenced on chest x-ray in some subjects) and were considered representative of middle-aged men in general. All had normal resting pulmonary function tests.

Table 12-2. Exercise parameters in 77 men during cycle ergometer exercise*

Parameter	Range
Age (years)	34 to 74
Weight (kg)	53 to 124
Percent of predicted weight	79 to 160
$\dot{V}_{O_2}$ max (l/min STPD)	2.24 ± 0.42
$\dot{V}_{O_2}$ at AT	1.23 ± 0.22
$\dot{V}_{O_2}$ at AT/$\dot{V}_{O_2}$ max (%)	56 ± 8
Maximal heart rate/min	159 ± 18
$\dot{V}_{O_2}$ max/maximal heart rate (ml/beat)	14.2 ± 2.5

From Hansen, J.E., Sue, D.Y., and Wasserman, K.: Am. Rev. Respir. Dis. Suppl. **129**:S49, 1984.
*AT, anaerobic threshold; STPD, standard temperature, pressure, dry

CLINICAL USE OF PHYSIOLOGIC EXERCISE TESTING

Physiologic exercise testing is a useful tool in several clinical situations (see box on p. 250).

Several points should be emphasized about physiologic exercise testing in the clinical setting.

1. Physiologic exercise testing is different from the standard cardiac 'stress test.' Although the two tests can be combined, in practice the cardiac stress test usually looks for evidence only of ECG abnormalities or of coronary insufficiency (chest pain or ST segment depression); it does not ordinarily assess oxygen uptake or make any attempt to diagnose noncardiac causes of dyspnea. Most hospitals maintain a facility for cardiac stress testing, but relatively few also provide for physiologic stress testing.
2. Physiologic exercise testing is only indicated after completion of a full clinical evaluation (history and physical examination, chest x-ray, hematocrit, resting pulmonary function tests, blood gas analysis, and electrocardiogram), and is used to provide information not otherwise available.
3. Exercise testing is only an adjunct to the clinical evaluation and, like any other test, should be interpreted in light of the full clinical picture. Just as a clinical diagnosis would not be made on the basis of a chest x-ray or blood gas analysis alone, a diagnosis should not be made based on the exercise test alone. Exercise measurements should never substitute for intelligent assessment of the history, physical examination, and other relevant laboratory data. Careful patient observation is also important during the test to gauge the level of cooperation and understanding, as well as for qualitative assessment of the patient's symptoms.
4. Before interpreting exercise test data, one should at least have available the following:
    a. Reason for the test (e.g., dyspnea on exertion)

COMMON CLINICAL INDICATIONS FOR PHYSIOLOGIC EXERCISE TESTING

1. Dyspnea during exertion without apparent organic basis (not explained by resting pulmonary function tests and full clinical evaluation)
2. Dyspnea that could be caused by either a cardiac or a pulmonary problem
3. When objective measurement of exercise ability is required, e.g., occupational lung disease evaluation or physical fitness evaluation
4. For evaluation or diagnosis of exercise-induced asthma.

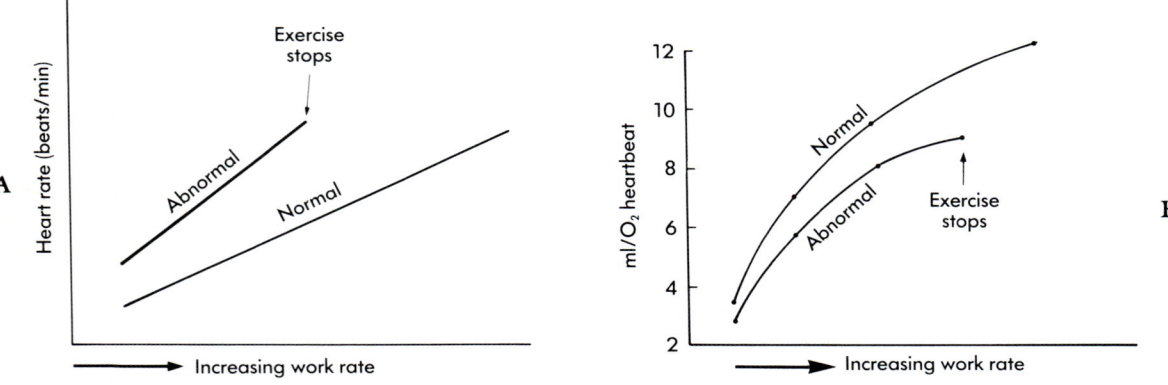

Fig. 12-6. Exercise limitation caused by heart disease. **A,** Heart rate. **B,** O_2-pulse.

b. Results of physical examination, particularly with regard to heart or lung disease, orthopedic impairment, and neuromuscular problems
c. Results of resting ECG, chest x-ray, hematocrit, and spirometry (including maximal voluntary ventilation)
d. Assessment of the patient's effort during the test. (A physician is always present or close by during the test, but data interpretation may be done by someone who was not present.)

CLINICAL INTERPRETATION OF PHYSIOLOGIC EXERCISE TESTING

All organic causes of dyspnea arise from interference with oxygen delivery to the exercising muscles. The following discussion concentrates on differentiating among cardiac disease, respiratory disease, and poor physical fitness as a cause for exercise limitation. The need to make this distinction is a common reason for physiologic exercise testing.

Cardiac disease. The heart limits exercise when cardiac output cannot meet the body's oxygen needs. This limitation can come about from either inadequate stroke volume (SV) or heart rate (HR). Cardiac output impairment is usually caused by inadequate stroke volume; to compensate for reduced stroke volume, heart rate and oxygen extraction will increase (see Equation 2). Since the heart rate is inappropriately high for the level of oxygen consumption, the O_2-pulse ($\dot{V}O_2/HR$) is reduced (Figs. 12-6, *A*, and 12-6, *B*). A lower-than-expected O_2-pulse is the hallmark of exercise limitation caused by heart disease.

As a result of cardiac limitation to oxygen delivery, the patient experiences an early anaerobic threshold; lactic acid production and hyperventilation (reduced $Paco_2$) begin at relatively low level of oxygen uptake. Severe dyspnea ensues, and the patient is unable to reach his maximal exercise capacity.

Respiratory disease. Respiratory impairment can generally limit exercise in one of two ways: (1) decrease in total or minute ventilation ($\dot{V}E$); and (2) impairment of gas transfer across the alveolar-capillary membrane.

A decrease in $\dot{V}E$ is seen in patients with severe restrictive or obstructive lung disease. $\dot{V}E$ during exercise is a useful measurement, in part because the patient can serve as his own control. The maximal total ventilation is usually measured before exercise testing as the maximal voluntary ventilation (MVV). If MVV is not measured, it can be closely approximated by multiplying the patient's forced expiratory volume, 1 sec (FEV_1) by 35. For example, if FEV_1 is 3 L, the patient's MVV should be approximately 105 L/min.

With an intact respiratory system, $\dot{V}E$ is never the limiting factor in exercise. Healthy subjects reach only approximately 60% to 70% of their ventilatory capacity (MVV) at the point of maximal oxygen consumption. A patient who stops exercising (because of dyspnea) when $\dot{V}E$ is close to his MVV has inadequate ventilatory reserve. Typically, with ventilatory impairment exercise stops well before the anaerobic threshold is reached (Fig. 12-7). If exercise continues beyond the patient's ventilatory limit, $Paco_2$ will likely rise, something that never happens in healthy patients.

Impairment of gas transfer across the alveolar-capillary membrane will cause an abnormal increase in the alveolar-arterial Po_2 difference during exercise. The most common cause of hypoxemia at rest is ventilation/perfusion (V/Q) imbalance (see Chapter 5), but resting V/Q imbalance does not predict hypoxemia during exercise. In many cases V/Q relationships improve during exercise, so the Pao_2 may actually increase (it normally remains unchanged). The change in Pao_2 is a distin-

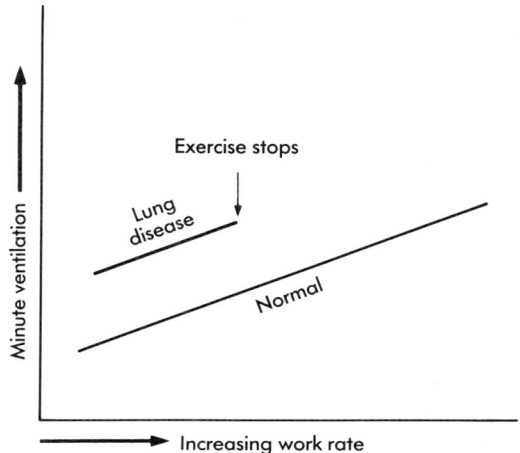

Fig. 12-7. Exercise limitation caused by ventilatory impairment.

guishing point between chronic bronchitis and emphysema; in the former, Pao_2 stays the same or improves with exercise, whereas in emphysema, Pao_2 characteristically falls.

The Pao_2 usually falls during exercise when there is diffusion impairment. Normally, as cardiac output speeds through the pulmonary capillaries, the large reserve for diffusion assures that end-capillary Po_2 is maintained at a normal level. Diffusion impairment causes a fall in end-capillary and arterial Po_2 during exercise (Fig. 12-8, p. 254). This fall in Pao_2 is seen in emphysema (loss of capillary vascular bed) and interstitial lung disease (thickening of alveolar capillary membrane).

Clinical problem 4

Provide a possible physiologic explanation for the following changes in blood gas values during exercise (all values are in mm Hg).

	Resting	*During exercise*
Patient A:	Pao_2, 65; $Paco_2$, 40	Pao_2, 50; $Paco_2$, 43
Patient B:	Pao_2, 71; $Paco_2$, 37	Pao_2, 77; $Paco_2$, 37
Patient C:	Pao_2, 80; $Paco_2$, 32	Pao_2, 65; $Paco_2$, 29

Poor physical fitness. Exercise limitation from poor physical fitness can usually be appreciated from the pattern of ventilatory and cardiac response in relation to the work load and oxygen uptake. Commonly the subject "poops out" well before anaerobic threshold, although the heart rate and $\dot{V}_E$ have increased appropriately for the level of exercise. Occasionally the heart rate or $\dot{V}_E$ will rise more than expected for the level of work because of anxiety or early (and inappropriate) hyperventilation, respectively. Nonetheless, by carefully analyzing the exercise data in light of the total resting evaluation, poor fitness can usually be distinguished from cardiac and respiratory limitation.

Based on the previous discussion, exercise test interpretation can be approached systematically. This approach is based on testing that includes Group 1, 2, and 3 measurements (see Table 12-1).

1. Determine if anaerobic threshold is reached. Generally, AT is determined from analysis of respiratory quotient, end-tidal partial pressure of carbon dioxide ($PetCO_2$), and ratio of slope of $\dot{V}_E$ to the slope of oxygen consumption ($\dot{V}O_2$) (see Fig. 12-4 and box on p. 246). Normally, anaerobic threshold (AT) should occur at an oxygen consumption near 20 ml/min/kg; for a 50-kg person, this is a $\dot{V}O_2$ of 1 L/min.
2. Determine if ventilatory limit has been reached by comparing the patient's exercise minute ventilation to his resting maximal voluntary ventilation (MVV). If MVV was not measured before the exercise test, use $35 \times FEV_1$ to estimate MVV.
3. If blood gas analysis is available, check for fall in PaO_2 and calculate the alveolar-arterial oxygen pressure difference ($P(A-a)O_2$) (see Chapter 5). Check for an early fall in $PaCO_2$; a decrease in $PaCO_2$ before AT may indicate hyperventilation from anxiety. Any increase in $PaCO_2$ during exercise is abnormal and indicates severe ventilatory limitation.

The following cases illustrate this approach.

Clinical problem 5

A 60-year-old man with a long history of smoking complains of dyspnea during exertion. When examined, the patient has a prolonged expiratory time and a systolic ejection murmur; he weighs 80 kg. Pulmonary function tests are consistent with moderate airways obstruction: FEV_1 equals 1.4 L and MVV equals 50.5 L/min, both approximately half of predicted normal.

A cardiac stress test is normal (no ischemic changes), and cardiac catheterization shows a mild degree of aortic stenosis. Coronary angiography reveals minimal narrowing of two coronary vessels. Because of concern about exercise dyspnea, the patient is referred for physiologic exercise testing. The following data are obtained.

	Rest	2 mph 0% grade	2.5 mph 0% grade	3 mph 5% grade	3 mph 10% grade
$\dot{V}O_2$, L/min	0.35	0.81	0.95	1.1	1.4
$\dot{V}CO_2$, L/min	0.30	0.61	0.76	0.91	1.2
$\dot{V}_E$, L/min	12	32	34	40	48
RQ	—	—	—	—	—
PaO_2, mm Hg	90	96	95	88	86
$P(A-a)O_2$	18	10	12	20	22
$PaCO_2$, mm Hg	32	34	33	34	34
Heart rate	72	94	99	108	117
Oxygen/pulse	—	—	—	—	—

a. Calculate the RQ and oxygen/pulse at rest and for each stage of exercise.
b. Immediately after the measurements were obtained at 3 mph, 10% grade, the patient stopped exercising because of severe dyspnea. Was anaerobic threshold reached? Was there a ventilatory limitation?
c. How do you interpret this patient's exercise test?

Exercise physiology

Clinical problem 6

A 57-year-old man was referred by the state Industrial Commission for evaluation of his dyspnea during exertion. The patient had a long history of industrial exposure to chemicals as a worker in the printing industry. During at least one prior evaluation, a physician had written "industrially-related asthma," although there was no documentation for this diagnosis. The patient complained mainly of dyspnea during slight exertion, such as stair climbing or walking uphill, and was convinced he had a valid industrial claim.

Physical examination revealed an obese man in no visible distress. Except for moderate obesity (205 lbs, 66 in tall), there were no remarkable findings. Electrocardiogram was within normal limits, and chest x-ray showed clear lung fields and normal heart size. Resting pulmonary function studies follow (percent predicted in parentheses).

FVC (L)	3.84 (95%)	Pao_2 (mm Hg)	73
FEV_1 (L)	3.20 (110%)	Sao_2 (%)	95
FEV_1/FVC	83 (115%)	$Paco_2$ (mm Hg)	39
MVV (L/min)	112 (99%)	pH	7.44
Diffusing capacity (ml/min/mm Hg)	23 (89%)		

Despite the normal results of the resting studies, the patient maintained that effort-related dyspnea was a real problem. Other doctors had told him he had an industrially related condition, and he wanted to "get to the bottom of it." For this reason physiologic exercise testing was performed, using a treadmill at zero elevation. The results follow.

Graded exercise test results for 57-year-old man

	At rest	Miles per hour				
		1	2	2.5	3	3.5
Time (min)	0	2	4	6	8	10
HR	80	110	123	134	142	154
$\dot{V}_E$ (L/min)	6.4	15.1	20.8	29	34.2	38.5
$\dot{V}_{O_2}$ (L)	0.230	0.640	0.920	1.15	1.32	1.39
$\dot{V}_{CO_2}$ (L)	0.175	0.470	0.690	0.930	1.2	1.35
RQ	0.76	0.73	0.75	0.81	0.91	0.97
METS						
$Petco_2$		28.6	30.8	31.9	32.6	32.5
$Peto_2$		118.5	116.7	117.9	120.4	122.4
V_D/V_T						
$Paco_2$	39	39	39	40	41	40
Pao_2	73	73	72	77	80	83
Sao_2	95	95	95	96	96	97
pH	7.44	7.44	7.43	7.42	7.41	7.42
HCO_3^-	26	26	25	25	25	25

The patient quit exercising after the last set of measurements was obtained. At this point he was very short of breath and just could not continue any longer.

   a. Calculate the patient's METS and V_D/V_T for each level of exercise.
   b. Was anaerobic threshold reached? Was there a ventilatory limitation?
   c. How do you interpret this patient's exercise test? Based on these data, should he receive compensation for an industrially related problem?

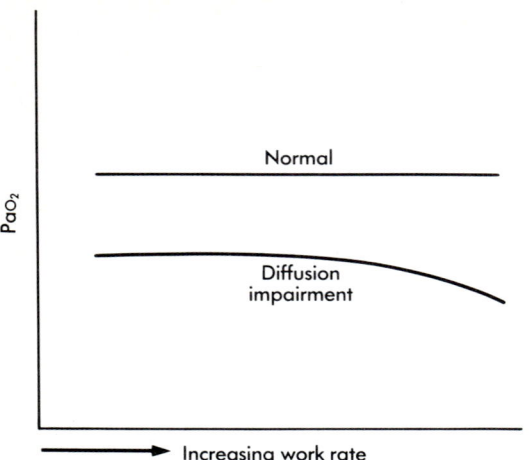

Fig. 12-8. Exercise limitation caused by diffusion impairment. Pa_{O_2} falls in the presence of diffusion impairment.

SUMMARY

During exercise much more oxygen and carbon dioxide are exchanged than at rest. This single metabolic fact accounts for the changes in cardiac, pulmonary, and circulatory physiology during exercise. When the cardiopulmonary system can no longer deliver enough oxygen for the increase in metabolism during exercise, the body turns to anaerobic metabolism to furnish energy. Whereas aerobic exercise can continue indefinitely, anaerobic metabolism leads to buildup of lactic acid and results in early dyspnea and fatigue.

Mild-to-moderate exercise, i.e., exercise done before anaerobic threshold is reached, does not lead to hyperventilation. Alveolar ventilation rises to meet the increase in carbon dioxide production so that Pa_{CO_2} stays fairly constant. At the point where anaerobic threshold begins, lactic acid increases and Pa_{CO_2} falls.

Many measurements can be made during exercise. Exercise measurements can be grouped according to the equipment required and range from totally noninvasive (no mouthpiece or needles) to highly invasive (right-sided heart catheter). The pattern of changes in heart rate, minute ventilation, expired gases, and many other measurements can be helpful in some clinical situations. Indications for physiologic exercise testing include dyspnea during exertion that is unexplained by resting studies and the need for evaluation of exercise-induced asthma.

Two common limitations to exercise are heart disease and lung disease. In heart disease, the heart rate often rises higher than predicted for the level of exercise; in lung disease, minute ventilation may not rise to the expected value for a given level of exercise. Diffusion impairment can also limit exercise. Although diffusion impairment does not generally lead to reduced Pa_{O_2} at rest, it can cause a fall in Pa_{O_2} during mild-to-moderate exercise.

REVIEW QUESTIONS

State whether each of the following is true or false.
1. Both oxygen uptake and carbon dioxide production increase during exercise.
2. Hyperventilation (reduction in Pa_{CO_2}) during exercise usually begins when pulse rate and respiratory rate rise by 20% to 25% above resting levels.
3. Anaerobic threshold can be identified by a rise in minute ventilation out of proportion to the rise in oxygen uptake.
4. Diffusion barrier that does not cause hypoxemia at rest will not lead to hypoxemia during exercise.
5. In the healthy individual, alveolar ventilation will always rise to meet any increase in carbon dioxide production so that hypercapnia never occurs during exercise.
6. Given a patient with chronic obstructive pulmonary disease, a fall in exercise Pa_{O_2} is more characteristic of emphysema than of chronic bronchitis.
7. With increasing amounts of exercise, the level of oxygen uptake also rises and never reaches a plateau.

8. One measure of fitness is the level of oxygen uptake for a given amount of exercise.
9. Daily aerobic exercise leads to improved air flow rates as measured by spirometry.
10. Daily aerobic exercise leads to a reduction of resting heart rate.

References

Hansen, J.E., Sue, D.Y., and Wasserman, K.: Predicted values for clinical exercise testing; Am. Rev. Respir. Dis. Suppl. **129**:S49, 1984.

Jones, N.L., and Campbell, E.J.M.: Clinical exercise testing, ed. 2, Philadelphia, 1982, W.B. Saunders Co.

Suggested readings

Exercise testing in the dyspneic patient, Am. Rev. Respir. Dis. Suppl. **129**(2), 1984.

Loke, J., editor: Exercise: physiology and clinical applications, Clin. Chest Med. **5**:1, 1984.

Nery, L.E., Wasserman, K., French, W., et al.: Contrasting cardiovascular and respiratory responses to exercise in mitral valve and chronic obstructive pulmonary disease, Chest **83**:446, 1983.

Wasserman, K.: Breathing during exercise, N. Engl. J. Med. **298**:780, 1978.

Wasserman, K.: Dyspnea on exertion: is it the heart or the lungs? JAMA **248**:2039, 1982.

Wasserman, K., and Whipp, B.J.: Exercise physiology in health and disease: state of the art, Am. Rev. Respir. Dis. **112**:219, 1975.

See also General References in Appendix G.

chapter 13
Pleural effusions

OUTLINE

Pleural fluid dynamics
Transudates vs. exudates
Diagnostic procedures
Determining cause of exudative effusion
Selected pleural fluid laboratory tests
Mechanism of pleural fluid acidosis
Use of laboratory tests in specific exudative effusions
Pneumothorax
Chest tube drainage
Obliteration of the pleural space
Pleural effusion, lung mechanics, and gas exchange

Pleural effusions constitute a major problem in all areas of clinical medicine, particularly internal medicine and surgery. Pleural effusions are commonly found in patients who have congestive heart failure, in states of hypoalbuminemia, and in a variety of pulmonary diseases such as lung cancer, pneumonia, tuberculosis, and pulmonary embolism. Although a large number of diseases may lead to pleural effusion, the majority of effusions are caused by heart failure, infection, malignancy, and pulmonary embolism (see Table 13-1).

Confirmation of pleural effusion is almost always made by chest x-ray, although an effusion may certainly be suspected by physical examination. The principal physical findings are dullness to percussion and decreased breath sounds in the lung base. Pleural effusions are often initially seen with a meniscus on standard posteroanterior and lateral chest x-rays (Fig. 13-1), although frequently a decubitus film may be necessary to demonstrate that the fluid is "free" and shifts with change in body position (Figs. 13-2 and 13-3).

Table 13-1. Approximate annual incidence of various types of pleural effusions in the United States

Cause of effusion	Incidence
Congestive heart failure	500,000
Pneumonia (bacterial)	300,000
Malignant disease	200,000
Lung	60,000
Breast	50,000
Lymphoma	40,000
Other	50,000
Pulmonary embolism	150,000
Pneumonia (viral)	100,000
Cirrhosis with ascites	50,000
Gastrointestinal disease	25,000
Collagen vascular disease	6,000
Tuberculosis	2,500
Asbestos exposure	2,000
Mesothelioma	450

Modified from Light, R.W.: Pleural diseases, Philadelphia, 1983, Lea & Febiger.

Pleural effusions

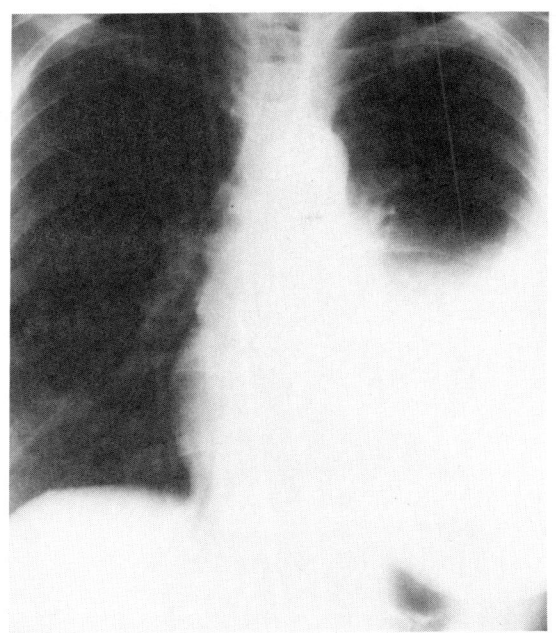

Fig. 13-1. Posteroanterior chest x-ray showing large left pleural effusion with a characteristic meniscus and a shift of the heart slightly to the right (viewer's left) by the fluid. This x-ray appearance is typical of large pleural effusions. The cause of this effusion was tuberculosis.

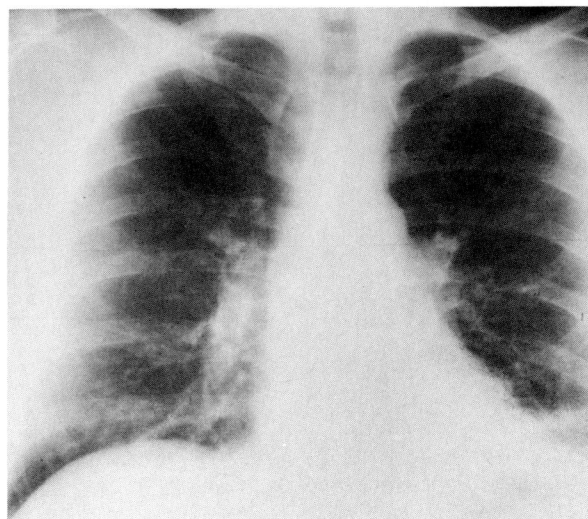

Fig. 13-2. **A,** Posteroanterior chest x-ray shows blunting of the patient's left costophrenic angle; this blunting could result from free or loculated pleural fluid or from scarring.

continued

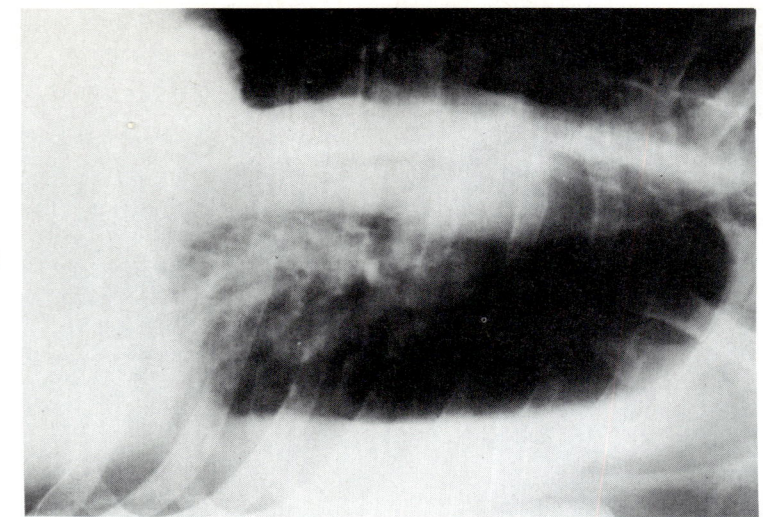

Fig. 13-2, cont'd. **B,** Decubitus x-ray shows layering of free pleural fluid. The cause of this effusion was lung cancer.

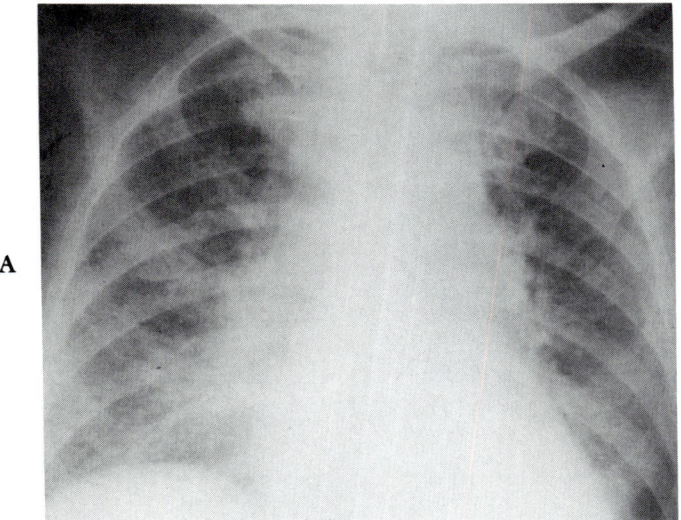

Fig. 13-3. **A,** X-ray taken with patient in supine position showing bilateral haziness that at first suggested congestive heart failure. This diagnosis was not confirmed clinically, and the patient was sent for another x-ray in the upright position.

continued

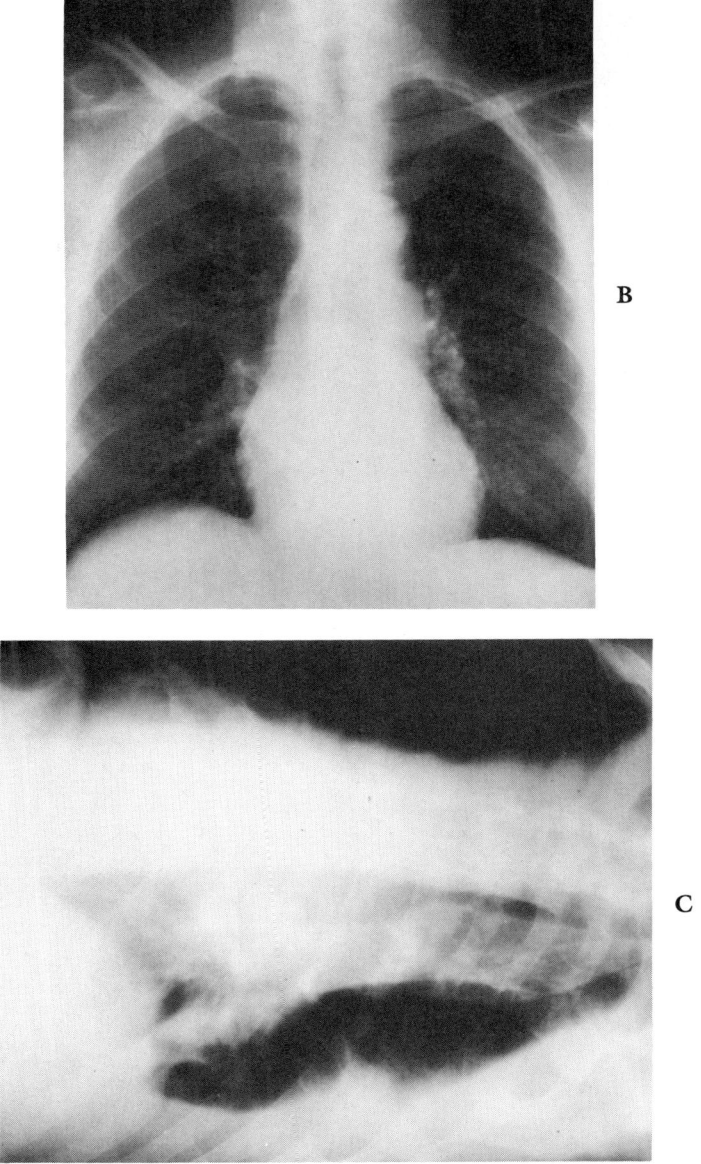

Fig. 13-3, cont'd. B, X-ray in upright position shows the unexpected finding of clear lung fields. However, note the slight blunting of the left costophrenic angle. **C,** X-ray with patient in decubitus position shows significant layering of fluid. All three x-rays were obtained the same day. The initial film represents free pleural fluid layering posteriorly. The x-ray obtained in the upright position shows that all the fluid has shifted below the lower margin of the lungs ("subpulmonic") so that what looks like the patient's diaphragm is actually the top margin of the subpulmonic pleural effusion. This pleural effusion was related to ascites and a low albumin state.

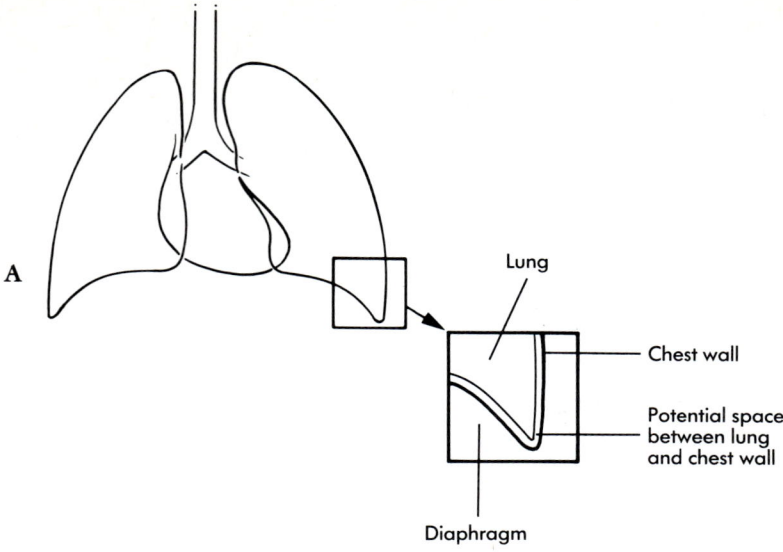

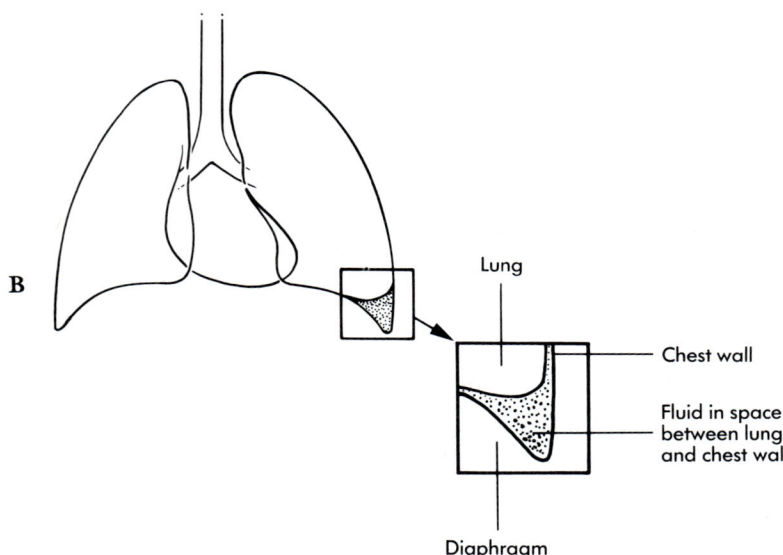

Fig. 13-4. The pleural space, which is a potential space until something accumulates between the pleural surfaces (e.g., fluid, air, or blood). **A,** Drawing representing posteroanterior chest x-ray without visible pleural fluid. *Right,* Enlargement of area in box. **B,** Drawing representing posteroanterior chest x-ray showing small left pleural effusion. *Right,* Enlargement of area in box.

PLEURAL FLUID DYNAMICS

An understanding of pleural effusions requires some discussion of normal pleural fluid dynamics. In healthy patients there is a continuous movement of pleural fluid from the systemic capillaries into the pleural space and then into the pulmonary capillaries. The pleural space is really a "potential" space because the pleural membranes touch as they slide up and down during breathing. It is only when something *accumulates* between the pleural layers (e.g., a pleural effusion) that a real space is appreciated (Fig. 13-4).

The *parietal pleura* is a smooth, glistening, semi-transparent membrane that lines the thoracic cavity and is supplied by systemic capillaries. The hydrostatic pressure in these capillaries is approximately $+30$ cm H_2O; the intrapleural hydrostatic pressure is approximately -5 cm H_2O so that a net hydrostatic pressure of approximately $+35$ cm H_2O tends to force fluid into the pleural space (Fig.

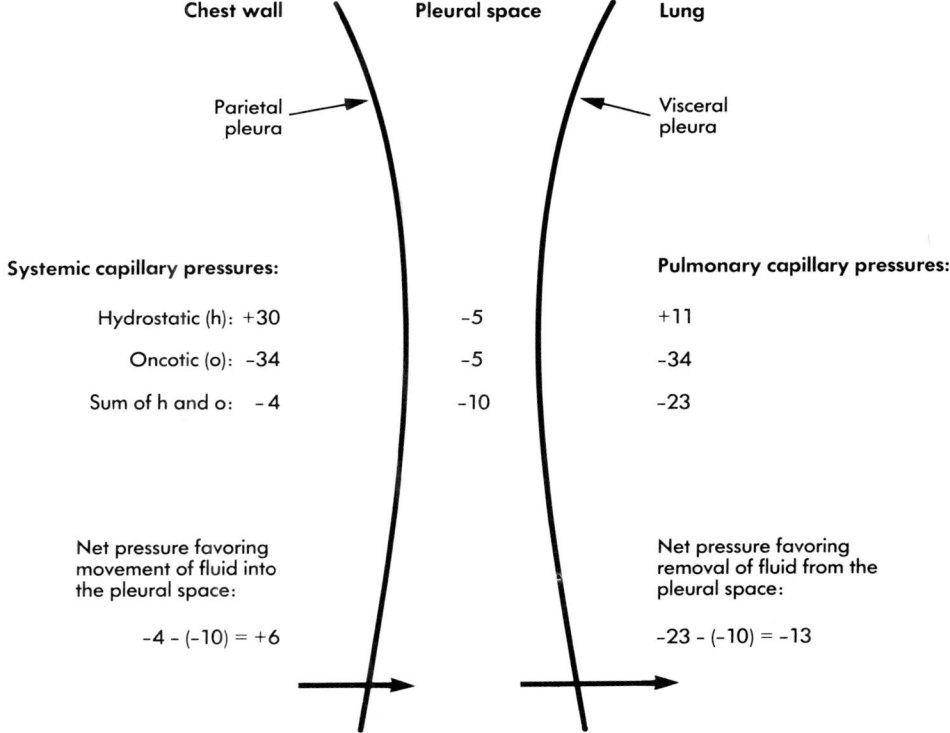

Fig. 13-5. Normal pleural fluid movement. A physiologic balance between the systemic and pulmonary capillaries provides for continuous movement of fluid from parietal pleura capillaries into the pleural space and then into visceral pleura capillaries. All pressures are in cm H_2O. Pressures that tend to force fluid out of the capillaries are shown by a plus sign ($+$); pressures that act to hold fluid in the capillary or pleural space are assigned a minus sign ($-$). There is a net $+6$ cm H_2O pressure favoring fluid movement into the pleural space and a net -13 cm H_2O pressure favoring removal of fluid from the pleural space. In this diagram the surfaces are shown apart, but in healthy people they touch, separated only by a thin (and radiologically invisible) film of pleural fluid.

13-5). At the same time, a net oncotic pressure of −29 cm H_2O, caused mainly by protein, acts to keep fluid in the systemic capillaries. The +6 cm H_2O difference between opposing hydrostatic and oncotic pressures results in fluid leaving the parietal pleura capillaries and entering the pleural space.

The *visceral pleura,* also a semitransparent membrane, lines the lungs and is supplied by capillaries that arise from the pulmonary circulation. Compared to parietal pleura, visceral pleura is much larger in surface area because it invaginates toward the hilum in both lungs to cover all five lobes.

The hydrostatic pressure in the visceral pleura capillaries is approximately +11 cm H_2O, and the total hydrostatic pressure favoring fluid leaving the visceral capillaries is +16 cm H_2O (Fig. 13-5). The net oncotic pressure affecting the visceral capillaries is approximately −29 cm H_2O (same as for the parietal pleura). The difference of −13 cm H_2O "pulls" pleural fluid into the visceral pleura capillaries.

The hydrostatic and oncotic pressures in the two vascular systems are responsible for the dynamic equilibrium of fluid formation and absorption.* A positive 6 cm H_2O pressure forces fluid into the pleural space, and a negative 13 cm H_2O acts to remove the fluid. The larger visceral pleura surface also favors fluid absorption. The result is a continuous movement of fluid from parietal to visceral pleura, creating a radiologically invisible fluid interface between the two surfaces.

TRANSUDATES VS. EXUDATES

The mechanism of pleural fluid formation determines whether or not the effusion is a transudate or an exudate. From the previous description one can see that abnormal amounts of fluid can accumulate whenever there is an *increase in hydrostatic pressure,* a *decrease in oncotic pressure,* or both. Fluid formed by either of these mechanisms is called a *transudate*. Compared to exudates, transudates have a relatively low-protein content.

Clinical causes of transudate include congestive heart failure (increased hydrostatic pressure), nephrosis, cirrhosis (decreased oncotic pressure) (see Table 13-2). Pleural surfaces are histologically normal in transudative processes.

Alteration of pleural surfaces caused by inflammation, tumor, or infiltrative disease can lead to pleural effusion without invoking a change in oncotic or hydrostatic pressure; such fluid is called

Table 13-2. Diseases associated with exudative and transudative pleural effusions*

Exudates	Transudates
Malignancy	Congestive heart failure
Carcinoma	Hypoproteinemic states, including
Mesothelioma	cluding
Lymphoma	Nephrotic syndrome
Infection	Liver cirrhosis
Parapneumonic	Pneumothorax
Tuberculosis	Atelectasis
Fungal	Pulmonary embolism (some cases)
Viral	cases)
Collagen-vascular	Peritoneal dialysis
Systemic lupus	Meigs' syndrome (benign ovarian tumor)
Rheumatoid arthritis	ovarian tumor)
Pulmonary embolism (some cases)	
Pancreatitis	
Subphrenic abscess	
Uremia	
Asbestosis	
Chylothorax	
Traumatic hemothorax	
Esophageal rupture	
Drug-induced effusion	
Postradiation therapy	
Sarcoidosis	
Idiopathic (undiagnosed)	

*The majority of diagnosed exudates are caused by malignancy, infection, or pulmonary embolism; approximately 20% of exudative effusions remain undiagnosed after the initial evaluation. The majority of transudates are caused by congestive heart failure and low-protein states.

---

*Fluid movement obeys Starling's law of transcapillary fluid exchange, which is discussed under "Pulmonary Edema" in Chapter 11.

an *exudate*. Compared to transudates, exudates have a relatively high-protein content.

Exudates occur when pleural surfaces are primarily involved with the disease process. Examples of conditions that may cause exudative effusions are tuberculous pleuritis, pneumonia, lung cancer, and collagen-vascular diseases (Table 13-2). In approximately 20% of exudative effusions, no cause will be found after the initial hospital workup (Hirsch, Ruffie, Bignon, et al., 1979; Leuallen and Carr, 1955; Storey, Dines, and Coles, 1976).

Although all pleural effusions can be classified as exudate or transudate, some fluids warrant special mention. Impaired lymphatic drainage of the pleural space, as seen in patients with mediastinal lymphoma or thoracic duct rupture, can cause a *chylous* pleural effusion (chylothorax) that is rich in triglycerides. Rupture of a blood vessel into the pleural space can lead to a *hemothorax*. Obstructed bile ducts or trauma to the gallbladder can lead to bile in the pleural space, a *bilithorax*. Chylous, bloody, and bilious effusions should have exudative characteristics.

Note that the true distinction between transudates and exudates is *not* a laboratory one but is a fundamental difference in the way the fluid is formed. However, pleural effusions that are clearly transudative or exudative in origin (based on clinical and therapeutic assessment, plus pathologic evaluation of tissues and fluid when necessary) correlate with certain laboratory values. There is a very good—but not perfect—laboratory distinction between transudates and exudates, accurate enough to be of help in the clinical situation.

At one time a pleural fluid protein content of 3 gm% was used to separate transudates from exudates. However, this criterion wrongly classified approximately 10% of pleural effusions. An important 1972 study showed that exudates and transudates, defined on strict pathophysiologic grounds, can be separated better by the *ratios* of pleural fluid to serum protein and lactate dehydrogenase (LDH), an enzyme present in blood and many other tissues (Light, MacGregor, Luchsinger, et al.). In this study, almost every exudate met at least one, and transudates none, of the following criteria:

1. $\dfrac{\text{LDH in pleural fluid}}{\text{LDH in serum}}$ More than 0.60

2. $\dfrac{\text{Protein in pleural fluid}}{\text{Protein in serum}}$ More than 0.50

3. Pleural fluid LDH greater than two thirds of the upper limit of normal for serum LDH

If a pleural fluid meets any one of these criteria, the chances are very good (over 95% confidence) that it represents an exudate. However, it cannot be overemphasized that the LDH and protein criteria are laboratory correlates only and do not, strictly speaking, define an exudate or transudate. On occasion, diseases that seemingly should cause exudates do not fit these laboratory correlations. For example, some pleural effusions from patients with a pulmonary embolism have been described with transudative characteristics, even when there was no clinical evidence for congestive heart failure (Bynum and Wilson, 1976). Also, *a patient may have more than one disease,* giving a confusing picture.

Clinical problem 1

Each of the following patients initially was seen with a pleural effusion that was aspirated for diagnostic reasons. Based on the clinical and laboratory information provided, state whether the effusion is an exudate or transudate and what is its most likely cause. For completeness, the pleural-fluid white blood cell (WBC) count is also provided.

a. A 56-year-old alcoholic man initially is seen because of dyspnea. Chest x-ray shows a large left pleural effusion, a very small right pleural effusion, and cardiomegaly. There is trace edema in both legs, and the patient has a sinus tachycardia of 110/min. He is afebrile. Laboratory values show the following:

Test	*Blood*	*Pleural fluid*
Albumin	3.6 gm%	—
Total protein	6.1 gm%	1.6 gm%
LDH	238 units	105 units
WBC count	8500/cu mm	800/cu mm (86% lymphocytes)

b. A 64-year-old woman is initially seen with weakness and weight loss of 6 weeks duration. She had a myocardial infarction 1 year earlier but was stable until her recent weight loss. Chest x-ray shows bilateral pleural effusions, which are greater on the right than the left. Laboratory values are as follows:

Test	Blood	Pleural fluid
LDH	150 units	210 units
Total protein	7.3 gm%	5.6 gm%
WBC count	6700/cu mm	2000/cu mm (98% mononuclears)
Cytology		No malignant cells

c. A 44-year-old man is hospitalized for multiple injuries following an automobile accident. The sixth hospital day the patient develops chest pain. Chest x-ray shows a small left pleural effusion that was not present at the time of admission. A perfusion lung scan is read as "indeterminate for pulmonary embolism." Fifty cc of yellowish pleural fluid is removed at thoracentesis.

Test	Blood	Pleural fluid
LDH	120 units	78 units
Total protein	7.1 gm%	4.2 gm%
WBC count	10,555 (with a normal differential)	2700/cu mm (55% segmented neutrophils, 45% lymphocytes)

DIAGNOSTIC PROCEDURES

Pleural fluid is aspirated with the aid of a syringe and a needle (usually 14- to 20-gauge in diameter) inserted into the pleural space (Fig. 13-6). The procedure is called a *thoracentesis*. Care must be taken not to let the pleural space communicate with atmospheric pressure since the latter is positive relative to the pleural space and any connection with the pleural space could result in a pneumothorax.

If pleural fluid is seen easily on chest x-ray, thoracentesis should be a safe procedure, and fluid can be removed for both diagnostic and therapeutic reasons. The therapeutic indication is especially important if the effusion is massive and the patient is dyspneic. Generally, several hundred cc of fluid can be removed safely without difficulty.

Attention has been called to the hypoxemia that develops following a thoracentesis (Brandstetter and Cohen, 1979). Fifteen patients undergoing thoracentesis had a fall in arterial partial pressure of oxygen (PaO_2) 20 minutes after the procedure was performed. There was a direct relationship between the volume of fluid removed and the degree of hypoxemia. Hypoxemia can be prevented by using supplemental oxygen during the procedure.

It has also been reported that the rapid removal of large amounts of pleural fluid can cause so-called "re-expansion" pulmonary edema. The physiologic mechanism is unknown but may be related to the generation of large negative intrapleural pressures during the procedure (Light, Jenkinson, Minh, et al., 1980). The complication can generally be prevented by removing less than 1500 cc at any one time. A post-thoracentesis chest x-ray should also be obtained to rule out a pneumothorax.

A *pleural biopsy* may be indicated when the pleural fluid itself is nondiagnostic and/or one suspects either malignancy or tuberculosis. Pleural biopsy is generally not helpful unless tuberculosis or malignancy is suspected since the characteristics of the pleura on microscopic examination are nondiagnostic for other causes of effusion.

A "closed" pleural biopsy can be done at the bedside using a special biopsy needle inserted at the time of thoracentesis; this instrument "hooks" onto and removes small portions of parietal pleural, which can then be examined under the microscope.

"Open" pleural biopsy can be done with either pleuroscopy or at the time of open lung biopsy. Pleuroscopy is a surgical procedure (requires a surgeon and operating room) whereby a fiberoptic or rigid scope is inserted into the pleural space, through which small biopsies can be taken under direct visualization. Although literature reports for pleuroscopy are favorable, the procedure is not universally practiced. For difficult-to-diagnose pleural effusions, some thoracic surgeons prefer instead to do a small thoracotomy and a lung biopsy.

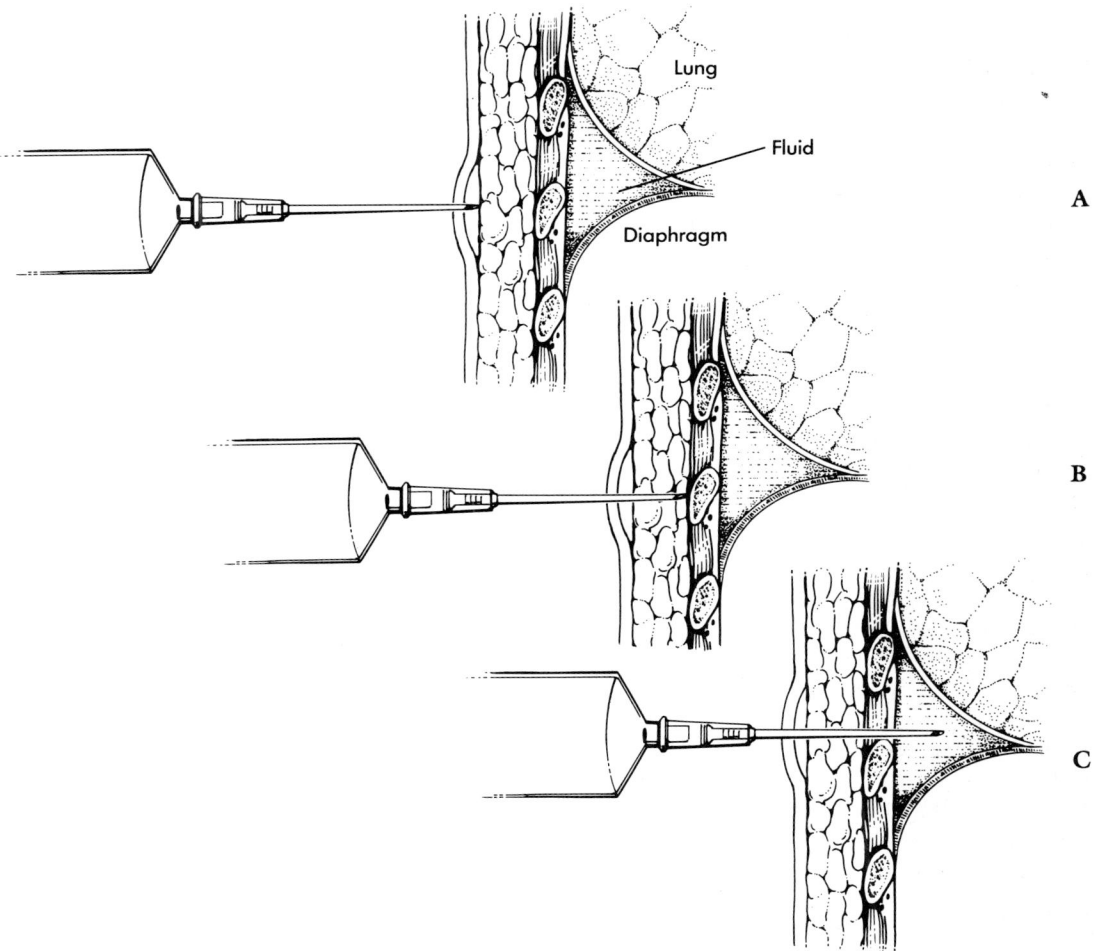

Fig. 13-6. Technique of thoracentesis. **A,** Using a small bore needle (0.25 gauge), the skin is injected with local anesthetic. **B,** With a larger needle (0.22 gauge), local anesthetic is injected into the periosteum of the rib. **C,** With the aspirating needle (0.22 gauge or larger), the pleural space is entered, and fluid is removed.

DETERMINING CAUSE OF EXUDATIVE EFFUSION

The major problem in clinical diagnosis of pleural effusions is not distinguishing transudates from exudates but is *determining the cause of effusion when it is an exudate*. For this reason many laboratory correlations have been made with various diseases known to cause exudative effusion. A list of some correlations is provided in Table 13-3.

Very few pleural fluid laboratory tests are potentially diagnostic. Tests that may actually make a diagnosis are the following:
- Cytologic examination of pleural fluid cells for malignancy
- Culture of organisms from the pleural fluid for diagnosis of infected pleural space
- Microbiologic stain for bacteria, also for diagnosis of infected pleural space
- Wright's stain of sediment for "lupus erythematosis" cells (polymorphonuclear leukocytes that have ingested nuclear material into their cytoplasm); these cells, in pleural fluid, are considered diagnostic of lupus pleuritis
- Pleural biopsy, which may demonstrate malignancy or granulomas with central necrosis (caseation), the latter considered diagnostic for tuberculosis

All the other tests in Table 13-3 may help in confirming a suspected diagnosis or in ruling it out but not in establishing a definitive cause.

The laboratory tests in Table 13-3 are among those most frequently requested for the fluid (and for the biopsy if one is obtained). Each test is ranked for the diagnostic possibilities shown. The numbers used in the ranking and their meaning are:
1. Test results will not be helpful in confirming the suspected diagnosis or in ruling it out.
2. Test results may be helpful in confirming the suspected diagnosis, in helping to rule it out, or in assessing its severity if present. Test results will not be diagnostic.
3. Test results may be diagnostic.

Despite the many available tests, a large percentage of effusions remain undiagnosed during the initial evaluation, which may include not only thoracentesis and pleural biopsy but a multitude of other studies. Many undiagnosed patients, when followed over a period of months to years, are ultimately found to have malignancy or collagen-vascular disease (Gunnels, 1978; Ryan, Rodgers, Unni, et al., 1981). There still remains a large group of patients who are initially seen with pleural effusion for which no diagnosis is ever made; in these patients the effusion either responds to nonspecific therapy, clears without treatment, or resolves leaving an area of scarring on the chest x-ray.

There is a minor controversy in the literature over what laboratory tests to order on pleural fluid (Dines, Pierre, and Franzen, 1975; Storey, Dines, and Coles, 1976; Light, 1983; Peterman and Speicher, 1984; Jay, 1985). Because a thoracentesis is usually performed only once, a test that might be helpful should not be omitted. On the other hand, there are many possible tests, and they can add up to a large expense. Ordering a laboratory test simply because it exists when the results cannot help the patient is a waste of money.

When the major differential is between transudate and exudate, it makes sense to first obtain pleural fluid protein and LDH, and only proceed with further laboratory tests if the fluid is exudative (Peterman and Speicher, 1984). Unfortunately, this approach is often impractical; it requires that sufficient fluid be retained by the laboratory, be properly stored, and then be analyzed or discarded depending on the LDH and protein values.

It is more difficult to decide what to order when an exudate is either confirmed or strongly suspected. Information such as that presented in Table 13-3 can serve as a guide. For example, if a parapneumonic effusion is suspected, then protein, LDH, glucose, pH, white blood cell count, WBC differential, culture, and Gram stain tests should always be obtained. An amylase, triglyceride, cholesterol, and CEA test will be of no help in making or ruling out this diagnosis.

Table 13-3. Relative usefulness of pleural fluid laboratory tests*

	Exudate vs. transudate	TB	Para-pneumonic	Malignancy	Collagen-vascular	Pulmonary embolism
Chemistry						
Protein†	3	2	2	1	2	1
LDH†	3	2	2	1	2	1
Glucose	1	2	2	2	2	1
Amylase	1	1	1	1	1	1
Trig/chol	1	1	1	1	1	1
Complement	1	1	1	1	2	1
CEA	1	1	1	2	1	1
pH	2	2	2	2	2	1
Cells						
Total WBC	2	1	2	1	1	1
WBC differential	1	2	2	1	1	1
% Mesothelials	1	2	1	1	1	1
% Eosinophils	1	1	1	2	1	1
Total RBC	1	2	1	2	1	2
Cytology	1	1	1	3	1	1
LE cells	1	1	1	1	3‡	1
Microbiology						
Gram stain	1	1	3	1	1	1
Routine culture	1	1	3	1	1	1
AFB stain	1	3	1	1	1	1
AFB culture	1	3	1	1	1	1
Pleural biopsy						
Histology	1	3	1	3	1	1
AFB culture	1	3	1	1	1	1

*TB, tuberculosis; LDH, lactate dehydrogenase; CEA, carcinoembryonic antigen; WBC, white blood cell; RBC, red blood cell; AFB, acid-fast bacilli; Trig, triglyceride; Chol, cholesterol; LE, lupus erythematosis
†When compared against simultaneous serum values, pleural fluid protein and LDH can separate transudates from exudates with greater than 95% confidence.
‡Diagnostic for lupus pleuritis only

By considering the most likely diagnoses before thoracentesis, laboratory tests can be ordered in a seemingly rational way. Indeed, some authors have advocated algorithms for test ordering that are based on the suspected diagnosis, the ultimate aim of which is to save money by not ordering useless laboratory tests (Storey, Dines, and Coles, 1976).

The major problem with this approach is that the diagnosis usually is not known or not enough is known to strongly suspect a particular diagnosis at the time of thoracentesis. Might a patient with fever have a malignancy as well as an infection? Might a suspected malignancy be a collagen-vascular process instead?

The best approach is to think carefully about why the thoracentesis is being done and to consider the most likely diagnoses. Take into account the capability of the laboratory (it does no good to order a test that is not available) and how the results will be interpreted. In general, err on the side of ordering a test if it might help. It is much cheaper to order a test than to repeat a thoracentesis or prolong the hospitalization because of an uncertain diagnosis. Also, remember that some effusions will remain undiagnosed after a complete workup.

SELECTED PLEURAL FLUID LABORATORY TESTS

Mention has been made of the potential diagnostic value of microbiologic staining, culture, and cytology. Table 13-3 lists many other tests that can be ordered on pleural fluid. Some, such as protein and lactate dehydrogenase (LDH), are obtained on virtually every pleural effusion because they serve to distinguish between transudates and exudates. Other tests, such as carcinoembryonic antigen, are obtained infrequently. Following is a brief discussion of selected laboratory tests and how they may be used in diagnosis of pleural effusion.

Glucose. Normal pleural fluid glucose has a range similar to serum, 70 to 120 mg/100 ml. Pleural fluid glucose tends to correlate with pH (low pH, low glucose) in parapneumonic, malignant, and rheumatoid effusions (Light, 1983). Pleural fluid glucose is most consistently reduced in rheumatoid arthritis effusions, where it is usually less than 50 mg/100 ml; a higher value should cast doubt on rheumatoid arthritis as the cause of effusion. Although both pH and glucose can be used for their correlative value in certain effusions, pH is available more quickly and seems to have more utility in diagnosis.

Amylase. Amylase is generally elevated in effusions from pancreatitis. High amylase levels (from salivary glands) may also be found in effusions due to esophageal rupture (Light, 1983).

Triglycerides and cholesterol. *Chylous* effusions, which occur from interruption or blockage of pleural lymphatic drainage, have elevated triglycerides and low cholesterol. *Chyliform* effusions occur in some long-standing infectious processes, neoplasms, and tuberculous effusions; they have elevated cholesterol and (usually) normal or low triglycerides. Lipoprotein electrophoresis is the definitive test for chylous effusions; it will demonstrate the characteristic chylomicron band that is always present in true chylous effusions (and absent in chyliform effusions). A pleural fluid triglyceride level of more than 110 mg/100 ml is also considered diagnostic of chylous effusion (Staats, Ellefson, Budahn, et al., 1980). Both types of effusion may appear milky or off-white in color, an appearance that always warrants measuring cholesterol and triglyceride in the pleural fluid. However, true chylous effusions may *not* appear milky.

Complement. Total pleural fluid complement is reduced in both rheumatoid and systemic lupus-induced pleural effusions, but not in other causes of exudates (Halla, Schrohenloher, and Volanakis, 1980). Except for helping to diagnose one of these two collagen-vascular diseases, measuring pleural fluid complement is not considered useful.

Carcinoembryonic antigen (CEA). In one study (Rittgers, Lowenstein, Feinerman, et al., 1978), carcinoembryonic antigen levels greater than 12 ng/ml were very suggestive of malignant etiology. Only 3 out of 121 patients with pleural fluid that was not eventually proven malignant had CEA levels above 12 ng/ml. The authors caution that CEA is not specific for malignancy and that proper use of CEA levels requires complete clinical and laboratory assessment of the patient.

Cells. All pleural effusions contain cells (Fig. 13-7). The number of cells and their morphology (cell cytology) can help in diagnosing pleural effusions. Some investigators believe the only useful test on pleural fluid cells is cytology, specifically to look for malignancy (Dines, Pierre, and Franzen, 1975). This is a narrow view. In fact the pleural fluid literature suggests several useful correlations from a complete cell count:

- A very bloody pleural effusion (greater than 100,000 red blood cells/cu mm) usually indicates one of three diagnoses—malignancy,

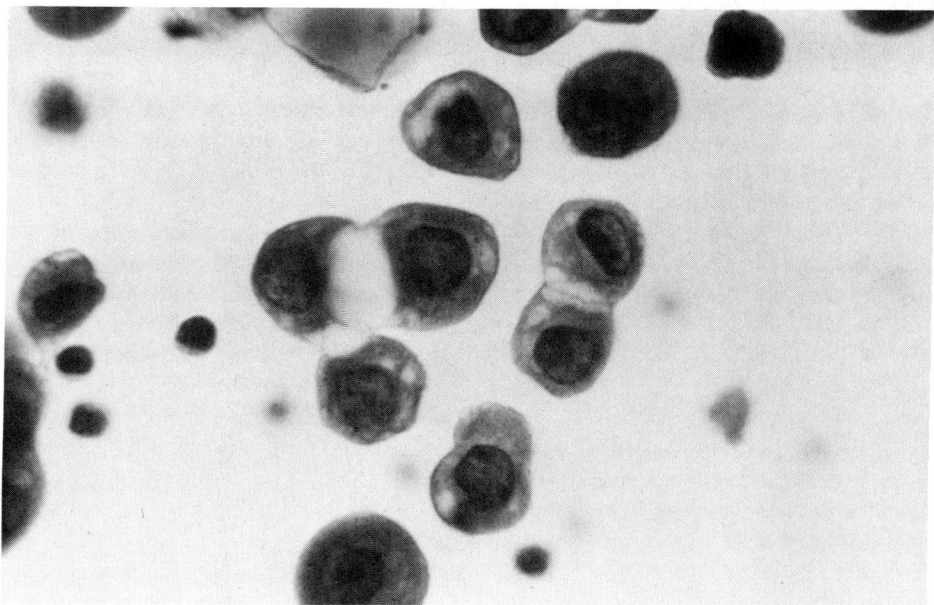

Fig. 13-7. Cells in the pleural fluid. All pleural effusions contain some cells, and the number and type of cells are often useful in characterizing the fluid. The small rounded mononuclear cells are lymphocytes. The much larger mononuclear cells are mesothelial cells. Although lymphocytes are common in tuberculous effusions, if more than 1% of non-red blood cells are mesothelial, a tuberculous cause is highly unlikely.

pulmonary embolism, or trauma (including iatrogenic laceration of intercostal blood vessels) (Light, Erozan, and Ball, 1973). Of course malignancy and pulmonary embolism may also cause a nonbloody pleural effusion.
- Greater than 10,000 white blood cells/cu mm is virtually diagnostic of an exudative effusion since transudates do not manifest this many white cells. A white cell count less than 10,000/cu mm may represent a transudate or exudate (Light, Erozan, and Ball, 1973).
- If more than 1% of the pleural fluid cells (excluding red blood cells) are mesothelial cells, the diagnosis of tuberculous effusion is considered unlikely (Spriggs and Boddington, 1960). Why tuberculous effusions do not show many mesothelial cells is unknown, but this correlation is more useful than the lymphocyte predominance often found in tuberculous effusions (see the section on tuberculosis later in this chapter).
- Pleural fluid eosinophils making up more than 10% of the pleural fluid white blood cell count, without concomitant blood eosinophilia, argues strongly against a malignant effusion. In a review of 245 cases of malignant pleural effusion, only 12 cases of pleural fluid eosinophilia were documented (Adelman, Albelda, Gottlieb, et al., 1984). Pleural fluid eosinophilia is also uncommon in tuberculous pleural effusions. Air previously introduced into the pleural space (as from prior thoracentesis) is one cause of eosinophilia in pleural fluid, although the mechanism is unknown.

Clinical problem 2

For each of the following clinical conditions, state which pleural fluid laboratory tests you would order and why.

  a. A 65-year-old woman is initially seen after 3 months of weight loss. Chest x-ray shows a large right pleural effusion and a right hilar mass. She is afebrile and has no other complaints. Physical examination reveals a palpable lymph node just above her right clavicle.

  b. A 24-year-old alcoholic man is initially seen with high fever, abdominal pain, and a left pleural effusion.

  c. A 58-year-old man is initially seen with progressive dyspnea, bilateral pleural effusions, and leg edema up to his knees. He is afebrile. Physical examination reveals an enlarged heart and an S_3 gallop (abnormal third heart sound).

  d. A 51-year-old woman is recovering from hip surgery. Before surgery her chest x-ray was normal. On the third postoperative day she develops sharp left-sided chest pain and coughs up a little blood. A chest x-ray reveals a small left-sided pleural effusion.

pH. For pH measurement a few cc of pleural fluid are collected anaerobically at the time of thoracentesis and analyzed like an arterial blood gas. Pleural fluid pH, compared to protein, glucose, and LDH, is a relatively new measurement. The value of pleural fluid pH is based on its correlation with several diagnoses and their clinical severity and on the test's rapid availability (just a few minutes, like a blood gas analysis).

Normally, pleural fluid is alkaline and has a pH close to 7.60. Pleural fluid pH values above 7.50 almost always represent a transudate; pH between 7.3 and 7.5 may represent a transudate or an exudate, and values below 7.30 invariably represent an exudate (Good, Taryle, Maulitz, et al., 1980). These correlations assume a normal arterial pH (7.36 to 7.44).

An acid pH has been used extensively to confirm the need for chest tube drainage in a parapneumonic effusion (see section on ''Parapneumonic Effusions''). Other causes of acidic pleural effusions (pH less than 7.30) include tuberculosis, rhematoid arthritis and lupus erythematosis, malignancy, hemothorax, and esophageal rupture (Good, Taryle, Maulitz, et al., 1980; Good, Antony, Reller, et al. 1983; Good, King, Antony, et al., 1983).

A very low pleural fluid pH is found in esophageal rupture; values near 6.0 or lower are common. A pleural fluid pH this low should make one consider ruptured esophagus, especially if the patient has been vomiting or is in shock.

MECHANISM OF PLEURAL FLUID ACIDOSIS

The pathogenesis of low pleural fluid pH has been worked out in a series of experiments over the past decade (Table 13-4). It seems to result from a combination of (1) too much acid generated by pleural membranes or cells in pleural fluid, and (2) blockage of acid leaving pleural space.

Table 13-4. Mechanisms of low pleural fluid pH

Condition	Typical pH	Predominant mechanism
Empyema	Less than 7.2	Acid generation by leukocytes and pleural fluid bacteria (Potts, Taryle, and Sahn, 1978; Potts, Willcox, Good, et al., 1978; Taryle, Good, and Sahn, 1979)
Esophageal rupture	6.0 or less	Pleural fluid leukocyte metabolism (Good, King, Antony, et al., 1983)
Rheumatoid arthritis	Less than 7.25	Blockage of hydrogen ions leaving the pleural space, caused by thickened pleural membrane (Sahn, 1985)
Malignancy	Any value; the lower the pH the more severe the condition	Impaired hydrogen ion efflux caused by abnormal pleural membrane (Good, Taryle, and Sahn, 1985)

Acid generation by cells in the pleural fluid is the predominant mechanism for low pH in infection and esophageal rupture. Leukocytes in these effusions generate lactic acid, which is metabolized to carbon dioxide and water (Potts, Willcox, Good, et al., 1978). Buffering aspects of pleural fluid are such that partial pressure of carbon dioxide (PCO_2) in the pleural fluid rises much more than bicarbonate falls, so that low pH effusions are characterized by an elevated PCO_2. In addition to excess generation of acid, there is limited diffusion of carbon dioxide out of the pleural space (Light, 1983).

Blockage of hydrogen ion leaving the pleural space appears to be the predominant mechanism in malignancy and rheumatoid arthritis. In these conditions a thick pleural membrane prevents carbon dioxide and hydrogen ions from leaving the pleural space. Good, Taryle, and Sahn (1985) have demonstrated that low pleural fluid pH in malignant effusions correlates with more extensive pleural involvement with the tumor and a shorter life expectancy.

Systemic acidosis will also lower the pH of all body fluids, so one must always correlate a low pleural fluid pH with a blood pH.

USE OF LABORATORY TESTS IN SPECIFIC EXUDATIVE EFFUSIONS

This section emphasizes laboratory test results in some common causes of exudates. For more extensive discussion of the various causes of pleural effusion, two recent monographs are recommended (Light, 1983; Light, 1985).

Tuberculosis. Definite diagnosis of tuberculous pleural effusion requires growing the tuberculosis organisms or finding caseating granulomas in a pleural biopsy (granulomas with central necrosis). However, the nature of tuberculous pleural effusions is so well-characterized that some laboratory tests can help *rule out* the diagnosis. For example, virtually all documented, uncomplicated (sole cause) tuberculous effusions show the following:
- High lactate dehydrogenase (LDH) and protein ratios typical of exudates
- Pleural fluid pH of 7.45 or lower when blood pH is normal (Good, Taryle, Maulitz, et al., 1980; Kokkola, Sahlstrom, and Vuorio, 1974; Funahashi, Sarkar, and Kory, 1973; Light, MacGregor, Ball, et al., 1973)
- Mesothelial cell count less than 1% of total pleural fluid white blood cell count (Spriggs and Boddington, 1960)
- Total red blood cell count less than 100,000/ cu mm (Light, Erozan, and Ball, 1973)

In addition, over 90% of tuberculous effusions manifest the following:
- Lymphocyte predominance, i.e., more than 50% of pleural fluid white blood cells are lymphocytes (Berger and Mejia, 1973)

Thus a pleural fluid with a high pH, more than a few percent mesothelial cells, absence of lymphocyte predominance, or transudative values for LDH and protein strongly suggests a nontuberculous cause.

In summary, although chemistry and cell count criteria cannot be used to diagnose a tuberculous effusion, they may be helpful in ruling it out.

Parapneumonic effusions. Pleural effusions that arise from pneumonia are called parapneumonic. They may be complicated or uncomplicated, the former meaning loculation and/or an empyema. An empyema can be defined as infected pleural space, diagnosed either by a positive bacterial culture or the presence of bacteria on Gram stain of the fluid. *Empyemas almost always have to be drained.* An undrained empyema may necrose the lung and prove fatal. Drainage is usually accomplished with a chest tube, one end of which is inserted into the pleural space with the other end connected to a suction device (discussed in a later section).

A loculated effusion is one that does not layer out (change position) on decubitus chest x-rays. A noninfected, loculated effusion of parapneumonic origin should also be drained; if undrained, it may result in pleural fibrosis and severe restrictive impairment.

Because empyemas almost always require drain-

Table 13-5. Recommendations for chest tube drainage in parapneumonic effusions

Criteria	Need for chest tube drainage
Gross, visible pus	Immediate drainage
pH less than 7.00 or glucose less than 40 mg/100 ml	Immediate drainage
pH between 7.00 and 7.20 or LDH* above 1000 units/L	Consider drainage (drain if no clinical improvement or if repeat thoracentesis shows declining pH)
pH above 7.20 and LDH less than 1000 units/L	Drainage not required

Modified from Light, R.W.: Clin. Chest Med. **6**:1, 1985, and Light, R.W., Girard, W.M., Jenkinson, S.G., et al.: Am. J. Med. **69**:507, 1980.

*The LDH criterion is based on a normal range for blood LDH of approximately 100 to 200 International units. Some laboratories have different ways of measuring LDH that yield larger numbers for the normal range; in such circumstances the LDH criterion should be revised accordingly.

age, it is important to know, given a parapneumonic effusion, whether or not the fluid is infected. Not all empyemas look like "pus," nor do they all show organisms when looked for under the microscope; in addition, cultures may take several days or longer to show bacterial growth. For these reasons a quickly available laboratory test would be helpful if it correlated with pleural space infection.

Pleural fluid pH has proved to be such a useful correlation. *When the fluid is of parapneumonic origin,* a pleural fluid pH of less than 7.20 (with normal arterial pH) strongly correlates with infected pleural space and the ultimate need for chest tube drainage (Light, Gerard, Jenkinson, et al., 1980; Light, 1985). Criteria have been developed using the pleural fluid pH in conjunction with the pleural fluid glucose and LDH values (Table 13-5).

There are other causes of low pleural fluid pH and glucose, including tuberculosis, malignancy, and rheumatoid arthritis. The recommendations in Table 13-5 apply only to *parapneumonic* effusions.

Clinical problem 3

In each of the following cases the patient initially had unilateral pleural effusion and fever. Which pleural fluid (A, B, or C) is least likely to be of tuberculous origin?

	Pleural fluid		
	A	B	C
Pleural fluid test			
pH	7.38	7.32	7.46
RBCs/cu mm	10,350	5,280	26,000
WBCs/cu mm	4,700	2,100	8,200
% neutrophils	62	15	13
% lymphocytes	37	78	80
% mesothelials	1	2	6
% eosinophils	0	5	1
Protein ratio	0.61	0.52	0.73
Glucose (mg/100 ml)	81	73	72

Clinical problem 4

A patient is initially seen with a moderate-sized pleural effusion of unknown cause. She is febrile, and her sputum shows many Gram negative organisms. Pleural fluid pH is 7.10, and glucose is 37 mg/100 ml. Gram and acid-fast stains of the fluid are negative. What treatment would you recommend for the pleural effusion?

Malignant effusions. There are no specific pleural fluid findings when the pleural membrane is involved with cancer except for positive cytology. The fluid is usually an exudate, and the main cell type is mononuclear. However, pleural effu-

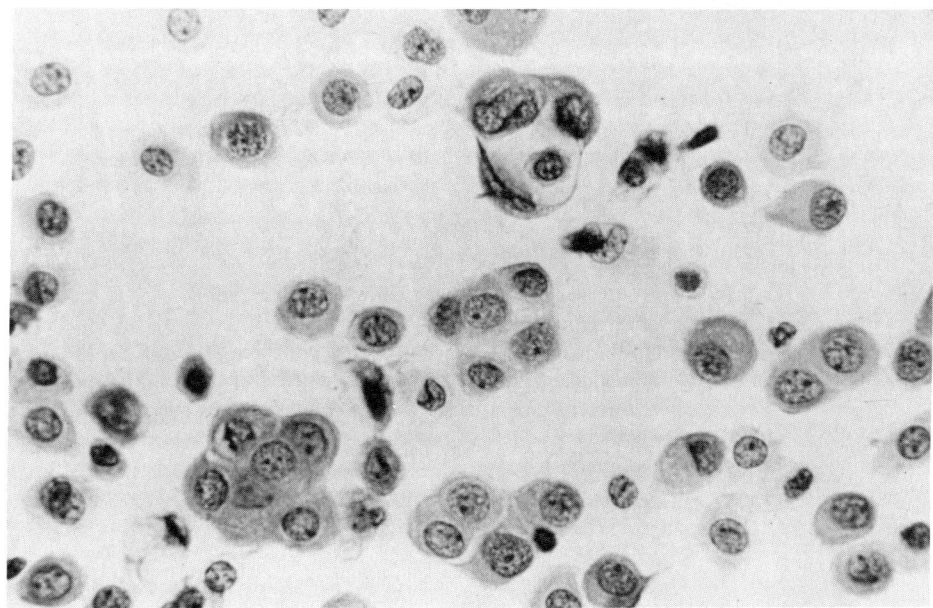

Fig. 13-8. Pleural effusion in malignancy. Malignant cells are easily distinguished from normal cells when seen under the microscope. The cells in this figure, many of which are shown in various stages of cell division, are cytologically malignant.

sions of malignant origin may be transudative if, for example, the tumor is causing intrathoracic vascular compression. Nothing in the pleural fluid except cytologically-malignant cells can be used to diagnose malignancy (Fig. 13-8).

Pleural effusions caused by carcinoma (as opposed to lymphoma) will manifest positive cytology on initial thoracentesis in about half the cases ultimately proven to be malignant. A concomitant pleural biopsy will increase the diagnostic yield significantly (Chernow and Sahr, 1977).

Pleural mesothelioma is an uncommon form of pleural malignancy that usually requires open lung biopsy for definite diagnosis (Taryl, Lakshminarayan, and Sahn, 1976; Legha and Muggia, 1977). Most cases of pleural mesothelioma are thought to arise from prior asbestos exposure.

Lymphoma is particularly difficult to diagnose in pleural fluid. Individual lymphoma cells tend to look like normal lymphocytes, and even clumps of them offer no cytologic clue as to their true origin. By contrast, carcinoma cells are individually highly abnormal and can be diagnosed by a trained cytologist as definitely malignant (Fig. 13-8).

Collagen-vascular. The principal collagen-vascular diseases associated with pleural effusions are systemic lupus erythematosus (SLE) and rheumatoid arthritis (RA).

In SLE the pleural fluid complement is generally low and the sugar content is normal. LE cells, when found, are diagnostic of lupus involvement of the pleura (Good, King, Antony, et al., 1983). Pleural fluid from lupus pleuritis is also characterized by an elevated antinuclear antibody titer of 1:160 or greater (Good, King, Antony, et al., 1983).

Pleural effusions from RA are characterized by

low complement levels and a *very low sugar content,* usually less than 50 mg/ml. In fact RA is the disease most consistently associated with a low pleural fluid glucose. The mechanism is thought related to a defect in transport of glucose across the pleural surfaces (Table 13-4).

Pleural fluid pH has also been studied in these two conditions. In one study all seven RA effusions had pH less than or equal to 7.20 while all five SLE effusions had a pH 7.35 or greater (Halla, Schrohenloher, and Volanakis, 1980). A later study found that two of fourteen patients with lupus pleuritis had pleural fluid pH less than 7.20, and in one patient it was 7.23; the others were all above 7.30 (Good, King, Antony, et al., 1983). Thus a low pleural fluid pH may be found in SLE or RA; a pleural fluid pH above 7.3 may be found in SLE but is unlikely in an effusion from RA.

Pulmonary embolism. Pulmonary embolism (PE) leads to pleural effusions in an estimated 30%-50% of cases (Brown and Light, 1985), but the pleural fluid findings are perhaps the least specific of any cause. PE-induced effusion may be a transudate or an exudate, bloody or nonbloody (Bynum and Wilson, 1976). The main reason to aspirate pleural fluid when PE is suspected is to look for some other cause, not to diagnose PE.

Finding a grossly bloody effusion is suggestive of PE, providing two other causes are ruled out—trauma (including laceration of a blood vessel during the thoracentesis) and malignancy. None of the other causes of exudate are commonly associated with a grossly bloody pleural fluid.

The diagnosis of PE is almost always made with the aid of lung scans and/or pulmonary angiogram. Because pleural effusion is so common in this con-

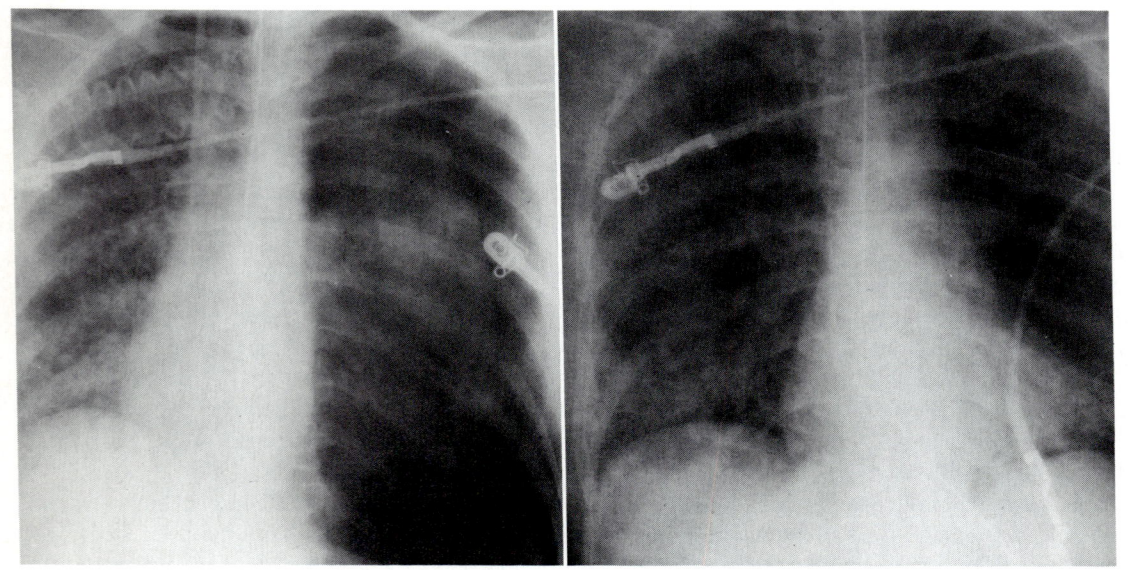

Fig. 13-9. Pneumothorax. **A,** Chest x-ray from a patient who was receiving positive pressure ventilation; a large left pneumothorax occurred during insertion of a central venous catheter. Note that the patient's heart is pushed over to the side opposite the pneumothorax. **B,** Chest x-ray after insertion of chest tube. The left lung has fully re-expanded. Note that the heart is now in its proper position.

dition, an undiagnosed effusion should always make one think of pulmonary embolism.

PNEUMOTHORAX

Pneumothorax is the term for air that enters the pleural space, either from inside the lungs through the airways or from outside the lungs through the chest wall (Fig. 13-9). The normally subatmospheric intrapleural pressure favors development of pneumothorax whenever there is an opening between the pleural space and either the airways or the outside atmosphere (see Chapter 3 for discussion of intrapleural pressures during breathing). Specific causes of pneumothorax are listed in the box below.

The clinical results of pneumothorax—patient symptoms, findings on examination, chest x-ray—depend on how quickly air entered the pleural space and the total volume of the accumulated air. There may be no symptoms when the amount of air in the pleural space is small. More commonly pain occurs at the time of the air leak, especially if the parietal pleura is irritated. Dyspnea occurs when the pneumothorax is relatively large and almost always represents an indication for chest tube insertion (see the next section). Auscultation over the area of a large pneumothorax will reveal decreased-to-absent breath sounds, and percussion will reveal increased resonance. The diagnosis is always confirmed by chest x-ray (Fig. 13-9).

Pneumothorax can be immediately life-threatening if it leads to tension in the pleural space. So-called tension pneumothorax occurs when the leak acts as a one-way valve, letting air in with each inhalation and none out during exhalation. The result is a rapid buildup of positive pressure in the pleural space, which can compress the mediastinum and great vessels and cause fatal shock. The tipoff for this desperate situation is a shocky patient whose hemithorax has absent breath sounds and marked hyperresonance to percussion. Treatment is immediate chest tube placement or insertion of a large-bore needle directly through the chest wall so that air can escape and relieve pressure on the great vessels. Fortunately, the tension variety of pneumothorax is relatively uncommon.

Many pneumothoraces resolve spontaneously with no specific treatment except supplemental oxygen therapy. Favoring spontaneous reabsorption is the fact that air pressure in a pneumothorax is higher than the gas pressure in the surrounding capillaries and venules; the resulting pressure gradient favors gradual reabsorption of the pneumothorax air. Supplemental oxygen enhances this reabsorption by denitrogenating the blood.

Consider a patient who suffers a small, spontaneous pneumothorax. Assuming the pneumothorax occurs at sea level, pressure in the collected pleural air will be 760 mm Hg minus intrapleural pressure of approximately -5 mm Hg or approximately 755 mm Hg. The pneumothorax will be reabsorbed by the surrounding capillaries and ven-

---

POTENTIAL CAUSES OF PNEUMOTHORAX

1. Air in the pleural space from the airways
   a. Idiopathic—occurs spontaneously without apparent reason; presumably caused by rupture of clinically inapparent bleb, cyst, or bulla
   b. Rupture or tear of esophagus or other mediastinal structure into the pleural space.
   c. Chronic lung disease (most commonly from severe emphysema, asthma, or interstitial fibrosis)
   d. Positive pressure ventilation, particularly with use of positive end-expiratory pressure (see Chapter 10)
   e. Infection, tumor, or foreign body causing a bronchopleural connection.
2. Air in the pleural space from outside the chest wall
   a. Trauma
   b. During thoracentesis or pleural biopsy
   c. During insertion of central venous catheter

ules because they contain gas pressures typical of mixed venous blood, which is always lower than the pneumothorax pressure.

Pneumothorax air pressure	Mixed venous blood gas pressures	
760 mm Hg	P_{O_2}	40 mm Hg
−5 mm Hg	P_{CO_2}	46 mm Hg
	P_{N_2}	573 mm Hg
	P_{H_2O}	47 mm Hg
755 mm Hg		706 mm Hg

As long as air does not continue to leak into the pleural space, the 49 mm Hg gradient for diffusion will eventually allow complete reabsorption of the air.

Clinical problem 5

In the previous example, assume that the patient is given 40% oxygen through a face mask, increasing his Pa_{O_2} to 200 mm Hg, and that his Pa_{CO_2} is 40 mm Hg. If his mixed venous P_{O_2} increases to 45 mm Hg, what will be the gradient for diffusion of the pneumothorax into the blood?

CHEST TUBE DRAINAGE

When large amounts of pleural fluid need to be drained completely or when there is a large pneumothorax, a wide-bore chest tube will often be inserted into the pleural space. A chest tube allows for the rapid and usually complete removal of fluid and air from the pleural space. A chest tube is more painful for the patient than a simple thoracentesis, and its insertion should not be taken lightly. Conversely, a chest tube should not be withheld if it may be beneficial.

Chest tubes are almost never inserted for purely diagnostic purposes but only when there is a therapeutic need to remove fluid and/or air. In most hospitals chest tubes are inserted by members of the surgical team. However, it is important for other physicians, as well as nurses and respiratory therapists, to have an understanding of chest tube drainage.

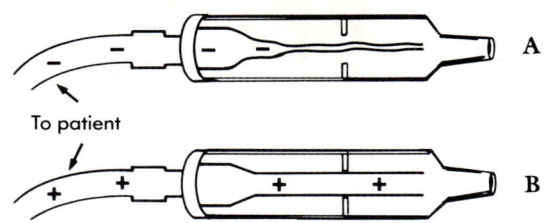

Fig. 13-10. Heimlich one-way valve used for evacuating a small pneumothorax. **A,** The negative intrapleural pressure during inspiration is transmitted to the flexible tubing, which collapses; thus prevents outside air from entering the thorax. **B,** Pleural pressure is positive during expiration; this opens up the flexible tubing and allows pneumothorax air to escape.

Because the purpose of the tube is to drain fluid and/or air from the pleural cavity, the tube is usually connected to some type of drainage system. All connections are sealed with tape to prevent air from entering the patient's pleural cavity. Several different types of drainage systems are described here briefly.

A one-way or *Heimlich valve* is the simplest type of drainage system, requiring no connection to wall suction or bottles. The Heimlich valve consists of a collapsible rubber tube connected to the chest tube (Fig. 13-10). When the patient inspires, negative pressure is transmitted through the chest tube, and the rubber tube collapses; during expiration positive airway pressure is transmitted and the tube opens up, allowing pleural space air to exit. This valve is adequate for a relatively small pneumothorax but is not usually helpful if the pneumothorax is large or if there is fluid to be drained.

The *one-bottle system* is the next simplest type of chest tube drainage system. It provides an underwater seal that lets air leave the patient's chest cavity but does not let air back into the pleural space. The distal end of the drainage tube is placed approximately 2 cm below the liquid surface (saline or water), and the bottle at all times remains vented to the atmosphere (Fig. 13-11). The air pressure that builds up in the pleural space is forced into the bottle when it exceeds the water pressure in the

Pleural effusions

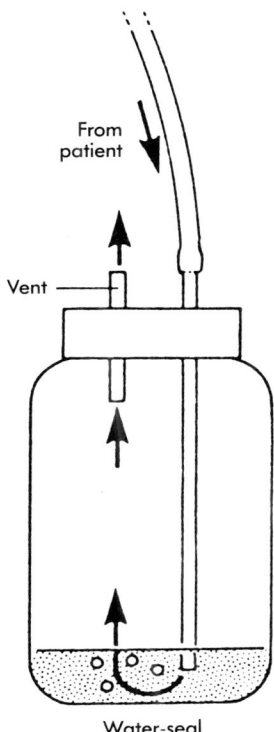

Fig. 13-11. One-bottle pleural drainage system. (From Luce, J.M.: Intensive respiratory care, Philadelphia, 1984, W.B. Saunders Co.)

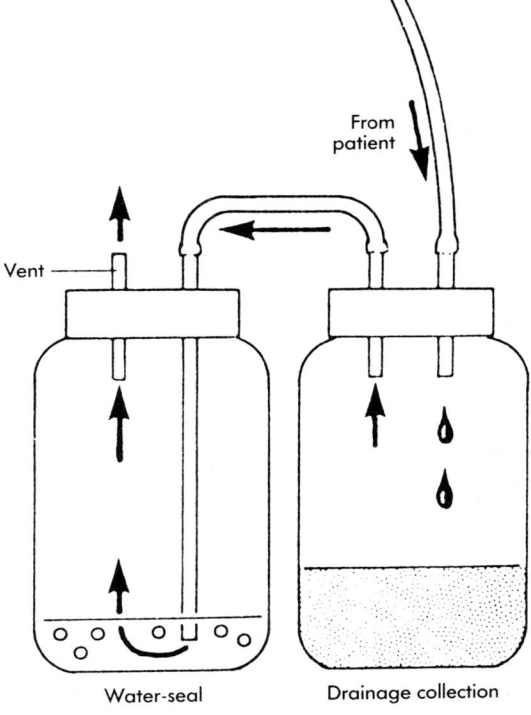

Fig. 13-12. Two-bottle pleural drainage system. (From Luce, J.M.: Intensive respiratory care, Philadelphia, 1984, W.B. Saunders Co.)

bottle (e.g., 2 cm H_2O). If the intrapleural pressure becomes negative, there is no danger of atmospheric air entering the tubing because the water creates a seal. Transmission of pleural pressure will force the water level to rise and fall, which confirms that the tube is functioning properly. The drainage bottle must be vented to air to prevent a pressure buildup in the bottle as gas or liquid accumulates.

Despite its simplicity the one-bottle system is seldom used. The drainage collecting in the bottle increases the length of the submerged tubing and therefore the amount of pressure that must be overcome to evacuate the pleural space. When used at all, it is mainly for pneumothorax and not for pleural effusion.

In the *two-bottle system* the underwater-seal bottle is connected to a collection bottle that traps fluid, allowing the fluid level to rise while the level in the water-seal bottle remains constant (Fig. 13-12). Although this system is adequate for draining small amounts of air and fluid, large amounts of pleural fluid usually require that suction be added.

The *three-bottle system* with added suction is the most popular method used in hospitals today (including commercial units based on the three-bottle system). An adequate amount of suction for most situations is -20 cm H_2O. To help regulate suction pressure, a suction-control bottle is placed between the water-seal bottle and the suction device (Fig. 13-13). The drainage bottle makes up the third bottle in this system.

A long, open tube in the suction-control bottle

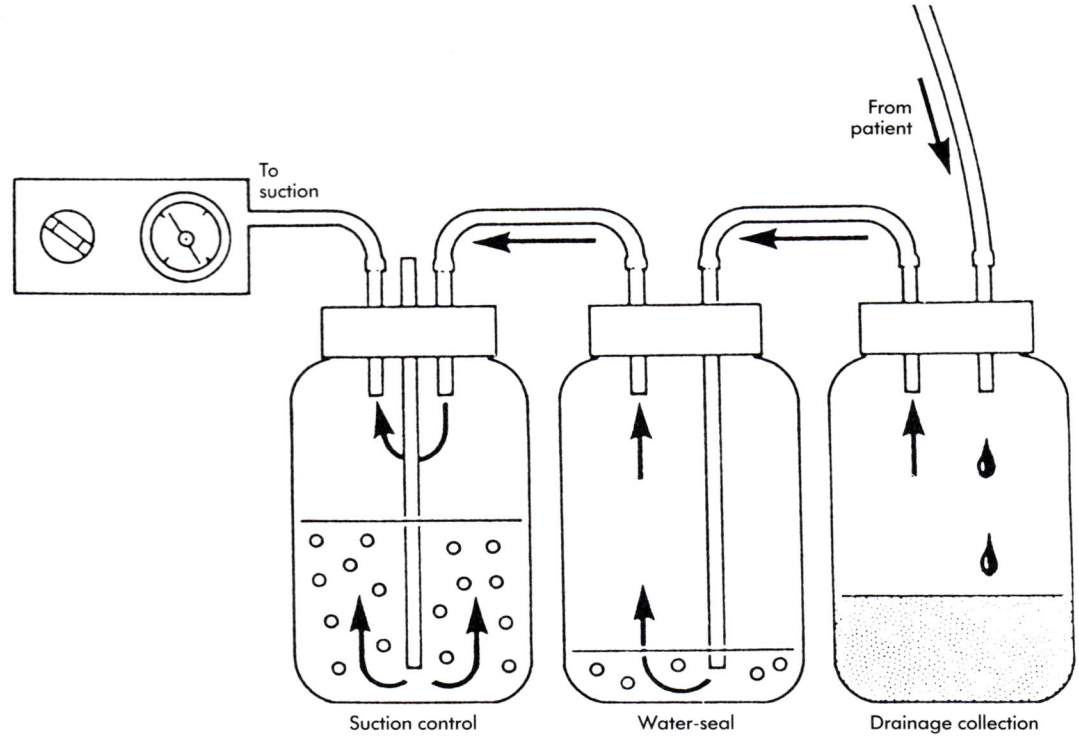

Fig. 13-13. Three-bottle pleural drainage system. (From Luce, J.M.: Intensive respiratory care, Philadelphia, 1984, W.B. Saunders Co.)

has one end under 20 cm of H_2O and the other end open to outside air (Fig. 13-13). The height of the water level in the suction-control bottle determines the maximal amount of negative pressure that can be exerted on the pleural space. If the amount of negative pressure applied to the suction control bottle exceeds the depth of the tube under water, outside air will be drawn in and the water will bubble. Bubbling in the suction-control bottle means only that suction exceeds the depth of the tube, not that drainage is occurring from the pleural space. When fluid in the suction-control bottle bubbles, the pressure inside the bottle equals the depth of the air vent, e.g., 20 cm H_2O. This pressure (i.e., -20 cm H_2O) will be transmitted to the water-seal bottle and (minus the fluid height in the water-seal bottle) to the drainage collection bottle and the pleural space.

When pleural space air is removed, bubbles will be seen in the water-seal bottle (middle bottle of Fig. 13-13). When there is no longer pleural space air to be drained, the water-seal bottle should not bubble. Continued bubbling in the water-seal bottle means an air leak is somewhere in the system.

The water in the water-seal bottle will fluctuate with the patient's respirations only when the suction is turned off. With the suction turned off, it is important that the suction-control bottle be vented to room air so that pressure will not build up in the system (in the two-bottle system the water-seal bottle is vented to room air).

These systems can be set up in any hospital using

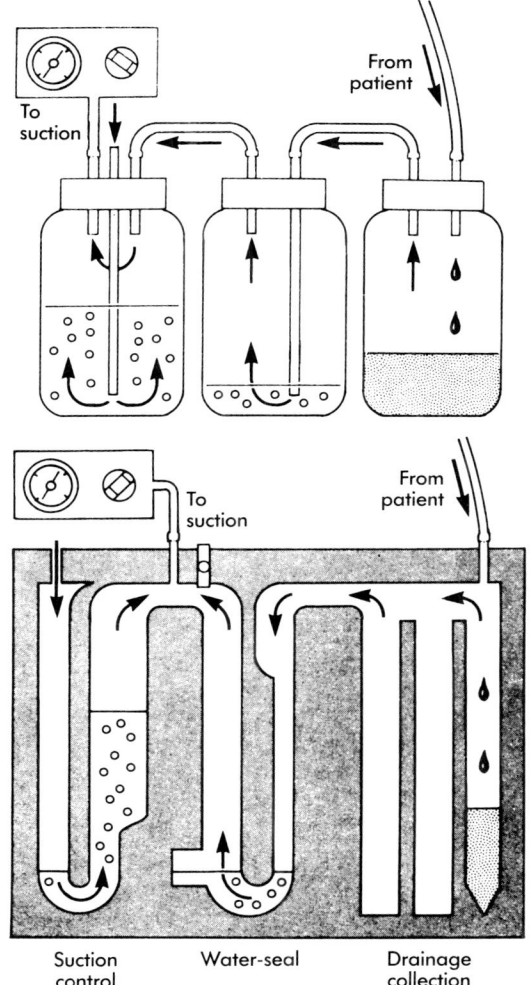

Fig. 13-14. Pleur-evac pleural drainage system, an example of a commercially available drainage system based on three-bottle system. (From Luce, J.M.: Intensive respiratory care, Philadelphia, 1984, W.B. Saunders Co.)

standard tubing and bottles. Several commercially available systems are based on the three-bottle system. Commercial systems come all in one piece and need only be connected to the patient's chest tube and the suction apparatus. A popular system is shown in Fig. 13-14.

Despite the seeming simplicity of chest tube drainage, the technique is fraught with many potential problems. The most common problem is inadequate drainage. Inadequate drainage usually arises from one of three factors: (1) kinking of the tube inside or outside the patient's chest; (2) misplacement of the chest tube within the thoracic cavity; and (3) slippage of the chest tube from the intrapleural space. To some extent adequate drainage can be maintained by meticulous attention to the chest x-ray (obtained immediately after placement and then at least daily) and to the drainage system apparatus.

The decision about when to pull a chest tube is a clinical one based on the adequacy of drainage, the patient's clinical course, and the underlying problem. Most chest tubes are left in for 3 to 5 days, except in patients who are receiving mechanical ventilation, in which case the tube may be left in much longer.

Some physicians prefer to clamp the chest tube before removing it; if no pneumothorax occurs after clamping (based on chest x-ray), the tube can be safely removed. Others do not clamp the tube but simply place it to water seal (no suction); if there is no pneumothorax after 12 to 24 hours, the tube is then removed.

OBLITERATION OF THE PLEURAL SPACE

Occasionally pleural fluid recurs so frequently or so easily that the pleural space must be obliterated to prevent pleural fluid from continuing to accumulate. This problem is most commonly encountered in pleural effusion caused by malignancy, although it occurs in other conditions, including intractable congestive heart failure. Many different pleural "sclerosing" agents have been instilled in attempts to obliterate the pleural space, including talc, nitrogen mustard, bleomycin, quinacrine (Atrabrine), and tetracycline hydrochlorine.

Tetracycline hydrochloride is now the most widely used pleural space sclerosing agent (Wallach, 1975; Lees and Hoy, 1979). Tetracycline powder (same as used for intravenous therapy) is dissolved in water and instilled into the pleural space. Proper technique requires that a chest tube be inserted and that the pleural space be fully evacuated (based on chest x-ray) before instilling the drug. A local anesthetic such as lidocaine (Xylocaine) should be mixed with the tetracycline before instillation to relieve the pain of sclerosis. After the tetracycline is instilled, the patient is turned to several different positions so the drug can cover most of the pleural surfaces. There may be a febrile reaction following instillation, but of all the drugs used for sclerosis, tetracycline seems to be the most effective and the best tolerated.

The mechanism by which tetracycline effects pleural adhesion is unknown. At one time it was thought to scar the pleura because of its very low pH, but this mechanism has not been confirmed.

When tetracycline (or some other drug) does not work, the patient may need a surgical procedure such as decortication (removing the pleura) or open scarification of the pleural surfaces. Either technique requires a thoracotomy. Fortunately, thoracotomy is rarely necessary today because of the good results achieved with tetracycline.

PLEURAL EFFUSION, LUNG MECHANICS, AND GAS EXCHANGE

Depending on the amount and the nature of pleural effusion or pleural disease, the patient may have impairment of pulmonary function. In some instances, the pleural surfaces are irritated in such a way as to cause significant pain, which may limit respirations or cause splinting. Splinting occurs when the patient inspires less than a full breath because of chest pain. If the diaphragm is involved, the pain may also be referred to the shoulder.

To a certain extent all patients with pleural effusion have *restrictive* respiratory impairment. When the pleural effusion is large in relation to the thoracic lung volume or there is underlying parenchymal lung disease, the patient may experience dyspnea. (Significant dyspnea at rest is the main reason for therapeutic thoracentesis.)

Restriction occurs because the lung is displaced from the pleural effusion and cannot expand normally. In the absence of other factors (pleural pain or underlying lung or chest wall disease), the amount of fluid determines the amount of pulmonary restriction. The total lung capacity should be reduced by at least the volume of pleural fluid.

Interestingly, major blood gas abnormality does not usually accompany pleural effusion (Brandstetter and Cohen, 1979). Severe hypoxemia or any hypercapnia in the presence of unilateral pleural effusion (or medium-sized bilateral effusions) invariably points to significant parenchymal lung disease. (In theory, massive bilateral pleural effusions could compromise almost all lung volume, causing respiratory failure. However, it seems that patients seek medical attention long before this point is reached).

Typical blood gas values from a patient with large pleural effusion (and no underlying lung disease) show hypocapnia (hyperventilation) and no or minimal hypoxemia. This preservation of blood gases can be explained by changes in ventilation-perfusion ratios. A large pleural effusion will displace and compress healthy lung, removing both alveolar ventilation and capillary perfusion. As a result there should be little venous admixture and, therefore, normal or near normal PaO_2. At the same time mechanical compression may lead to a hyperventilation response (probably through reflex receptors). The remaining lung tissue (even if only one lung) will then be overventilated. Since ventilation-perfusion ratios are not greatly disturbed, PaO_2 should remain normal or nearly so.

Clinical problem 6

A 55-year-old man with a long history of smoking is initially seen with a pleural effusion that occupies two thirds of his right hemithorax. The patient is dyspneic at rest and is breathing 36 times/min. Arterial blood gas analysis shows pH, 7.47; $PaCO_2$, 55 mm Hg; and PaO_2, 51 mm Hg (FIO_2, 0.21). How do you explain these blood gas values?

Clinical problem 7

A patient is hospitalized with a large pleural effusion. Blood gas analysis shows $Paco_2$, 25 mm Hg; Pao_2, 67 mm Hg; and pH, 7.51. Thirty minutes after a liter of fluid is removed, arterial blood gas analysis shows $Paco_2$, 25 mm Hg; Pao_2, 59 mm Hg; and pH, 7.49. Both blood gas samples are obtained while the patient is breathing room air. How do you explain the difference in Pao_2?

SUMMARY

Pleural effusions are found in many clinical conditions. The most common causes are congestive heart failure, pneumonia, malignancy, and pulmonary embolism; together these diseases account for over one million new cases of pleural effusion each year in the United States. Transudates occur from an imbalance of hydrostatic or oncotic forces affecting normal pleural fluid (PF) movement. Exudates occur from direct involvement of pleural surfaces with a disease process.

Exudates, and not transudates, almost always manifest one of three laboratory findings: (1) a PF/serum lactate dehydrogenase (LDH) ratio more than 0.6; (2) a PF/serum protein ratio more than 0.5; or (3) a PF LDH greater than two thirds of the upper normal value for serum LDH. Many other laboratory tests are available for pleural fluid, but only a few are potentially diagnostic for a specific disease, such as cytology, which may diagnose a malignant effusion. Other laboratory tests are helpful in confirming or eliminating certain conditions. Pleural fluid pH is an example of a test that is never diagnostic alone but is helpful in characterizing many conditions, empyema in particular.

When a large pleural effusion has to be evacuated completely or a large pneumothorax is present, a chest tube is inserted and is connected to suction. The most popular chest tube drainage system is based on three interconnected bottles. When fluid recurs despite chest tube drainage, a situation common to malignant effusions, a sclerosing agent may be inserted to cause pleural adhesion; the most widely used sclerosing agent is tetracycline.

REVIEW QUESTIONS

State whether each of the following is true or false.
1. The difference between exudates and transudates is primarily determined by pleural fluid to serum ratios of lactate dehydrogenase (LDH) and protein.
2. Pleural fluid normally flows from parietal pleura to visceral pleura.
3. Pleural fluid glucose is usually low in effusions caused by rheumatoid arthritis.
4. Pleural fluid pH above 7.40, with normal systemic pH, rules out an infectious cause.
5. Pleural fluid pH below 7.20, with normal blood pH, suggests a need for chest tube drainage when the cause of the effusion is pneumonia.
6. Chylous pleural effusions usually have elevated cholesterol and low triglyceride levels.
7. Air pressure in a tension pneumothorax is above atmospheric pressure.
8. In ordering laboratory tests on pleural fluid when malignancy is suspected, the only test of true diagnostic value is cell cytology.
9. Pleural effusions caused by pulmonary embolism are invariably exudative by established LDH and protein criteria.
10. If more than 5% of pleural fluid cells are mesothelial cells, a tuberculous cause of the effusion is unlikely.

References

Adelman, M., Albelda, S.M., Gottlieb, J., et al.: Diagnostic utility of pleural fluid eosinophilia, Am. J. Med. **77**:915, 1985.

Berger, H.W., and Mejia, E.: Tuberculous pleurisy—critical review, Chest **63**:88, 1973.

Brandstetter, R.D., and Cohen, R.P.: Hypoxemia after thoracentesis, JAMA **242**:1060, 1979.

Brown, S.E., and Light, R.W.: Pleural effusion associated with pulmonary embolization, Clin. Chest. Med. **6**:77, 1985.

Bynum, I.J., and Wilson, J.E.: Characteristics of pleural effusions associated with pulmonary embolism, Arch. Intern. Med. **136**:159, 1976.

Chernow, B., and Sahn, S.A.: Carcinomatous involvement of the pleura: an analysis of 96 patients, Am. J. Med. **63**:695, 1977.

Dines, E.D., Pierre, R.V., and Franzen, S.J.: The value of cells in the pleural fluid in the differential diagnosis, Mayo Clin. Proc. **50:**571, 1975.

Funahashi, A., Sarkar, T.K., and Kory, R.: Measurements of respiratory gases and pH of pleural fluid, Am. Rev. Resp. Dis. **108:**1266, 1973.

Good, J.T., Jr., Antony, V.B., Reller, L.B., et al.: The pathogenesis of the low pleural fluid pH in esophageal rupture, Am. Rev. Respir. Dis. **127:**702, 1983.

Good, J.T., Jr., King, T.E., Antony, V.B., et al.: Lupus pleuritis: clinical features and pleural fluid characteristics with special reference to pleural fluid antinuclear antibodies, Chest **84:**714, 1983.

Good, J.T., Jr., Taryle, D.A., Maulitz, R.M., et al.: The diagnostic value of pleural fluid pH, Chest **78:**55, 1980.

Good, J.T., Jr., Taryle, D.A., and Sahn, S.A.: The pathogenesis of low glucose, low pH malignant effusions, Am. Rev. Respir. Dis. **131:**737, 1985.

Gunnels, J.J.: Perplexing pleural effusion, Chest **74:**390, 1978.

Halla, J.T., Schrohenloher, R.E., and Volanakis, J.E.: Immune complexes and other laboratory features of pleural effusions: a comparison of rheumatoid arthritis, systemic lupus erythematosus, and other diseases, Ann. Intern. Med. **92:**748, 1980.

Hirsch, A., Ruffie, P., Bignon, N., et al.: Pleural effusion: laboratory tests in 300 cases, Thorax **34:**106, 1979.

Jay, S.J.: Diagnostic procedures for pleural disease, Clin. Chest Med. **6:**33, 1985.

Kokkola, K., Sahlstrom, K., and Vuorio, M.: Oxygen and carbon dioxide tensions in the pH of pleural effusion, Scand. J. Respir. Dis. Suppl. **89:**195, 1974.

Lees, A.W., and Hoy, W.: Management of pleural effusions in breast cancer, Chest **75:**51, 1979.

Legha, S.S., and Muggia, F.M.: Pleural mesothelioma: clinical features and therapeutic implications, Ann. Intern. Med. **87:**613, 1977.

Leuellan, E.C., and Carr, D.T.: Pleural effusion: a statistical study of 436 patients, N. Engl. J. Med. **252:**79, 1955.

Light, R.W., Erozan, Y.S., and Ball, W.C., Jr.: Cells in pleural fluid: their value in differential diagnosis, Arch. Intern. Med. **132:**854, 1973.

Light, R.W., Girard, W.M., Jenkinson, S.G., et al.: Parapneumonic effusions, Am. J. Med. **69:**507, 1980.

Light, R.W., Jenkinson, S.G., Minh, V., et al.: Observations on pleural pressures as fluid is withdrawn during thoracentesis, Am. Rev. Respir. Dis. **121:**799, 1980.

Light, R.W., MacGregor, M.I., Ball, W.C., Jr., et al.: Diagnostic significance of pleural fluid pH and P_{CO_2}, Chest **64:**591, 1973.

Light, R.W., MacGregor, M.I., Luchsinger, P.C., et al.: Pleural effusions: the diagnostic separation of transudates and exudates, Ann. Intern. Med. **77:**507, 1972.

Light, R.W.: Parapneumonic effusions and empyema, Clin. Chest Med. **6:**55, 1985.

Light, R.W.: Pleural diseases, Philadelphia, 1983, Lea & Febiger.

Light, R.W., editor: Pleural diseases, Clin. Chest Med. **6:**1, 1985.

Peterman, T.A., and Speicher, C.E.: Evaluating pleural effusions: a two-stage laboratory approach, JAMA **252:**1051, 1984.

Potts, D.E., Taryle, D.A., and Sahn, S.A.: The glucose-pH relationship in parapneumonic effusions, Arch. Intern. Med. **138:**1378, 1978.

Potts, D.E., Willcox, M.A., Good, J.T., Jr., et al.: The acidosis of low-glucose pleural effusions, Am. Rev. Respir. Dis. **117:**665, 1978.

Rittgers, R.A., Lowenstein, M.S., Feinerman, A.E., et al.: Carcinoembryonic antigen levels in benign and malignant pleural effusions, Ann. Intern. Med. **88:**631, 1978.

Ryan, C., Rodgers, R., Unni, K., et al.: The outcome of patients with pleural effusion of indeterminate cause at thoracotomy, Mayo Clin. Proc. **56:**145, 1981.

Sahn, S.A.: Immunologic diseases of the pleura. In Light, R.W., editor: Clinics in chest diseases, Philadelphia, 1985, W.B. Saunders Co.

Spriggs, A.I., and Boddington, M.M.: Absence of mesothelial cells from tuberculous pleural effusions, Thorax **15:**169, 1960.

Staats, B.A., Ellefson, R.D., Budahn, L.L., et al.: The lipoprotein profile of chylous and nonchylous pleural effusions, Mayo Clin. Proc. **55:**700, 1980.

Storey, D.D., Dines, D.E., and Coles, D.T.: Pleural effusion: a diagnostic dilemma, JAMA **236:**2183, 1976.

Taryle, D.A., Good, J.T., and Sahn, S.A.: Acid generation by pleural fluid: possible role in the determination of pleural fluid pH, J. Lab. Clin. Med. **93:**1041, 1979.

Taryle, D.A., Lakshminarayan, S., and Sahn, S.A.: Pleural mesotheliomas: an analysis of 18 cases and review of the literature, Medicine **55:**153, 1976.

Wallach, H.W.: Intrapleural tetracycline for malignant pleural effusion, Chest **68:**510, 1975.

Wallach, H.W.: Letter to the editor, Chest **73:**246, 1978.

See also General References in Appendix G.

chapter 14
Sleep Disorders

OUTLINE

The study of sleep disorders
Polysomnography
Normal sleep
Sleep apnea
Obstructive sleep apnea
Pickwickian syndrome
Ondine's curse
Treatment of sleep apnea
Cheyne-Stokes breathing

THE STUDY OF SLEEP DISORDERS

Roughly one third of our lives is spent asleep. What happens during sleep can affect our performance while awake, yet the study of sleep disorders is a relatively new field. It is a multidisciplined, growing area of research with articles generated from many different specialties, including psychiatry, internal medicine, pediatrics, neurology, and pulmonary medicine. This research has made physicians more aware of sleep disorders, and has led to the general realization that many people do indeed experience respiratory problems during sleep.

There is a wide range of sleep disorders. Insomnia, sleep-walking, recurring bad dreams, excessive snoring, and nocturnal leg cramps are some of the most familiar disorders. This chapter concentrates on respiratory disorders during sleep, most of which have been elucidated with the technique of polysomnography. Polysomnography is the continuous recording of several physiologic variables during sleep. For some patients, determining the pattern of a nighttime breathing disorder has been helpful in diagnosing specific daytime medical problems.

Just the fact that we spend so much time sleeping justifies research into this activity. Although sleep research is still a relatively young field, the following benefits are already apparent:

1. The sudden infant death syndrome (SIDS) is the most common cause of death in the first year following the neonatal period. Research suggests that many victims have a central nervous system problem that either causes them to stop breathing or makes them unable to overcome obstruction of the upper airways. As an outgrowth of this research, apnea monitors have been developed for infants at risk. The monitor sounds an alarm when breathing slows or stops, waking the baby and summoning the parents.

2. Many obese patients suffer prolonged episodes of apnea during sleep, usually as a result of upper airways obstruction. Repeated episodes of sleep apnea can lead to hypoxemia and pulmonary hypertension. Losing weight is one treatment, but some patients have required a tracheostomy to bypass the obstructed upper airways. Recent research has shown that drugs may be just as effective

> **CLUES SUGGESTING A RESPIRATORY SLEEP DISORDER**
>
> 1. Excessive daytime sleepiness, including instances of falling asleep when the person should be awake (e.g., when driving a car, operating machinery, talking on the phone)
> 2. Marked obesity, particularly when accompanied by excessive snoring at night
> 3. Any irregular breathing pattern detected by a bed partner (e.g., gasping respirations, irregular snoring interrupted by silent periods)
> 4. Repeated episodes of sudden awakening during the night; confusion or disorientation when awakening
> 5. Evidence of cor pulmonale not easily explained by routine clinical evaluation, including daytime blood gas values
> 6. Unexplained polycythemia (hematocrit exceeding 55%)
> 7. Abnormal cardiac rhythm during sleep (as detected by continuous monitoring)

as tracheostomy in treating selected patients. Newer methods of keeping the airways open, such as nasal continuous positive airway pressure, are also being investigated as alternatives to tracheostomy.

3. Some patients with chronic obstructive pulmonary disease have severe hypoxemia at night; their oxygen saturation (SaO_2) falls, increasing the risk of cardiac arrhythmias and sudden death. This drop in SaO_2 can occur even without episodes of sleep apnea. After identifying high-risk patients with nocturnal oxygen monitors (usually oximeters), oxygen therapy can be instituted, possibly prolonging life (see Chapter 9).

Although polysomnography is required to diagnose a respiratory sleep disorder, some clues from a basic clinical evaluation can suggest the problem (see the box above).

POLYSOMNOGRAPHY

Many patients with respiratory sleep disorders have normal or near normal pulmonary function tests and blood gas values while awake. Accurate diagnosis of respiratory sleep disorders requires that several measurements be made during sleep (polysomnography).

For the polysomnography examination, the patient is brought to the sleep laboratory before bedtime and is connected, by way of wires, to a variety of recording instruments. Although the test is usually performed at night, it may be done anytime the patient can enter a natural sleep. Recording instruments include electroencephalogram (EEG), electrocardiogram (ECG), thermistors to measure air flow through the mouth and nostrils, chest wall sensors, an oximeter, and a device to measure ocular movements (see box that follows).

> **POLYSOMNOGRAPHY**
>
> 1. Electroencephalogram (EEG)
> 2. Electrocardiogram (ECG)
> 3. Electro-oculogram (EOG)
> 4. Electromyelogram (EMG)—usually a single electrode is connected to the chin
> 5. Breathing pattern
>   a. Airflow at mouth and nose
>   b. Thoracoabdominal movement (with a strain gauge or an inductance pneumograph)
> 6. Oxygen saturation (with ear or finger oximeter)

All measurements are continuously recorded on graph paper while the patient sleeps (Fig. 14-1). By the end of the sleep period, the polysomnography record will show what breathing problems occurred and how long they lasted.

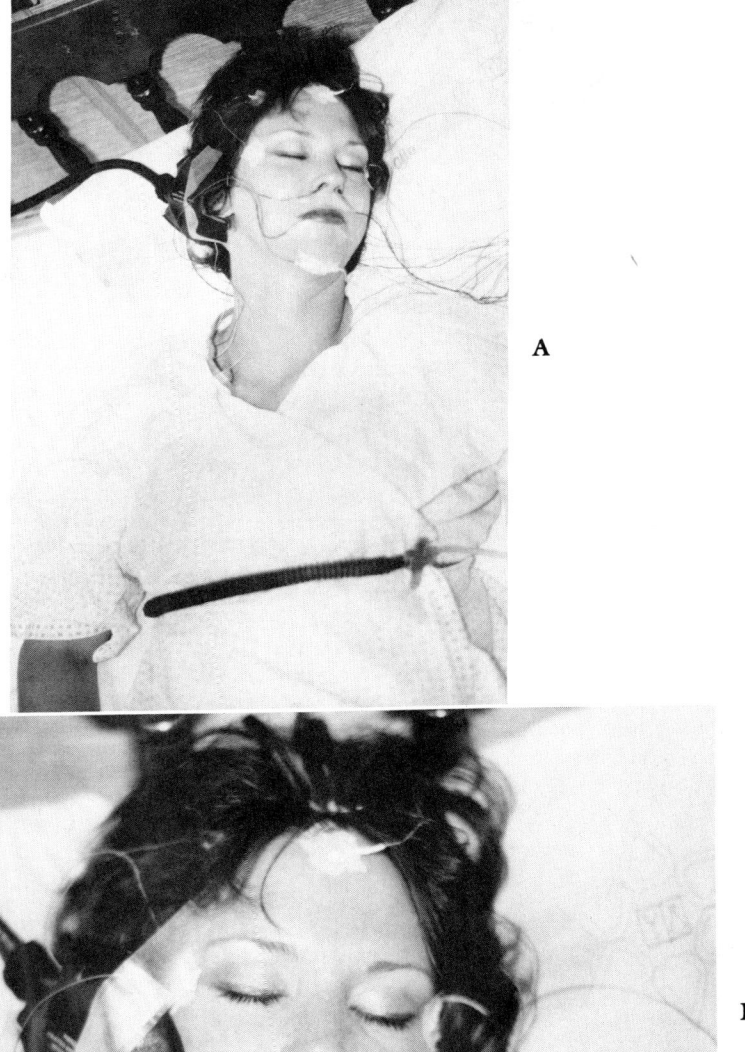

Fig. 14-1. Polysomnography. The patient is connected, by wires, to several recording instruments. **A,** The black band around patient's waist is a strain gauge used to record chest wall excursions. **B,** Close-up of face. On her right ear is an ear oximeter, used to measure oxygen saturation (see also Fig. 12-2). The electrode taped under her chin records chin muscle movement (electromyogram [EMG]). Electrodes taped on either side of her eyes record rapid eye movement (electro-oculogram [EOG]). Thermistors taped to her nostrils and mouth record air flow. Leads for recording brain waves (electroencephalogram [EEG]) are also placed around the scalp area.

In contrast to blood gas values or spirometry, polysomnography is available in relatively few hospitals. Nonetheless, studies using polysomnography have shed light on many respiratory disorders and have helped increase our understanding of breathing during sleep. Furthermore, by appreciating the incidence and variety of sleep disorders from polysomnography, physicians are better able to study patients without a completely equipped sleep laboratory. For example, respiratory rate ECG, and oxygen saturation monitoring can be performed in a regular hospital room. Even a few hours of such limited monitoring may shed light on a particular patient's problem.

Clinical problem 1

A 46-year-old man was referred to the pulmonary function laboratory because of polycythemia (hematocrit 57%). At the time of referral he weighed 312 lbs and stood 5 feet and 9 inches. By history he occasionally fell asleep during the day but never while driving a car. Below are the resting blood gas values, obtained with the patient in the sitting position and breathing room air, and pulmonary function results.

Blood gas values	Lung volume/ capacity	Liters	% Predicted
Pa_{O_2}, 69 mm Hg	Forced vital capacity	4.2	89%
Sa_{O_2}, 94%	FEV_1	3.2	85%
Pa_{CO_2}, 35 mm Hg	Functional residual capacity	1.4	78%
pH, 7.44	Expiratory reserve volume	0.3	35%

A few days later, again as an outpatient, the patient was placed in a hospital bed and was connected to a portable heart monitor and ear oximeter. Within approximately 30 minutes he fell asleep. Within another half hour his oxygen saturation decreased from 92% to 47% and was associated with continued chest wall movement but cessation of air flow at the mouth and nose. During this period the patient's heart rate increased from 92 to 108 beats/minute and two premature ventricular contractions were seen. Because of severe hypoxemia he was awakened and the test was terminated.

How would you interpret this test and what would you advise?

NORMAL SLEEP

There are definite electroencephalogram (EEG), electromyogram (EMG), and electro-oculogram (EOG) changes during sleep, and these changes are used to divide the normal sleep period into two distinct categories: nonrapid eye movement (NREM) and rapid eye movement (REM) sleep (Table 14-1).

NREM sleep is also known as "quiet sleep." After falling asleep we progress through four stages of NREM sleep that are diagnosed from the EEG. Each deeper stage is characterized by further reduction in muscle tone. In terms of sensory awareness, quiet sleep has been compared to that of a lightly anesthetized patient. Sleep apnea occurs most commonly during light NREM sleep (stages I and II) and in REM sleep.

After 70 to 100 minutes of NREM sleep, the first period of *REM sleep* begins. REM sleep, also known as "active sleep," is a deeper level of sleep and is marked by jerky body movements and irregular, occasionally rapid, respirations. In REM sleep the cough reflex is depressed, and there is a general depression of response to mechanical and chemical stimuli.

REM sleep occurs intermittently throughout the night, alternating with NREM sleep (Fig. 14-2). On average, a young adult spends approximately one quarter of sleep time in REM sleep; this percentage is higher in children and lower in the elderly.

Unfortunately there is no universal agreement on what happens to breathing during sleep, in part because detailed studies have been done on relatively few patients. Also, the techniques used to make respiratory measurements often vary from study to study, making comparison difficult. Compounding the problem is the fact that techniques of measurement can affect what is being measured. For example, an oral airway, sometimes used in the measurement of tidal volume, is known to in-

Table 14-1. Physiologic characteristics of NREM and REM Sleep*

Characteristics	NREM Sleep	REM Sleep
Synonyms	Quiet sleep Synchronized sleep Slow wave sleep (III-IV)	Active sleep Desynchronized sleep Dreaming sleep
Metabolism	Decrease in oxygen consumption and carbon dioxide production Decrease in minute ventilation	Decrease in oxygen consumption and carbon dioxide production Decrease in minute ventilation
Respiration	Stage-dependent; during I and II respirations are periodic, with waxing and waning of tidal volume and frequency, resembling Cheyne-Stokes breathing; during III and IV respirations are smooth, regular, and automatic	Irregular and occasionally rapid
Upper airway muscles	Tone preserved	Tone depressed
Response to inhaled carbon dioxide	Normal increase in minute ventilation	Subnormal increase in minute ventilation
Response to hypoxemia	Normal increase in minute ventilation	Normal increase in minute ventilation

*I, II, III, IV refer to stages of NREM sleep.

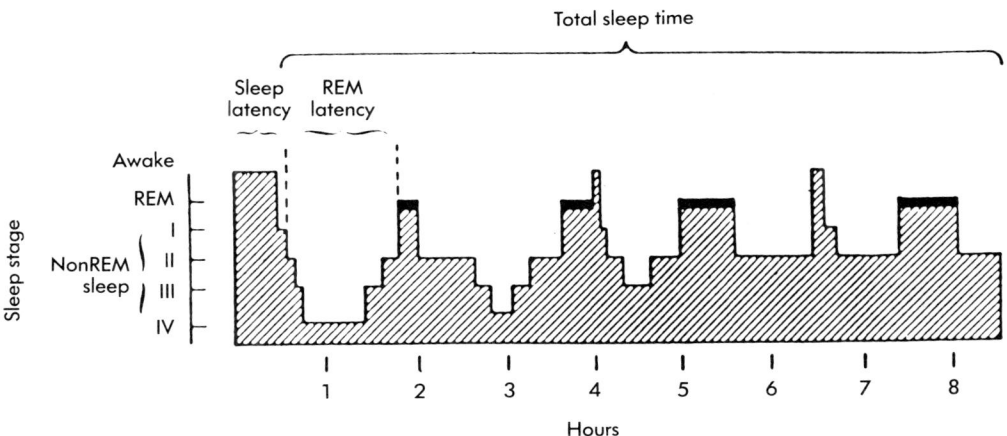

Fig. 14-2. REM and non-REM sleep. All night sleep recording of a healthy young volunteer showing rapid eye movement (REM) sleep and nonREM sleep stages I, II, III, and IV. Sleep latency is the time from "lights out" to the onset of sleep (defined as the beginning of stage II). REM latency is the time from the onset of sleep until the onset of the first REM period. (From Gillin, J.C.: Sleep and dreams. In Michaels, R., editor: Psychiatry, vol. 3, Philadelphia, 1985, J.B. Lippincott Co.)

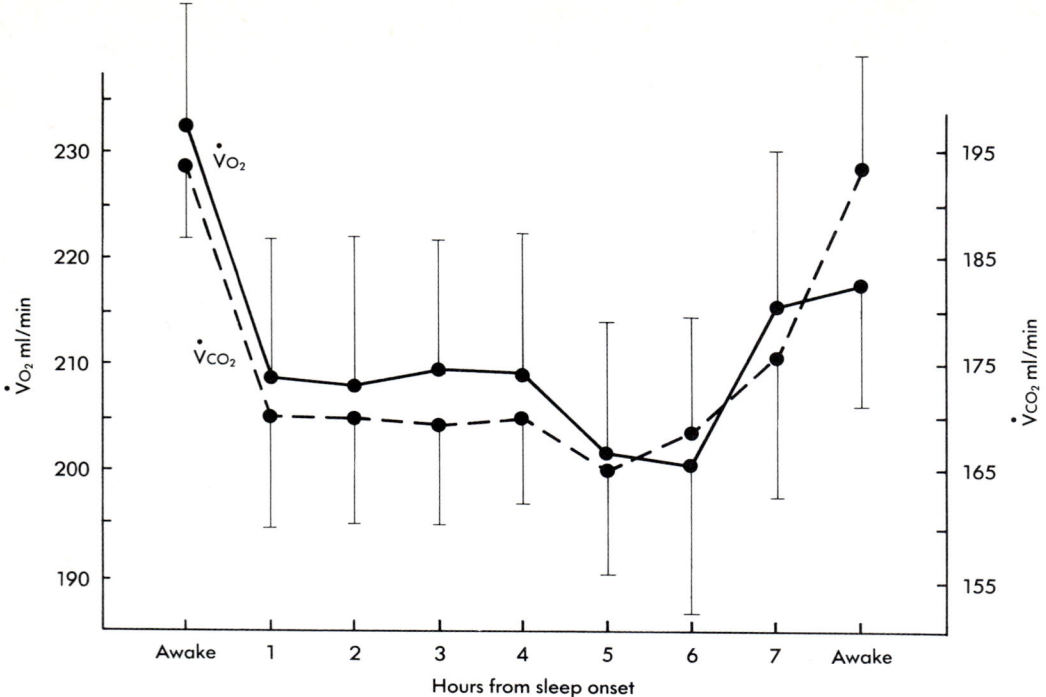

Fig. 14-3. Changes in oxygen consumption and carbon dioxide production during sleep. Effect of time (hours from sleep onset) on oxygen consumption ($\dot{V}_{O_2}$) and carbon dioxide production ($\dot{V}_{CO_2}$) is shown. $\dot{V}_{O_2}$ and $\dot{V}_{CO_2}$ decreased rapidly after sleep onset, remained fairly constant through the night, and began to rise toward morning. $\dot{V}_{O_2}$ and $\dot{V}_{CO_2}$ were lower during sleeping hours 1 through 6 than the mean awake value. However, the $\dot{V}_{O_2}$ and $\dot{V}_{CO_2}$ values at hour 7 rose and were not statisically different from the mean awake value. (Standard error is demonstrated by vertical lines.) (From White, D.P., Weil, J.V., and Zwillich, C.W.: J. Appl. Physiol. **59**:384, 1985.)

crease tidal volume and slow respirations in sleeping subjects.

Regardless of the differences in methodology, all studies find that metabolism slows during sleep. One study of 21 healthy individuals (11 men and 10 women) found a fall in both oxygen consumption ($\dot{V}_{O_2}$) and carbon dioxide production ($\dot{V}_{CO_2}$) during sleep (White, Weil, Zwillich, et al., 1985) (Fig. 14-3). This decrease in metabolsim was accompanied by a fall in minute ventilation ($\dot{V}_E$), resulting mainly from a fall in tidal volume; the respiratory rate remained approximately the same as when the patients were awake (Fig. 14-4). These changes in metabolism and ventilation were not related to either age or sex.

Although breathing during REM sleep may be irregular, the degree of reduction in $\dot{V}_{CO_2}$, $\dot{V}_{O_2}$, and $\dot{V}_E$ does not change significantly between REM and NREM sleep. Reductions in metabolism and ventilation are more related to how long someone has been asleep than to the specific stage of sleep (White, Weil, Zwillich, et al., 1985).

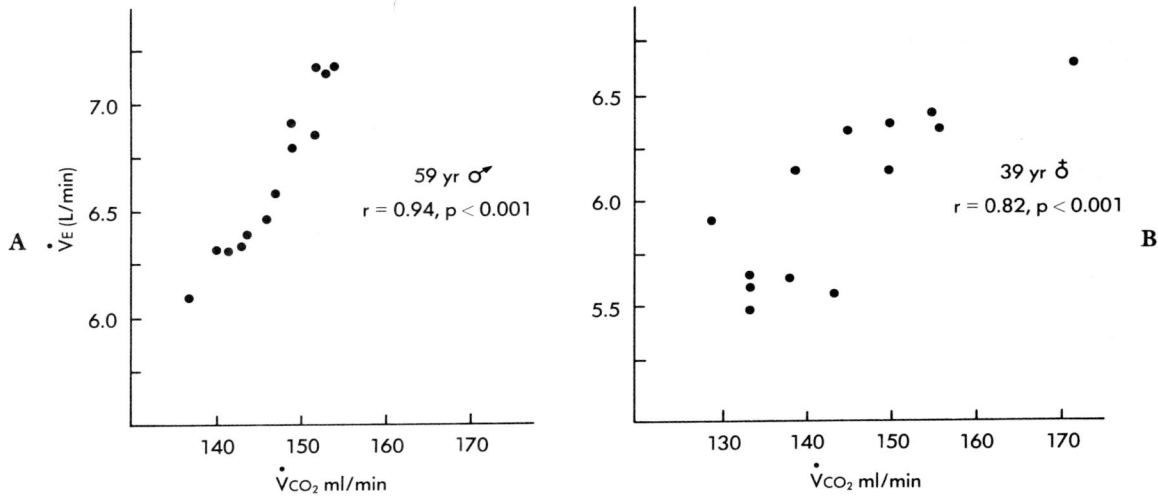

Fig. 14-4. Correlation between ventilation ($\dot{V}E$) and carbon dioxide production ($\dot{V}CO_2$) during sleep in a 59-year-old man, **A,** and a 39-year-old woman, **B.** Points are the mean values for a single recording period (3 to 25 minutes) in that individual. All stages of sleep are included for each subject. Ventilation correlates closely with $\dot{V}CO_2$ during sleep. (From White, D.P., Weil, J.V., and Zwillich, C.W.: J. Appl. Physiol. **59**:384, 1985.)

Clinical problem 2

$PaCO_2$ has been shown to rise slightly during sleep (Douglas, White, Pickett, et al., 1982). For this to occur, the fall in alveolar ventilation must be greater than the fall in carbon dioxide production (see Chapter 4). Based on information provided by White, Weil, Zwillich, et al. (discussed above), how would you explain the slight hypercapnia that occurs during normal sleep?

SLEEP APNEA

A variety of abnormal breathing patterns may occur during sleep, but the most important clinically is apnea—literally cessation of all air movement. It is normal to have brief apneic periods throughout sleep, usually lasting only a few seconds each. An apneic period that lasts 10 seconds or longer is considered abnormal. The sleep apnea syndrome is diagnosed by two criteria, using both clinical and polysomnography information:

1. More than 30 apneic episodes (of 10 seconds or more each) per night or at least five apneic episodes per 1 hour of sleep
2. Symptoms or signs of impairment from sleep apnea (e.g., daytime hypersomnolence or polycythemia)

Patients must satisfy both criteria to warrant the diagnosis of sleep apnea syndrome. At one time only the first criterion was thought sufficient to diagnose the syndrome, but studies have since demonstrated that clinically healthy people, particularly older subjects, can have more than five apneic episodes per 1 hour of sleep (Block, Boysen, Wynne, et al., 1979; Berry, Webb, Block, et al., 1984); these people are asymptomatic and warrant no treatment.

In some patients breathing does not stop but slows. Hypopnea is defined as a reduction in airflow sufficient to cause a drop in oxygen saturation of 4% to 5% from baseline. Hypopnea is probably caused by partial airways obstruction, the same mechanism responsible for loud snoring.

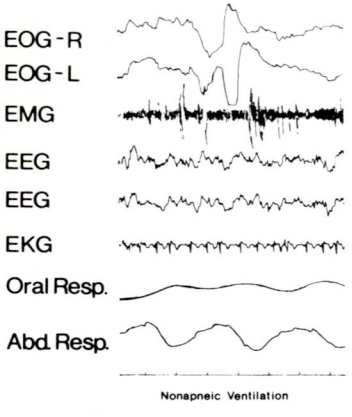
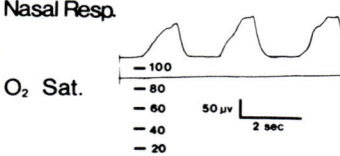

Fig. 14-5. Polysomnography pattern in central sleep apnea. *Left,* Normal sleep ventilation. *Below,* Absent respiratory effort (abdominal respiration) without oral or nasal airflow. Because of the circulation time from the lungs to the ear, there is a time lag in the decrease of the O_2 Sat related to the apnea. *EOG-R* and *EOG-L,* right and left electro-oculogram; *EMG,* chin electromyogram; *EEG,* electroencephalogram; *ECG,* electrocardiogram. (From Mitchell, R.S., and Petty, T.L.: Synopsis of clinical pulmonary diseases, ed. 3, St. Louis, 1982, The C.V. Mosby Co.)

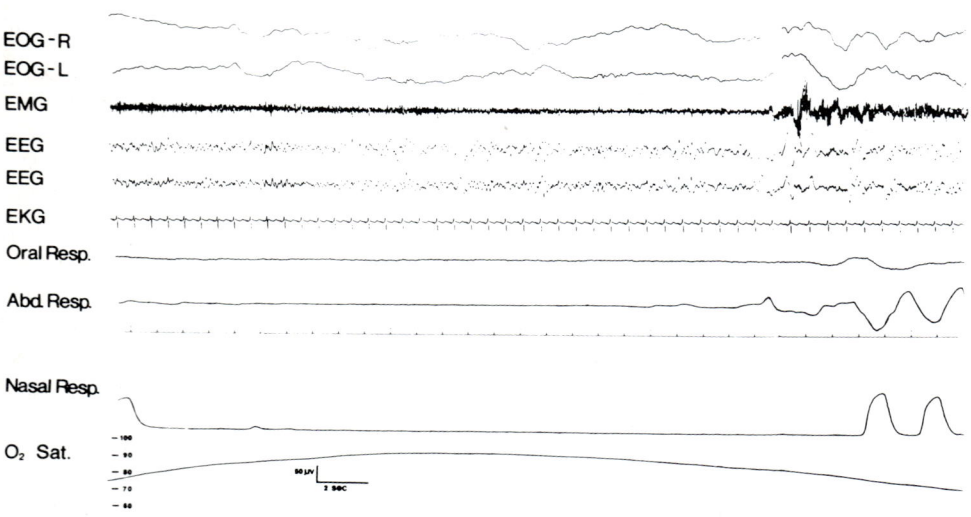

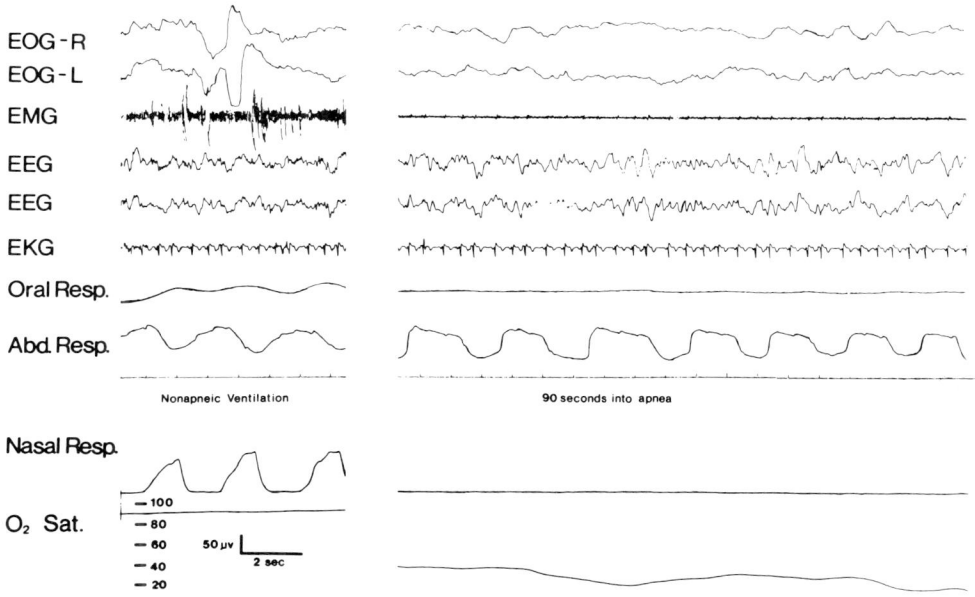

Fig. 14-6. Polysomnography pattern in obstructive sleep apnea. *Left,* Normal sleep ventilation. *Right,* Absent nasal and oral flow but continual abdominal respirations. Note that oxygen saturation (O_2 Sat) falls to extremely low levels. (From Mitchell, R.S., and Petty, T.L.: Synopsis of clinical pulmonary diseases, ed. 3, St. Louis, 1982, The C.V. Mosby Co.)

Sleep apnea is easy to diagnose during polysomnography since there is no airflow at the mouth or nose. Sleep apnea is now generally classified into two broad types—central and obstructive.

The defect in *central sleep apnea* is somewhere in the central nervous system, presumably affecting the brainstem respiratory neurons. During apnea of central origin no effort is made to breathe, so there is no movement of the chest cage (Fig. 14-5). These patients may have associated neurologic diseases such as poliomyelitis, spinal cord injuries, or central nervous system tumors. Patients suffering from central sleep apnea may be of any age and weight and of either sex. Central sleep apnea is much less common than obstructive sleep apnea.

Obstructive sleep apnea is characterized by occlusion of the upper airways. In obstructive sleep apnea there is breathing effort (the chest cage moves in and out), but there is no movement of air in and out of the lungs (Fig. 14-6). Obstructive sleep apnea is a relatively common finding in patients referred for polysomnography.

A small number of patients have both types of sleep apnea; so-called *mixed sleep apnea* is characterized by an initial episode of central apnea followed by an obstructive component. The treatment of mixed sleep apnea is the same as for purely obstructive sleep apnea.

In a multicenter review, sleep apnea was found in 857 of 1983 patients (43.2%) who underwent polysomnography for excessive daytime sleepiness, and most of these patients had obstructive sleep apnea (Coleman, Roffwarg, Kennedy, et al., 1982). Another polysomnographic study of 48 patients referred for evaluation to one hospital found obstructive apnea in 18 patients, central apnea in

Table 14-2. Sleep study of 48 patients referred for evaluation

Findings on polysomnography	Number of patients	Reason for referral
Obstructive apnea	17	Somnolence
	1	Carotid body resection
Central apnea	2	Somnolence
	1	Polycythemia
Hypopnea with low SaO_2	9	Polycythemia
	1	Mild chronic airflow obstruction
Normal study	5	Somnolence
	5	Polycythemia
	4	Mild chronic airflow obstruction
	3	Miscellaneous

From Kryger, M.H., Mezon, B.J., Acres, J.C., et al.: Diagnosis of sleep breathing disorders in a general hospital, Arch. Intern. Med. 142:956, 1982. Copyright 1982, American Medical Association.

3, hypopnea with low oxygen saturation in 10, and a normal polysomnogram in 17 (Table 14-2). The two main reasons for referral were excessive daytime sleepiness (somnolence) and unexplained polycythemia. All but two of the patients with demonstrated sleep apnea were men.

OBSTRUCTIVE SLEEP APNEA

Many studies have confirmed upper airways obstruction as the most common cause of sleep apnea (Coleman, Roffwarg, Kennedy, et al., 1982, Kryger, Mezon, Acres, et al., 1982). In the general population obstructive sleep apnea is a relatively common disorder, affecting from 1% to 4% of all adults (Sullivan and Issa, 1985). Factors that increase the risk for obstructive sleep apnea are listed in the following box. The existence of so many potentially predisposing factors emphasizes the importance of a thorough history and physical examination before any polysomnographic study.

FACTORS THAT INCREASE RISK FOR OBSTRUCTIVE SLEEP APNEA

1. Obesity (particularly in men)
2. Alcohol (only in men and when consumed before bedtime)
3. Irregular work shift (e.g., night shift)
4. Chronic obstructive pulmonary disease
5. Large tonsils
6. Craniofacial deformities (e.g., acromegaly)
7. Enlarged tongue
8. Hypothyroidism
9. Chest wall deformities
10. Tranquilizers (particularly when added to any other risk factor)

Snoring is a classical finding in obstructive sleep apnea. Snoring is the result of air flowing past a *partially occluded* upper airway and is often heard immediately before and after total airway occlusion. Of course not all snorers manifest obstructive sleep apnea, but very loud or persistent snoring may indicate the need for polysomnography, particularly if the snoring is punctuated by episodes of total silence (no air flow).

Although the presence of any risk factor cannot be used to predict obstructive sleep apnea, it may provide a clue to treatment if sleep apnea syndrome is diagnosed. For example, alcohol has been found to aggravate sleep apnea by decreasing the tone of the upper airway musculature (Remmers, DeGroot, Sauerland, et al., 1984), an effect seen in men but not women (Block, Boysen, Wynne, et al., 1985). Any man suffering from documented sleep apnea should therefore be advised to curtail his alcohol intake, particularly before bedtime.

Most patients with obstructive or mixed sleep apnea are obese. Obesity per se appears to weaken upper airway muscles and to aggravate the in-

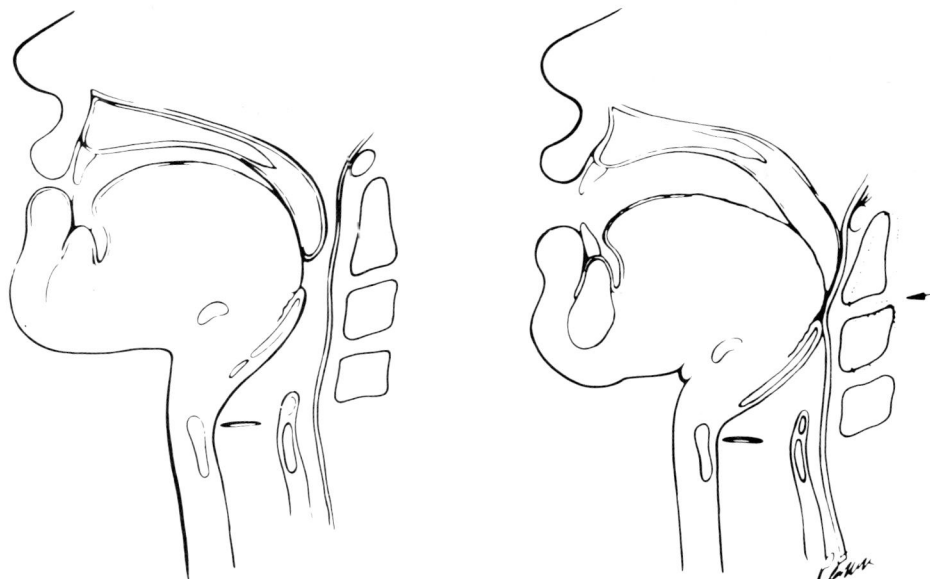

Fig. 14-7. Occlusion of the upper airway in obstructive sleep apnea. Lateral views of the head. *Left,* Upper airway is patent. *Right,* Note obstruction *(arrow)* when the posterior pharynx and base of the tongue approach one another. (From Suratt, P.M., Dee, P., Atkinson, R.L., et al.: Am. Rev. Respir. Dis. **127**:487, 1983.)

creased airways resistance that occurs during sleep. Despite the clear association with obesity, the severity of obstructive sleep apnea cannot be predicted by body weight nor in fact by daytime breathing tests or clinical history.

Chronic obstructive pulmonary disease (COPD) also predisposes a patient to obstructive sleep apnea, but the severity of the COPD (including carbon dioxide retention) does not predict either its presence or severity. Conversely, most patients with obstructive sleep apnea do not retain carbon dioxide; indeed, except for those with underlying lung disease, daytime blood gas values in patients with obstructive sleep apnea are usually normal or near normal. (Patients with hypercapnia, obesity, and daytime hypersomnolence are described in the section on Pickwickian syndrome later in this chapter.)

Obstructive sleep apnea is basically the result of occlusion of the oropharyngeal airway. This occlusion can be related to *physiologic* factors, *anatomic* factors, or both.

Physiologic factors include reduced upper airway muscle tone and negative airway pressure generated during inspiration. For various reasons, pharyngeal and genioglossus muscles can lose their tone to the point of slowing or preventing air flow (Fig. 14-7). Even in healthy, nonobese, nonsnoring men, upper airway resistance during sleep was found to increase two to three times compared to the awake period (Hudgel, 1984). In men with obstructive sleep apnea, there appears to be a correlation between collapsibility of the nasopharyngeal airway while awake and the degree of sleep-disordered breathing (Suratt, Mctier, Wilhoit, et al., 1985). The normal increase in airways resistance during sleep, in addition to the abnormal collapsibility of the pharyngeal muscles, explains (on a physiologic basis) many cases of sleep apnea.

Factors that affect the collapsibility of pharyngeal muscles include alcohol, sedatives, and obesity.

When pharyngeal muscle tone is reduced, negative upper airway pressure can cause the airway to narrow or occlude completely. Normally, inspiration causes negative airway pressure throughout the airways, resulting in inspiratory air flow (see Chapter 3). Despite negative airway pressure, normal pharyngeal muscle contraction is able to maintain patency of the upper airway. However, in obstructive sleep apnea, negative airway pressure *overcomes* the ability of weakened pharyngeal muscles to keep the airway patent. In addition, the negative upper airway pressure can be heightened by nasal obstruction, which increases (makes more negative) the oropharyngeal pressure during inspiration.

Several anatomic factors can narrow the upper airway and predispose the patient to obstructive sleep apnea. Tonsillar enlargement, an enlarged tongue, a small jaw, and certain craniofacial deformities can all narrow the airway; in children the most common predisposing factor to obstructive sleep apnea is hypertrophied tonsils and adenoids. Of course obstructive sleep apnea is more likely to occur if anatomic narrowing is accompanied by hypotonic airway muscles.

PICKWICKIAN SYNDROME

Pickwickian syndrome refers to a condition where there is marked obesity, hypercapnia, and daytime hypersomnolence. Pickwickian syndrome does not refer to a specific disease but is merely a descriptive term used for this group of patients. Most, if not all, patients with Pickwickian syndrome suffer from obstructive sleep apnea, which is probably the cause of their hypersomnia. Sleep is so disturbed by cycles of apnea and partial arousal that patients are sleep-deprived on "awakening" in the morning and so tend to fall asleep throughout the day.

A patient with these characteristics was described in a 1956 paper under the title "Extreme obesity associated with alveolar hypoventilation—a Pickwickian syndrome" (Burwell, Robin, Whaley, et al., 1956). The authors made reference to a much earlier description by Charles Dickens in his first novel *The Posthumous Papers of the Pickwick Club* (1837)—hence the name of the syndrome. At the beginning of Chapter 54 Dickens describes the appearance of a character named Joe:

The object that presented itself to the eyes of the astonished clerk, was a boy—a wonderfully fat boy—habited as a serving lad, standing upright on the mat, with his eyes closed as if in sleep. He had never seen such a fat boy, in or out of a travelling caravan; and this, coupled with the calmness and repose of his appearance, so very different from what was reasonably to have been expected in the inflicter of such knocks, smote him with wonder.

"What's the matter?" inquired the clerk.

The extraordinary boy replied not a word; but he nodded once, and seemed, to the clerk's imagination, to snore feebly.

"Where do you come from?" inquired the clerk.

The boy made no sign. He breathed heavily, but in all other respects was motionless.

The clerk repeated the question thrice, and receiving no answer, prepared to shut the door, when the boy suddenly opened his eyes, winked several times, sneezed once, and raised his hand as if to repeat the knocking. Finding the door open, he stared about him with astonishment, and at length fixed his eyes on Mr. Lowten's face.

"What the devil do you knock in that way for?" inquired the clerk, angrily.

"Which way?" said the boy, in a slow and sleepy voice.

"Why, like forty hackney-coachmen," replied the clerk.

"Because master said, I wasn't to leave off knocking till they opened the door, for fear I should go to sleep," said the boy.

Much has been learned about the Pickwickian syndrome since the 1956 paper. We now know that a decreased drive to breathe and not the obesity is the major underlying problem. (Compared to the number of obese people, Pickwickian syndrome is uncommon; most obese people do not suffer hypercapnia.) The decreased breathing drive seems to be aggravated by the obesity, and the clinical symptoms can often be reversed by losing weight.

Also, some patients have benefited from the drug medroxyprogesterone acetate, which stimulates their drive to breathe and has been shown to improve daytime blood values.

ONDINE'S CURSE

Ondine's curse refers to a condition where the lungs and chest bellows are normal but where patients stop breathing, usually during sleep; the sleep apnea is of central and not obstructive origin. The name is appropriately applied to those patients in whom "the only explanation for alveolar hypoventilation is failure of automatic control of ventilation by the central nervous system" (Mellins, Balfour, Turino, et al. 1970). Like the Pickwickian syndrome, Ondine's curse does not refer to a specific disease but is merely a descriptive term used for certain patients. In approximately half of these patients a central nervous system abnormality can be identified, but for the others there is no apparent lesion.

The name comes from a legend about an ondine or water nymph. This ondine married a mortal man with the understanding that he would never marry a mortal woman. However, when the ondine later returned to the sea, her husband did remarry. His punishment for this act has varied according to different accounts of the legend so that there are now several versions of the story (Comroe, 1975; Sugar, 1982). The play *Ondine*, by Jean Giraudoux (1939), seems to be the basis for naming the medical syndrome. In Giraudoux's play the husband's name is Hans:

Ondine: Live, Hans. You too will forget.
Hans: Live! It's easy to say. If at least I could work up a little interest in living—but I'm too tired to make the effort. Since you left me, Ondine, all the things my body once did by itself, it does now only by special order. The grass doesn't look green to my eyes unless I order them to see it green. And it's not very gay, you know, when the grass is black. It's an exhausting piece of management I've undertaken. I have to supervise five senses, two hundred bones, a thousand muscles. A single moment of inattention, and I forget to breathe.

He died, they will say, because it was a nuisance to breathe. . . .*

TREATMENT OF SLEEP APNEA

Many therapies have been tried for sleep apnea. The large number of treatments reflects the heterogeneity of causes (e.g., obesity, hypertrophied tonsils, brain stem disease) and also the fact that no single drug or procedure is both well tolerated and uniformly successful. Table 14-3 lists most of the available therapeutic measures.

For obese patients, losing weight is probably the most beneficial therapy, but this is more easily said than done. Weight reduction, which should be the cheapest and most effective treatment for many sleep apnea patients, is notoriously difficult to achieve *and* sustain. Nonetheless, this should be the first line of treatment in any obese patient suffering the effects of sleep apnea.

Before embarking on specific therapy all underlying problems that could predispose to hypoventilation should be corrected, e.g., stopping all sedatives, correcting metabolic alkalosis, optimizing underlying lung or heart disease, and treating hypothyroidism if present.

Clinical problem 3

An obese, 52-year-old woman is referred for possible sleep apnea syndrome. She gives a history of daytime hypersomnolence and admits to being tired and fatigued "all the time." Her medications include a diuretic for high blood pressure, a benzodiazepine tranquilizer, and a nonsteroidal drug for arthritis. During clinical examination there is no evidence for hypothyroidism. Pulmonary function studies show mild restrictive impairment. Blood gas values (at rest, and while breathing room air) are: Pa_{O_2} 68 mm Hg; Sa_{O_2}, 92%; Pa_{CO_2}, 51 mm Hg; pH, 7.49; and HCO_3^-, 37 mEq/L.

What would you recommend, either as the next test or as treatment?

---

*From Giraudoux, J.: Ondine, 1939. (Translated by M. Valency, New York, 1954, Random House, Inc.)

Table 14-3. Specific therapies used for sleep apnea syndrome

Type of therapy	Mechanism(s)	Primary efficacy in
Weight reduction	Removal of fat around upper airway; improved pharyngeal muscle tone	Both central and obstructive sleep apnea
Drug (each taken by mouth)		
Protriptyline—5-30 mg, 1 hour before bedtime	REM sleep inhibitor	Obstructive sleep apnea
Acetazolamide—250 mg, 2-4 times/day	Respiratory stimulant	Central sleep apnea
Medroxyprogesterone—20-40 mg, 3 times/day	Respiratory stimulant	Pickwickian syndrome
Theophylline (to achieve a serum level of 10-20 mg/L in adults)	Respiratory stimulant	Central sleep apnea
Methylphenidate—10 mg, 3 times/day	Respiratory stimulant	Both central and obstructive sleep apnea
Surgery		
Tracheostomy	Bypass obstruction	Obstructive sleep apnea
Uvulopalatopharyngoplasty	Keep airway open	Obstructive sleep apnea
Mandibular advancement	Remove obstruction	Obstructive sleep apnea
Tonsillectomy	Remove obstruction	Obstructive sleep apnea
Mechanical ventilation		
Intermittent positive pressure	Keep airway open; maintain ventilation	Both central and obstructive sleep apnea
Negative pressure	Maintain ventilation	Central sleep apnea
Miscellaneous		
Nasal continuous expiratory positive airway pressure	Keep airway open	Obstructive sleep apnea
Tongue retractor	Keep airway open	Obstructive sleep apnea
Nasopharyngeal airway	Keep airway open	Obstructive sleep apnea
Phrenic nerve pacing	Stimulate diaphragm	Central sleep apnea

Drugs. Several drugs are now available for treatment of sleep apnea. Discussion of specific drugs is beyond the scope of this chapter, but it must be emphasized that no single drug is considered "best" for sleep apnea. Indeed, much work needs to be done on how these drugs work. Their success in therapy depends on accurate diagnosis, which is not always easy. Probably the most widely used sleep apnea drug is medroxyprogesterone acetate, which is indicated mainly for the Pickwickian-type patient.

Surgery. Although tracheostomy has been shown effective in bypassing the obstruction and relieving symptoms, it is now rarely performed for

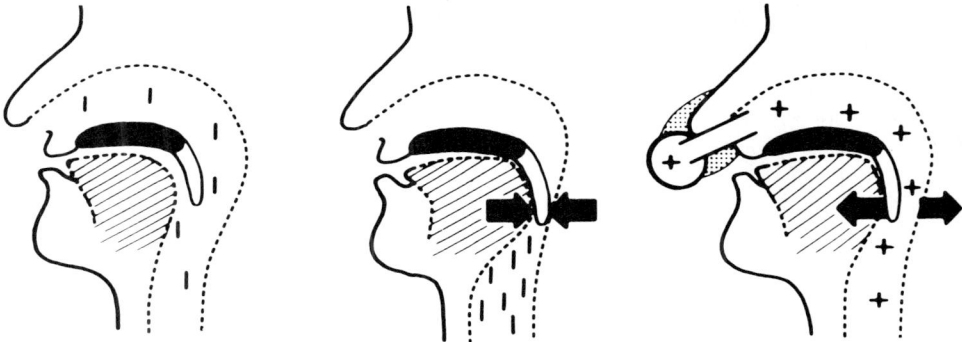

Fig. 14-8. Nasal constant positive airway pressure for obstructive sleep apnea. The positive airway pressure can prevent pharyngeal collapse *(arrows).* (From Sullivan, C.E., Berthon-Jones, M., Issa, F.G., et al.: Lancet **1**:862, 1981.)

obstructive sleep apnea, mainly because of its morbidity. Tracheostomy is reserved for patients with truly debilitating or life-threatening obstructive sleep apnea (Guilleminault, Simmons, Motta, et al., 1981).

Uvulopalatopharyngoplasty (UPPP) involves shortening the soft palate and removing the uvula, tonsils, and any redundant peritonsillar tissue. This operation is reserved for patients with obstructive sleep apnea who have obvious excess oropharyngeal tissue; in one series this meant patients 125% or more above ideal body weight (Conway, Fujita, Zorick, et al., 1985). In this study 33 of 66 patients undergoing UPPP were judged to have benefited clinically and by polysomnography. In 20 of the 33 patients improvements were maintained after 1 year (Conway, Fujita, Zorick, et al., 1985).

Mechanical ventilation. This procedure is not a realistic option for patients with obstructive sleep apnea. Negative pressure ventilation has been used for selected cases of severe central sleep apnea; it works on the same principle as the old iron lung (see Chapter 10).

Miscellaneous. One promising nondrug, nonsurgical treatment for obstructive sleep apnea is nasal continuous positive airway pressure (CPAP). (For a general discussion of CPAP see Chapter 9.) The first report on the use of CPAP for treating obstructive sleep apnea found good results using a small tube inserted through the nares, through which was applied low levels of positive air pressure (4.5 to 10 cm H_2O) (Sullivan, Berthon-Jones, Issa, et al., 1981; Fig. 14-8). By providing a constant positive airway pressure in the pharyngeal airway, CPAP completely prevented upper airways occlusion during sleep in five patients and allowed each patient "an entire night of uninterrupted sleep." Sullivan and Issa (1985) remain strong proponents of CPAP for obstructive sleep apnea.

Others have found that expiratory positive airway pressure (EPAP) applied through a face mask is also beneficial for obstructive sleep apnea (Mahadevia, Onal, and Lopata, 1983). The main physiologic difference between EPAP and CPAP is on inspiration; inspiratory pressure is negative with EPAP and positive with CPAP. The fact that EPAP reduced both the frequency and the duration of apneas suggests that *any* positive airway pressure applied during sleep can be beneficial for obstructive sleep apnea. Although procedures using positive pressure are beneficial in carefully performed studies, the techniques require considerable apparatus and patient compliance and for that reason are not yet widely employed.

A variety of other miscellaneous techniques have been used for obstructive sleep apnea, including tongue-retaining devices (Cartwright and Samelson, 1982) and an orthodontic appliance (Soll and George, 1985). However, the only treatment that can be universally recommended is weight loss (for obese patients); beyond that, treatment for sleep apnea must be tailored carefully to each patient and undertaken with the realization that several methods might have to be tried before the patient is helped.

Clinical problem 4

A 50-year-old man is examined because of hypercapnia and daytime hypersomnolence. He no longer drives a car because of falling asleep at the steering wheel. He smokes one pack of cigarettes per day.

Physical examination is unremarkable except for massive obesity and swelling of both legs. His chest x-ray shows small lung volumes and no infiltrates. The patient's blood gas values (obtained while breathing room air and in the upright position) are shown below:

Pa_{O_2}, 65 mm Hg
Sa_{O_2}, 86%
Hb_{CO}, 4.9%
Pa_{CO_2}, 51 mm Hg
pH, 7.38

Pulmonary function studies reveal moderate restrictive impairment with no evidence of airways obstruction. A formal sleep study reveals many episodes of obstructive sleep apnea, consistent with the sleep apnea syndrome. During the study the patient desaturates to 52%.

How would you approach his therapy? Be specific.

CHEYNE-STOKES BREATHING

There are many abnormal breathing patterns besides classic sleep apnea; some are associated with neurologic impairment, such as Biot's breathing (two or three rapid deep breaths in a row followed by long periods of apnea).

One of the most common and best studied abnormal breathing patterns is Cheyne-Stokes breathing,* also known as periodic breathing. Cheyne-Stokes breathing is characterized by alternately in-

---

*Named after John Cheyne, Scottish physician (1777-1836), and William Stokes, Irish physician (1804-1878).

creasing and decreasing tidal volumes that are punctuated by periods of apnea that may last from a few seconds to 2 minutes (Fig. 14-9). In his classic monograph *Diseases of the Heart and the Aorta,* Dr. Stokes wrote (1854):

A form of respiratory distress, peculiar to this affection (fatty degeneration of the heart), consisting of a period of apparently perfect apnoea, succeeded by feeble and short inspirations, which gradually increase in strength and depth until the respiratory act is carried to the highest pitch of which it seems capable, when the respirations, pursuing a descendent scale, regularly diminish until the commencement of another apnoeal period.

This description cannot be improved on today, except that it is now known that Cheyne-Stokes breathing also occurs in conditions other than heart failure. It is often seen in patients with a variety of central nervous system problems, uremia, and other metabolic disorders and in some older, healthy people.

Cheyne-Stokes breathing represents an example of a defect in ventilatory control, specifically in its feedback (Cherniack and Longobordo, 1973). Arterial partial pressure of carbon dioxide (Pa_{CO_2}) is normally fine-tuned by the brainstem controlling system. For example, if Pa_{CO_2} increases as a result of lung disease, the brainstem controlling system will send a signal to increase alveolar ventilation and thus return Pa_{CO_2} to normal. This response might alter the breathing pattern (e.g., to rapid and shallow), but as long as the controlling system is intact there will be an attempt to regulate Pa_{CO_2}.

In Cheyne-Stokes breathing caused by congestive heart failure, a prolonged circulation time causes a delay of blood reaching the brain so that changes at the alveolar level are not sensed by the brainstem in the normal time span; as a result, Pa_{CO_2} sensed by the chemoreceptors is out of phase with alveolar P_{CO_2} (Fig. 14-9). The patient is apneic when alveolar P_{CO_2} is elevated and hyperpneic when alveolar P_{CO_2} is reduced.

Circulation time delay does not explain Cheyne-Stokes breathing in patients without heart failure, most of whom have some type of central nervous

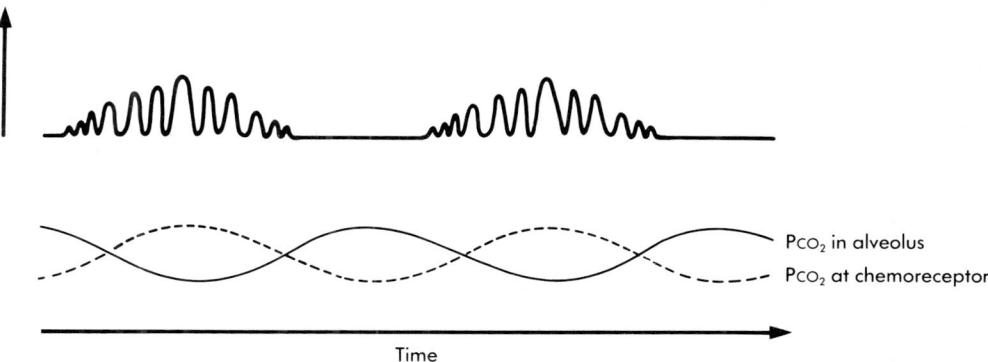

Fig. 14-9. Pattern of respirations in Cheyne-Stokes breathing. In patients with prolonged circulation time (heart failure), the pattern of breathing—alternating periods of apnea and hyperpnea—is out of phase with the P_{CO_2} in the alveolus.

system disorder. Furthermore, most patients with congestive heart failure do not manifest Cheyne-Stokes breathing, so there must be some defect in the brainstem controlling system for Cheyne-Stokes breathing to occur.

Although the presence of Cheyne-Stokes breathing implies a definite disorder of the central nervous system controlling system, the actual change in blood gas values may be relatively minor. When apneic periods are associated with cardiac arrhythmias or are judged to be life-threatening for other reasons, intravenous aminophylline is recommended. The mechanism by which aminophylline corrects or ameliorates Cheyne-Stokes breathing is unknown.

SUMMARY

We spend approximately one third of our lives asleep, but this activity has only recently come under intensive study. Polysomography is the measurement of several physiologic variables during sleep, including electroencephalogram, air flow in and out of the lungs, and chest wall movement. Normal sleep can be divided into alternating phases of nonrapid eye movement (NREM) and rapid eye movement (REM). In NREM sleep, upper air muscle tone is preserved, and breathing tends to be regular. In REM sleep, upper airway muscle tone is depressed, and breathing tends to be irregular. During all stages of sleep, metabolism slows as manifested by declines in both oxygen consumption and carbon dioxide production; at the same time minute ventilation falls, and Pa_{CO_2} rises slightly.

Sleep apnea is defined as an absence of breathing for 10 seconds or more. Diagnosis of sleep apnea syndrome requires at least 30 apneic episodes per night plus symptoms or signs of impairment from the sleep apnea, such as secondary polycythemia or daytime hypersomnolence. Sleep apneas can be obstructive or central in origin. Obstructive sleep apnea is far more common than central sleep apnea. Within each catagory are several potential causes. Pickwickian syndrome and Ondine's curse are terms used to describe specific groups of patients who suffer from obstructive and central sleep apnea, respectively.

Obesity seems to be the most prevalent predisposing factor to obstructive sleep apnea, and any treatment program must include weight reduction if the patient is obese. Several drugs and surgical procedures have been used to treat sleep apnea syndrome, but no drug or procedure is uniformly successful or applicable to all patients.

REVIEW QUESTIONS

State whether each of the following is true or false.

1. REM sleep accounts for less than half of all sleep time.
2. Aminophylline is the treatment of choice for obstructive sleep apnea.
3. Pharyngeal muscles normally occlude the airways during inspiration.
4. Nasal blockage makes upper airway pressure more negative.
5. Cheyne-Stokes breathing is characterized by a pattern of even breathing interrupted by periods of apnea lasting 5 to 10 seconds.
6. Polysomography should include continuous measurement of Pao_2.
7. Obstructive sleep apnea is far more common than central sleep apnea.
8. Medroxyprogesterone acetate is the drug of choice for Pickwickian syndrome patients.
9. Pickwickian syndrome patients usually hyperventilate while awake.
10. Ondine's curse is characterized by seizures during stage IV of NREM sleep.

References

Berry, D.T.R., Webb, W.B., and Block, A.J.: Sleep apnea syndrome—a critical review of the apnea index as a diagnostic criterion, Chest **86**:529, 1984.

Block, A.J., Boysen, P.G., Wynne, J.W., et al.: Sleep apnea, hypopnea and oxygen desaturation in normal subjects: a strong male predominance, N. Engl. J. Med. **300**:513, 1979.

Burwell, C.S., Robin, E.D., Whaley, R.D., et al.: Extreme obesity associated with alveolar hypoventilation—a Pickwickian Syndrome, Am. J. Med. **21**:811, 1956.

Cartwright, R.D., and Samelson, C.F.: The effects of nonsurgical treatment of obstructive sleep apnea: the tongue-retaining device, JAMA **248**:705, 1982.

Cherniack, N.S., and Longobordo, G.S.: Cheyne-Stokes breathing: an instability in physiological control, N. Engl. J. Med. **288**:952, 1973.

Coleman, R.M., Roffwarg, H.P., Kennedy, S.J., et al.: Sleep-wake disorders based on a polysomnographic diagnosis: a national cooperative study, JAMA **247**:997, 1982.

Comroe, J.H., Jr.: Frankenstein, Pickwick, and Ondine, Am. Rev. Dis. **111**:689, 1975.

Conway, W., Fujita, S., Zorick, F., et al.: Uvulopalatopharyngoplasty: one-year follow-up, Chest **88**:385, 1985.

Dickens, C.: The posthumous papers of the Pickwick Club, London, 1837, Chapman & Hall Ltd.

Douglas, N.J., White, D.P., Pickett, C.K., et al.: Respiration during sleep in normal man, Thorax **37**:840, 1982.

Gillin, J.C.: Sleep and dreams. In Michael, R., editor: Psychiatry, vol. 3, Philadelphia, 1985, J.B. Lippincott Co.

Giraudoux, J.: Ondine, 1939. Translated by M. Valency, New York, 1954, Random House, Inc.

Guilleminault, C., Simmons, F.B., J., et al.: Obstructive sleep apnea syndrome and tracheostomy, Arch. Intern. Med. **141**:985, 1981.

Hudgel, D.W.: Sleep Apnea. In Mitchell, R.S., and Petty, T.L.: Synopsis of clinical pulmonary disease, St. Louis, 1982, The C.V. Mosby Co.

Hudgel, D.W., Martin, R.J., Johnson, B., et al.: Mechanics of the respiratory system during sleep in normal man, J. Appl. Physiol. **56**:133, 1984.

Kryger, M.H., Mezon, B.J., Acres, J.C., et al.: Diagnosis of sleep breathing disorders in a general hospital, Arch. Intern. Med. **142**:956, 1982.

Mahadevia, A.K., Onal, E., and Lopata, M.: Effects of expiratory positive airway pressure on sleep-induced respiratory abnormalities in patients with hypersomnia-sleep apnea syndrome, Am. Rev. Respir. Dis. **128**:708, 1983.

Mellins, R.B., Balfour, H.H., Turino, G.M., et al.: Failure of automatic control of ventilation (Ondine's curse), Medicine **49**:487, 1970.

Remmers, J.E., DeGroot, W.J., Sauerland, E.K., et al.: Pathogenesis of upper airway occlusion during sleep, J. Appl. Physiol. **44**:931, 1978.

Soll, B.A., and George, P.T.: Treatment of obstructive sleep apnea with a nocturnal airway-patency appliance (letter), N. Engl. J. Med. **313**:386, 1985.

Stokes, W.: Diseases of the heart and the aorta, Dublin, 1854, Hodges & Smith.

Sugar, O.: In search of Ondine's curse, JAMA **240**:236, 1978.

Sullivan, C.E., Berthon-Jones, M., Issa, F.G., et al.: Reversal of obstructive sleep apnea by continuous positive airway pressure applied through the nares, Lancet **1**:862, 1981.

Sullivan, C.E., and Issa, F.G.: Obstructive sleep apnea. In Kryger, M.H., editor: Symposium on sleep disorders, Clin. Chest Med. **6**:633, 1985.

Suratt, P.M., Dee, P., Atkinson, R.L., et al.: Fluoroscopic and computed tomographic features of the pharyngeal airway in obstructive sleep apnea, Am. Rev. Respir. Dis. **127**:487, 1983.

Suratt, P.M., Mctier, R.F., and Wilhoit, S.: Collapsibility of the nasopharyngeal airway in obstructive sleep apnea, Am. Rev. Respir. Dis. **132**:967, 1985.

White, D.P., Weil, J.V., and Zwillich, C.W.: Metabolic rate and breathing during sleep, J. Appl. Physiol. **59**:384, 1985.

See also General References in Appendix G

chapter 15
Newborn and Infant

OUTLINE

Changes at birth
Apgar score
The pediatric history
Vital signs
Physical examination
Chest x-ray examination
Pulmonary function tests
Blood gases
Ventilation-perfusion imbalance
Oxygen therapy
Hemodynamic assessment
Sudden infant death syndrome
Infant respiratory distress syndrome

The preceding chapters have been written in reference to adult patients. All the case examples, as well as all values for normal physiology, have been about adults. The respiratory system of the newborn and infant differs in several ways from that of the adult, hence this chapter. No attempt is made to cover this field completely, only to highlight those aspects unique to the newborn and infant. The reader is also referred to several excellent texts on the subject (listed at the end of the chapter).

An infant's age can be defined as either chronologic or gestational. *Chronologic* age is computed from the date of birth, e.g., 18 months old. *Gestational* age is computed from the date of conception, e.g., 28 weeks old. A *term* infant at birth is between 38 and 42 weeks gestational age. Infants born at 37 or fewer weeks gestational age are *preterm,* and those infants born at 43 or more weeks, *postterm.*

CHANGES AT BIRTH

The fetus undergoes profound changes within hours of birth. A few of the changes in cardiopulmonary physiology are briefly discussed here.

In the fetus the right and left sides of the heart pump blood in parallel to the aorta (Fig. 15-1). The fetal heart receives oxygenated blood from the placenta by way of the vena cava. Most of this placental blood is shunted through a patent foramen ovale into the left atrium, and from there it goes to the left ventricle and aorta. Venous return from the head is not shunted through the foramen ovale but goes directly from the right atrium to the right ventricle. However, because the fetus also has a ductus arteriosus connecting the pulmonary artery to the aorta, most of the right-sided cardiac output is shunted to the aorta, either directly or indirectly. Shortly after birth the ductus arteriosus and foramen ovale close, and the flow pattern changes to that of the adult (see Fig. 2-12).

The fetal organ of gas exchange is the placenta. At the moment of birth and for the rest of life this function is transferred to the lungs. At birth the lungs inflate, and pulmonary vascular resistance falls. As the arterial partial pressure of oxygen (PaO_2) increases with air breathing, the foramen ovale and ductus arteriosus begin to close, and all venous blood flows through the lungs. (If the infant

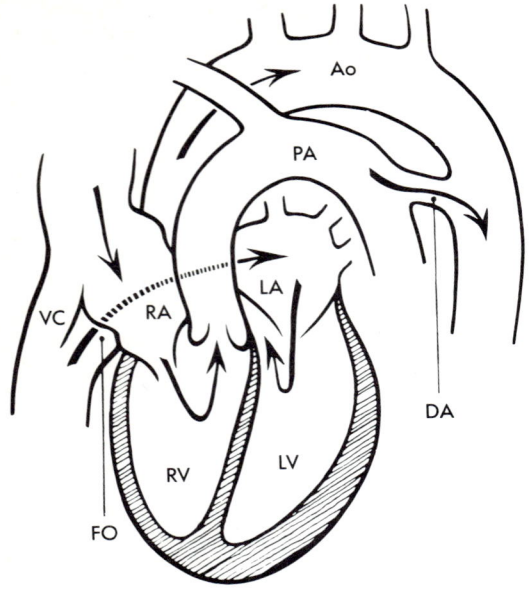

Fig. 15-1. Fetal circulation. Blood from the placenta enters the right atrium and is preferentially shunted through the patent foramen ovale *(FO)* into the left atrium, where it enters the left ventricle and aorta. Blood received from the head enters the right atrium, right ventricle, and pulmonary artery, where it is shunted to the aorta through the ductus arteriosus *(DA)*. These shunts close shortly after birth. (From Slonim, N.B., and Hamilton, L.H.: Respiratory Physiology, ed. 4, St. Louis, 1981, The C.V. Mosby Co.)

becomes hypoxic after birth, blood flow may be re-established through the ductus arteriosus.)

Before birth the lungs are filled with fluid. At birth the lungs fill with air and remain open with the help of surfactant. Surfactant is a phospholipid that lowers surface tension and keeps alveoli from collapsing at low lung volumes. Premature infants lack normal amounts of surfactant and for this reason are at risk for developing respiratory distress syndrome (discussed later in this chapter).

The healthy newborn infant has a transient respiratory acidosis. Initiation of ventilation with the first breath results in a rapid fall in arterial partial pressure of carbon dioxide ($Paco_2$) (Fox, 1983), and within an hour Pao_2 rises to near normal levels (Fig. 15-2, *A*). When there is asphyxia with delayed onset of breathing, normalization of blood gases is delayed (Fig. 15-2, *B*).

Fetal hemoglobin (Hgb F) has a higher affinity for oxygen than adult hemoglobin (Hgb A); as a consequence the Hgb F oxygen dissociation curve is shifted to the left (Fig. 15-3). As with any dissociation curve shifted to the left, less oxygen will be released to the tissues for a given Po_2 (more will stay bound to the hemoglobin). Also, the higher the proportion of Hgb F, the lower the Po_2 at which cyanosis can be detected (Fig. 15-3).

Table 15-1. Oxygen transport in term infants

No. of infants	Age	Total hemoglobin (g/dl blood)	O_2 capacity (ml/dl blood)	P_{50} at pH 7.40 (mm Hg)	2,3-DPG mmol/ml RBC	Fetal hemoglobin (% of total)
19	1 day	17.8 ± 2.0	24.7 ± 2.8	19.4 ± 1.8	5433 ± 1041	77.0 ± 7.3
18	5 days	16.2 ± 1.2	22.6 ± 2.2	20.6 ± 1.7	6850 ± 996	76.8 ± 5.8
14	3 weeks	12.0 ± 1.3	16.7 ± 1.9	22.7 ± 1.0	5378 ± 732	70.0 ± 7.33
10	6-9 weeks	10.5 ± 1.2	14.7 ± 1.6	24.4 ± 1.4	5560 ± 747	52.1 ± 11.0
14	3-4 months	10.2 ± 0.8	14.3 ± 1.2	26.5 ± 2.0	5819 ± 1240	23.2 ± 16.0
8	6 months	11.3 ± 0.9	14.7 ± 0.6	27.8 ± 1.0	5086 ± 1570	4.7 ± 2.2
8	8-11 months	11.4 ± 0.6	15.9 ± 0.8	30.3 ± 0.7	7381 ± 485	1.6 ± 1.0

From Oski, F.A.: Hematologic problems. In Avery, G.B., editor: Neonatology: Pathophysiology and management of the newborn, ed. 2, Philadelphia, 1981, J.B. Lippincott Co.

Newborn and infant

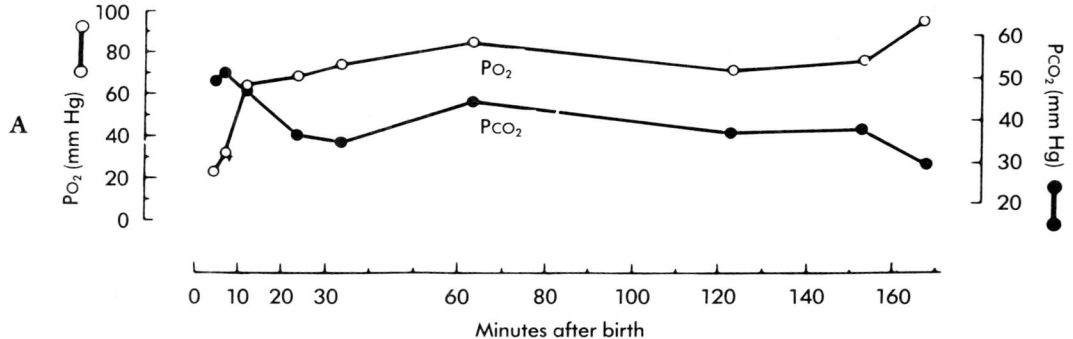

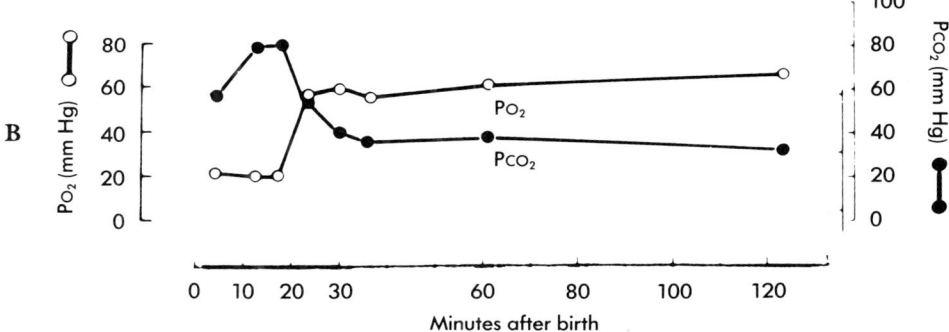

Fig. 15-2. Changes in Pao₂ and Paco₂ after birth in a full term infant, **A**, and in an infant suffering from asphyxia, **B**. From Fanaroff, A.A., and Martin, R.J.: Behrman's neonatal-perinatal medicine: diseases of the fetus and infant, ed. 3, St. Louis, 1983, The C.V. Mosby Co.)

Clinical problem 1

Explain how persistence of fetal hemoglobin after birth can result in tissue hypoxia even though Pao_2 and Sao_2 are normal.

The reason that Hb F has a higher oxygen affinity is not because of its different molecular structure *per se,* but because it binds less 2,3-diphosphoglycerate (DPG) than Hgb A. The organic phosphate 2,3-DPG lowers hemoglobin's oxygen affinity (see Chapter 6). Since Hgb F does not bind 2,3-DPG to the extent of Hgb A, the P_{50} of Hgb F is lower (its dissociation curve is shifted to the left of adult hemoglobin).

Total hemoglobin content in the newborn is normally approximately 18 gm%, and the oxygen capacity is approximately 25 ml O_2/100 ml—values that are higher than the mother's. The percent of Hgb F is highest at birth and falls to insignificant amounts by the end of the first year (Table 15-1).

Note that the P_{50} also rises as the content of Hb F falls. In some cases of severe anemia Hb F will persist beyond the first year, and in some adult anemias Hb F will reappear in significant quantities.

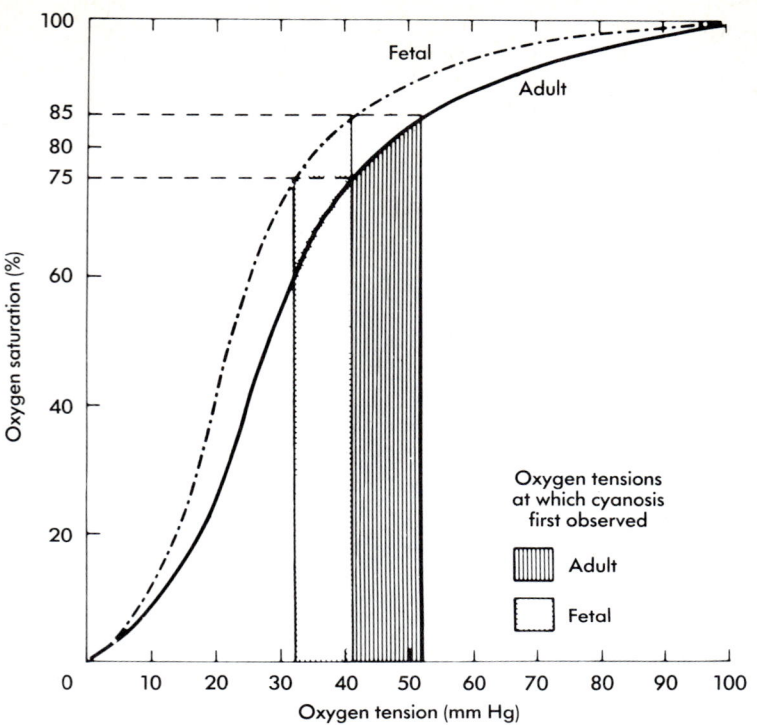

Fig. 15-3. Fetal hemoglobin dissociation curve compared to normal adult curve. The P_{50} of fetal hemoglobin is lower than that of adult hemoglobin. With a normal hemoglobin content, central cyanosis is detectable at an oxygen saturation of approximately 85%. With adult hemoglobin (Hgb A) this level of oxygen saturation represents a PaO_2 of just over 50 mm Hg (at normal pH); with fetal hemoglobin (Hgb F) the corresponding PaO_2 is just over 40 mm Hg. Thus the higher the percentage of Hgb F, the lower the PaO_2 at which central cyanosis is detectable. (From Fanaroff, A.A., and Martin, R.J.: Behrman's neonatal-perinatal medicine: diseases of the fetus and infant, ed. 3, St. Louis, 1983, The C.V. Mosby Co.)

Clinical problem 2

What is the arterial oxygen content in an infant with the following laboratory values? Hemoglobin content, 18 gm% (50% fetal and 50% adult hemoglobin); PaO_2, 95 mm Hg; SaO_2, 98%.

APGAR SCORE

The most widely accepted objective assessment of an infant's status immediately after birth is the Apgar score, which is the sum of points assigned for specific physical criteria at the time of delivery (Table 15-2). This system was developed by Dr. Virginia Apgar, a pediatrician (Apgar, 1953). The Apgar score focuses on immediate assessment of skin color, respiratory effort, cardiac function, body tone, and responsiveness to painful stimuli at the moment of birth.

An Apgar score of 8 to 10 indicates no asphyxia. The infant is considered to have mild asphyxia at a score of 5 to 7, moderate asphyxia at a score of

Table 15-2. Apgar scoring

Sign	Score 0	Score 1	Score 2
Color	Body pale or blue; extremities blue	Body pink; extremities blue	Completely pink
Heart rate	Absent	Less than 100/min	Above 100/min
Reflex irritability	No response	Some motion	Cry
Muscle tone	Limp	Some flexion	Good flexion
Respiratory effort	Absent	Weak cry; irregular respirations	Strong cry

3 to 4, and severe asphyxia at a score of 0 to 2. Each lower level demands increased monitoring and resuscitative efforts.

Most infants are assigned Apgar scores at 1 and 5 minutes after birth. If the infant is in any distress, Apgar scores are determined more often and over a longer time span. For instance, a sick infant may have Apgar scores recorded 1, 2, 5, 10, 15, and 20 minutes after delivery.

Clinical problem 3

What is the Apgar score of an infant who is acrocyanotic at birth and who has crying on painful stimulus, irregular respirations, some flexion in the arms, and a heart rate of 90 beats per minute?

THE PEDIATRIC HISTORY*

The infant's history is usually obtained from several sources, including the parents, the mother's labor and delivery record, and the infant's own medical record. The particularly important aspects follow.

Mother's history. Was the infant's mother healthy before pregnancy? Is she taking any medications? Does she have any chronic diseases? Infants born to diabetic mothers may be physically premature for their gestational age and are therefore susceptible to diseases of prematurity, such as infant respiratory distress syndrome.

Family history. Is there a family history of prematurity or of infant respiratory problems? The severity of diseases like respiratory distress syndrome tend to be similar among siblings. Cystic fibrosis, an inherited disease that may cause early respiratory problems, should always be suspected if another sibling has it.

Pregnancy history. Did the mother have any illness during pregnancy? Viral infections that cause only mild respiratory symptoms in the mother may profoundly affect the infant. Did the mother have any vaginal bleeding? The source of vaginal bleeding is usually the mother but occasionally is the baby. Infants born of mothers with a bleeding history may suffer from hypovolemia.

Was there evidence of amniotic or urinary tract infection? An infant delivered in the presence of maternal infection is at a greater than normal risk for infection. Did the mother have any traumatic injury that might have affected transfer of oxygen and other nutrients to the baby? Did the mother's uterus grow appropriately during pregnancy? If the uterus does not grow normally, the infant could develop pulmonary hypoplasia or severe malformations. Any of these problems of pregnancy can lead to newborn respiratory distress.

Labor history. Newborn infection should be suspected if there is maternal fever, high-maternal white blood cell count, a tender uterus, a his-

---

*This and the next two sections (Vital Signs and Physical Examination) are based on information presented by Deming, 1985 (see references).

tory of amniotic membrane rupture for more than 24 hours, foul-smelling amniotic fluid, or fetal tachycardia. Neonatal asphyxia should be suspected if there is a history of maternal hypotension, abnormal fetal heart rate, decreased fetal movement, presence of meconium in the amniotic fluid, a long labor, or abnormal vaginal bleeding.

Delivery history. The incidence of respiratory disease varies with gestational age. By history, the mother's last menstrual period (LMP) can be dated and the date of delivery can be estimated (this appears as the estimated date of confinement [EDC] on the mother's chart).

Other important questions concern the method of delivery, e.g., vaginal vs. cesarean, spontaneous vs. forceps, and low-forceps vs. mid- or high-forceps. Spontaneous or low-forceps vaginal delivery suggests a normal delivery and, by inference, a healthy baby. High-forceps, or an unplanned cesarean delivery, suggests some difficulty during labor or delivery; infants delivered in this manner are at increased risk for respiratory disease. It is also helpful to know the mode of anesthesia, e.g., intravenous or intramuscular narcotic, local, epidural, spinal, or general. Narcotics and general anesthetics may enter the infant's blood and produce respiratory depression. Spinal anesthetics may lower the mother's blood pressure and compromise the infant's oxygen supply.

Postnatal history. For the majority of infants the postnatal history is "normal." However, all infants require some form of respiratory aid at birth, if nothing more than clearing the airway. Did the infant have only this simple intervention, or was supplemental oxygen, bagging, or intubation necessary? If so, how quickly did the infant respond? As a general part of the history it should be noted how long the infant was in the hospital, the condition at discharge, and any medical problems since delivery.

VITAL SIGNS

Vital signs, which include temperature, heart and respiratory rate, and blood pressure, are an integral part of any clinical examination. Normal pediatric values are given in Table 15-3. As might be expected, the small size of the pediatric patient warrants a special approach to vital signs, either in their measurement or interpretation.

Body temperature in the newborn is normally in the same range as in the adult. An infant's temperature is usually measured in the axilla or rectum. Compared to the oral temperature, the axillary temperature is approximately 1° F lower and the rectal temperature is approximately 1° F higher (Table 15-3).

The newborn maintains body temperature by balancing heat production with heat loss. However, the newborn has a much greater heat loss than the older child or adult, because heat loss is largely determined by the ratio of body surface area to body weight (Table 15-4).

The average term infant has a body surface area of 0.25 m² and a body weight of 3.5 kg, resulting in a surface area/weight ratio more than three times that of an adult man (Table 15-4). For preterm infants the ratio is even more striking—over 7 times that of an adult man. Because of the relatively large surface area/mass ratio, preterm infants lose heat easily and are heavily dependent on the environment to help contain body heat.

Hyperthermia in the newborn is usually caused by environmental factors, such as too many clothes, a heater that is too close to the infant, or an overheated isolette. Less commonly, hyperthermia in infants is the result of infection. *Hypothermia* is a more frequent sign of infection in newborns than in the older child or adult. Hypothermia probably occurs because the infant is unable to maintain normal heat production during the acute infection. In contrast to adults, infants do not shiver when hypothermia is present.

The environmental temperature is extremely important for infants. Most infants that are sick are placed in a neutral thermal environment (NTE),

Table 15-3. Normal range of vital signs in infants and children

Vital sign	Newborn (term)	Older infant and child
Temperature	98-99 (oral)	Same
	97-98 (axillary)	Same
	99-100 (rectal)	Same
Heart rate (beats/min)	120-200	100-180 (up to 3 yr)
		70-150 (above 3 yr)
Respiratory rate (breaths/min)	35-55	20-30 (up to 6 yr)
Blood pressure (mm Hg)		
Systolic	60-90	75-130 (up to 3 yr)
		90-140 (above 3 yr)
Diastolic	30-60	45-90 (up to 3 yr)
		50-80 (above 3 yr)

Table 15-4. Ratio of surface area/body weight

	Surface area (m^2)	Weight (kg)	Surface area/weight (m^2/kg)
Adult male	1.7	80	0.02
Term infant	0.25	3.5	0.07
Infant with gestational age of 28 weeks	0.15	1.0	0.15

which is the environmental temperature at which oxygen consumption is lowest. Fig. 15-4 shows the relation between oxygen consumption, body temperature, and environmental temperature. If the environmental temperature leaves the neutral thermal range, the infant can usually maintain a stable body temperature but at the cost of a significant increase in oxygen consumption. Neutral thermal environments are defined for an infant based on body weight plus gestational and chronologic age.

Heart rate is normally a function of gestational age (the lower the gestational age the higher the heart rate) and chronologic age (Table 15-3). Ranges for tachycardia and bradycardia must take into account the gestational age (for newborns) or the chronologic age (for infants). The mean heart rate of a healthy term infant is approximately 175 beats per minute, but it normally falls considerably after birth. Tachycardia in the newborn can be the result of crying, pain, a decrease in circulating blood volume, drugs, hyperthermia, and heart disease.* Bradycardia can be caused by hypoxia, Valsalva's maneuver that frequently occurs during crying, heart disease, and certain drugs.

Because of the small size of the radial arteries, the pulse of an infant or newborn is usually felt at the brachial or femoral artery, using the fingerpads. The brachial pulse can be felt over the brachial artery as it passes on the medial superior surface of the arm, just proximal to the medial epicondyle of the elbow with the infant in the supine position. The femoral artery is found in the groin about halfway across the thigh and just below the inguinal ligament.

Respiratory rate in the normal newborn depends on the gestational age and whether it is measured

---

*Tachycardia is the only way of increasing cardiac output in the newborn: stroke volume at rest is normally greater than 90% of maximal stroke volume.

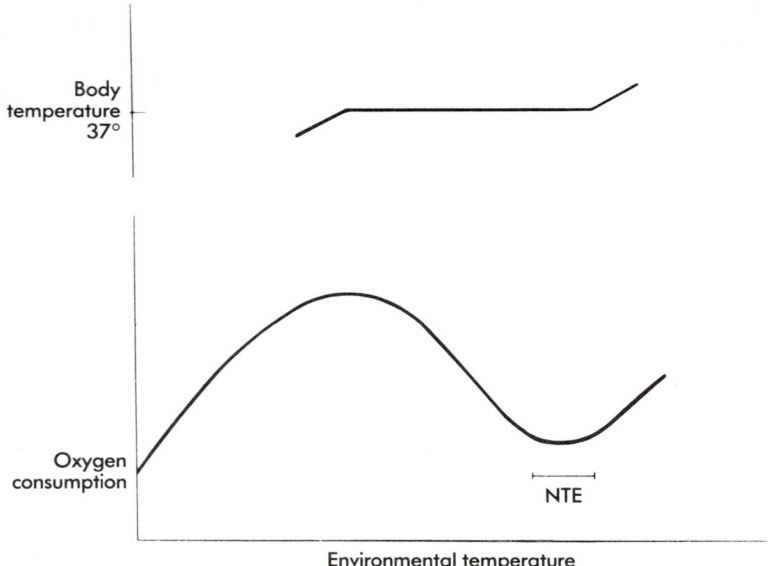

Fig. 15-4. Relation between oxygen consumption, body temperature, and environmental temperature. Outside of the neutral thermal environment (NTE), oxygen consumption will rise as the infant tries to maintain a stable body temperature. (From Wilkins, R.L., Sheldon, R.L., and Krider, S.J., editors: Clinical assessment in respiratory care, St. Louis, 1985, The C.V. Mosby Co.)

during sleep or while the infant is awake; the awake rate tends to be higher than the rate during sleep. Normal term infants breathe between 35 and 55 times per minute. The lower the gestational age, the higher is the observed respiratory rate.

Tachypnea can be caused by hypoxemia, metabolic and respiratory acidosis, anxiety, pain, hyperthermia, and crying. Bradypnea (a slow respiratory rate) is usually caused by certain medications such as narcotics, but in the newborn bradypnea may also herald respiratory decompensation. Initially, infants in respiratory distress usually have tachypnea with marginally acceptable blood gas values. As the disease progresses and as the infant tires from the increasing work of breathing, bradypnea can appear just before respiratory collapse.

Apnea is the cessation of respiratory effort. Arbitrarily, long apnea is the cessation of breathing for more than 20 seconds, and short apnea is the cessation of breathing for 10 to 20 seconds. Cessation of breathing for 5 to 10 seconds is a *respiratory pause*. Newborns can also manifest a phenomenon known as periodic respiration—respiratory pauses or short apneas interspersed with normal breathing. This respiratory pattern may last from several minutes to several hours.

Long apnea is always abnormal. Short apnea and respiratory pauses may be normal, depending on the gestational age of the infant. Short apnea and respiratory pauses are common in preterm infants and may be present in normal term infants up to 3 months of age. Apneic periods may precede episodes of sudden infant death. The sudden infant death syndrome is discussed later in this chapter.

Respiratory rate can be counted by visually observing chest wall motion or by counting respirations while listening with a stethoscope. Visual observation gives a respiratory rate closer to the infant's true resting rate. However, because the normal infant breathes fast with a relatively small tidal volume, it may be difficult to appreciate each breath visually. In such situations the respiratory rate should be counted by auscultation with the stethoscope, although the infant may respond to the touch of the stethoscope with a slight increase in respiratory rate.

The infant's respirations should also be checked for regularity and depth. Many immature infants will have a normal respiratory rate but an irregular breathing pattern, e.g., periodic respirations or apneas interspersed between periods of normal breathing. Also, infants with lung disease may have a normal respiratory rate but their tidal volumes may be so small that they have decreased alveolar ventilation.

Normal values for *blood pressure* depend on the size of the infant; the larger the infant, the higher the blood pressure. A term infant's systolic blood pressure should be no higher than 90 mm Hg, with a diastolic pressure no higher than 60 mm Hg. As in adults, blood pressure in newborns can be measured with a blood pressure cuff or by way of an indwelling arterial cannula.

PHYSICAL EXAMINATION

The physical examination of a newborn and an older infant is based on three of the four classic methods—inspection, palpation, and auscultation. (The fourth classical method, percussion, is rarely used in newborns and infants.)

Probably the single most important aspect of the infant physical examination is *inspection*. The infant should be nude and in a supine position initially. The examiner should first look at the infant's overall appearance to assess the level of illness, check for malformations, and note if the body position is appropriate for the gestational age (Fig. 15-5). The term infant at rest flexes the arms and legs into a "fetal" position. Infants at earlier gestational ages have less muscle tone, and their extremities are not flexed during rest.

The infant's lungs are situated in the chest much like those of the adult. The infant's chest has a greater anteroposterior diameter than an adult's chest. With growth the anteroposterior diameter decreases and becomes more like the adult configuration (Fig. 15-6). The imaginary lines and the thoracic cage landmarks are the same in infants and adults.

The infant's skin should be examined for cyanosis, although this assessment can be difficult, especially in the newborn. Central cyanosis depends not only on the oxygen saturation in arterial blood (SaO_2) and on the hemoglobin content (as in adults), but also on the ratio of fetal to adult hemoglobin (see Table 15-1 for normal ranges).

Infants with hypothermia or with a hematocrit greater than 65% have bluish extremities (acrocyanosis) but are not truly cyanotic. Preterm infants with thin skin can look quite pink when they are really hypoxemic. Color in the tongue, nail beds, and mucous membranes of the mouth give the most reliable visual clues of the overall level of oxygenation.

Clinical problem 4

How much *deoxygenated* hemoglobin must be in the capillaries in order to appreciate cyanosis?
   a. At least 20% of the total hemoglobin content
   b. At least 50% of the total hemoglobin content
   c. 5 gm of hemoglobin per 100 ml blood
   d. 10 gm of hemoglobin per 100 ml blood
   e. None of the above

The breathing pattern of the infant should also be observed. An infant in respiratory distress characteristically has tachypnea, intercostal retractions, nasal flaring, and, on occasion, grunting. Retractions occur as the lungs become less compliant than the chest wall. During inspiration the infant has strong diaphragmatic contractions in an attempt to inflate the lung. This creates a large negative intrapleural pressure; as a result the chest wall collapses inward at points of least resistance. These points of collapse are usually *intercostal* (between the ribs), *subcostal* (below the lower rib margins),

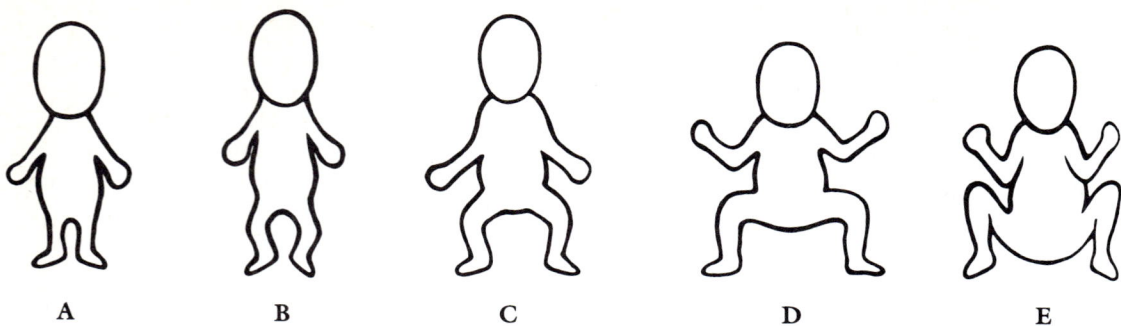

Fig. 15-5. Body position of infant at different gestational ages, **A** through **E**. A premature infant born at 28 weeks (**A**) through a full term infant (**E**). (From Wilkins, R.L., Sheldon, R.L., and Krider, S.J., editors: Clinical assessment in respiratory care, St. Louis, 1985, The C.V. Mosby Co.)

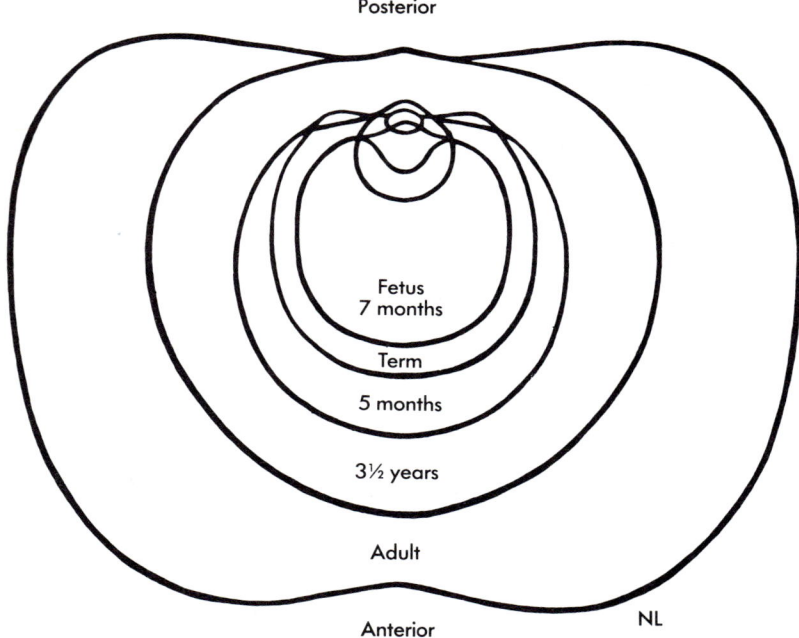

Fig. 15-6. Changes in anteroposterior chest configurations with age. (From Wilkins, R.L., Sheldon, R.L., and Krider, S.J., editors: Clinical assessment in respiratory care, St. Louis, 1985, The C.V. Mosby Co.)

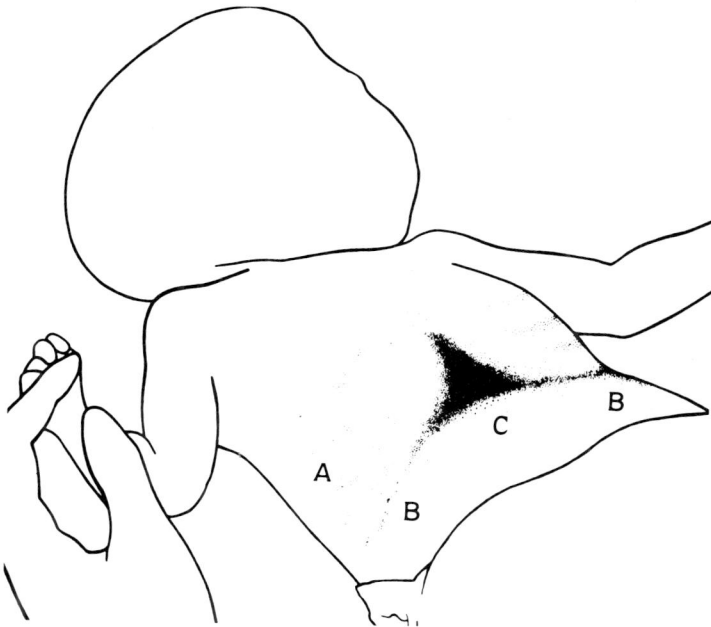

Fig. 15-7. Points of chest wall collapse. Retractions occur in the intercostal (**A**), subcostal (**B**), and substernal (**C**) areas. (From Wilkins, R.L., Sheldon, R.L., and Krider, S.J., editors: Clinical assessment in respiratory care, St. Louis, 1985, The C.V. Mosby Co.)

or *substernal* (below the bottom of the sternum) (Fig. 15-7). Infants with lung disease tend to have greater retractions toward the center of the body (substernal and subcostal). Infants with heart disease as the cause of respiratory distress tend to have intercostal retractions on the sides of their thorax because the large heart prevents backward motion of the sternum.

Infants are obligate nose breathers, and the minute ventilation they require must be achieved through their noses. Nasal flaring (dilation of the nostrils during inspiration) is an attempt to achieve airway dilation, decrease airway resistance, and increase air flow.

Grunting may be heard at the end of expiration just before rapid inspiration. Grunting is the infant's attempt to increase the gas volume in the lung; it is typically present in diseases that decrease lung volume (e.g., infant respiratory distress syndrome). At the end of inspiration the infant occludes his airway glottis and actively exhales against the closed glottis. The grunting sound is produced when the infant suddenly opens his glottis and quickly exhales, inhales, and recloses the glottis.

While observing the respiratory pattern and breathing effort, the precordium should be observed for any increase in wall motion, i.e., lifting or shifting motion of the chest wall as the heart contracts (hyperdynamic precordium). Such chest wall motion indicates increased heart volume on the right side and is usually the result of left-to-right shunting across the ductus arteriosus. When the ductus arteriosus remains patent after birth, blood from the aorta will flow directly to the pulmonary artery, resulting in pulmonary edema and congestive heart failure. The presence of a hyperdynamic precordium is a clue that the infant's respiratory distress may not be solely of pulmonary origin but may also be the result of cardiac abnormality.

In infants *palpation* is directed less at the lungs and more at the abdomen. Infants use their diaphragms as the major source of power for respiration. Because their abdominal wall musculature is relatively weak, abdominal contents move a great deal with respiration. Anything that impedes abdominal motion can affect breathing, including intra-abdominal organomegaly (e.g., liver, spleen) and intra-abdominal tumors. Distention of the abdomen by fluid or air can also impede abdominal movement. It is important to be gentle when palpating an infant's abdomen; the masses may not be felt if vigorous palpation pushes the mass away from the examining fingers.

Auscultation can yield helpful information if the infant is quiet. For optimal conditions, auscultation is usually done right after inspection. Although most infants adopt the supine position or lie on one side, auscultation is best accomplished with the infant prone. The majority of the auscultation should be completed before moving the infant. If the infant's position does not allow an adequate examination, the infant should be gently moved to a more desirable position.

The types of breath sounds are the same as in the adult (see Chapter 1). A decrease in breath sounds implies a decrease in air flow, a typical finding in respiratory distress syndrome. Wheezing implies air flow through constricted airways, e.g., bronchopulmonary dysplasia or asthma. Crackles (rales) usually imply excess fluid in the lung (pulmonary edema) or alveolar air space infection (pneumonia).

The abdomen should be auscultated when there is a question as to whether an infant is properly intubated. If the endotracheal tube is in the esophagus, there will be loud breath sounds over the stomach.

A technique frequently used in examining infants but not older patients is *transillumination*. Because the infant chest wall is relatively thin, a bright fiberoptic light placed against the chest in a dark room produces a lighted halo around the point of skin contact. In the presence of a pneumothorax or pneumomediastinum, the entire hemithorax "lights" up. Transillumination is rapid and safe and allows quick diagnosis of some serious conditions.

CHEST X-RAY EXAMINATION

X-ray views and the methods used to obtain chest x-rays differ considerably between infants and older patients. In the older patient the x-ray beam passes from the back to the front (posteroanterior). This minimizes any distortion from the divergence of the x-ray beam as it passes through the body. Also, the preferred position for taking x-ray films in adults is with the patient upright. Infants cannot easily be placed upright, and they dislike being forced to lie on their stomachs; thus most x-ray examinations are performed with the infant in the supine position, lying on the x-ray film. The x-ray beam then passes from the front of the infant to the back (anteroposterior) (Fig. 15-8).

As in the older patient, anteroposterior and lateral views allow the examiner to see all areas of the lung in a standard presentation. X-ray interpretation is approached systematically, as it is for adults. Particular attention should be paid to the large airways (larynx, trachea, and major bronchi) for normal location in the chest, deviation from external masses or pressure, filling defects from internal masses, or hypoplasia.

Occasionally, decubitus films of the chest and abdomen are helpful in detecting the presence of fluid or air in the pleural space and in checking for foreign body obstruction. In older patients, such an obstruction is assessed with a combination of inspiratory and expiratory chest films. When the obstruction is not complete (i.e., some air passes the obstruction during inspiration), the obstructed lung appears relatively overinflated on expiration when compared with the nonobstructed lung.

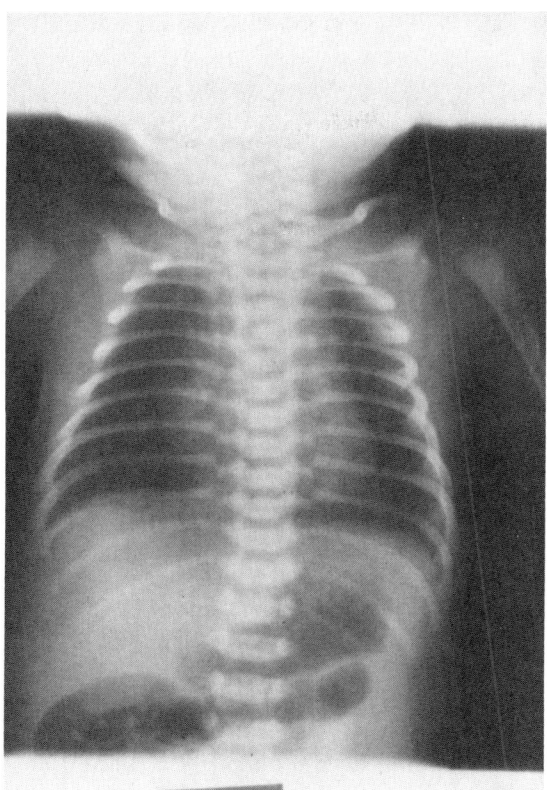

Fig. 15-8. Normal infant chest x-ray.

Because newborns cannot cooperate for inspiratory and expiratory views, right and left lateral decubitus views are often obtained to detect partial bronchial obstruction. For example, if the infant has a partial mechanical obstruction in the right main bronchus, the left lung will shrink or collapse when the infant is lying with the left side down, but the right lung will stay inflated when the infant is lying with the right side down.

Generally, a chest x-ray should be obtained if an infant has unexplained tachypnea, cyanosis, abnormal breath sounds, malformations of the chest or airway, or a very ill appearance.

PULMONARY FUNCTION TESTS

Fig. 15-9 shows the newborn's total lung capacity (TLC) contrasted with the TLC of an adult man and woman. The subdivisions (tidal volume [VT], functional residual capacity, [FRC], residual volume [RV], and vital capacity [VC]) are reduced proportionately.

Pulmonary function can be tested in infants and newborns. However, standardized equipment for these tests is not available. Nurseries that measure pulmonary function are usually found in major teaching and research institutions that have the capability of custom designing equipment to fulfill their needs. Thus the majority of newborn nurseries that take care of sick infants cannot measure pulmonary function.

The fundamental difference between newborn and adult pulmonary function testing is the patient's ability to cooperate. Pulmonary function tests in adults and older children depend on the patient's ability to follow simple commands. Pulmonary tests in infants must be performed without patient cooperation.

Three lung volumes can be measured relatively easily in newborns: functional residual capacity (FRC), thoracic gas volume (TGV), and crying vital capacity (CVC). All three of these volumes are measured independently of the infant's cooperation. However, a certain degree of caution must be exercised when interpreting results of these tests. The range of normal values is great, and all three tests are subject to error. To compare results between different infants or between the same infant at different times, the values must be standardized based on weight or length, e.g., cubic centimeter of gas per kilogram body length or cubic centimeter of gas per centimeter body length.

The FRC is measured by one of two methods: closed system helium dilution (the most common method) and open system nitrogen washout method. The TGV, which is measured with a plethysmograph, includes all gas in the thoracic cavity, whether it is communicating with the airway or not.

The CVC is the measurement of tidal volume

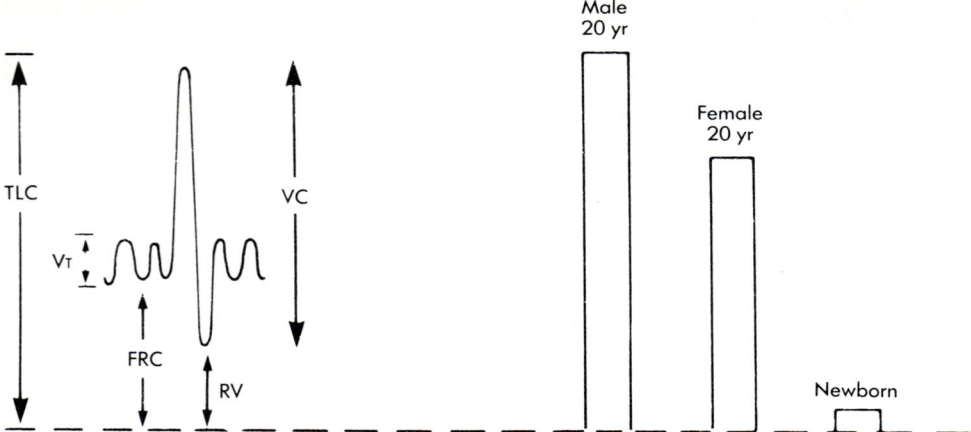

Fig. 15-9. Total lung capacity of a newborn compared with that of young adults. *Left,* A normal adult spirogram. RV + VC = TLC. Bars on right represent TLC. TLC is approximately 6 L in an average adult male, 4.2 L in an average adult female, and 160 ml in a newborn of average size (3 kg). *TLC,* total lung capacity; V_T, tidal volume; *FRC,* functional residual capacity; *RV,* residual volume; *VC,* vital capacity. (From O'Brodovich, H.M., and Chernick, V.: The functional basis of respiratory pathology. In Kendig, E.L., and Chernick, V., editors: Disorders of the respiratory tract in children, Philadelphia, 1983, W.B. Saunders Co.)

while the infant is crying. It is useful in following infants who have lung diseases that cause changes in FRC (e.g., infant respiratory distress syndrome) and in whom it is difficult to measure FRC. The CVC does require that the infant be able to cry vigorously, which may be difficult in sick infants.

Other pulmonary measurements, such as compliance and resistance are possible but not practical in most clinical settings.

Clinical problem 5

An infant 100 cm long (approximately 39 inches) has a TLC of 1.15 L. Approximately what value would you expect for the infant's vital capacity?
- a. 525 ml
- b. 650 ml
- c. 725 ml
- d. 870 ml
- e. 960 ml

BLOOD GASES

Newborn blood gases are monitored either by analysis of blood samples or by transcutaneous monitoring. Blood for partial pressure of oxygen (P_{O_2}), partial pressure of carbon dioxide (P_{CO_2}), and pH may be obtained from either arterial, capillary, or venous samples. Normal values in newborns depend on exactly when the blood is drawn (see Fig. 15-2). After the transitional period shown in Fig. 15-2, blood gas values are similar to those in adults.

Arterial samples are the most reliable source for blood gas analysis in newborns and small children. This fact must be weighed against the problems associated with arterial puncture in this age group. The procedure requires good technique and often extra assistance. Newborns and young infants have small arteries, and they cannot be expected to hold still; when they move about, the risk of arterial

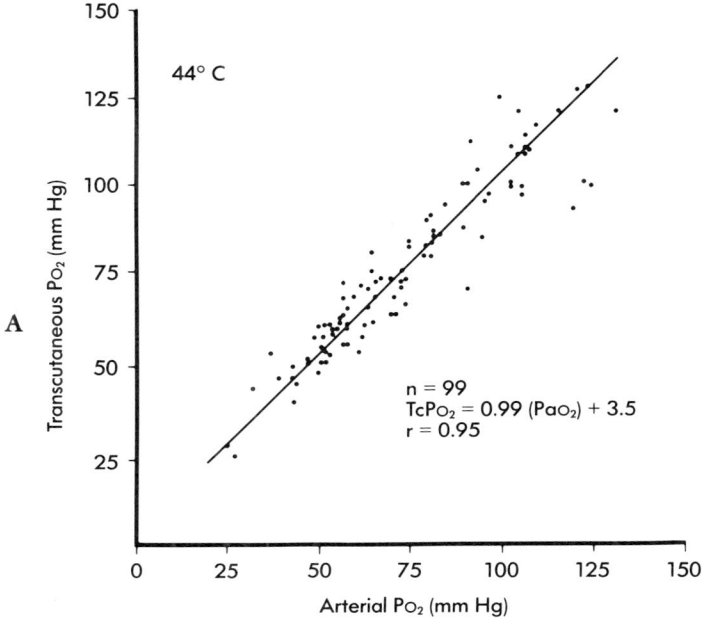

Fig. 15-10. Correlations between transcutaneous and arterial measurements of Po_2 and Pco_2. **A,** Correlations in preterm infants with respiratory distress syndrome. *continued*

damage is increased. Also, arterial blood may not reflect the resting state if the procedure causes the infant to cry. Crying can change the pattern of ventilation in one of two ways; infants can either hyperventilate or hold their breath and stop ventilating. Either effect can rapidly alter Po_2 and Pco_2.

Because of the problems associated with arterial puncture, capillary samples are widely used. Capillary sampling requires less technical expertise and effort than does arterial puncture. Capillary samples are generally obtained by puncturing the skin of the infant's heel, although the fingers and earlobes can also be used.

When the values of capillary Pco_2 and pH are compared with those from an arterial sample, Pco_2 is 2 to 5 mm Hg higher, and pH is 0.01 to 0.03 units lower. These small differences are not important in most clinical situations. Differences between capillary Po_2 and arterial Po_2 (Pao_2) are more significant. Unfortunately, there is no fixed ratio of capillary to arterial Po_2. An infant with a capillary Po_2 of 50 mm Hg may have a Pao_2 anywhere from 50 to 90 mm Hg or higher. However, Pao_2 should be no lower than capillary Po_2.

To obtain a capillary sample that closely reflects arterial blood, the extremity must be warmed to approximately 103° F. Caution must be used in warming so that the infant does not get burned and so that the warming device does not get cold and secondarily cool the extremity. All values will be unreliable if the extremity is edematous, cyanotic, cool, or if the infant has poor peripheral circulation. Also, since capillary puncture is painful, the sample reflects the infant's condition during crying, which may differ from the resting condition.

One of the most significant advances in the field of monitoring sick patients has been development

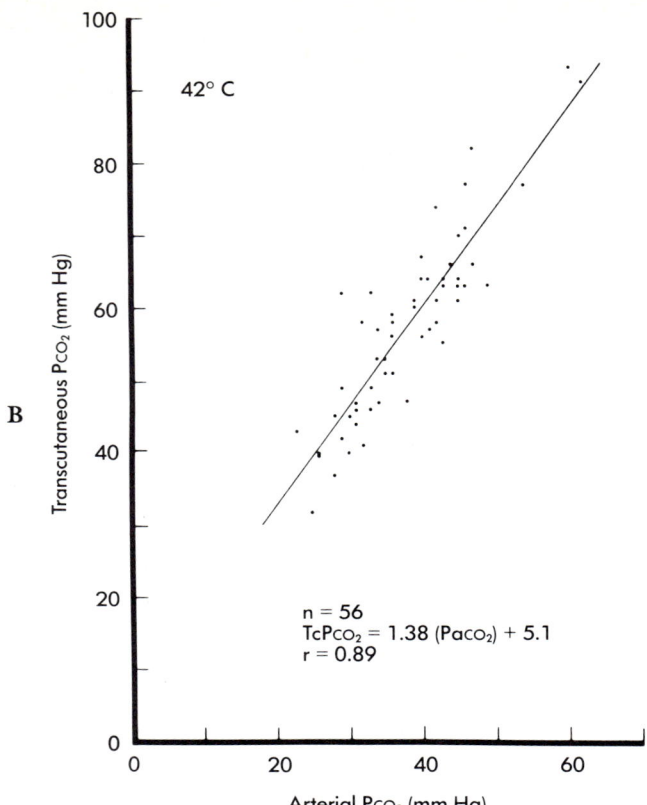

Fig. 15-10, cont'd. **B,** Correlation in preterm and term infants with cardiopulmonary disease. (From Fanaroff, A.A., and Martin, R.J.: Behrman's neonatal-perinatal medicine: diseases of the fetus and infant, ed. 3, St. Louis, 1983, The C.V. Mosby Co.)

of transcutaneous oxygen and carbon dioxide electrodes. The transcutaneous oxygen ($tcPO_2$) electrode measures oxygen in the skin capillaries; it does not measure arterial PO_2 (PaO_2). However, $tcPO_2$ closely approximates PaO_2, providing there is no decrease in blood flow under the electrode (Fig. 15-10, *A*). A decrease in blood flow can occur in conditions such as acidosis, shock, hypovolemia, hypoglycemia, and inadequate warming of the skin. In such conditions $tcPO_2$ can significantly underestimate PaO_2.

A $tcPO_2$ monitor can provide a good method of evaluating the physiologic changes that occur with arterial blood sampling. The person obtaining the sample should note the $tcPO_2$ value three times: before disturbing the infant, at the beginning of blood flow into the syringe, and approximately 1 minute after the sample is obtained. These three $tcPO_2$ values can be used to assess the infant's resting condition, the physiologic changes caused by the arterial sampling procedure, and the correlation between PaO_2 and $tcPO_2$.

Transcutaneous carbon dioxide (tcP_{CO_2}) electrodes are also available. Like the tcP_{O_2} electrode, tcP_{CO_2} is a measure of the gas present in the skin and not in the blood (Fig. 15-10, B). Although tcP_{CO_2} may not always be the same as arterial partial pressure of carbon dioxide (Pa_{CO_2}), it can be used to monitor trends in Pa_{CO_2}, analogous to using expired P_{CO_2} (Chapter 4).

VENTILATION-PERFUSION IMBALANCE

As in adults, ventilation-perfusion (V/Q) imbalance is the most common cause of hypoxemia in infants. However, there is one striking difference in its manifestation. Clinical Problem 8 in Chapter 5 discusses a 54-year-old man with right-sided pneumonia whose Pa_{O_2} improved when positioned with his left side (good lung) down. The principle, at least in adults, is that oxygenation improves when the good lung is dependent because gravity results in increased blood flow and ventilation to dependent lungs. Since the good lung does not have a disturbance in ventilation (it is disease-free), the result is favorable V/Q relationships and better blood gases than when the diseased lung is dependent.

In infants the opposite appears to be the case (Heaf, Helms, Gordon, et al., 1983). In infants with unilateral lung disease, oxygenation improves when the good lung is uppermost, i.e., when the *diseased* lung is dependent. This finding has been confirmed in infants ages 11 days to 27 months who suffered from unilateral lung disease (Davies, Kitchman, Gordon, et al., 1985). Using ventilation scans, the authors found that the distribution of ventilation was consistently away from the dependent lung, a reversal of the adult pattern. Infants in this study had a higher Pa_{O_2} when the diseased lung was dependent.

This difference in ventilation is explained by differences in lung mechanics and diaphragmatic function between infants and adults (Davies, Kitchman, Gordon, et al., 1985). Because the infant's chest wall is floppier (more compliant) than an adult's, the resting pleural pressure is less negative (closer to atmospheric). For this reason dependent airways are most likely to close at low lung volumes, and air is preferentially distributed to the upper lung. The authors also postulate that the greater weight of abdominal contents in adults increases the contractility of the dependent diaphragm, resulting in relatively more ventilation to the dependent lung.

Note that the major difference is in distribution of ventilation—not perfusion. As in adults, perfusion in infants should preferentially go to the bases, although the shorter distance for blood to travel suggests that the difference between apical and basilar (or uppermost and lowermost) blood flow is not as great as in adults.

It is not known at what age the infant distribution of ventilation changes to the adult pattern, but it seems that infants with unilateral lung disease should be placed so that the normal lung is uppermost.

OXYGEN THERAPY

The principles of oxygen therapy discussed in Chapter 9 also apply to pediatric patients. The fundmental rule—give the lowest feasible fraction of inspired oxygen (FI_{O_2}) that will maintain adequate oxygenation—is vitally important in premature infants. Low-birthweight infants who are given supplemental oxygen are at greatest risk for developing retrolental fibroplasia (retinopathy of prematurity [ROP]) and subsequent blindness. In two large studies retrolental fibroplasia correlated with low birth weight and the length of time supplemental oxygen was delivered but not with arterial partial pressure of oxygen (Pa_{O_2}) (Kinsey, Arnold, Kalina, et al., 1977; Campbell, Bull, Ellis, et al., 1983).

As in adults, clinical findings are an unreliable guide to hypoxemia or to oxygen therapy. It must be remembered that cyanosis may not appear if the infant is anemic; conversely, cyanosis may be present if the infant is polycythemic even though there is no decrease in arterial oxygen content.

The methods of oxygen administration discussed in Chapter 9 also apply to the pediatric population. In addition to nasal cannulas and face masks, infants may also receive oxygen by way of oxygen tents and oxygen hoods. Oxygen tents are no longer used in adult medicine because of their large size and requisite need for large amounts of supplemental oxygen. However, an infant or small child may tolerate a tent better than a facial appliance. In infants, more so than in adults, it is imperative to monitor the fraction of inspired oxygen (FIO_2) closely; in neonatal intensive care units the FIO_2 is monitored continuously.

HEMODYNAMIC ASSESSMENT

Hemodynamic monitoring in the infant is in some ways easier and in other ways more difficult than in the adult. The presence of patent umbilical vessels makes cannulation of the aorta and inferior vena cava relatively simple. However, cannulation of the pulmonary artery is quite difficult and usually must be done in a cardiac catheterization laboratory. Also, in the presence of a patent ductus arteriosis and foramen ovale, the newborn may have varying amounts of right-to-left shunt depending on the pulmonary vascular resistance. These shunts make accurate calculation of cardiac output difficult if not impossible.

Cannulation of the umbilical artery and vein is a routine procedure in most neonatal units. The technique is done under sterile conditions with close physiologic monitoring. Fig. 15-11 shows a lateral x-ray film of an infant with both an arterial and venous umbilical catheter in place.

Indications for umbilical *artery* catheterization include:

1. The need for frequent arterial sampling for blood gases
2. Continuous blood pressure monitoring
3. Large scale blood replacement (e.g., exchange transfusion)

Indications for umbilical *vein* catheterization include:

1. Central venous pressure monitoring

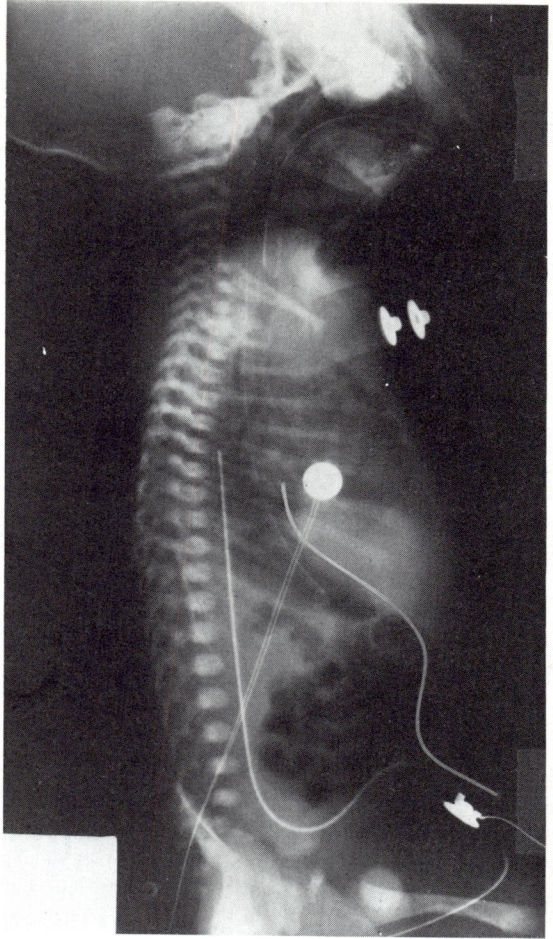

Fig. 15-11. Lateral x-ray showing umbilical venous and arterial catheters in place. The arterial catheter (lowermost in this x-ray) enters through the umbilicus, passes through the umbilical artery and other arterial branches, and ends in the thoracic aorta. The venous catheter (uppermost in x-ray) enters through the umbilicus, passes through the umbilical vein and other venous branches, and ends in the right atrium. (From Wilkins, R.L., Sheldon, R.L., and Krider, S.J., editors: Clinical assessment in respiratory care, St. Louis, 1985, The C.V. Mosby Co.)

2. Large scale blood replacement

These two methods of hemodynamic monitoring are susceptible to many of the same problems that exist in adults and older children. Infection, hemorrhage, thrombus formation, embolization, and arteriospasm are major concerns in infant hemodynamic monitoring.

SUDDEN INFANT DEATH SYNDROME

Approximately 8,000 to 10,000 times a year in the United States, an infant dies suddenly and unexpectedly before his or her first birthday. Autopsy does not reveal any apparent cause of death, although changes characteristic of hypoxemia are often found. This condition used to be called "crib death" or "cot death."

Like sleep apnea syndrome, sudden infant death syndrome (SIDS) has many potential causes and is appropriately classified a syndrome rather than a specific disease. In some studies, autopsied SIDS victims showed thickening of the smooth muscle in the small pulmonary arteries and right ventricle, indicators of recurrent or chronic hypoxemia (Shannon and Kelly, 1982). This does not indicate a cause but rather suggests that hypoxemia accompanied or preceded whatever condition led to apnea.

Many infants suffer potentially lethal "near miss" episodes, whereby they stop breathing but are revived in time for full recovery. Near-miss patients have provided researchers with much information about what may happen to SIDS victims. Sleep apnea has been a common finding in infants who have suffered one or more near misses (Shannon and Kelly, 1982). Causes similar to adult sleep apnea have been identified, such as upper airways obstruction (adenoid hypertrophy) and central hypoventilation. In addition, cardiac conduction defects, seizures, brain malformations, poisoning (botulism, organophosphate), and infantile myasthenia have been found. In many near-SIDS infants arterial partial pressure of carbon dioxide is elevated to 45 to 50 mm Hg during quiet sleep, and abnormal breathing patterns are present.

The fact that sleep apnea is the most frequent abnormality found in near-miss infants has lead to an exciting area of clinical applicability, i.e., identifying infants at risk for SIDS and attempting to prevent the next episode of apnea. Apnea monitors are being used to detect prodromes of SIDS (Shannon and Kelly, 1982; Avery and Frantz, 1983). Although these instruments are not infallible, when used under the supervision of trained medical personnel with round-the-clock support for any questions or complications, the outcome is usually excellent (Shannon and Kelly, 1982).

Table 15-5. Comparisons between ARDS and IRDS

	IRDS	ARDS
Incidence (estimate)	40,000 per year	150,000 per year
Setting	Low gestational age; prematurity	Trauma, sepsis, etc.
Basic cause	Lack of normal surfactant activity	Unknown; probably multifactorial
Prevention	Pregnancy to term; prepartum steroids	Avoid precipitating event
Physiology	Severe ventilation/perfusion imbalance; low lung compliance	Severe ventilation/perfusion imbalance; low lung compliance
Pathology	Hyaline membranes; fibrosis	Hyaline membranes; fibrosis
Treatment	Ventilator support; high FIo_2; PEEP; conventional volume ventilation	Ventilator support; high FIo_2; PEEP; jet ventilation
Overall mortality	Variable*	50% to 60%
Lung function in survivors	Good	Good

*Depends on gestational age: approximately 50% mortality when IRDS develops in infants born between 26 and 28 weeks gestation.

INFANT RESPIRATORY DISTRESS SYNDROME

Historically, infant respiratory distress syndrome (IRDS) was characterized well before the adult respiratory distress syndrome (ARDS). In fact ARDS was so-named because it seemed to resemble the catastrophic respiratory failure seen in many premature infants (Fig. 15-12). Although the two conditions manifest similar changes in lung physiology (severe shunting and low compliance), their cause is much different (Fig. 15-13 and Table 15-5). Basically, IRDS is the result of a lack of normal surfactant activity in premature lungs; the greatest risk factor is thus low gestational age. IRDS occurs in more than 70% of newborns at 28 to 30 weeks of gestation but only rarely at 37 weeks or beyond (Martin, et al., 1983). ARDS, on the other hand, is the result of a specific precipitating event, such as sepsis or trauma, that causes pulmonary capillaries to leak a cellular exudate (see Chapter 11); surfactant activity is reduced in ARDS as a result of this alveolar flooding.

One exciting aspect of IRDS is the potential for its prevention with prepartum administration of corticosteroids; this treatment decreases both the incidence and severity of IRDS. Steroids appear to be effective only when given before 34 weeks gestation and between 24 hours and 7 days before delivery.

Fig. 15-14 contrasts lung volumes and capacities in a normal infant and in an infant with IRDS. Qualitatively the changes are similar to those of ARDS (Chapter 11).

The treatment goals in IRDS are also the same as in ARDS—reversal of the severe shunting and improvement of lung compliance. The administration of steroids to the infant is of no proven benefit.

Methods of monitoring and ventilation differ somewhat from those in ARDS. High-frequency ventilation and transcutaneous measurement of P_{O_2} and P_{CO_2} are more apt to be used in IRDS than in ARDS (Fig. 15-10). When conventional volume ventilation is used, the frequency of spontaneous ventilation compared to mechanical ventilation is

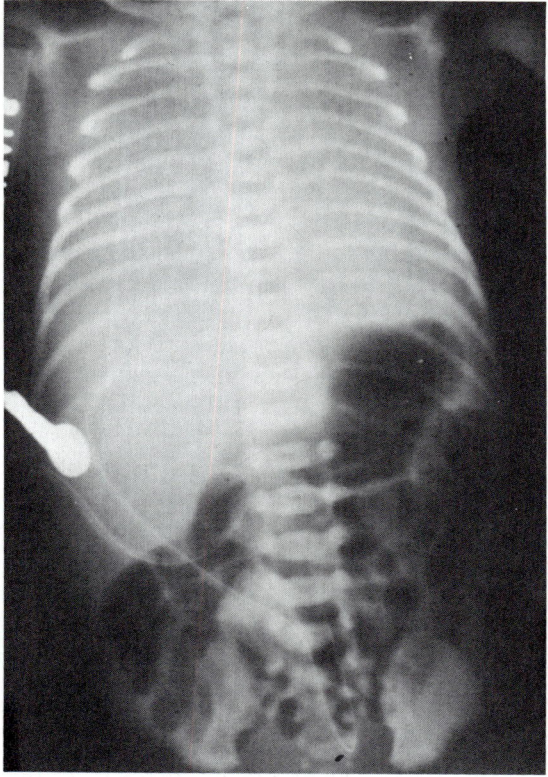

Fig. 15-12. Chest x-ray of infant with respiratory distress syndrome.

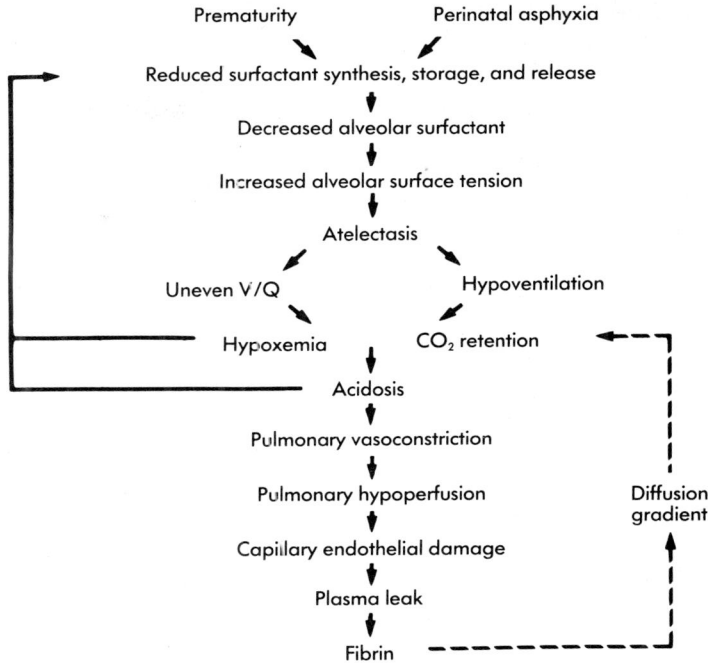

Fig. 15-13. Schema for the infant respiratory distress syndrome. (From Fanaroff, A.A., and Martin, R.J.: Behrman's neonatal-perinatal medicine: diseases of the fetus and infant, ed. 3, St. Louis, 1983, The C.V. Mosby Co.)

not as important as in adults. More crucial is the *synchrony* of spontaneous to mechanical ventilation. For example, an infant who exhales during the inspiratory cycle of the ventilator can generate tremendous intrathoracic pressures, resulting in lung damage. The infant's chest wall motion should be observed while listening to the ventilator cycle. An inward motion of the chest or even absence of an outward motion during mechanical inspiration may indicated that breathing is not synchronized with the ventilator.

Airway pressures used in assessing intubated infants include peak and mean airway pressure and end-expiratory pressure when positive end-expiratory pressure is used. These pressures are interpreted as they are in the adult. Static airway pressure, airways resistance, lung compliance, intrapleural pressure, lung volume, and expired gas analysis are not generally measured in the clinical management of newborns. However, the fraction of inspired oxygen (FIO_2) must be accurately measured. In a closed system, such as with mechanical ventilation, FIO_2 should be measured on the inspiratory side of the ventilator circuit. For an infant breathing spontaneously, the FIO_2 should be measured close to the infant's nose.

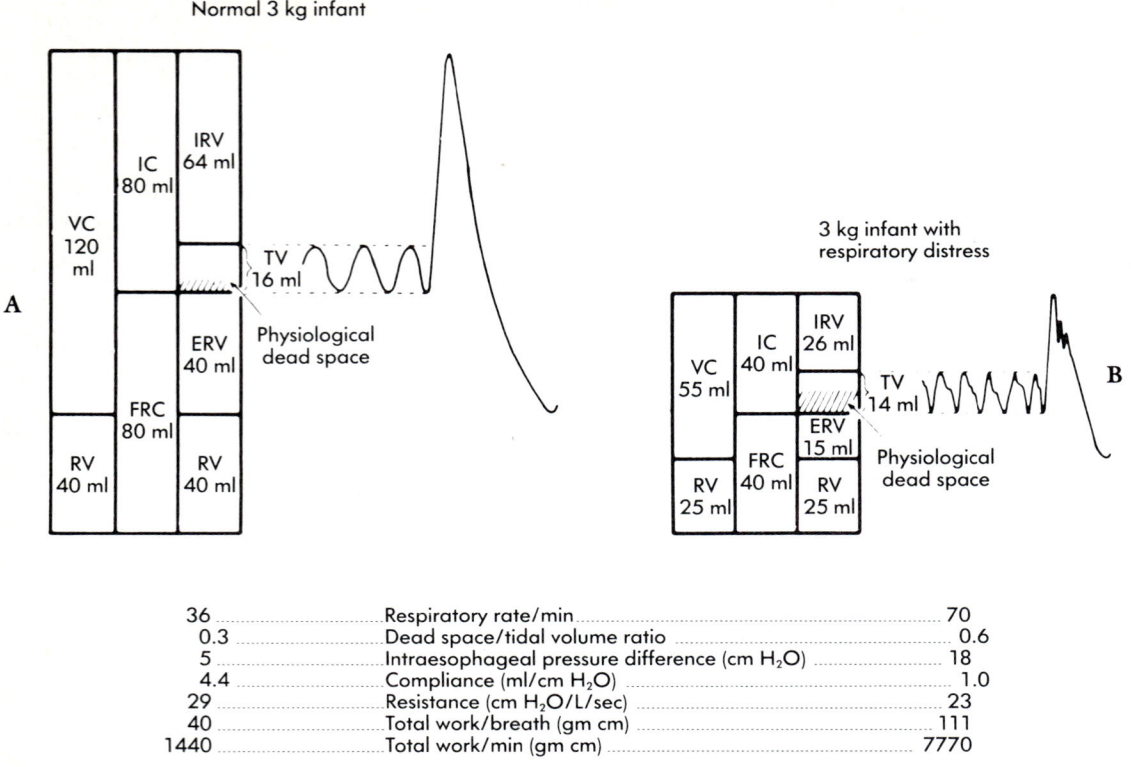

Fig. 15-14. Lung volumes in normal infant and infant with respiratory distress syndrome. (Figure is from Fanaroff, A.A. and Martin, R.J.: Behrman's Neonatal-perinatal medicine: diseases of the fetus and infant, ed. 3, St. Louis, 1983, The C.V. Mosby Co.; originally from Cook, C.D.: Respiration and metabolism of newborn infants. Exhibited at VIII International Congress of Pediatrics, Copenhagen, 1956.)

SUMMARY

At birth the fetus undergoes profound changes in cardiopulmonary physiology. The gas exchange function is transferred from the placenta to the lungs, which inflate with air at the moment of birth. As the newborn's arterial partial pressure of oxygen (PaO_2) rises, the foramen ovale and ductus arteriosus begin to close, routing all venous return through the lungs. In the first few hours after birth the infant experiences hypoxemia and respiratory acidosis; after approximately 3 days, blood gas values are similar to those in children and adults. At birth the Apgar score provides a quick, objective assessment of the newborn's overall condition.

Respiratory assessment of the newborn and the infant differs in several important aspects from the adult. Emphasis in the medical history is placed on information about the mother's health, pregnancy, labor, and delivery; family illnesses; and the postnatal period. The newborn's body temperature is normally in the same range as the adult's, but the child has a greater heat loss because of much larger surface area to weight ratio. Normal newborn heart and respiratory rates are much higher than in the adult.

Pulmonary function is often difficult to measure in infants and small children since they cannot cooperate for effort-dependent tests. In place of traditional vital capacity, a crying vital capacity and a functional residual capacity can be determined, but these measurements are subject to error and must be interpreted cautiously. Easier to obtain and interpret are arterial or capillary blood gas values. Transcutaneous monitoring has proved useful as a substitute for blood sampling and is widely used to measure PO_2 ($tcPO_2$) and PCO_2 ($tcPCO_2$) in neonatal intensive care units.

Infant respiratory distress syndrome (IRDS) has the same physiologic problems as adult respiratory distress syndrome. The cause of IRDS is the lack of normal surfactant activity that results from prematurity. Treatment goals of IRDS are the same as in ARDS, but high-frequency ventilation and transcutaneous monitoring are more often employed in management of IRDS.

REVIEW QUESTIONS

State whether each of the following is true or false.

1. The Apgar score includes postnatal measurement of thigh blood pressure.
2. The ratio of body surface area to body weight is about the same in term infants as in infants 7 months old.
3. A newborn heart rate of 95 beats per minute is subnormal.
4. Normal term infants breathe between 40 and 60 breaths per minute.
5. Infants with unilateral lung disease should be positioned with their good lung uppermost.
6. The prevalence of IRDS correlates inversely with gestational age at birth.
7. Fetal hemoglobin has a lower affinity for oxygen than does adult hemoglobin.
8. Normal newborn blood gas measurements show a low $PaCO_2$ and an elevated pH.
9. PO_2 measured by the transcutaneous method is identical to PO_2 measured on an arterial blood sample.
10. One indication for catheterizing the umbilical artery is frequent arterial blood gas measurement.

References

Apgar, V.: A proposal for a new method of evaluation of the newborn infant, Anesth. Analg. **32:**260, 1953.
Avery, M.E., and Frantz, I.D.: To breathe or not to breathe: what have we learned about apneic spells and sudden infant death? N. Engl. J. Med. **309:**107, 1983.
Campbell, P.B., Bull, M.J., Ellis, D.F., et al.: Incidence of retinopathy of prematurity in a tertiary newborn intensive care unit, Arch. Ophthalmol. **101:**1686, 1983.
Davies, H., Kitchman, R., Gordon, I., et al.: Regional ventilation in infancy: reversal of adult pattern, N. Engl. J. Med. **313:**1626, 1985.
Deming, D.D.: Respiratory assessment of the newborn and the child. In Wilkins, R.L., Sheldon, R.L., and Krider, S.J., editors: Clinical assessment in respiratory care, St. Louis, 1985, The C.V. Mosby Co.
Fanaroff, A.A., and Martin, R.J.: Behrman's neonatal-perinatal medicine, ed. 3, St. Louis, 1983, The C.V. Mosby Co.
Heaf, D.P., Helms, P., Gordon, I., et al.: Postural effects on gas exchange in infants, N. Engl. J. Med. **308:**1505, 1983.
Kendig, E.L., and Chernick, V.: Disorders of the respiratory tract in children, Philadelphia, 1983, W.B. Saunders Co.
Kinsey, V.E., Arnold, H.J., Kalina, R.E., et al.: PaO_2 levels and retrolental fibroplasia: a report of the cooperative study, Pediatrics **60:**655, 1977.
Martin, R.J., Fanaroff, A.A., and Skalina, M.: The respiratory distress syndrome and its management. In Fanaroff, A.A., and Martin, R.J.: Behrman's neonatal-perinatal medicine, ed. 3, St. Louis, 1983, The C.V. Mosby Co.
Oski, F.A.: Hematologic problems. In Avery, G.B., editor: Neonatology: pathophysiology and management of the newborn, ed. 2, Philadelphia, 1981, J.B. Lippincott Co.
Shannon, D.C., and Kelly, D.H.: SIDS and near-SIDS, N. Engl. J. Med. **306:**959, 1982.
Slonim, N.B., and Hamilton, L.H.: Respiratory physiology, ed. 4, St. Louis, 1981, The C.V. Mosby Co.

Suggested readings

Golden, S.M., and Peters, D.: Handbook of neonatal intensive care, St. Louis, 1985, The C.V. Mosby Co.
Lough, M.D., Doershuk, C.F., and Stern, R.C.: Pediatric respiratory therapy, ed. 3, Chicago, 1985, Year Book Medical Publishers, Inc.
Lough, M.D., Williams, T.J., and Rawson, J.E.: Newborn respiratory care. Chicago, 1981, Year Book Medical Publishers, Inc.
See also General References in Appendix G.

APPENDICES

A Answers to clinical problems
B Normal values for FVC and FEV_1
C Basic equations and formulas
D Abbreviations and symbols
E Glossary
F Common clinical conditions
G General references
H Microcomputer programs

appendix A
Answers to clinical problems

CHAPTER 1

1. PITFALL. Many patients interpret the question "Do you smoke?" literally, and they honestly answer "no" if they quit just one day, one week, or 2 weeks ago. This is a common response and is not meant to be deceptive. This physician should have followed up with "Did you ever smoke?" or some other question to elicit a more detailed smoking history. A patient with a lung mass likely has a carcinoma if he has smoked; carcinoma is far less likely if the patient has never smoked.

2. PITFALL. There is often a wide discrepancy between prescribed medications and what the patient is actually taking. In fact, this patient had *not* been taking the medication as instructed on the drug labels. The list copied by the intern in no way represented this patient's true drug history. Had the intern questioned the patient directly, he would have learned she was confused about the drugs and had taken them only sporadically and ineffectively for the past month. Undertreatment was contributing to her asthma problem.

   A thorough drug history is more than just a list. It includes uncovering what drugs the patient actually uses, how and when they are taken, and what is the patient's understanding of the medication. For various reasons, many patients do not take drugs the way they are prescribed.

3. PITFALL. This patient had pulmonary asbestosis, a diagnosis that is usually made on the basis of an abnormal chest x-ray and a "positive" work history. This patient certainly had a positive history for occupational asbestos exposure; had the intern pursued this line of questioning, he would have learned that, for at least 10 years, the patient had stripped asbestos lining from boilers. An occupational history is sometimes very important in making the right diagnosis. At the very least, one should not assume that a job title conveys anything about occupational exposure. For example, a patient who worked "in the coal mines" could have done anything from paperwork in the office to emptying coal from the rail cars at the mine entrance to blasting at the coal face. Each job obviously presents a different hazard and risk of exposure.

4. PITFALL. The physical examination as a guide to asthma severity is often unreliable. The pitfall is in not recognizing this fact and in not obtaining some objective measurement of air flow. The reason this patient was not wheezing had more to do with lack of adequate airflow than with recovery from her attack. Wheezing is sometimes not heard during an asthma attack unless the patient takes in a deep breath and exhales forcefully.

5. PITFALL. Asthma can occur at any age. However, lack of reversibility should make one

doubtful of this diagnosis, particularly if the patient is a nonsmoker. Other conditions can cause wheezing, including upper airways obstruction, which this patient had. Part of a thyroid goiter had been removed 5 years earlier; now her remaining thyroid was again enlarging, compressing her trachea. Since this enlargement was mainly in the substernal region, it was not obvious on physical examination. A flow-volume loop or chest x-ray would have revealed an abnormality inconsistent with asthma and would have suggested the proper diagnosis.

6. PITFALL. Tachypnea is an important clinical sign, just like fever and tachycardia. It should not be attributed to "anxiety" and "pain," unless other causes have been ruled out. In a postoperative patient, pneumonia, atelectasis, pulmonary embolism, sepsis, and many other conditions could be heralded by tachypnea. This patient, in fact, had pneumonia, which was diagnosed later in the day when he developed a temperature of 102° F.

7. Answer. Patient *a* has a history consistent with an upper respiratory infection, for which a chest x-ray is seldom necessary.

   Patient *b* is a man who smokes and who has had a recent onset of a chronic cough. He is at risk for lung cancer and many other pulmonary problems, so a chest x-ray is clearly indicated.

   Patient *c* has a new onset of asthma. A chest x-ray should always be obtained when asthma is newly diagnosed in order to rule out complicating or coexisting pulmonary conditions.

   Patient *d* has emphysema. Clinical diagnosis of congestive heart failure (i.e., using only the patient's history and the physical examination) is notoriously unreliable in chronic lung disease patients. The chest x-ray is the best noninvasive test to diagnose or rule out congestive heart failure in such patients.

TRUE-FALSE ANSWERS

1. True
2. False
3. False
4. False
5. True
6. False
7. True
8. False
9. False
10. False

CHAPTER 2

1. Atmospheric P_{O_2} = $F_{I_{O_2}}$ ×
   $$\text{Barometric pressure} = 0.21 \times 253 = 53.13 \text{ mm Hg}$$

   The climber's *alveolar* P_{O_2} at the top of Mt. Everest will depend on his or her degree of hyperventilation, the respiratory quotient, and the barometric pressure (P_B) at the summit. During the 1981 American Medical Expedition to the summit of Mt. Everest, alveolar P_{CO_2} was measured on an expired air sample as 7.5 mm Hg.

   Could a climber make it to the top of this mountain without supplemental oxygen? The alveolar P_{O_2} ($P_{A_{O_2}}$) can be calculated using the alveolar air equation (this equation is formally introduced in Chapter 5):

   $$P_{A_{O_2}} = F_{I_{O_2}} \times (P_B - 47 \text{ mm Hg H}_2\text{O vapor pressure}) - \frac{(P_{CO_2})}{R}$$

   Assuming an R value (respiratory quotient) of 0.85:

   $$P_{A_{O_2}} = 0.21 (253-47) - \frac{7.5}{0.85} = 34.5 \text{ mm Hg}$$

   If alveolar-arterial P_{O_2} difference is only 6 mm Hg (a normal value for a young climber), $P_{a_{O_2}}$ will be approximately 28 mm Hg. A highly conditioned individual could survive with this $P_{a_{O_2}}$; in fact, several climbers have made it to the top of Mt. Everest without supplemental oxygen.

2. Both values are correct in their proper context. The vital capacity measured by the student is the volume collected under ATPS conditions.

Answers to clinical problems

The same amount of air occupies a greater volume inside her lungs where it is exposed to a higher temperature (BTPS conditions). The computer program accounts for this difference and multiplies the measured ATPS value by 1.074, the correction factor when the test was performed.

3. STPD, standard temperature and pressure; dry, 0° C, 760 mm Hg, 0 water vapor pressure. Oxygen uptake is measured under ATPS conditions. To convert from ATPS to STPD, use the general gas law.

   STPD   ATPS

   $$\frac{V_1 P_1}{T_1} = \frac{V_2 P_2}{T_2}$$

   $$\frac{V_1 (760)}{273} = \frac{327 (747 - 47)}{298}$$

   $$V_1 = \frac{(327)(700)(273)}{(298)(760)}$$

   = 276 ml, the STPD volume of oxygen per min.

4. If there is no barrier to gaseous diffusion, P_{O_2} in plasma will be the same as in the air:

   P_{O_2} in air = 0.21 (760 − 27) = 154 mm Hg
   O_2 content = 0.003 × (P_{O_2})/100 ml plasma
   = 0.003 (154)/100 ml plasma
   = 0.462 ml O_2/100 ml plasma

   Adding hemoglobin to plasma allows much more oxygen to enter the blood since oxygen can bind chemically without affecting P_{O_2}. The new oxygen content is

   Amount O_2 bound to Hgb + Amount O_2 dissolved in plasma

   Each gram of hemoglobin is capable of holding 1.34 cc of oxygen, so 10 gm% can hold 13.4 cc per 100 ml of blood. Although oxygen content is greatly increased by the addition of hemoglobin, *P_{O_2} remains the same:* 154 mm Hg. Since there is no barrier to diffusion, more oxygen molecules enter the blood from the air to replace those binding to hemoglobin.

   The amount of oxygen dissolved in the plasma is a function of the gaseous phase partial pressure, not the hemoglobin content. As long as the blood is freely exposed to the same oxygen partial pressure in the air, the blood P_{O_2} will be unchanged. Adding another 5 gm% hemoglobin (to total 15 gm%) will increase the oxygen content but will not change the P_{O_2}.

5. Oxygen uptake will rise very little since the amount of oxygen used by the respiratory muscles is relatively small, even during hyperventilation or physical exercise. For the same reason, metabolic carbon dioxide production will rise only slightly. However, since minute ventilation has doubled, carbon dioxide output for the lungs will almost double. In this example, metabolic $\dot{V}_{O_2}$ will equal lung $\dot{V}_{O_2}$, but metabolic $\dot{V}_{CO_2}$ will be only approximately one half the lung $\dot{V}_{CO_2}$.

6. a. Blood gases in this example are feasible, since Pa_{O_2} is greater than Pv_{O_2} and since Pa_{CO_2} is less than Pv_{CO_2}.
   b. Some part of these blood gas values must represent either a measurement or a technical error since Pa_{O_2} cannot be less than Pv_{O_2}.
   c. There must also be an error in this set of blood gas values since Pa_{CO_2} cannot be greater than Pv_{CO_2}.

TRUE-FALSE ANSWERS

1. True   6. False
2. False   7. False
3. True   8. False
4. False   9. True
5. True   10. True

CHAPTER 3

1. Compliance is the change in volume per change in pressure. For the problem as stated:

   Lung compliance (C_L) = $\dfrac{3000 \text{ ml}}{\text{Change in intrapleural pressure}}$

In the problem, intrapleural pressure is -30 cm H_2O during breath-holding. However, at the beginning of inspiration, intrapleural pressure is not 0 but -5 cm H_2O (intrapleural pressure is always subatmospheric at rest). Thus the *change* in intrapleural pressure is only 25 cm H_2O, not 30 cm H_2O.

$$C_L = \frac{3000 \text{ ml}}{[-30 - (-5)]} = \frac{3000}{25} = \frac{120 \text{ ml}}{\text{cm } H_2O}$$

This is a normal lung compliance.

2. The tidal volume is 10 L/40 breaths or 250 ml. The patient has rapid, shallow breathing, a pattern typical of severe pulmonary restriction. Since she cannot take a deep breath (she is "restricted"), rapid, shallow breathing is her attempt to maintain adequate alveolar ventilation. As will be discussed in Chapter 4, this breathing pattern is less efficient than normal breathing and results in increased dead space ventilation.

3. Airways resistance (R_{aw}) is driving pressure divided by airflow. In this example R_{aw} is 1 cm H_2O/0.5 L/sec or 2 cm H_2O/L/sec, a value within the normal range. With the same airflow and a driving pressure of 5 cm H_2O, R_{aw} is 10 cm H_2O/L/sec.

4. Normal ratio of inspiratory/expiratory time (I/E) is approximately 1. Typically, patients with airways obstruction (e.g., patients with asthma or chronic bronchitis) have prolonged expiratory time; it takes longer to exhale because of the increased airways resistance and, as a consequence, I/E is reduced.

5. Residual volume is the amount of air in the lungs at the end of a forced vital capacity maneuver:

$$RV = TLC - VC = 5.4 - 3.5 = 1.9 \text{ L}$$

Functional residual capacity equals expiratory reserve volume plus residual volume:

$$FRC = 1.9 + 1.3 = 3.2 \text{ L}$$

6. If TLC = 6 L and if FVC = 4.2 L, residual volume = 1.8 L. Reduction of FVC by one third will give an FVC of 2.8 L; if TLC is unchanged, the new RV must be 6 − 2.8, or 3.2 L. The initial RV/TLC ratio was 1.8/6.0 = 0.30, a normal value; the new ratio is 3.2/6.0 = 0.53. Such a markedly increased RV/TLC, with reduced FVC, is characteristic of severe obstructive lung disease (TLC may be normal or increased, depending on the underlying cause of airways obstruction).

7. On a time-volume plot it is difficult to draw an exact tangent at the point of peak flow; for this reason a peak flow meter is preferable for peak flow measurement. On this FVC curve, a tangent at the point of peak flow (see following figure) traverses approximately 5.6 L/half second or 11.2 L/sec (672 L/min).

Shown on p. 329 is Fig. 3-8, with lines drawn to demonstrate peak flow (Clinical Problem 7) and maximal midflow between 25% and 75% of the FVC (Clinical Problem 10).

8. Patient A. $FEV_1/FVC = 4.0/5.5 = 73\%$
—the lower limit of normal
Patient B. $FEV_1/FVC = 1.4/4.6 = 30\%$
—very severe airways obstruction
Patient C. $FEV_1/FVC = 2.0/2.3 = 87\%$
—no significant airways obstruction

Note that Patient C *may* have airways obstruction, but it is not apparent from the FEV_1/FVC. Sometimes patients with severe asthma can have a normal FEV_1/FVC when both FEV_1 and FVC are markedly but proportionately reduced. Also note that a normal FEV_1/FVC does not rule out small airways obstruction.

9. The physiologic purpose behind "pursed lip breathing" is to increase airway pressure toward the alveoli and to reduce the tendency of the airways to collapse during expiration. Any increase in airway pressure will oppose the tendency of pleural pressure to collapse the airways. With increased airway pressure on expiration, the EPP will move toward the mouth.

10. The maximal midflow between 25% and 75%

Answers to clinical problems

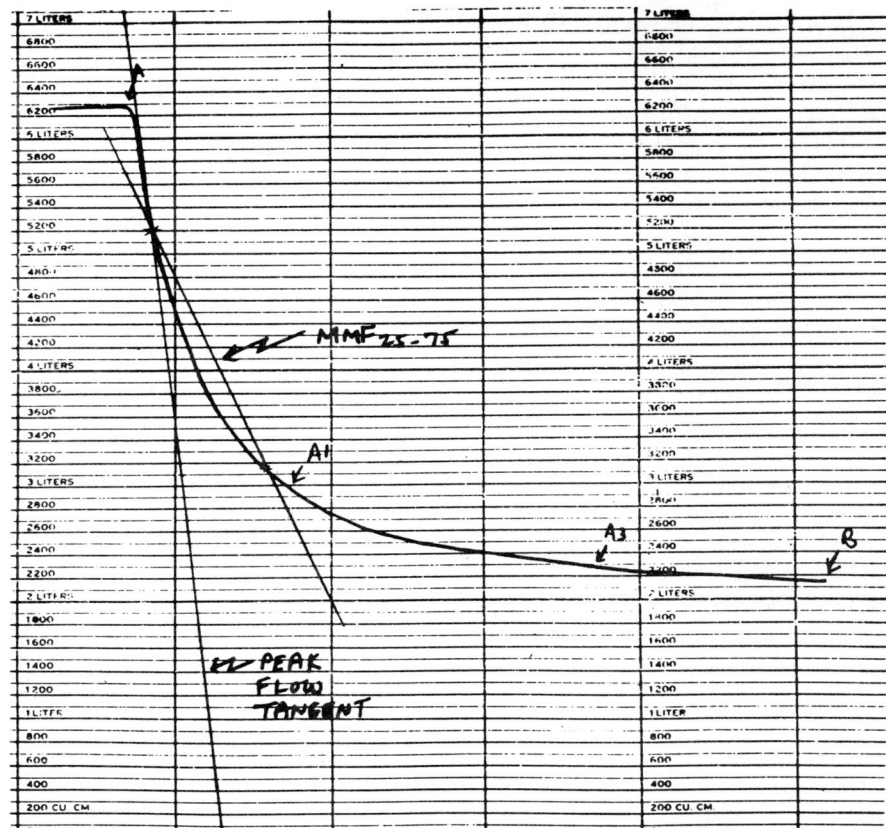

Fig. 3-8.

of the FVC is shown in Fig. 3-8; it is the line drawn between the points at 25% and 75% of the FVC (approximately 1 and 3 L from the beginning of forced expiration, respectively). The slope of this line is the MMF_{25-75} and is approximately 3.2 L/sec.

11. These spirometric curves are redrawn from actual tracings. Without correcting to BTPS conditions, values close to the following should have been calculated:

Measurements	Normal	Before bronchodilator	After bronchodilator
FVC (L)	4.00	1.95	2.80
FEV_1 (L)	3.15	1.10	1.50
FEV_1/FVC (%)	79	56	54
Peak flow (L/min)	≃480	≃80	≃150

Two points warrant further clarification. First, the patient's spirometry clearly improved, but the FEV_1/FVC *decreased*, meaning that the FVC improved relatively more than the FEV_1. It is best to look at FVC and FEV_1 independently when checking for a bronchodilator response. Second, the peak flow can only be approximated from spirometric tracings since the steepest slope is difficult to draw and extrapolate for the full 60 sec.

12. Interpretation. Before the use of bronchodilators, all spirometric parameters are markedly reduced. In addition, the ratio of FEV_1 to FVC is only 60% (80% of the predicted ratio), so the patient has moderate-severe airways obstruction.

After the use of bronchodilators, the FVC, FEV_1, and peak flow improved, the $MMF_{25\text{-}75}$ increased only slightly, and the FEV_1/FVC went down. As in the previous problem, this represents a true bronchodilator response, but the FVC increased relatively more than the FEV_1. These results are consistent with the clinical diagnosis of bronchial asthma.

13. Interpretation. Before the use of bronchodilators, there is a slight decrease in FEV_1/FVC compared to the minimal predicted amount of 75%. Also, the $MMF_{25\text{-}75}$ is reduced. This study indicates mild airways obstruction, a definite improvement over the study 2 weeks earlier.

    After the use of bronchodilators, the FEV_1/FVC and $MMF_{25\text{-}75}$ both increase to near normal. The patient has essentially recovered from his asthma attack. Although he still demonstrates a bronchodilator response, his impairment is minimal and does not warrant continuation of the medication.

TRUE-FALSE ANSWERS

1. False
2. True
3. False
4. False
5. True
6. False
7. True
8. False
9. True
10. True

CHAPTER 4

1. This patient might be diagnosed as "hyperventilating from anxiety." Unfortunately, this asssessment could be disastrous if, for example, a sedative is ordered and the patient is actually hypoventilating. First, of course, the patient may *not* be moving a lot of air; tidal volume (V_T) is difficult to estimate. More importantly, even if V_T is known and hence the patient's minute ventilation ($f \times V_T$), the status of alveolar ventilation cannot possibly be known since dead space ventilation and carbon dioxide production are unknown. The adequacy of alveolar ventilation can only be assessed by measuring Pa_{CO_2}.

2. The same reasoning used in the first answer holds here. Depth of breathing is difficult to assess clinically. As long as the patient has *some* respiratory movement, one cannot reliably assess alveolar ventilation. Comatose patients may (and frequently do) hyperventilate. If there is a question about adequacy of alveolar ventilation (always the case in comatose patients), Pa_{CO_2} should be checked.

3. b. Pa_{CO_2} 40, $\dot{V}_A$ 8.6, $\dot{V}_{CO_2}$ 400. The Pa_{CO_2} reflects a ratio of carbon dioxide production to alveolar ventilation. If carbon dioxide production goes up (as in a runner), the level of $\dot{V}_A$ will rise to meet it; as a result, the runner increases her minute ventilation, but the *ratio* of $\dot{V}_{CO_2}$ to $\dot{V}_A$ stays the same. Answer *a* makes no sense since the ratio is unchanged but the Pa_{CO_2} is low. Answer *c* is incorrect since Pa_{CO_2}, $\dot{V}_A$ and $\dot{V}_{CO_2}$ sould change during exercise. As for answer *d*, if $\dot{V}_A$ doubles with no change in $\dot{V}_{CO_2}$, then Pa_{CO_2} should be 20 mm Hg, not 40. Finally, in answer *e* the ratio of $\dot{V}_{CO_2}/\dot{V}_A$ is normal, so Pa_{CO_2} should not be elevated.

4. d. The Pa_{CO_2} is neither age-dependent nor sex-dependent, and these characteristics are not in the P_{CO_2} equation. Pregnancy causes hyperventilation, but this is a result of increased $\dot{V}_E$ and a resultant increase in $\dot{V}_A$. Answer c is also incorrect; oxygen consumption is nowhere in the P_{CO_2} equation. Although oxygen consumption and carbon dioxide production both go up in certain states (e.g., exercise), the former does not lead to an elevated Pa_{CO_2}. Minute ventilation could explain differences in Pa_{CO_2} answer e, but since tidal volume and respiratory rate are the same, minute ventilation ($V_T \times f$) is also the same. Thus answer d is the best answer by elimination. More importantly, for the same $\dot{V}_E$ to give different Pa_{CO_2} values, there must be a difference in either $\dot{V}_{CO_2}$ or $\dot{V}_D$.

5. c. It is not necessary to know the level of carbon dioxide production ($\dot{V}_{CO_2}$) to assess if $\dot{V}_A$ is appropriate for the clinical situation. The

$\dot{V}CO_2$ is the numerator of the PCO_2 equation; thus $PaCO_2$ gives the adequacy of $\dot{V}A$ for $\dot{V}CO_2$. It *is* important to know if $\dot{V}A$ is adequate for whatever $\dot{V}CO_2$ the patient has. Whether or not $PaCO_2$ is appropriate for the clinical situation does require knowing the patient's mental status, respiratory pattern, PaO_2, pH. This information is amplified by the answers to the next question.

6. a. The patient is hyperventilating; the low $PaCO_2$ is explained by the appropriate compensation for metabolic acidosis.
   b. The patient has normal alveolar ventilation with respect to the amount of carbon dioxide production, since $PaCO_2$ is in the normal range (38 mm Hg). But given the respiratory effort exerted by the patient, $PaCO_2$ should be lower; i.e., the patient should be hyperventilating. "Normal" $PaCO_2$ in this case is explained by *severe* airways obstruction.
   c. This patient is hypoventilating as defined by the elevated $PaCO_2$. This elevation is compensated for by renal retention of bicarbonate (resulting in near normal pH), and the patient is in no acute distress. In this case hypercapnia is an adaptive mechanism for a patient with severe lung disease; he does not have to work as hard to maintain normal $PaCO_2$.
   d. Despite the appearance of his moving a lot of air, this patient is hypoventilating. What does this tell about the patient's dead space? If the minute ventilation is, in fact, normal or elevated, then dead space ventilation must be quite large.
   e. This patient has normal alveolar ventilation for the amount of carbon dioxide production, but is it appropriate in this situation? No. This low a PaO_2 (40 mm Hg) should elicit a hyperventilation response. Perhaps the patient is also suffering from a drug overdose that affects his central nervous system's drive to breathe. Without knowing the cause of blunted ventilatory response, the clinical picture is insufficient to explain the $PaCO_2$; more information is needed.

In summary, $PaCO_2$ in the normal range indicates only that alveolar ventilation is adequate for carbon dioxide production. It does not mean that the level of alveolar ventilation is necessarily good or bad for the patient; this level can only be assessed by explaining $PaCO_2$ in the clinical context. Conversely, a high or low $PaCO_2$ means too little or too much alveolar ventilation, respectively, for carbon dioxide production, but it may also reflect an appropriate clinical response.

7. Alveolar ventilation can be calculated from the PCO_2 equation.

$$\dot{V}_A = \frac{\dot{V}CO_2 \times 0.863}{PaCO_2} = \frac{200 \times 0.862}{80} = 2.16 \text{ L/min}$$

This result is approximately half the normal $\dot{V}A$. Since she is breathing 10 times/min, each breath is delivering approximately 216 ml to the gas-exchanging alveoli. Assuming an anatomic dead space of 150 ml, this would give a tidal volume of approximately 366 ml and a minute ventilation of 3.66 L. The sleeping pills have led to a reduction of $\dot{V}E$ and an inadequate $\dot{V}A$ for her $\dot{V}CO_2$.

8. In this patient $\dot{V}E$ is fixed at 700 cc/breath $\times$ 10 breaths/min, or 7 L/min. With a fixed $\dot{V}E$, $\dot{V}A$ depends on $\dot{V}D$. If there is no change in the pulmonary condition, $\dot{V}D$ (and hence $\dot{V}A$) should remain steady.

$$\dot{V}_A = \frac{200 \text{ ml/min} \times 0.863}{38 \text{ mm hg}} = 4.54 \text{ L}$$

Since $\dot{V}A$ is fixed, the new $PaCO_2$ is easily calculated.

$$PaCO_2 = \frac{300 \text{ ml/min} \times 0.863}{4.54 \text{ L}} = 57 \text{ mm Hg}$$

Several conditions can increase metabolic carbon dioxide production; fever, hyperthyroidism, exercise, and dietary changes are among the most common. When an intubated patient begins to receive hyperalimentation, carbon dioxide production can increase significantly; if $\dot{V}_A$ is limited or fixed, Pa_{CO_2} will also increase. This scenario has been well documented in critically ill, intubated patients.

9. This patient's $\dot{V}_E$ is 550 × 16 = 8.8 L/minute, slightly above normal. As explained previously, hypercapnia is caused by decreased $\dot{V}_A$ for carbon dioxide production. Note that even if carbon dioxide production is increased, $\dot{V}_A$ is *still* reduced. However, since the patient is at rest, his $\dot{V}_{CO_2}$ is likely normal. Since each tidal volume (V_T) breath is 550 ml, the explanation for hypercapnia must be that a larger percent of V_T is going to dead space. The result is reduced $\dot{V}_A$ despite the elevated $\dot{V}_E$. This is the explanation for hypercapnia in most COPD patients.

10. Based on her history and a prior pulmonary function study, this patient does not have chronic lung disease. The major changes have been a weight gain of 120 lbs over 12 months, a chest x-ray film suggesting congestive heart failure, and the onset of hypercapnia. The elevated Pa_{CO_2} must be a result of decreased $\dot{V}_E$, increased $\dot{V}_D$, or both.

    Her current tidal volume (300 ml) and respiratory rate (28) give a $\dot{V}_E$ of 8.4 L/min, less than half that of a year earlier. Considering her massive obesity and consequent increased carbon dioxide production, 8.4 L/minute is a low value; hence $\dot{V}_A$ is reduced, at least in part, for this reason.

    The low tidal volume also means that the proportion of each breath going to dead space is increased (increased V_D/V_T). Since her respiratory rate is now higher than it was a year earlier, her $\dot{V}_D$ is also increased.

    In summary, she has both physiologic reasons for hypercapnia: decreased $\dot{V}_E$ and increased $\dot{V}_D$. Clinically, they are related to her massive obesity (with impairment of chest bellows) and her congestive heart failure.

11. Answer: $V_D/V_T = 56 - 26/56 = 0.54$. This is a very high V_D/V_T and suggests that early weaning from the ventilator may be difficult. The higher the V_D/V_T is, the more air that has to be inhaled to satisfy $\dot{V}_A$ and the greater the work of breathing. A high V_D/V_T might make the difference between successful weaning and prolonged artificial ventilation, especially if there are other complicating problems (e.g., chest muscle weakness and electrolyte imbalance).

12. The Pa_{CO_2}s resulting from a 1 L/min decrease in $\dot{V}_A$ can be charted from Fig. 4-3 or calculated from the P_{CO_2} equation,

$$Pa_{CO_2} = \frac{\dot{V}_{CO_2} \times 0.863}{\dot{V}_A}$$

Patient A will increase Pa_{CO_2} 5.5 mm Hg, to 34.5 mm Hg; patient B will increase Pa_{CO_2} almost 29 mm Hg, to 86.3 mm Hg. The same net decrease in $\dot{V}_A$ has a greater effect on P_{CO_2} in hypercapnic patients than in patients with normal or reduced P_{CO_2}.

Note that a rise in $\dot{V}_{CO_2}$, when $\dot{V}_A$ is fixed, will also result in increased Pa_{CO_2} (see Fig. 4-3). This increase can occur during exercise in patients with severe COPD and in artificially ventilated patients receiving a sudden increase in carbohydrate load (see Problem 8). In such cases $\dot{V}_{CO_2}$ rises, but $\dot{V}_E$ and $\dot{V}_A$ are not able to rise proportionately; as a result Pa_{CO_2} goes up, again demonstrating the fundamental reason for all clinical hypercapnia—a level of alveolar ventilation that is inadequate for carbon dioxide production.

TRUE-FALSE ANSWERS

1. False
2. True
3. True
4. False
5. True
6. False
7. True
8. True
9. False
10. True

Answers to clinical problems 333

CHAPTER 5

1. More information is needed. With an FIO_2 of 0.21 at sea level, a PaO_2 of 90 mm Hg is normal. This PaO_2 at higher FIO_2s would not be normal. In a patient receiving 100% inspired oxygen, a PaO_2 of 90 mm Hg would indicate severe respiratory failure. Only by comparing PaO_2 against PAO_2 can one know if the lungs are transferring oxygen properly.

2. The adequacy of oxygen transfer is to be determined. In each case $PaO_2 = 85$ mm Hg. Values are at sea level where barometric pressure = 760 mm Hg. For each example, calculate $P(A-a)O_2$.

   a. $PAO_2 = 0.21 (760 - 47) - 1.2 (25)$
   $= 150 - 30 = 120$ mm Hg
   $P(A-a)O_2 = 120 - 85 = 35$ mm Hg

   This is an elevated $P(A-a)O_2$; the lungs are not transferring oxygen properly.

   b. $PAO_2 = 102$ mm Hg (calculated as above)
   $P(A-a)O_2 = 17$ mm Hg

   This is a borderline elevated value; the patient may have a slight pulmonary problem.

   c. $PAO_2 = 90$ mm Hg
   $P(A-a)O_2 = 5$ mm Hg

   Despite hypercapnia, there is no impairment in oxygen transfer from the alveoli into the blood.

   d. $PaO_2 = 0.40 (713) - 1.2(30)$
   $= 285 - 36 = 249$ mm Hg
   $P(A-a)O_2 = 164$ mm Hg

   $P(A-a)O_2$ is markedly elevated. Although PaO_2 is adequate, there is definite impairment of lung oxygen transfer.

3. a, c, e, f. Elevated PCO_2 (b) does not, per se, increase $P(A-a)O_2$ since both PAO_2 and PaO_2 will be decreased the same amount. Anemia (d) and carbon monoxide (h) have no direct effect on either PAO_2 or PaO_2. High altitude (g) lowers both PAO_2 and PaO_2 because of decreased barometric pressure.

4. a. $PAO_2 = 0.40 (760-47) - 1.2 (50)$
   $= 225$ mm Hg
   $P(A-a)O_2 = 225 - 150 = 75$ mm Hg

   Because the $P(A-a)O_2$ is elevated this patient most likely has lung disease.

   b. $PAO_2 = 0.28 (713) - 1.2 (75)$
   $= 200 - 90 = 110$ mg Hg
   $P(A-a)O_2 = 110 - 95 = 15$ mm Hg

   Despite severe hypoventilation, there is no evidence for lung disease. Hypercapnia is most likely a result of disease involving the central nervous system or chest bellows.

   c. $PAO_2 = 0.21(713) - 1.2(15)$
   $= 150 - 18 = 132$ mm Hg
   $P(A-a)O_2 = 132-120 = 12$ mm Hg

   Hyperventilation can easily raise PaO_2 above 100 mm Hg when the lungs are normal as in this case.

   d. $PAO_2 = 0.80(713) - 40 = 530$ mm Hg

   (Note that the factor 1.2 is dropped since FIO_2 is close to 100%.)

   $P(A-a)O_2 = 530 - 350 = 180$ mm Hg

   Despite very high PaO_2, the lungs are not transferring oxygen normally.

   e. $PAO_2 = 0.21(713) - 1.2(72)$
   $= 150 - 80 = 64$ mm Hg
   $P(A-a)O_2 = 64 - 80 = -16$ mm Hg

   A negative $P(A-a)O_2$ is incompatible with life. This is a not uncommon laboratory result and can be explained by: (1) incorrect FIO_2; (2) incorrect blood gas measurement; (3) transcription error.

5. Calculate PAO_2, using the barometric pressure for Leadville (Table 5-2).

   $PAO_2 = 0.21(517 - 47) - 1.2(27)$
   $= 99 - 32 = 67$ mm Hg

Then,

$$P(A-a)O_2 = 67 - 40 = 27 \text{ mm Hg}$$

Even though PaO_2 is much lower in Leadville than at sea level, the $P(A-a)O_2$ is elevated at 27 mm Hg, indicating a problem with oxygen transfer, i.e., V/Q imbalance. This patient was suffering from altitude-induced pulmonary edema.

6. During hemodialysis with an acetate bath, carbon dioxide diffuses out of the blood and into the dialysate bath. You are asked to calculate PaO_2 during dialysis, when $P(A-a)O_2$, $PaCO_2$, and pH remain the same and when 50 ml of carbon dioxide enters the dialysate per minute. The PaO_2 can be calculated by first determining $P(A-a)O_2$ before and during dialysis; to do this correctly, use the actual R values and the long form of the alveolar air equation:

Before dialysis

$$R = \frac{200}{250} = 0.80$$

$$P_{AO_2} = 0.21(713) - 38\left[0.21 + \frac{(1 - 0.21)}{0.80}\right]$$

$$= 150 - 46 = 104 \text{ mm Hg}$$

$$P(A-a)O_2 = 103 - PaO_2 \text{ (measured)}$$

$$= 104 - 84 = 20 \text{ mm Hg}$$

During dialysis

$$R = \frac{150}{250} = 0.60$$

$$P_{AO_2} = 0.21(713) - 38\left[0.21 + \frac{(1 - 0.21)}{0.60}\right]$$

$$= 150 - 58 = 92 \text{ mm Hg}$$

$$P(A-a)O_2 = 20 \text{ mm Hg (same as before dialysis)}$$

$$PaO_2 = P_{AO_2} - P(A-a)O_2$$

$$= 92 - 20 = 72 \text{ mm Hg}$$

Thus the PaO_2 falls from 84 to 72, a difference of 12 mm Hg, during dialysis.

7. $P_{AO_2} = 0.21(713) - 1.2(74)$
   $= 150 - 89 = 61 \text{ mm Hg}$
   $P(A-a)O_2 = 61 - 42 = 19 \text{ mm Hg}$

Since $P(A-a)O_2$ is in the normal range for a 73-year-old woman, it can be assumed PaO_2 is reduced from hypercapnia. It is likely she does not have pneumonia or any other acute pulmonary problem.

8. Although increased $P(A-a)O_2$ is almost always caused by V/Q imbalance, it is often a challenge to explain how the imbalance leads to venous admixture. This patient developed worsening hypoxemia while lying on his right side—the side with pneumonia. Since blood flow is gravity-dependent, there is increased blood flow to the right lung while that lung is dependent. Although ventilation is also influenced by gravity, ventilation is reduced to the right lung because of the pneumonia. Thus the blood flow is increased relative to the ventilation, resulting in increased venous admixture.

When the patient lies on his left side, there is increased blood flow to his normal lung and decreased blood flow to the diseased lung. The result is less venous admixture than when the right lung is dependent.

Because of the effect of gravity on perfusion, it is generally recommended that adults with hypoxemia from unilateral lung disease keep their diseased lung dependent. However, the opposite is recommended in infants (see Chapter 15).

9. Pulmonary embolism commonly causes hypoxemia. The mechanism is V/Q imbalance—but exactly how? A blood clot in the pulmonary artery should lead to decreased perfusion to a large group of alveoli, converting the alveolar space to dead space. Increased dead space alone should *not* cause hypoxemia. Furthermore, the fact that patients suffering from pulmonary embolism classically *hyperventilate* indicates adequate compensation for the

increased dead space. Instead, hypoxemia must be caused by increased venous admixture, i.e., shunting or low V/Q ratios. There are at least two possible mechanisms by which this increase in venous admixture may occur.
1. Blood is shunted away from the clotted vessel(s) to the nonembolized circulation. This rerouted blood flow exceeds the oxygenation capacity of the alveoli serving the nonembolized circulation. The result is the *overperfusion* of normal alveolar-capillary units creating units with low V/Q ratios, and hence an increase in venous admixture.
2. The pulmonary clot causes local release of kinins and other peptides that affect the architecture of surrounding alveolar-capillary units. As a result, normal V/Q units are converted to low V/Q units, either by localized atelectasis or by bronchoconstriction, and alveolar ventilation is decreased relative to perfusion.

There is experimental evidence for the occurrence of both mechanisms in pulmonary embolism, and both likely play a role clinically. The main point is that hypoxemia manifested by increased $P(A - a)O_2$ is invariably caused by V/Q imbalance and therefore represents a pulmonary problem. Regardless of the clinical setting, an understanding of basic pulmonary physiology should help explain the mechanism.

TRUE-FALSE ANSWERS

1. False
2. True
3. True
4. True
5. True
6. False
7. False
8. False
9. True
10. True

CHAPTER 6

1. Arterial oxygen content =
$$(0.98 \times 15 \times 1.34) + (0.003 \times 92)$$
$$= 19.7 + 0.28$$
$$= \frac{19.98 \text{ ml } O_2}{100 \text{ ml blood}}$$

2. Calculate the oxygen content of each patient.

Patient A:

$0.85 \times 1.34 \times 15 + (0.003 \times 50) =$
$17.09 + 0.15 = 17.24$ ml O_2/100 ml blood

Patient B:

$0.94 \times 1.34 \times 8 + (0.003 \times 80) =$
$10.08 + 0.24 = 10.32$ ml O_2/100 ml blood

Based on oxygen content, Patient B is more hypoxemic despite having a much higher PaO_2 than patient A. This result illustrates the importance of hemoglobin and of not relying solely on PaO_2 and SaO_2 in assessing oxygenation.

3. b. This patient has a normal PaO_2 but a markedly reduced SaO_2. The most common cause of such a disparity is that something is preventing oxygen from binding to hemoglobin; *carbon monoxide must be considered the cause until proved otherwise.* None of the other situations will explain such a disparity. Anemia does not affect the SaO_2 for a given PaO_2. Hypothermia shifts the oxygen dissociation curve to the left and would therefore *elevate* the SaO_2 for a given PaO_2. Severe parenchymal lung disease can reduce SaO_2 only by the reduction of the PaO_2; it does not cause a disparity between the two values. Finally, of course, these blood gas values are not normal for any age.

4. b. The oxygen content is calculated as in Clinical Problem 1:

Oxygen content = $(0.50 \times 1.34 \times 13) +$
$(0.003 \times 85) = 8.97$ ml O_2/100 ml blood
(or 9.0 when rounded off)

Again note that the PaO_2 is normal in carbon monoxide poisoning but that SaO_2 and oxygen content are reduced.

5. The PaO_2 is 85 mm Hg and the SaO_2 is 60%; the latter measurement is much reduced from the expected SaO_2 of more than 95%. Since

the pH and the $Paco_2$ are normal, it is likely that something is preventing the normal saturation of hemoglobin. This blood gas result could represent either methemoglobinemia, severe carbon monoxide poisoning, or, alternatively, a genetically altered hemoglobin.

Normally, almost all adult hemoglobin is in the reduced state, whether or not combined with oxygen, since the reduced state refers only to the fact that iron is Fe^{++}. When iron is Fe^{+++}, the hemoglobin is said to be oxidized (*not* oxyhemoglobin); hemoglobin containing Fe^{+++} is methemoglobin, and is unable to carry oxygen.

The 60% of hemoglobin that is saturated with oxygen is *oxyhemoglobin* (reduced, Fe^{++}). Normal hemoglobin not combined with oxygen is *deoxygenated* (reduced, Fe^{++}); this deoxygenated hemoglobin most commonly is a result of a reduced Pao_2, which is not a problem here. The 40% of the hemoglobin that is not saturated with oxygen may represent *carboxyhemoglobin* (Fe^{++} combined with carbon monoxide), methemoglobin (Fe^{+++}), or hemoglobin of an abnormal amino acid sequence that has an extremely high P_{50}.

Cyanosis is present if the 40% of unoxygenated hemoglobin is either methemoglobin (Fe^{+++}) or normal hemoglobin (reduced, Fe^{++}); there will be no cyanosis if it is carboxyhemoglobin.

6. Oxygen delivery equals cardiac output times oxygen content

= 5000 ml blood/min × 8.97 ml O_2/100 ml blood
= 448.5 ml O_2/min

Oxygen delivery is reduced solely because of a reduction in Sao_2 (causing reduced Cao_2); the cardiac output is normal. In carbon monoxide poisoning, reduced oxygen delivery is one of two major causes of hypoxia; the other is a leftward shift of the oxygen dissociation curve. As a result of the leftward shift, oxygen that is bound to hemoglobin is held more tightly than normal and is not released to the tissues as readily.

7. Oxygen uptake ($\dot{V}o_2$) equals cardiac output times ($Cao_2 - Cvo_2$) (Equation 3). The cardiac output is given (5.2 L/min). From the information provided, Cao_2 and Cvo_2 need to be calculated. Since only the Pao_2 is provided, the standard oxygen dissociation curve is used to calculate the Sao_2. At a pH of 7.5 and a Pao_2 of 80 mm Hg, Sao_2 is 94%. Hence,

Cao_2 = (0.94 × 15 × 1.34) +
(0.003 × 80) = 9.13 ml O_2/100 ml blood

Since the Pvo_2 is not given the same oxygen dissociation curve is used to work backward to calculate the Pvo_2; an Svo_2 of 75% at pH 7.5 gives a Pvo_2 of approximately 38 mm Hg. Hence,

Cvo_2 = (0.75 × 15 × 1.34) +
(0.003 × 38) = 15.19 ml O_2/100 ml blood

and

$\dot{V}o_2$ = 5200 × (19.13 − 15.19) =
205 ml O_2/min

8. $\dot{V}o_2 = QT \times (Cao_2 - Cvo_2)$

$$(Cao_2 - Cvo_2) = \frac{\dot{V}o_2}{QT} = \frac{250 \text{ ml } O_2/\text{min}}{7500 \text{ ml blood/min}} = 3.33 \text{ ml } O_2/100 \text{ ml blood}$$

This patient has arterial hypoxemia which can be appreciated from the calculation of the Cao_2:

Cao_2 = (6 gm% Hgb × 1.34 $\frac{\text{ml } O_2}{\text{gm Hgb}}$ ×
0.97) + (0.003 × 125)
= 7.80 ml O_2/100 ml blood +
0.38 ml O_2/100 ml blood
= 8.18 ml O_2/100 ml blood

The major compensation for arterial hypoxemia is increased cardiac output.

9. a. $\dot{V}O_2 = QT \times (CaO_2 - CvO_2)$ (Equation 3).

$$(CaO_2 - CvO_2) = \frac{250 \text{ ml } O_2/\text{min}}{5000 \text{ ml blood/min}} = 5 \text{ ml } O_2/100 \text{ ml blood}$$

At sea level, a 30-year-old patient breathing room air with normal lungs should have a PaO_2 above 90 mm Hg and an SaO_2 of approximately 97%. Thus

$CaO_2 = (0.97 \times 1.34 \times 15) + (0.003 \times 90) = 19.77$ ml O_2/100 ml blood

$CvO_2 = 19.77 - 5 = 14.77$ ml O_2/100 ml blood

$CvO_2 = (SvO_2 \times 1.34 \times Hgb) + (0.003 \times PvO_2)$

$$SvO_2 = \frac{CvO_2 - (0.003 \times PvO_2)}{(1.34 \times Hgb)}$$

For this calculation, ignore $(0.003 \times PvO_2)$ since it is a very small number. Hence,

$$SvO_2 = \frac{14.77}{20.1} = 0.73 \text{ (or 73\%)}$$

Using the arterial oxygen dissociation curve, an SvO_2 of 73% gives a PvO_2 of approximately 39 mm Hg. Since venous pH is more acidic than arterial pH, an SvO_2 of 73% will actually give a PvO_2 slightly higher than 39 mm Hg.

b. Perform the calculations in 9a, using a cardiac output of 2.5 L/min.

$(CaO_2 - CvO_2) = 10$ ml O_2/100 ml blood
$CvO_2 = 9.5$ ml O_2/100 ml blood
$SvO_2 = 47\%$
$PvO_2 = 26$ mm Hg (approximate)

c. Calculate PaO_2, using FIO_2 of 1.00. Since it is assumed the patient has normal lungs, the alveolar PO_2 will be approximately 673 mm Hg and the PaO_2, approximately 650 mm Hg. (This assumes a $P(A-a)O_2$ of 23 mm Hg; $P(A-a)O_2$ increases when 100% oxygen is breathed, see Chapter 5.) The SaO_2 will be 100% at this PaO_2. Performing the same calculation as in 9a,

$$SvO_2 = \frac{17.05}{20.10} = 0.85, \text{ or } 85\%$$

At this SvO_2, the PvO_2 is approximately 50 mm Hg.

d. If hemoglobin content is 8 gm%, then the CaO_2 equals 10.45 ml O_2/100 ml blood. Performing the calculation as in 9a,

$$SvO_2 = \frac{5.45}{1.34 \times 8} = 0.51, \text{ or } 51\%$$

From the dissociation curve, $PvO_2 = 27$ mm Hg (approximate).

Physiologic adjustments, especially increased cardiac output, are made to prevent severe hypoxemia in anemia. For this reason, the PvO_2 is usually normal in chronic anemia.

10. The PaO_2 and the SaO_2 appear adequate before and after dobutamine therapy, although the CaO_2 is slightly reduced. However, both SvO_2 and PvO_2 are much lower than one might expect knowing only the arterial measurements. The reduced mixed venous values reflect an inadequate oxygen delivery for the body's needs; this inadequacy in turn is a result of a reduced cardiac output.

After dobutamine therapy, the cardiac output increased. As a result, oxygen delivery improved, resulting in significantly higher SvO_2 and PvO_2.

This case represents an example of how assessment of overall oxygenation may require sophisticated measurements, including those for cardiac output and for mixed venous oxygen saturation. Without such measurements, the PaO_2 and the SaO_2 could have given false reassurance about this patient's state of oxygenation.

TRUE-FALSE ANSWERS

1. False 6. True
2. False 7. True
3. False 8. True
4. True   9. True
5. True   10. False

CHAPTER 7

1. This patient was admitted with dehydration and cellulitis. Her serum HCO_3^- was elevated on all 3 hospital days, indicating a definite acid-base disorder. As an isolated finding, elevated HCO_3^- suggests primary metabolic alkalosis or compensation for respiratory acidosis.

    Blood gas measurements were not obtained until the third hospital day. They revealed a pH of 7.20, a $Paco_2$ of 92 mm Hg, and a HCO_3^- of 35 mEq/L.

    In retrospect, when admitted she had an undiagnosed *respiratory acidosis;* the clue was a high HCO_3^- that was present on day 1. Meperidine and diazepam further depressed her breathing and worsened her carbon dioxide retention to the point of decompensation on day 3. This patient required intubation and artificial ventilation and eventually recovered.

2. There is a 10 mEq/L discrepancy between the calculated and the measured HCO_3^-. To the extent that the pH and the $Paco_2$ are correct, so is the calculated HCO_3^-. Of course either the pH or the $Paco_2$ may be incorrect; if so, the HCO_3^- will also be incorrect. In this patient, the blood gas values suggest a state of metabolic alkalosis (elevated HCO_3^-); the venous HCO_3^- is normal and therefore does not agree with the blood gas results. Possible reasons for this difference are outlined in the box on p. 133.

    In the event of such discrepancy, both the blood gas results *and* the serum HCO_3^- cannot be accepted. If the $Paco_2$ and the pH are believed, the calculated arterial HCO_3^- should also be believed, and the venous HCO_3^- should be ignored.

3. Assume the venous bicarbonate and the arterial bicarbonate are equal. Calculate the venous bicarbonate:

    $$\text{Anion gap} = Na^+ - (Cl^- + HCO_3^-)$$
    $$20 \text{ mEq/L} = 145 - (104 + HCO_3^-)$$
    $$HCO_3^- = 21 \text{ mEq/L}$$

    Then

    $$pH = 6.1 + \log \frac{21}{0.03(50)} = 7.25$$

4. Acute CO_2 retention leads to reduced pH, a state of acute respiratory acidosis. However, is it *only* acute respiratory acidosis, or is there some other process present? Acute CO_2 retention causes a drop in pH of approximately 0.07 units for every 10 mm Hg increase in $Paco_2$. The patient's pH is down 0.26, or 0.05 more than is expected for a 30 mm Hg increase in $Paco_2$, suggesting an additional, metabolic problem.

    In addition the calculated HCO_3^- is low normal. With acute CO_2 retention, the HCO_3^- should be raised 2 to 3 mEq/L. A low-normal HCO_3^- is another piece of evidence to suggest an additional metabolic disorder. Decreased vascular perfusion leading to mild lactic acidosis would explain the metabolic component.

5. The HCO_3^- and the pH are low, suggesting a state of metabolic acidosis. With fully compensated metabolic acidosis, the $Paco_2$ should be reduced. The fact that the $Paco_2$ is low normal suggests two possibilities. Either the metabolic acidosis is early in its development (less than 12 hours since its onset) or it is chronic and the patient is unable to hyperventilate for compensation. The latter case represents a state of *relative respiratory acidosis* since the inability to lower the $Paco_2$ contributes to the acidemia (pH would be higher if $Paco_2$ were lower). The latter situation is also more ominous since it indicates a respiratory disorder in addition to the metabolic problem.

    Only by detailed clinical evaluation and fol-

low-up can one decide between the two possible mechanisms.
6. The patient's blood gas values fall into the band of chronic respiratory acidosis. Considering the patient's history, he has likely been retaining carbon dioxide for several days. (However, the acid-base map cannot diagnose chronic respiratory acidosis definitively; there is more than one way to arrive at a particular point on the acid-base map.)
7. The young woman's blood gas values fall into the band of acute respiratory acidosis. She has retained carbon dioxide acutely, probably for less than several hours. This retention is often seen in drug overdose, although several other clinical causes are possible. Since she is comatose and severely hypoventilating, intubation and artificial ventilation are required.
8. Part A. d., indeterminate without more information. If, based on blood gas values and other laboratory data, an acid-base disorder is found, the next logical step is to determine the clinical cause(s). Elevated Pa_{CO_2}, pH, and HCO_3^- certainly suggest metabolic alkalosis, but there are other possibilities. Isolated blood gas values should be viewed as one point, on a two-dimensional plot, that can be arrived at from various pathways and not as diagnostic of any particular acid-base disorder. Diagnosing metabolic alkalosis solely on the basis of blood gas values has two potential pitfalls:
   1. Using blood gas values alone is clinically insufficient since there are several causes of metabolic alkalosis; the *clinical cause* has to be found and corrected. Acidosis and alkalosis, with their adjectives metabolic and respiratory, are analagous to "anemia" or "fever." As physiologic changes, they are manifestations of an underlying clinical problem and not clinical diagnoses in themselves.
   2. The patient may in fact *not* have metabolic alkalosis or may have metabolic alkalosis *plus* another serious acid-base disorder.

This patient's initial blood gas values represent several clinical possibilities—simple metabolic alkalosis, chronic respiratory acidosis followed by acute hyperventilation (acute respiratory alkalosis), and respiratory acidosis complicated by metabolic alkalosis. For example, suppose the patient's pulmonary function tests and blood gas values were normal one week earlier and in the interval the patient had taken diuretics; a *primary metabolic alkalosis* would then be the most likely diagnosis. On the other hand, he could be a patient with chronic CO_2 retention, e.g., a Pa_{CO_2} of 60 mm Hg and a pH of 7.41, who then develops pneumonia, which causes a lowering of the Pa_{CO_2} from 60 to 50 mm Hg and a rise in pH above normal. This last scenario would reflect a state of chronic respiratory acidosis plus an acute increase in ventilation (respiratory alkalosis), not a primary metabolic alkalosis. Thus the patient could have either a metabolic problem alone, a respiratory problem alone, or both. *Only by the use of a detailed clinical and laboratory history (including previous blood gas data if available) can the actual cause be determined.*

Part B. The clinical history for this patient included chronic obstructive pulmonary disease and CO_2 retention. Subsequently he developed heart failure. After receiving treatment he returned to his baseline blood gas values. In retrospect, his blood gas values on admission were the result of acute hyperventilation and chronic respiratory acidosis.

9. d. A patient suffering from severe vomiting (causing metabolic alkalosis) as well as uremia (causing metabolic acidosis) can have both metabolic disorders at the same time. This patient has renal failure, with a blood urea nitrogen value of 121 mg%. The presence of metabolic acidosis is confirmed by the elevated anion gap (25 mEq/L) even though the pH is alkaline at 7.51.

From the information provided, one cannot completely rule out a primary respiratory acidosis as an additional problem. (After this patient recovered, he showed no evidence of underlying lung disease. Sometimes it requires days or weeks of follow-up to fully characterize acid base disorders.)

With multiple disorders, the resulting pH can be *low, high* or *normal,* depending on the relative severity of each process. An isolated blood gas analysis does not diagnose or separate the different conditions; they can only be discerned by knowing the patient's detailed history and clinical course, including other laboratory data.

10. This patient's blood gas values fall into the band of chronic respiratory alkalosis. However, this information does not provide the diagnosis for the disorder but only suggests the possibilities. Diagnosis must be made in conjunction with the clinical picture, plus other laboratory studies. Could she have a mixed problem—respiratory alkalosis plus metabolic acidosis?

    Calculating her anion gap,

    $$AG = Na^+ - (Cl^- + HCO_3^-) = 142 - 118 = 24 \text{ mEq/L}.$$

    This is an elevated AG, indicating a metabolic acidosis. However, it is not *just* metabolic acidosis since the blood gas values fall way outside the band for that disorder. There is good evidence she has *both* metabolic acidosis *and* respiratory alkalosis. The latter is probably a result of excessive artificial ventilation. The cause of metabolic acidosis must be looked for since it is not apparent from the information provided. Since the AG is elevated, the possibilities include lactic acidosis from hypoperfusion or drug-induced metabolic acidosis (see box on p. 136).

11. This patient initially had chronic respiratory alkalosis, resulting from several days of hyperventilation, during which time her kidneys had a chance to excrete bicarbonate and return the pH toward normal. Now her asthmatic condition has worsened; plotting both sets of blood gas values on the acid-base map shows that she has acutely *hypoventilated*. The second set of blood gas values falls between the bands of acute respiratory acidosis and metabolic acidosis.

    She has only "apparent" metabolic acidosis because her problems are really respiratory—initial respiratory alkalosis (with renal compensation) followed by acute respiratory acidosis. The distinction is important. Treatment is for respiratory processes, not metabolic ones. Adequate ventilation must be restored either by intubation or by other aggressive respiratory treatment. She does not have a primary metabolic process.

    This case shows how the acid-base map can be used to rule out a primary disorder as the sole cause of a patient's disturbance. It should also reinforce the idea that acid-base maps do not diagnose acid-base disorders. Diagnosis is properly completed only after full clinical and laboratory evaluation, including arterial blood gas analysis.

12. Plotting his blood gas values on the acid-base map reveals that the patient has more than a respiratory acidosis. The gases fall way outside the expected band for acute respiratory acidosis; the patient also has metabolic acidosis. If acute respiratory acidosis were the only process, a pH of 7.2, not 7.1, would be expected. In this patient the elevated anion gap helps confirm a metabolic acidosis. He has two reasons for metabolic acidosis—shock and severe hypoxemia. After being intubated, he is ventilated down to a "normal" Pa_{CO_2} of 40 mm Hg, yet remains acidemic because his metabolic process (lactic acidosis) has not been corrected. The last set of blood gas values still shows metabolic and respiratory acidosis, although to a lesser extent than was shown initially.

Answers to clinical problems

TRUE-FALSE ANSWERS
1. False
2. True
3. True
4. False
5. True
6. True
7. True
8. False
9. True
10. False

CHAPTER 8

1. This is a case of severe cor pulmonale and right-sided heart failure. The presence of lung disease, arterial hypoxemia, right ventricular enlargement, pulmonary artery enlargement (seen on the chest x-ray), right ventricular strain pattern (seen on ECG), increased second heart sound (pulmonic valve closure), and absence of pulmonary infiltrates (ruling out left ventricular congestive heart failure), all secure this diagnosis *without the need for invasive measurements*. Appropriate treatment is low supplemental oxygen therapy (see Chapter 9) and diuretics.

2. d. The dry skin, normal chest x-ray, and low blood pressure (with postural changes) all point to severe dehydration. In this patient serum electrolyte measurements helped confirm dehydration, showing low serum sodium and potassium concentration. The cause of the dehydration was nausea and vomiting for 1 to 2 days, presumably related to excessive alcoholic intake.

   In such an obvious case, hemodynamic monitoring by invasive methods is not indicated. Proper treatment is the administration of intravenous fluids, with careful monitoring of urine output, mental status, serum electrolytes, and vital signs. Only if there is no improvement or if treatment causes intractable heart failure will hemodynamic monitoring be indicated.

3. Based on the information provided, *all* listed diagnoses are possible. However, the most likely diagnoses are ARDS and cardiogenic shock. The patient's chest x-ray shows pulmonary edema, which could be caused by leaky pulmonary capillaries (ARDS) or left-sided heart failure. In someone who has suffered trauma and major surgery and who has received copious intravenous fluids, either condition is distinctly possible.

   For the proper management the patient's cardiac output and pulmonary artery wedge pressure should be measured. Obtaining the information requires bedside cardiac catheterization.

4. $$\text{Cardiac index} = \frac{3.1 \text{ L/min}}{1.8 \text{ m}^2} = 1.72 \text{ L/min/m}^2$$

   $$\text{Stroke volume} = \frac{3100 \text{ ml/min}}{120 \text{ beats/min}} = 26 \text{ ml/beat}$$

   $$\text{Stroke index} = \frac{26 \text{ ml/beat}}{1.8 \text{ m}^2} = 14 \text{ ml/beat/m}^2$$

   $$\text{SVR} = \frac{(66 - 5) \text{ mm Hg}}{3.1 \text{ L/min}} = 20 \text{ mm Hg/L/min}$$

   $$\text{PVR} = \frac{(31 - 24) \text{ mm Hg}}{3.1 \text{ L/min}} = 2.26 \text{ mm Hg/L/min}$$

   (Note that since a mixed venous oxygen measurement was not obtained, % shunt and oxygen uptake are not calculated.)

   This patient is suffering from cardiogenic shock—inadequate systemic perfusion caused by low cardiac output. Both the stroke volume and the stroke index are very low. The increased heart rate cannot make up for the small amount of blood that is pumped with each heartbeat. The patient is hypotensive because of the inadequate cardiac output, and as partial compensation, the systemic vascular resistance is increased. Pulmonary vascular resistance is within the normal range, indicating that the increased pulmonary artery pressure is caused by left-sided heart failure. From the data presented, there is no evidence of right-sided heart failure in this patient.

5. Patient A. Both PAP and PAWP are normal, and PAWP is the same as PAP; if necessary, diastolic PAP could be monitored as a guide to left-sided pressures in lieu of PAWP.

Patient B. PAP is elevated and PAWP is normal, a pattern often seen with severe chronic lung disease. When PAWP is normal, pulmonary hypertension cannot be attributed to left-sided heart failure. Because of the disparity in the two measurements, diastolic PAP cannot be used to reflect PAWP.

Patient C. Both PAP and PAWP are increased; since both pressures are almost the same, the elevated PAP is likely caused by the increase in left-sided heart pressures and not from lung disease per se. In such cases one cannot reliably monitor PAWP by measuring only diastolic PAP since the latter may not change in tandem with PAWP.

6. The PAWP provides information on both the pulmonary capillary hydrostatic pressure and the left heart filling pressure. You are asked to interpret PAWP in relation to capillary hydrostatic pressure and to assess the latter's role in pulmonary edema.

Patient A is hypotensive, with a low PAWP and a normal serum albumin level. In this case pulmonary edema is unlikely to be caused by hydrostatic or oncotic forces. Pulmonary edema in the face of a low PAWP and normal oncotic pressure is the picture of the adult respiratory distress syndrome (discussed in Chapter 11).

Patient B is normotensive, with a serum albumin level slightly below normal. The PAWP is definitely elevated and is likely the major, if not sole, physiologic mechanism of the patient's pulmonary edema. These findings suggest left-sided congestive heart failure as the cause of the pulmonary edema.

In Patient C the PAWP is elevated above normal but is *not* the sole reason for the pulmonary edema. The serum albumin level is very low, indicating a low serum oncotic pressure. In cases such as this it is difficult to gauge the relative contribution of each factor.

A third factor that can contribute to pulmonary edema is increased capillary permeability, which is discussed in Chapter 11.

7. Patient A has a low PAWP, reflecting a low left ventricular filling pressure (LVEDP). Treatment is the administration of large amounts of intravenous fluids.

Patient B has an elevated PAWP, so the low urine output cannot be attributed to low filling pressure. More likely the elevated PAWP is caused by low cardiac output. Treatment should be directed toward augmenting the cardiac output.

8. This is the picture of septic shock, i.e., hypotension caused by systemic infection. Cardiac output is high, systemic vascular resistance is low, and wedge pressure is normal (Table 8-5). The infiltrates in the patient's lungs are most likely a manifestation of adult respiratory distress syndrome (leaky pulmonary capillaries) and not congestive heart failure. Treatment of her hemodynamic problem includes more intravenous fluids (despite the presence of pulmonary infiltrates) plus appropriate antibiotics.

9. Among other problems, this patient has developed congestive heart failure. The elevated wedge pressure indicates elevated left ventricular end-diastolic pressure and a failing left ventricle. Although his cardiac index is within the normal range, it should be higher to handle the extra volume of fluid the patient has received. Without wedge pressure measurement, one could only use a trial and error method of treatment. Because of the elevated wedge pressure measurement, the patient received diuretics, and his intravenous fluids were restricted. On this regimen the patient slowly improved.

10. 1 PM. Initially the pulmonary arterial pressure (PAP) is elevated, and pulmonary arterial wedge pressure (PAWP) is normal. The patient is hypotensive (95/65), and the cardiac index is at the lower limit of the normal range. Blood gas measurements reflect improvement in both oxygenation and ventilation (compared with those measurements obtained in the emergency room). This is the picture of pulmonary

hypertension caused by an underlying lung disease and/or severe hypoxemia/acidosis. The systemic hypotension is probably caused by dehydration or underhydration; treatment at this point includes intravenous fluids, along with hemodynamic and blood gas monitoring.

3 PM. Two hours later, PAWP is up by 5 mm Hg, and both systemic arterial pressure and cardiac output have increased. PAP is down only slightly, and blood gas measurements have improved. Clearly, intravenous fluids are having a beneficial effect.

11 PM. Blood gas measurements now show a normal pH and adequate oxygenation. PAWP has increased to 16 mm Hg, and cardiac output is well within the normal range, reflecting improvement in left-ventricular filling pressure. PAP is still elevated at 48/24. These changes suggest a picture of pulmonary hypertension caused by an underlying lung disease (and not just transient hypoxemia/acidosis). At this point intravenous fluids can be tapered and consideration can be given to weaning the patient from the ventilator.

TRUE-FALSE ANSWERS

1. False
2. False
3. False
4. True
5. False
6. True
7. False
8. True
9. True
10. True

CHAPTER 9

1. Since virtually no oxygen is stored in the body's tissues, in the absence of breathing, the total oxygen available is the amount in the functional residual capacity (FRC) plus the amount in the blood.

    FRC oxygen supply = 0.21×3 L = 630 ml O_2

    Blood supply oxygen =
    $$\frac{5000 \text{ ml} \times 20 \text{ ml } O_2}{100 \text{ ml}} = 1000 \text{ ml } O_2$$

    Total oxygen supply = 1630 ml O_2

    Since 250 ml O_2 is taken up by the tissues per minute, a little over 3 minutes is needed to use half the oxygen supply. At this point the Pa_{O_2} is critically reduced. Although some adaptive mechanisms come into play (e.g., acidosis causing rightward shift of the oxygen dissociation curve), after 3 to 4 minutes of apnea most patients will manifest some hypoxic organ damage or will have died.

2. a. Although comfortable at rest, this patient is severely hypoxemic. Physiologically he should benefit from supplemental oxygen, especially when he is ambulatory.
    b. This person is also hypoxemic but mainly from severe anemia. Although the Sa_{O_2} is slightly reduced (91%), supplemental oxygen can improve the Sa_{O_2} by no more than a few percent. Generally such a modest improvement does not warrant prescribing supplemental oxygen unless the patient is acutely ill or symptomatic at rest.
    c. Although the Sa_{O_2} is adequate, this patient has pneumonia and is tachypneic; this clinical situation warrants supplemental oxygen.
    d. There is no indication for supplemental oxygen in this patient.
    e. This patient is hypoxemia, hyperventilating, and tachypneic, and she should benefit from supplemental oxygen.

3. All three patients are using nasal oxygen at 2 L/min, but the resulting FI_{O_2} varies because of differences in tidal volume.

    a. A flow rate of 2 L/min equals 33.3 ml/sec and is the amount of 100% oxygen inspired from the nasal cannula.

    50 ml (1.00) + 33.3 ml (1.00) +
    (Anatomic   (nasal cannula
    reservoir   oxygen)
    oxygen)

    216.7 (0.21) = 300 (0.xx)
    (Remaining   (Full tidal
    tidal volume volume
    oxygen)   oxygen)

    $$0.\text{xx} = \frac{128.9}{300} = 0.43$$

b. 50 ml (1.00) + 33.3 ml (1.00) +
$$416.7 (0.21) = 500 (0.xx)$$
$$0.xx = \frac{171.44}{500} = 0.34$$

c. Here the inspiratory time is 1.5 seconds; since 2 L/min equals 33.3 ml/sec, during each breath this patient will inspire 50 ml from the nasal catheter.

50 ml (1.00) + 50 ml (1.00) +
$$500 (0.21) = 600 (0.xx)$$
$$0.xx = \frac{205}{600} = 0.34$$

If this patient kept the same tidal volume (600 ml) but inspired each breath in 1 second, the FIO_2 would be:

50 (1.00) + 33.3 (1.00) +
$$516.7 (0.21) = 600 (0.xx)$$
$$0.xx = \frac{191.81}{600} = 0.32$$

4. Since the FIO_2 is increased, it is unlikely the patient's $PaCO_2$ would decrease. More likely his $PaCO_2$ would rise because of the blunting of the hypoxic breathing stimulus, ruling out answers *c* and *e*. It is also unlikely that the $PaCO_2$ would rise to 62 mm Hg when the PaO_2 is increased by only 3 mm Hg (choice *b*). Answer *a* is unlikely since pH would not increase if the $PaCO_2$ went from 50 to 55 mm Hg.

By this reasoning, the correct answer is *d*. The blood gas values in answer *d* are fully explained by the improvement in oxygenation leading to the raising of the $PaCO_2$ and the reduction of pH.

5. In contrast to oxygen, carbon dioxide is stored in the body, mainly in the form of bicarbonate. For this reason, it takes longer to eliminate the excess carbon dioxide than to use the available oxygen. While the supplemental oxygen was inhaled, excess carbon dioxide was accumulating in the body. When the supplemental oxygen is removed, the PaO_2 will fall *much faster* than the excess carbon dioxide will be excreted.

Although the hypoxic breathing stimulus should eventually cause the patient to hyperventilate, this result can only follow the lowering of the PaO_2. During this period of declining PaO_2, the $PaCO_2$ will remain higher than it was before the supplemental oxygen was given. From the alveolar air equation ($PAO_2 = PIO_2 - PaCO_2$), one can appreciate that the PaO_2 will fall *below* the room air value.

Since the $PaCO_2$ in blood gas value 2 is 12 mm Hg higher than in blood gas value 1, the PaO_2 could well fall 12 mm Hg below the room air value (48 mm Hg), to as low as 36 mm Hg. Eventually, the excess carbon dioxide may be blown off but not before the patient is exposed to a level of hypoxemia more severe than that before the oxygen was inhaled.

Reduction of PaO_2 by this mechanism is the principal physiologic reason why intermittent oxygen therapy is potentially dangerous in patients with chronic carbon dioxide retention.

6. At 2.5 atmospheres, the PO_2 atm is $FIO_2 \times PB$ or:
$$1.00 \times 1900 = 1900 \text{ mm Hg}$$

Alveolar PO_2 (PAO_2) equals:

$FIO_2 \times (PB - 47) - PaCO_2 =$
$$1.00 \times (1900 - 47) - 37 =$$
$$1816 \text{ mm Hg}$$

Assuming the patient has healthy lungs, the PaO_2 should be above 1700 mm Hg. The SaO_2 would be 1.00 if there was no carboxyhemoglobin present. Since HbCO = 4%,
$$SaO_2 = 1.00 - 0.04 = 0.96, \text{ or } 96\%$$

TRUE-FALSE ANSWERS

1. True
2. False
3. True
4. False
5. True
6. True
7. False
8. True
9. True
10. False

CHAPTER 10

1. a. This comatose man is retaining carbon dioxide and requires artificial ventilation. Worsening of mental status in a patient already comatose cannot be assessed. Without clinical warning, P_{CO_2} may continue to rise, leading to severe acidemia and hypoxemia. This patient should receive artificial ventilation to improve alveolar ventilation rather than for oxygenation.
    b. This young patient is alert but severely hypoxemic and in respiratory distress. He is on the verge of tiring out since, breathing at a rate of 42/min, his Pa_{CO_2} is only 38 mm Hg and his Pa_{O_2} is only 47 mm Hg. He should be intubated and receive artificial ventilation to improve his Pa_{O_2}.
    c. This woman has emphysema and, although alert, is in moderate respiratory distress. However, her Pa_{O_2}, Pa_{CO_2}, and pH do not pose imminent danger; the hypercapnia is well-compensated, and the Pa_{O_2} is adequate. Treating the patient conservatively and avoiding intubation is best. Little will be gained by artificial ventilation at this point.
    d. This woman has diabetic metabolic acidosis and is appropriately hyperventilating to compensate for the metabolic acidosis (see Chapter 7). There is no reason to artificially ventilate this patient.
    e. This drug addict responds to the narcotic antagonist but then lapses into a semistupor. However, she is able to hyperventilate (Pa_{CO_2} of 31 mm Hg) and oxygenation is adequate, so artificial ventilation is not needed at this point. The patient's mental status should continue to improve with repeated injections of the narcotic antagonist.
2. Minute ventilation on the assist-control mode is

    $$16 \times 700 = 11.2 \text{ L/min.}$$

    On IMV the minute ventilation is

    $(12 \times 700) + (8 \text{ spontaneous breaths} \times \text{tidal volume}) = 8.4 \text{ L/min} + ?$

    Important information (not provided in the problem) is the spontaneous tidal volume, which was measured at approximately 200 cc. For all practical purposes his spontaneous breathing was ineffective and contributed little or nothing to alveolar ventilation. The IMV mode resulted in a net *decrease* in both his minute ventilation (from 11.2 to approximately 10 L/min) and alveolar ventilation. The latter decrease resulted in a rise in Pa_{CO_2} to 47 mm Hg and in the manifestation of respiratory distress. This patient needed the full 16 ventilator breaths to maintain adequate alveolar ventilation.

3. a. This patient was intubated because of respiratory failure. Blood gas analysis indicates both respiratory and metabolic acidosis, as well as severe hypoxemia. To improve the Pa_{O_2} as quickly as possible, it is best to give 100% oxygen, initially. To preserve as much myocardium as possible, the best course is to increase the Pa_{O_2} quickly. The F_{IO_2} can then be lowered if blood values are adequate.
    b. Initial tidal volume should be large—approximately 15 cc/kg or 750 cc.
    c. Inspiratory pressure limit will depend on the peak inspiratory pressure needed for the tidal volume. If peak inspiratory pressure is 40 cm H_2O, an inspiratory pressure limit of 60 mm H_2O is appropriate.
    d. Initial respiratory rate should be 12 to 14 breaths per minute. The patient should be hyperventilated but not so quickly that pH rapidly changes from low (acidemia) to high (alkalemia).
    e. Peak inspiratory flow rate is adjusted to achieve an inspiratory time of approximately 0.5 to 1.5 sec. Usually, this is achieved at a rate of approximately 40 L/min.
    f. Inspiratory sensitivity depends on whether the assist-control or control mode of ventilation is used. If the patient is able to

trigger the machine on her own, then the assist-control mode can be used, in which case the inspiratory sensitivity dial will be turned "on."

At this point PEEP is not used because the patient may be adequately oxygenated without it. Also, the higher the mean airway pressure, the more likely it is that cardiac output will be impaired. PEEP should be a last resort in a patient suffering from left ventricular failure.

4. This patient has COPD and respiratory acidosis. His main physiologic threat is not so much hypoxemia as it is respiratory acidosis and acidemia. Alveolar ventilation must be augmented to improve this patient's status.
   a. It is likely that administration of 40% oxygen will be adequate.
   b. The tidal volume should be large because the patient has severe COPD, but not large enough to damage what are likely high-compliance lungs. A large tidal volume is needed both to ventilate the extra dead space and to achieve adequate alveolar ventilation. Initial tidal volume is set at 800 cc with careful observation of the peak inspiratory pressure.
   c. The inspiratory pressure limit is set at 20 cm above the peak pressure, or 60 cm H_2O and 40 cm H_2O, respectively.
   d. The respiratory rate is set at 10/min.
   e. The peak inspiratory flow rate is set at 40 L/min.
   f. The inspiratory sensitivity is turned off. The ventilatory mode chosen is intermittent mandatory ventilation.
   PEEP is contraindicated in patients with high-compliance lungs (see answer b).

5. This young patient overdosed on sleeping pills. Initial blood gas analysis while breathing with a ventilator showed a pH of 7.25 and a $PaCO_2$ of 56 mm Hg—both values definitely improved over the preintubation blood gas values. The patient is not yet in a ventilatory steady state and needs further time on this minute ventilation to achieve a steady state. At this point only the FIO_2 should be changed, and it can be decreased to 0.40.

6. The change in airway pressure is that between plateau (not peak pressure) and end-expiratory pressure:

   System compliance =
   $$\frac{\text{Tidal volume}}{\text{Change in airway pressure}} = \frac{800 \text{ cc}}{20 - 0} = \frac{40 \text{ cc}}{\text{cm } H_2O}$$

   Normal system compliance (e.g., in a patient intubated for a nonpulmonary reason who has no prior history of lung disease), ranges from approximately 40 to 80 cc/cm H_2O.

   Very low system compliance (15 to 25 cc/cm H_2O) is found in states of fibrosis and pulmonary edema. A low compliance that does not improve with treatment of the underlying condition is a bad prognostic sign.

7. a. The system compliance is plateau pressure minus PEEP (35 cm H_2O), divided into a tidal volume of 900 cc. System compliance equals 26 cc/cm H_2O.
   b. The system compliance is plateau pressure (64 cm of H_2O) minus PEEP (5 cm H_2O), or 59 cm H_2O, divided into a tidal volume of 900 cc. System compliance equals 15 cc/cm H_2O.

   This patient's compliance has decreased, i.e., greater pressure is now needed to achieve the same tidal volume. This change can be explained by any condition that impairs the distensibility of the lungs or the chest wall. In this patient the endotracheal tube had slipped into the right main stem bronchus; after the tube was pulled back, the compliance returned to its previous value.

8. This patient with severe emphysema was intubated because of progressive ventilatory failure. Emphysema is a high-compliance condition, i.e., the lungs are relatively more dis-

tensible than normal. Excessive airway pressure can overdistend the alveoli and can compress the pulmonary capillaries, creating extra (physiologic) dead space. This mechanism explains the rise in $Paco_2$. Although minute ventilation increased from 6 to 7.2 to 8.4 L/min over the course of several hours, the increase was not enough to satisfy the extra dead space created by the increased airway pressure. (This explanation assumes no significant change in the patient's carbon dioxide production).

9. The ratio of dead space to tidal volume is calculated by the Bohr dead space equation (Chapter 4):

$$V_D/V_T = \frac{Paco_2 - Peco_2}{Paco_2} = 0.57$$

where $Peco_2$ is the mean expired Pco_2. This is a high ratio (normal is approximately 0.30) and predicts weaning will not be easy. Generally, the higher the V_D/V_T, the more difficult it is to wean a patient from artificial ventilation.

10. The patient's blood gas analysis (ABG #4) on an IMV of 8/min is close to his baseline (ABG #1). Although he has carbon dioxide retention, it is well-compensated and he is comfortable. Weaning can be continued by decreasing the number of IMV breaths per minute. Weaning parameters (as outlined in the box on p. 216) could be obtained, but they should not preclude a further weaning attempt. It is best to continue with weaning and carefully observe the patient, as well as to check blood gas values intermittently.

(Note: An alternative weaning technique allows for removing the patient from the ventilator for 5 to 10 minutes at a time while preserving the same Fio_2 and observing his respiratory rate and level of distress. Although IMV is the more popular method, no proof exists that it is a better weaning technique than the older "trial and error" method.)

TRUE-FALSE ANSWERS

1. False   6. False
2. False   7. False
3. False   8. True
4. True   9. True
5. True   10. False

CHAPTER 11
A case of oxygenation respiratory failure

1. d. The most common cause of hypoxemia is V/Q imbalance—the altered distribution of ventilation to perfusion among the millions of alveolar-capillary units. Answer a is not correct because the patient is not hypoventilating; answer b is incorrect because a left-shifted oxygen dissociation curve would give a *higher* Sao_2 at this Pao_2 and in any case would not explain the low Pao_2; answer c is not correct because the patient's %HbCO is within normal limits. Finally, there is no evidence to support answer e.

2. c. O_2 content = Sao_2 × hemoglobin (gm%) × $\frac{1.34 \text{ ml } O_2}{\text{gram Hg}}$
   = 0.78 × 14 × 1.34 =
   14.63 ml O_2/100 ml blood

3. c. $P(A-a)o_2 = Pao_2 - Pao_2$
   $Pao_2 = Fio_2 (P_B - 47 \text{ mm Hg}) - 1.2 (Pco_2)$
   = 0.21 (760 − 47) − (1.2)(25)
   = 120 mm Hg
   Pao_2 = 38 mm Hg

   Hence,

   $P(A-a)o_2$ = 120 − 38 = 82 mm Hg

4. d. The low $Paco_2$ indicates that the patient is hyperventilating. On the acid-base map (Chapter 7) the blood gas value falls within the band for acute respiratory alkalosis.

5. c. There is no reason for low-supplemental

FIO_2 since the patient is not a carbon dioxide retainer; hence answers a, b, and e are inappropriate. Furthermore, transfusion is not indicated since the patient is not anemic. Answer d is incorrect since this mixture will raise the $PaCO_2$, increase the work of breathing, and do nothing to treat the underlying pneumonia.

6. c. The patient is shunting; i.e., blood is flowing through his lungs but is not being ventilated. Answer a is incorrect since he is not hypoventilating; answer b is incorrect since changes in the oxygen dissociation curve would not affect the PaO_2; answer d is incorrect since 100% oxygen should overcome a diffusion barrier; finally, answer e is incorrect since shunting is evident from the information given. While breathing inspired oxygen, without significant right-to-left shunting, PaO_2 will rise to above 600 mm Hg.

7. b. O_2 content = SaO_2 × Hg × 1.34
 = 0.85 × 13 × 1.34 =
 $$\frac{14.81 \text{ ml } O_2}{100 \text{ ml blood}}$$

 Since PaO_2 is low (60 mm Hg), the contribution from dissolved oxygen can be ignored.

8. e. While breathing 100% oxygen:

 $$PaO_2 = FIO_2 (P_B - 47) - PaCO_2$$

 Note that the factor *1.2* in the alveolar air equation becomes *1.00* when breathing 100% oxygen because nitrogen is removed from the lungs. (If you work through the long form of the alveolar air equation, you will note that as FIO_2 is increased, the bracket factor decreases toward 1.00.)

 $PaO_2 = FIO_2 (P_B - 47) - PCO_2 =$
 1.0 (713) − 25 = 688 mm Hg

 $P(A-a)O_2 = 688 - 60 = 628$ mm Hg

9. b. Compliance is change in lung volume per change in pressure; static compliance on a ventilator is

$$\frac{\text{Tidal volume}}{\text{Plateau pressure } - \text{ End-expiratory pressure}}$$

Since end-expiratory pressure is zero,

$$\frac{\text{Static}}{\text{compliance}} = \frac{700 \text{ cc}}{35 \text{ cm } H_2O} = \frac{20 \text{ cc}}{\text{cm } H_2O}$$

This is a low-static compliance; with reasonably healthy lungs, static compliance on a ventilator is in the range of 40 to 60 cc/cm H_2O. A value of only 20 cc/cm H_2O gives further evidence that the patient is suffering from very stiff lungs.

10. d. You are asked to calculate oxygen uptake per minute ($\dot{V}O_2$) given the cardiac output (Q_T) and SvO_2. This is possible using the Fick equation since you already know the arterial oxygen content (CaO_2) and can easily calculate the venous oxygen content (CvO_2).

$\dot{V}O_2 = Q_T \times (CaO_2 - CvO_2)$

$\dot{V}O_2 = 7000$ ml blood/min ×
$$\left(\frac{14.8 \text{ ml } O_2}{100 \text{ ml}} - \frac{11.3 \text{ ml } O_2}{100 \text{ ml}} \right)$$

$\dot{V}O_2 = 7000$ ml/min ×
3.50 ml O_2/100 ml = 245 ml O_2/min

11. d. $\frac{Q_S}{Q_T} = \frac{CcO_2 - CaO_2}{CcO_2 - CvO_2}$

CcO_2 is the end-capillary oxygen content; CaO_2 is the arterial oxygen content; CvO_2 is the mixed venous oxygen content. The CcO_2 is estimated by assuming that the end-capillary PO_2 is the same as the alveolar PO_2 (688 mm Hg) and that end-capillary blood is 100% saturated (a valid assumption on 100% inspired oxygen). When calculating the %shunt, it is important to include dissolved oxygen.

$$\frac{Q_S}{Q_T} = \frac{([13 \times 1.00 \times 1.34] + [0.003 \times 688]) - ([13 \times 1.34 \times 0.85] + [0.003 \times 60])}{([13 \times 1.00 \times 1.34] + [0.003 \times 688]) - ([13 \times 1.34 \times 0.65] + [0.003 \times 34])} = \frac{(19.48 - 14.99)}{(19.48 - 11.42)} = \frac{4.49}{8.06} = 0.56$$

A 56% right to left pulmonary shunt is not compatible with survival.

12. c. Either process alone (metabolic acidosis or respiratory alkalosis) would not give a pH of 7.40; combined, they act to cancel out the respective pH changes (low for acidosis, high for alkalosis) and give a normal pH. Note that the patient is hyperventilating more than is customary for this degree of acidosis and thus has a primary respiratory alkalosis, probably caused by the ventilator.

13. b. One of the advantages of PEEP is to allow FIO_2 to be lowered to an acceptable level. FIO_2 should be the first change made on the ventilator once an adequate PaO_2 is reached. It is best not to change two settings at once; otherwise, you have no way of knowing which setting is responsible for observed changes in the blood gas values. There is no point in continuing the same settings since the PaO_2 is now acceptable and the FIO_2 is too high.

14. c. A common complication of PEEP is to lower the cardiac output even though the PaO_2 may continue to rise. Since oxygen transport equals cardiac output times oxygen content, the result may be lowered oxygen transport. PEEP does not (at least commonly) result in answers a, b, d, or e.

A case of combined oxygenation and ventilatory failure in COPD

1. d. The patient is clearly hypoventilating ($PaCO_2$ is 60 mm Hg), constituting at least one reason for the low PaO_2. Assuming barometric pressure equals 760 mm Hg, the $P(A-a)O_2$ is 37 mm Hg, which is an elevated value and indicates ventilation-perfusion imbalance. Finally, note that at this PaO_2, the SaO_2 should be over 60%, not 51%. The lower SaO_2 indicates something else is binding to hemoglobin besides oxygen. In a heavy smoker, excess carbon monoxide is the most likely culprit.

2. c. This patient is a carbon dioxide retainer; giving too high an FIO_2 runs the risk of turning off his hypoxic drive to breathe and causing further hypoventilation. Thus low supplemental FIO_2 is the optimal initial treatment.

3. b. Look at the oxygen dissociation curve to appreciate that the patient's PaO_2 is on the so-called steep part of the curve. Hence, a small increment in the PaO_2 will lead to a relatively large increment in SaO_2 (when compared with the flat part of the oxygen dissociation curve). As a result, oxygen content can increase without cutting off the hypoxic drive to breathe.

4. b. If the patient's problem were only respiratory acidosis, the pH at this $PaCO_2$ would be approximately 7.15, not 7.10 (see the band for acute respiratory acidosis, Fig. 7-3). Since his pH is lower than predicted for uncomplicated acute respiratory acidosis, he must have another condition contributing to low pH, i.e., metabolic acidosis.

5. e. After 1 hour on the ventilator, the patient's $PaCO_2$ has decreased from 80 mm Hg to 50 mm Hg. Clearly the patient is in a transient situation and has not reached a steady state in terms of ventilation. Another hour may show further reduction of his $PaCO_2$. Thus it is best to leave the settings alone and especially not do anything that will lower the $PaCO_2$ any faster (as it may from answers c and d). The step in answer a

is unnecessary since the pH is increasing from reduction of $PaCO_2$; extra HCO_3^- may actually cause an unwanted alkalosis once $PaCO_2$ decreases further. The step in answer b is unwarranted since his PaO_2 is adequate while breathing 40% inspired oxygen.

6. e. or c. See answer to question 7.
7. e. Your goal should be to return the patient's acid-base and ventilatory status close to what it will be while breathing room air off the ventilator. He now has a metabolic alkalosis, caused by the diuretics and steroids, that is manifested by high pH and normal $PaCO_2$ (with resulting high HCO_3^-). The compensation for metabolic alkalosis is hypoventilation; once the patient is extubated, hypoventilation may occur rapidly, at least partly to compensate the alkalosis. Another reason the patient may hypoventilate once extubated relates to his chronic lung disease. Based on his history and presenting arterial blood gas values, he is most likely a chronic carbon dioxide retainer.

One danger of hypoventilation is the resultant hypoxemia. What you would like to do is (1) allow the patient to achieve his "normal" state of hypoventilation while being artificially ventilated so that he does not acutely hypoventilate once extubated; and (2) remove any *metabolic* cause for further hypoventilation by aggressively treating the metabolic alkalosis.

One approach is to decrease the number of IMV breaths per minute while correcting the alkalosis. This should allow the patient to gradually hypoventilate while assuring adequacy of oxygenation and, at the same time, correcting the metabolic process. Another 24 hours of such management might assure a more successful extubation.

There are many approaches to weaning such patients from the ventilator; of the answers provided here, e seems the most rational for the reasons given above. However, other physicians might opt for answer c, another reasonable approach. In managing such cases it is more important to be aware of the physiologic principles involved and of the clinical response to treatment than it is to follow rigid rules.

8. d. Since the patient has metabolic alkalosis, you want to evaluate his serum K^+; none of the other tests seem particularly indicated at this time.
9. d. Most likely the patient is hypokalemic because of the metabolic alkalosis.
10. b. Answer a is incorrect since the patient would not have a PaO_2 of 80 mm Hg with a $PaCO_2$ of 60 mm Hg (if he did, it would constitute a negative $P(A-a)O_2$, which is not compatible with life). Answer c is unlikely since we know he is a chronic carbon dioxide retainer; these gas measurements show not only a slightly reduced $PaCO_2$, but a normal PaO_2, both unlikely in a patient with such severe disease. Answer d is unlikely since the PaO_2 is too low for him to be "doing well." On a physiologic basis, this PaO_2 would give an SaO_2 less than 75%, not one of 80%. Answer e is unlikely since these gas values suggest a metabolic acidosis, which he has no reason to have. Also, it is unlikely he could hyperventilate to this degree and be considered "doing well."

TRUE-FALSE ANSWERS

1. True	6. False
2. True	7. True
3. False	8. False
4. True	9. False
5. False	10. False

CHAPTER 12

1. Carbon dioxide production during aerobic metabolism comes from the chemical combination of carbohydrate or fatty acid with oxygen and

the consequent production of carbon dioxide and water (see Fig. 12-1). During anaerobic metabolism, carbon dioxide is produced from the buffering of lactic acid. When anaerobic metabolism occurs along with aerobic metabolism, such as during the graded exercise test, lactate-generated carbon dioxide adds to the carbon dioxide from aerobic metabolism. At this point (anaerobic threshold), the total carbon dioxide load presented to the lungs increases, as can be appreciated from the rise in slope of $\dot{V}_{CO_2}$ (Fig. 12-1).

2. You are asked to determine alveolar and arterial P_{O_2} of a well-trained jogger who has been running on a treadmill. Resting $P_{ET CO_2}$ was 40 mm Hg and RQ was 0.8; after 5 minutes on the treadmill, the patient's RQ is still 0.8 ($\dot{V}_{CO_2}$ = 800; $\dot{V}_{O_2}$ = 1000), but minute ventilation has increased to 30 L/min. Despite the fivefold increase in $\dot{V}_E$, $P_{ET CO_2}$ is essentially unchanged at 30 mm Hg. $P_{ET CO_2}$ reflects $P_{A CO_2}$, which in turn reflects $P_{a CO_2}$ (see Chapter 4). Despite the large increase in minute ventilation, the jogger's $P_{a CO_2}$ is thus unchanged, and he is not hyperventilating.

3. This 40-year-old man had the following predicted and achieved $\dot{V}_{O_2}$ max and heart rate:

	Equation	Predicted	Achieved
$\dot{V}_{O_2}$ max (L/min)	4.2 − (0.032 × age)	2.92	2.80
Max heart rate	210 − (0.65 × age)	184	176

He achieved a $\dot{V}_{O_2}$ max and a maximal heart rate close to his predicted values and was pronounced physically fit for the expedition.

4. Patient A has low $P_{a O_2}$ and normal $P_{a CO_2}$ at rest. During exercise, the patient's $P_{a O_2}$ falls and $P_{a CO_2}$ rises slightly; this suggests both diffusion impairment *and* severe ventilatory limitation and is compatible with severe emphysema. (Regardless of exercise level, alveolar ventilation normally rises to match carbon dioxide production, so $P_{a CO_2}$ should normally never rise.) The severely emphysematous patient has lost pulmonary capillary vessels and so has less membrane area for diffusion. The severe airways obstruction of emphysema makes the patient unable to augment minute (and hence alveolar) ventilation to meet exercise needs.

Patient B has a slightly low $P_{a O_2}$ and a normal $P_{a CO_2}$ at rest. During exercise, the patient's $P_{a CO_2}$ is unchanged (a normal finding), and his $P_{a O_2}$ has increased by 6 mm Hg. Normally, $P_{a O_2}$ remains fairly constant during exercise. An increase of $P_{a O_2}$ over a low resting value without a change in $P_{a CO_2}$ indicates improvement in ventilation-perfusion distribution within the lungs. Such improvement is commonly seen during exercise in patients with chronic bronchitis.

Patient C has a low normal $P_{a O_2}$ and a reduced $P_{a CO_2}$ at rest. During exercise, the patient's $P_{a O_2}$ drops 15 mm Hg, and $P_{a CO_2}$ also falls slightly indicating further hyperventilation. The drop in $P_{a O_2}$ is best explained by a severe diffusion impairment, such as occurs from interstitial fibrosis. As pulmonary blood flow increases, there is less time for equilibration of oxygen, so $P_{a O_2}$ falls.

5. This case exemplifies a common problem for which patients are referred for exercise testing. The patient has mild heart disease but not enough to cause symptoms at rest. He also has airways obstruction. What causes his dyspnea?

   a. Respiratory quotient is $\dot{V}_{CO_2}$ divided by $\dot{V}_{O_2}$. O_2-pulse is oxygen uptake in cc/min divided by heart rate; units are cc O_2/heart beat. RQ and O_2-pulse are given below.

	Rest	2 mph	2.5 mph	3 mph	3 mph
RQ	0.86	0.75	0.80	0.83	0.86
O_2-pulse	4.86	8.62	9.60	10.19	11.97

   b. One way anaerobic threshold (AT) can be determined is by measuring the rise in blood lactate, but lactate was not measured in this patient. Another way of determining AT is by comparing the rise in minute ventilation ($\dot{V}_E$) to the rise in carbon dioxide producton ($\dot{V}_{CO_2}$); when the rise in $\dot{V}_E$ exceeds that for $\dot{V}_{CO_2}$, AT has been reached. In this patient, minute ventilation and carbon dioxide production each increased fourfold, so anaerobic threshold was not achieved.

How about ventilatory limitation? His MVV at rest was 50.5 L/min; shortly before he quit exercising, total minute ventilation was up to 48 L/min. Normally, maximal exercise ventilation reaches approximately 65% of the resting ventilatory capacity (MVV), leaving approximately 33% in reserve. This patient's exercise ventilation was over 90% of his MVV. Thus one can assume that ventilatory limitation was the reason he quit exercising.

c. The patient quit exercising because of dyspnea, which was likely related to ventilatory limitation. His heart rate increased appropriately, as did his O_2-pulse. He did not reach his predicted maximal heart rate and showed no evidence of a cardiac limitation to exercise. His dyspnea on exertion is most likely related to ventilatory impairment and not to any heart problem.

6. This patient had been seen by several physicians in the past but had not had formal exercise testing. His resting pulmonary function studies were normal. However, he had a clear history of dyspnea during exertion.

a. METS are multiples of the resting oxygen uptake. V_D/V_T is calculated from the Bohr equation (see Chapter 4):

$$V_D/V_T = \frac{P_{aCO_2} - P_{ECO_2}}{P_{aCO_2}}$$

The calculated METS and V_D/V_T follow:

	Miles per hour				
	1	2	2.5	3	3.5
METS	2.7	3.9	4.8	5.5	5.8
V_D/V_T	0.27	0.21	0.20	0.20	0.19

b. This patient came close to anaerobic threshold but did not reach it; there was no fall in P_{aCO_2}, and RQ did not go above 1. Also, the patient maintained a steady pH, and bicarbonate did not fall. There was no ventilatory limitation; his MVV at rest was 112 L/min, and maximal exercise ventilation was only 38.5 L, well below his MVV. His heart rate increased appropriately, and there was no wheezing after the completion of exercise.

c. This test was interpreted as showing poor fitness caused by obesity and a sedentary life style. He had neither ventilatory nor cardiac limitation to exercise, but he simply could not continue after 10 minutes because of fatigue and dyspnea. In the final analysis, he had no industrially-related problem that could account for his symptoms.

TRUE-FALSE ANSWERS

1. True
2. False
3. True
4. False
5. True
6. True
7. False
8. True
9. False
10. True

CHAPTER 13

1. a. Bilateral pleural effusions in the presence of cardiomegaly suggests congestive heart failure (CHF). Fluid from a patient with CHF should have transudative characteristics (low protein and LDH ratios). Alcoholics are also at increased risk for pneumonia, which causes an exudative effusion. However, the patient is afebrile and no mention is made of pneumonia on chest x-ray.

Both the pleural fluid/serum ratio for protein (1.6/6.1 = 0.26) and for LDH (105/238 = 0.44) correlate with a transudative mechanism. Thus by clinical evaluation and laboratory values, the pleural fluid is a transudate caused by CHF. Low pleural fluid white cell count and predominance of lymphocytes are also consistent with this cause.

b. This woman is first seen with bilateral pleural effusions. The most common cause of bilateral *exudative* effusions is malignancy, a diagnosis suggested by the history of recent weight loss and weakness. The most common cause of bilateral *transudative* effusions is CHF, also a possibility because of the myocardial infarction. No malignant cells were seen in fluid removed by thoracentesis, and the predominance of lymphocytes is consistent with either malignancy or CHF.

Pleural fluid/serum ratios clearly point to an exudative cause (protein ratio, 5.6/7.3 = 0.77; LDH ratio, 150/210 = 0.71) indicating that the bilateral effusions are not caused by CHF. Because of these findings, the patient had a repeat thoracentesis with closed pleural biopsy, which revealed carcinoma metastatic to the pleura.

c. The clinical history of this patient is strongly suggestive of pulmonary embolism. Pulmonary embolism is a common cause of pleural effusions, but the fluid characteristics are notoriously nonspecific—e.g., the fluid may be transudate or exudate, bloody or nonbloody. This pleural fluid has exudative characteristics and a predominance of polymorphonuclear leukocytes—findings also consistent with an infectious cause. In summary, although pulmonary embolism is strongly suspected, the pleural fluid in this example is not helpful in either ruling for or against the diagnosis.

2. a. Malignancy is strongly suspected. The most important pleural fluid laboratory test is cytology, which alone can confirm the diagnosis. Additional pleural fluid laboratory tests should include the following:

LDH and protein. These will determine if the fluid is likely an exudate or transudate. An exudate would suggest that the pleura is directly involved with the tumor; a transudate would suggest that the pleura is not directly involved and that another mechanism is causing fluid formation (e.g., vascular compression by tumor).

pH. The lower the pH, the more widespread is the tumor and/or the longer it has been present.

Cell count and differential. Malignant effusions usually manifest lymphocyte or mononuclear cell predominance. Finding numerous polymorphonuclear leukocytes would suggest another cause of the effusion; a large number of eosinophils would cast doubt on a malignant cause; and a large number of mesothelial cells would argue strongly against tuberculosis.

CEA. An elevated CEA would help confirm a malignant cause, but a low value would not rule it out.

Triglyceride. A triglyceride value above 110 mg/100 ml would point to a chylous effusion (even if the fluid is not milky in color) and a problem with the thoracic duct.

Culture and microbiologic stain. It can be argued (in this case) that bacteriologic studies are a waste of money. Nonetheless, most patients who are initially seen with effusions of uncertain cause will have their fluid sent for culture if for no other reason than habit. If one is sure the problem is noninfectious, these tests can be omitted. Tuberculous patients with effusion are invariably febrile, but if tuberculosis is suspected, the fluid should always be sent for tuberculous studies.

In summary, there should be some rationale for each laboratory test ordered. One should consider how the test result, normal or abnormal, will help in making a diagnosis.

b. This patient's story suggests either an infectious or inflammatory cause of effusion (e.g., pancreatitis). The following tests should be obtained on the pleural fluid:

Protein, LDH. These tests help differentiate exudate from transudate.

Culture and microbiologic stain. These tests diagnose infection.

Cell count, pH, glucose. These tests provide useful correlations with infection.

Amylase. This test helps diagnose pancreatitis.

As presented, cytology would be of low priority since malignancy is highly unlikely.

c. This is a case of congestive heart failure. Depending on the severity of the effusion and on the index of suspicion for other causes, a thoracentesis might or might not be done. If a thoracentesis is done, the following laboratory tests would be appropriate:

Protein, LDH. These tests confirm that the fluid is a transudate.

pH and cell count. These tests help characterize the fluid.

d. Clinically, the most likely diagnosis is pulmonary embolism, and the pleural effusion should probably not be tapped. Other diagnostic studies, e.g., perfusion lung scan, will have better yield.

3. Pleural fluid C is least likely to be of tuberculous origin. The high pH (7.46) and mesothelial cell count (6%) both argue against TB effusion. These two tests can never be used to definitely rule out the diagnosis, but the results do suggest some other cause. This patient had carcinoma metastatic to the pleura. (Patient A had pneumonia, and Patient B had a collagen-vascular cause of the effusion.)

4. This patient should have a chest tube placed. The pH and glucose are both very low, and clinically the patient has a parapneumonic effusion. Even though organisms are not seen in initial Gram and AFB stains, the effusion is in need of immediate drainage.

5. An increase in Pa_{O_2} will lower the P_{N_2} and thus the total gas pressure in blood. P_{N_2} should fall by the same amount as the P_{O_2} increases. If we assume total gas pressure in arterial blood is the same as atmospheric pressure:

Arterial blood

P_{O_2}	200 mm Hg
P_{CO_2}	40 mm Hg
P_{H_2O}	47 mm Hg
P_{N_2}	473 mm Hg
TOTAL	760 mm Hg

P_{N_2} will be the same in venous blood, but P_{O_2} will be much lower, in this case 45 mm Hg. Thus pleural space air is surrounded by capillaries and venules with the following gas pressures:

Mixed venous blood

P_{O_2}	44 mm Hg
P_{CO_2}	46 mm Hg
P_{H_2O}	47 mm Hg
P_{N_2}	473 mm Hg
TOTAL	611 mm Hg

Supplemental oxygen has increased the gradient for diffusion of the pneumothorax air from 49 mm Hg (755 − 706) to 144 mm Hg (755 − 611).

In theory, the higher the FI_{O_2} is, the bigger the gradient will be and the faster will reabsorption take place. The potential for oxygen toxicity must be considered so that in practice either a high FI_{O_2} is given for a few hours or a lower FI_{O_2} (e.g., 0.40 or less) is given for longer periods.

6. This patient's arterial blood gas values (pH, 7.47; Pa_{CO_2}, 55 mm Hg; Pa_{O_2}, 51 mm Hg) are best explained by underlying pulmonary disease, *not* by the large pleural effusion. The dyspnea is a sign that the patient is trying to hyperventilate. Even though two thirds of one lung is compressed by fluid, the remaining one third, plus the other lung, should be more than sufficient to eliminate carbon dioxide.

7. The $P(A-a)_{O_2}$ fell after thoracentesis, which can only be explained by increasing ventilation-perfusion imbalance. The exact mechanism is unknown, but presumably fluid removal increases perfusion to the affected lung more than alveolar ventilation.

Answers to clinical problems

TRUE-FALSE ANSWERS

1. False   6. False
2. True   7. True
3. True   8. True
4. False   9. False
5. True   10. True

CHAPTER 14

1. While awake, this patient's blood gas values and pulmonary function tests show only modest impairment. The low Pa_{O_2} is probably related to morbid obesity and basilar atelectasis; Sa_{O_2} is adequate. Expiratory reserve volume is very low, but the other lung volumes are normal or only slightly reduced—a pattern typical of obesity. Limited polysomnography (EEG, EMG, and EOG not included) was able to establish the diagnosis of obstructive sleep apnea (cessation of air flow with continued chest wall movement). The single observed apneic episode was accompanied by severe oxygen desaturation.

    Repeated episodes of desaturation during sleep can account for this patient's polycythemia. His daytime sleepiness probably results from recurrent apneic episodes and partial awakening throughout the night; he simply does not get a good night's sleep.

    As a minimum this patient should begin a weight reduction program. Because of severe oxygen desaturation, he should also be referred to a sleep center for complete polysomnography and appropriate specific therapy.

2. Hypercapnia results from insufficient alveolar ventilation ($\dot{V}A$) for the amount of CO_2 production. Decreased $\dot{V}A$ can only arise from decreased minute ventilation ($\dot{V}E$) or increased dead space ventilation (or a combination of the two). The fall in $\dot{V}E$ during sleep leads to a decrease in $\dot{V}A$. If $\dot{V}A$ falls proportionately the same as $\dot{V}_{CO_2}$, Pa_{CO_2} will remain unchanged. A slight rise in Pa_{CO_2} during sleep indicates a fall in $\dot{V}A$ greater than the fall in $\dot{V}_{CO_2}$; although this explains the hypercapnia, the reason for disproportionate change is unknown.

3. The blood gas values suggest metabolic alkalosis, a potential cause of carbon dioxide retention. It would be prudent to obtain serum electrolytes. If the patient's serum potassium is low, she should receive replacement with potassium chloride. The diuretic is most likely responsible for the alkalosis; it should be discontinued and some other drug used for hypertension. Finally, the benzodiazepine tranquilizer should be stopped.

    If after a few weeks the patient's alkalosis is corrected and she still complains of daytime sleepiness, polysomnography is indicated.

4. This patient has features characteristic of the Pickwickian syndrome—obesity, hypercapnia, and daytime hypersomnolence. The following steps are recommended:
    1. Stop smoking completely.
    2. Immediate weight reduction, in a supervised environment if possible.
    3. No driving until daytime sleepiness is corrected.
    4. Medroxyprogesterone acetate, 20 mg, 3 times a day.

    The first three measures are easy to recommend but are generally difficult to implement. Their success requires a cooperative and compliant patient, a concerned family, and a physician interested in the problem. If the patient is unwilling to give up smoking and enter a weight reduction program, it is unlikely that drug therapy will be successful.

TRUE-FALSE ANSWERS

1. True   6. False
2. False   7. True
3. False   8. True
4. True   9. False
5. False   10. False

CHAPTER 15

1. The amount of oxygen available to the tissues is less than normal since fetal hemoglobin holds

oxygen more tightly than does normal adult hemoglobin. This quality of fetal hemoglobin does not affect PaO_2, which is a function of the alveolar-capillary interface (see Chapter 5). For a given PaO_2, the increased oxygen affinity of fetal hemoglobin will actually raise SaO_2 slightly in the pulmonary capillary.
2. Fetal hemoglobin has the same capacity for oxygen as adult hemoglobin (1.34 ml O_2/gm Hb). Thus arterial oxygen content (CaO_2) is calculated as discussed in Chapter 6:

$$Ca O_2 = 1.34 \frac{ml\ O_2}{gm\ Hgb} \times \frac{18\ gm\ Hgb}{100\ ml} \times 0.98 + (0.003 \times 95)$$

$$= 23.64 + 0.29$$

$$= 23.93\ ml\ O_2/100\ ml\ blood$$

3.

	Points
Acrocyanotic	1
Crying on stimulus	2
Irregular respirations	1
Some flexion	1
Heart rate 90	1
Apgar score	6

An Apgar acore of 6 is considered indicative of mild asphyxia. Such a score warrants oxygen administration by bag and mask and stimulation by slapping the infant's feet or drying the infant with a warm towel.
4. c. For normal adult hemoglobin, cyanosis is usually detectable when there is at least 5 gm of deoxygenated hemoglobin per 100 ml blood *in the capillaries*. Cyanosis is not based on the percentage of deoxygenated hemoblogin, only on the total amount.
5. d. Fig. 15-9 shows that, in the adult, VC is approximately three fourths of TLC. This same proportion holds for the infant, so 870 ml is the correct answer. See also Fig. 15-14.

TRUE-FALSE ANSWERS

1. False
2. False
3. True
4. True
5. True
6. True
7. False
8. False
9. False
10. True

appendix B

Normal values for FVC and FEV_1

The two most useful spirometric values are forced vital capacity (FVC) and forced expiratory volume in the first second (FEV_1). Normal values for FVC and FEV_1 are provided in this appendix.* These values apply to a white population. Normal values are 10% to 15% lower for adult black men and women and for Asians. (For more information regarding race and pulmonary function see the references that follow this Appendix.)

NORMAL FEV_1 AND FVC IN MALES

Fig. 1 provides two age scales for FEV_1 and two scales for FVC. For older boys and men, align a straight edge from the person's age to their standing height, which is obtained with the subject's shoes off. The straight edge crosses the FEV_1 or FVC scale at the mean value for a white person of that age and height. For younger boys, the FEV_1 and FVC are horizontal to the height ordinate since age does not affect variability in this group. By subtracting the age-specific 95% confidence interval from the mean value, the lower limit of normal for the white male is obtained.

Example

The patient is a 40-year-old man who stands 5'10" tall (approximately 178 cm). A line connecting age 40 with 178 cm gives an FEV_1 of 4.2 L and an FVC of 5.1 L. These are mean values for a 40-year-old white male. To find the lower limit of normal, subtract 0.86; this gives 3.34 for FEV_1 and 4.05 for FVC. In a non-white male, the mean and lower limit of normal are approximately 10% to 15% less than the values obtained from this nomogram.

---

*These nomograms are reproduced with permission from Corre, K.A., Hansen, J.E., and Rothstein, R.J.: Nomograms for predicted FEV_1 and FVC in children, adolescents, and adults, Mt. Sinai J. Med. **52**:515-318, May 1985.

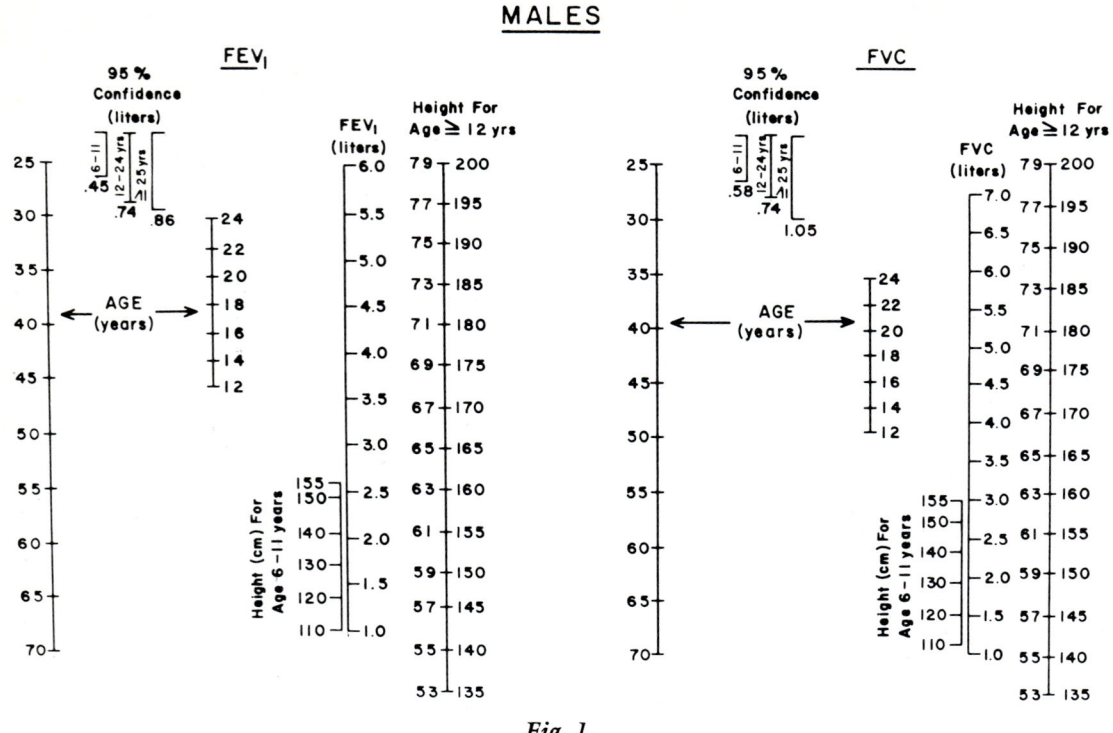

Fig. 1.

NORMAL FEV$_1$ AND FVC IN FEMALES

Fig. 2 provides two age scales for both FEV$_1$ and FVC. For older girls and women, align a straight edge from the person's age to their standing height, which is obtained with the subject's shoes off. The straight edge crosses the FEV$_1$ and FVC scale at the mean value for a white female of that age and height. For younger girls, the FEV$_1$ and FVC are horizontal to the height ordinate since age does not affect variability in this group. By subtracting the age-specific 95% confidence interval from the mean value, the lower limit of normal for the white female is obtained.

Example

The patient is a 9-year-old girl who is 54″ tall (approximately 137 cm). A horizontal line connecting 137 cm with the FEV$_1$ scale gives a mean value of approximately 1.9 L. A horizontal line to the FVC scale gives a mean value of approximately 2.2 L. Subtracting 0.45 gives a lower limit of normal for FEV$_1$ of 1.45 L and for FVC of 1.75 L. In a non-white female, the mean and lower limit of normal are approximately 10% to 15% less than the values obtained from this nomogram.

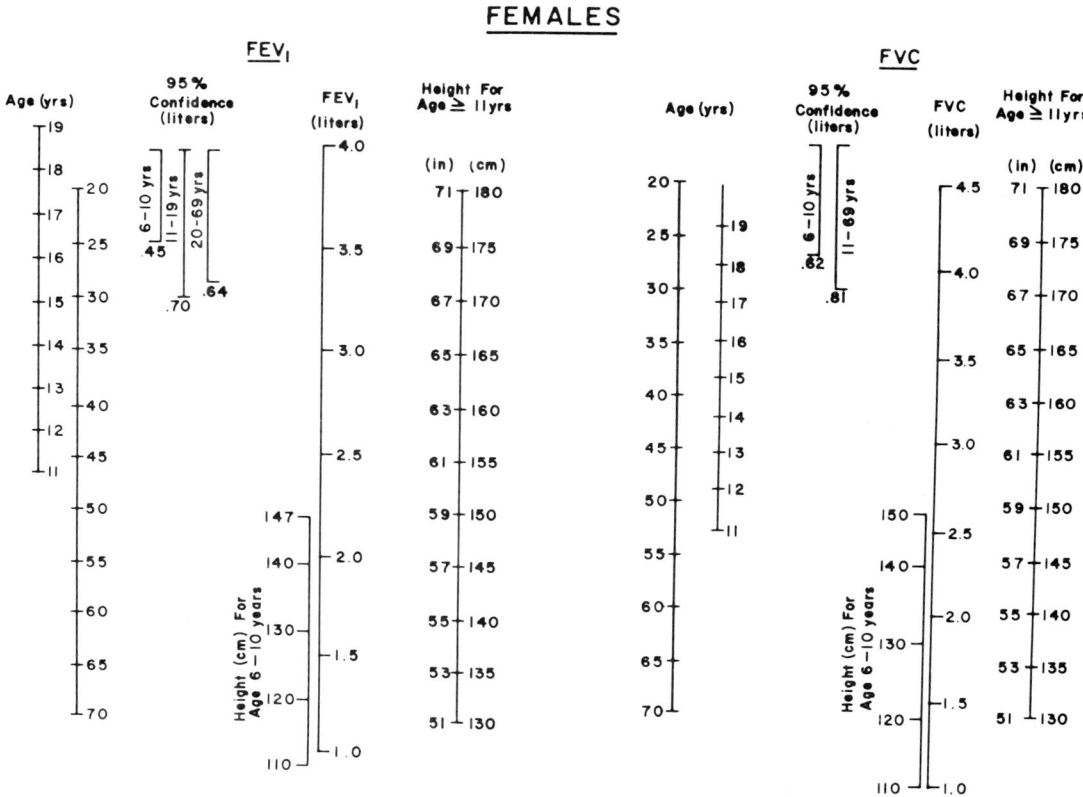

Fig. 2.

References

Damon, A.: Negro-white difference in pulmonary function, Hum. Biol. **38**:380-393, 1966.

Miller, C.J., Cotes, J.E., Hall, A.M., et al.: Lung function and exercise performance of healthy Caribbean men and women of African ethnic origin, Q.J. Exp. Physiol. **57**:325-341, 1972.

Oscherwitz, M., Edlavitch, S.A., Baker, T.R., et al.: Differences in pulmonary functions in various racial groups, Am. J. Epidemiol. **96**:319-327, 1972.

Schoenberg, J.B., Beck, G.J., and Bouhuys, A.: Growth and decay of pulmonary function in healthy blacks and whites, Respir. Physiol. **33**:367-393, 1978.

Seltzer, C.C., Siegelaub, A.B., Friedman, G.D., et al.: Differences in pulmonary function related to smoking habits and race, Am. Rev. Respir. Dis. **110**:598-608, 1974.

Woolcock, A.J., Colman, M.H., and Blackburn, C.R.B.: Factors affecting ventilatory lung function, Am. Rev. Respir. Dis. **106**:692-709, 1972.

appendix C
Basic equations and formulas

Pulmonary physiology cannot be taught or understood without reference to a few basic equations and formulas. This appendix lists the relationships I consider most important, in the order in which they were first introduced. (The chapter and page numbers are given in parentheses.)

Dalton's law of partial pressures:

$$P_T = P_1 + P_2 + P_3 + \ldots + P_n$$

(Chapter 2, Page 30)

Ideal general gas law:

$$\frac{P_1 V_1}{T_1} = \frac{P_2 V_2}{T_2}$$

(Chapter 2, Page 31)

Lung compliance:

$$C_L = \frac{\text{Change in volume}}{\text{Change in pressure}}$$

(Chapter 3, Page 46)

Airway resistance:

$$R_{aw} = \frac{\text{Driving pressure}}{\text{Air flow}}$$

(Chapter 3, Page 48)

Total lung capacity:

$$TLC = VC + RV = IRV + TV + ERV + RV$$

(Chapter 3, Page 50)

Minute ventilation:

$$\dot{V}_E = f \times V_T$$

(Chapter 4, Page 74)

$$\dot{V}_E = \dot{V}_A + \dot{V}_D$$

(Chapter 4, Page 75)

Alveolar P_{CO_2} equation*:

$$P_{ACO_2} = \frac{\dot{V}_{CO_2} \times 0.863}{\dot{V}_A}$$

(Chapter 4, Page 77)

Respiratory quotient:

$$RQ = \frac{\dot{V}_{CO_2}}{\dot{V}_{O_2}}$$

(Chapter 4, Page 78)

Steady state relationship:

$$RQ \text{ (metabolic)} = RQ \text{ (pulmonary)}$$

(Chapter 4, Page 78)

Bohr dead space equation:

$$\frac{V_D}{V_T} = \frac{P_{ACO_2} - P_{ECO_2}}{P_{ACO_2}}$$

(Chapter 4, Page 82)

Short form of alveolar P_{O_2} equation:

$$P_{AO_2} = F_{IO_2}(P_B - 47) - 1.2 (P_{ACO_2})$$

(Chapter 5, Page 92)

Alveolar-arterial P_{O_2} difference:

$$P(A-a)O_2 = P_{AO_2} - P_{aO_2}$$

(Chapter 5, Page 93)

Arterial O_2 content:

$$C_{aO_2} = (S_{aO_2} \times Hgb \times 1.34) + (0.003 \times P_{aO_2})$$

(Chapter 6, Page 115)

---

*The alveolar P_{CO_2} equation is perhaps the single most important equation in clinical practice of respiratory medicine. Its derivation is provided at the end of this appendix.

Basic equations and formulas

Arterial O_2 delivery:

$$O_2 \text{ delivery} = Q_T \times C_{aO_2}$$

(Chapter 6, Page 123)

Fick equation for oxygen uptake:

$$\dot{V}_{O_2} = Q_T \times (C_{aO_2} - C_{vO_2})$$

(Chapter 6, Page 123)

Henderson-Hasselbalch equation:

$$pH = pK + \log \frac{HCO_3^-}{0.03(P_{aCO_2})}$$

(Chapter 7, Page 131)

Anion gap (unmeasured anions):

$$AG = Na^+ - (Cl^- + HCO_3^-)$$

(Chapter 7, Page 137)

Relationship between cardiac output (Q_T), stroke volume (SV), and heart rate (HR):

$$SV = \frac{Q_T}{HR}$$

(Chapter 8, Page 160)

Systemic vascular resistance:

$$SVR = \frac{MSAP - CVP}{Q_T}$$

(Chapter 8, Page 160)

Relationship between pulmonary hydrostatic and oncotic pressures:

$$Qf = K(P_{hyd_c} - P_{hyd_i}) - K@(P_{onc_c} - P_{onc_i})$$

(Chapter 11, Page 223)

Percent of cardiac output shunted past the lungs:

$$\frac{Q_S}{Q_T} = \frac{C_{cO_2} - C_{aO_2}}{C_{cO_2} - C_{vO_2}}$$

(Chapter 11, Page 224)

Difference between aerobic and anaerobic metabolism of glucose:

Aerobic
Glucose + 6 O_2 → 6 CO_2 + 6 H_2O + 36 ATP

(Chapter 12, Page 241)

Anaerobic
Glucose + 2 ADP → Lactic acid + 2 ATP

(Chapter 12, Page 241)

DERIVATION OF P_{CO_2} EQUATION:

$$\dot{V}_{CO_2} = F_{ECO_2} \times \dot{V}_A$$
$$= F_{ACO_2} \times \dot{V}_A$$

Step 1

$$F_{ACO_2} = \frac{P_{ACO_2}}{P_B - P_{H_2O}}$$

Step 2

$$\dot{V}_{CO_2} = \frac{P_{ACO_2} \times \dot{V}_A}{P_B - P_{H_2O}}$$

Step 3

$$P_{ACO_2} = \frac{\dot{V}_{CO_2} \text{ (STPD)} \times (P_B - P_{H_2O})}{\dot{V}_A \text{ (BTPS)}}$$

Step 4

$$P_{ACO_2} = \frac{\dot{V}_{CO_2} \text{ (ml/min STPD)} \times (P_B - P_{H_2O})}{\dot{V}_A \text{ (L/min BTPS)} \times CF \times 1000 \text{ ml/L}}$$

Step 5

where CF represents the correction factor to convert STPD to BTPS. When barometric pressure is equal to 760 mm Hg and P_{H_2O} is equal to 47 mm Hg, CF is equal to 0.826.

$$P_{ACO_2} = \frac{\dot{V}_{CO_2} \times 713}{\dot{V}_A \times 0.826 \times 100}$$

Step 6

$$P_{ACO_2} = \frac{\dot{V}_{CO_2} \times 0.863}{\dot{V}_A}$$

Step 7

Note: Any correction factor will give the same result for the constant in this equation (0.863). Calculation of BTPS correction factor (CF in Step 5):

$$\frac{V_1 P_1}{T_1} = \frac{V_2 P_2}{T_2}$$

V_1, P_1, and T_1 are STPD conditions; V_2, P_2, and T_2 are BTPS conditions.

$$\frac{V_1(760)}{273} = \frac{V_2(760 - 47)}{310}$$

$$V_1 = V_2 \times (760 - 47) \times \frac{273}{310}$$

$$V_1 = V_2 \times 0.826$$

0.826 is the CF in Step 5.

appendix D
Abbreviations and symbols

ELEMENTS AND COMPOUNDS

O_2	Oxygen
CO_2	Carbon dioxide
N_2	Nitrogen
He	Helium
H_2O	Water
Na^+	Sodium ion
K^+	Potassium ion
Cl^-	Chloride ion
HCO_3^-	Bicarbonate ion
$NaHCO_3$	Sodium bicarbonate
H_2CO_3	Carbonic acid
CO	Carbon monoxide
CN	Cyanide
CA	Carbonic anhydrase
Hgb	Hemoglobin
HbCO	Carboxyhemoglobin
HbO_2	Oxyhemoglobin

GAS CONTENTS, FRACTIONS, PRESSURES, AND SATURATIONS

Ca_{O_2}	Content of oxygen in arterial blood
Cv_{O_2}	Content of oxygen in mixed venous blood
Cc_{O_2}	Content of oxygen in end-capillary blood
$C(a - v)_{O_2}$	Arterial-mixed venous oxygen content difference
FI_{O_2}	Fraction of inspired oxygen
FE_{O_2}	Fraction of expired oxygen
P_B	Barometric (atmospheric) pressure
P_{O_2}	Partial pressure of oxygen
PI_{O_2}	Partial pressure of oxygen in inspired gas
PA_{O_2}	Partial pressure of oxygen in alveolar gas
Pa_{O_2}	Partial pressure of oxygen in arterial blood
$P(A-a)_{O_2}$	Alveolar-arterial oxygen pressure difference
$P(a-A)_{CO_2}$	Arterial-alveolar carbon dioxide pressure difference
Pv_{O_2}	Partial pressure of oxygen in mixed venous blood
Pc_{O_2}	Partial pressure of oxygen in end-capillary blood
P_{CO_2}	Partial pressure of carbon dioxide
PI_{CO_2}	Partial pressure of carbon dioxide in inspired gas
PA_{CO_2}	Partial pressure of carbon dioxide in alveolar gas
Pa_{CO_2}	Partial pressure of carbon dioxide in arterial blood
Pv_{CO_2}	Partial pressure of carbon dioxide in mixed venous blood
P_{50}	P_{O_2} at which hemoglobin content is 50% saturated with oxygen
Sa_{O_2}	Percent saturation of oxygen in arterial blood
Sv_{O_2}	Percent saturation of oxygen in mixed venous blood

SYMBOLS FOR VOLUME AND VENTILATION

V	Volume
V_D	Dead space volume
V_A	Alveolar volume
V_T	Tidal volume
V_D/V_T	Dead space/tidal volume
$\dot{V}$	Ventilation
$\dot{V}_D$	Dead space ventilation
$\dot{V}_E$	Minute ventilation
$\dot{V}_A$	Alveolar ventilation

SYMBOLS FOR PERFUSION, DIFFUSION, AND GAS EXCHANGE

Q	Blood perfusion (flow)
Q_S	Shunt flow
Q_T	Cardiac output
Q_S/Q_T	Shunt fraction
DL_{CO}	Diffusing capacity for carbon monoxide
DL_{O_2}	Diffusing capacity for oxygen
V/Q	Ventilation/perfusion
$\dot{V}_{O_2}$	Oxygen consumption, either by the lungs or by body metabolism
$\dot{V}_{CO_2}$	Carbon dioxide elimination, either by the lungs or from body metabolism
R or RQ	Respiratory quotient: $\dot{V}_{CO_2}/\dot{V}_{O_2}$

appendix E
Glossary

a/A ratio Ratio of measured arterial P_{O_2} (Pa_{O_2}) to calculated alveolar P_{O_2} (PA_{O_2}). The a/A ratio remains relatively stable when lung conditions are stable but FI_{O_2} changes.

acid-base The acidity or alkalinity of the blood. A patient's acid-base status is reflected by changes in components of the bicarbonate buffer system, which is the largest of all the blood buffers. These components (pH, HCO_3^-, and Pa_{CO_2}) are related by the Henderson-Hasselbalch equation.

acidemia Arterial blood pH below 7.36.

acidosis A physiologic process that tends to cause an acidemia; it may be metabolic or respiratory in origin. *Metabolic acidosis* is manifested by a primary decrease in blood bicarbonate. *Respiratory acidosis* is manifested by a primary increase in blood P_{CO_2}.

adult respiratory distress syndrome (ARDS) Acute, fulminant, noncardiac pulmonary edema, that is accompanied by severe hypoxemia.

alkalemia Arterial blood pH above 7.44.

alkalosis A physiologic process that tends to cause an alkalemia; it may be metabolic or respiratory. *Metabolic alkalosis* is manifested by a primary increase in blood bicarbonate. *Respiratory alkalosis* is manifested by a primary decrease in blood P_{CO_2}.

alveolar air equation The equation used to calculate mean alveolar P_{O_2}. In its most practical and abbreviated version, the equation states: $PA_{O_2} = FI_{O_2}(P_B - 47 \text{ mm Hg}) - 1.2 (Pa_{CO_2})$.

alveolar ventilation ($\dot{V}_A$) Air that reaches the alveoli *and* takes part in gas exchange. It is not defined anatomically but by its relationship to alveolar P_{CO_2}: $\dot{V}_A = \dot{V}_{CO_2} \times k/PA_{CO_2}$, where $\dot{V}_A$ equals alveolar ventilation, $\dot{V}_{CO_2}$ equals CO_2 excretion per minute, Pa_{CO_2} equals alveolar P_{CO_2}, and k has a value of 0.863.

alveolar-arterial P_{O_2} difference The difference between calculated alveolar P_{O_2} and measured arterial P_{O_2}. Also called the $A - a$ *gradient*. An increase in the difference indicates gas exchange impairment and is usually the result of ventilation-perfusion imbalance. Abbreviated $P(A-a)_{O_2}$.

alveoli Terminal units of the airways. Alveoli are surrounded by a meshwork of capillaries. Alveolar-capillary units are the site of gas exchange.

aminophylline A methylxanthine drug used to treat asthma and reversible airways disease. (See the section on asthma in Appendix F.)

anaerobic exercise Exercise that does not use oxygen as an energy substrate.

anemia A decrease in the number of circulating red blood cells. Anemia is quantitated by measurement of the hematocrit or hemoglobin content.

anion gap The difference between measured cations and anions: $AG = (Na^+ + K^+) - (Cl^- + HCO_3^-)$. K^+ is usually ignored in this calculation, so normal AG is 8 to 16 mEq/L. Elevated AG usually indicates a state of metabolic acidosis.

apnea Absence of breathing. Sleep apnea is characterized by many apneic periods during a night's sleep, each lasting more than 10 seconds.

arterial Pertaining to the arteries. After birth, systemic arterial blood is oxygenated whereas pulmonary arterial blood is relatively deoxygenated. (Compare venous.)

asbestosis Interstitial lung disease resulting from inhalation of asbestos dust. (See Appendix F.)

asthma Reversible airways obstruction. (See Appendix F.)

atelectasis Collapse of part of the lung. It may involve only a small number of alveoli or an entire lobe. *Absorption atelectasis* occurs in low V/Q units from high FIO_2 therapy; nitrogen is washed out, and after the alveolar oxygen is absorbed into the blood, the alveoli collapse.

ATPS Abbreviation for ambient temperature and pressure, saturated. Used to express volume of gases collected under atmospheric or room air conditions.

Avogadro's law A law stating that equal volumes of different gases at the same pressure and temperature contain the same number of molecules.

Avogadro's number The number of molecules in a mole of gas—6.02×10^{23}. For an ideal gas, a gram molecular weight occupies 22.4 L at standard pressure and temperature dry and contains 6.02×10^{23} molecules.

barometric pressure (P_B) The pressure exerted by the atmosphere; also called *atmospheric pressure*. At sea level the barometric pressure is 760 mm Hg; it decreases with altitude.

base excess Technically, the amount of strong acid or alkali necessary to titrate a 1 L sample of blood to pH 7.40. Often used to indicate a state of metabolic alkalosis (positive base excess) or metabolic acidosis (negative base excess). Base excess is an in vitro measurement and does not take into account complex in vivo buffering mechanisms.

beta-adrenergic drugs Drugs that act by stimulating the beta-adrenergic system (the portion of the autonomic nervous system that causes bronchodilation). Epinephrine is a beta-adrenergic drug. (See the section on asthma in Appendix F.)

bicarbonate (HCO_3^-) A component of the major blood buffer system—the bicarbonate system. Low HCO_3^- is found in states of metabolic acidosis and respiratory alkalois; high HCO_3^- is found in states of metabolic alkalosis and respiratory acidosis.

Bohr dead space equation An equation used to calculate the ratio of dead space to tidal volume: $V_D/V_T = P_{aCO_2} - P_{eCO_2}/P_{aCO_2}$, where P_{aCO_2} is arterial P_{CO_2} and P_{eCO_2} is the mean expired P_{CO_2}.

Bohr effect The effect of P_{CO_2} on hemoglobin affinity for oxygen; also used to describe the effect of H^+ on this affinity. Increases in P_{aCO_2} or H^+ decrease oxyhemoglobin saturation, shifting the oxygen dissociation curve to the right. Decreases in P_{CO_2} or H^+ have the opposite effect.

Boyle's law A law stating that at constant temperature, the volume of a given quantity of gas varies inversely with the pressure of that gas: $P_1V_1 = P_2V_2$, where P_1 and V_1 are the initial pressure and volume and where P_2 and V_2 are the final pressure and volume. This law is the basis for body plethysmography measurements of lung volumes.

breathing The act of rhythmic inspiration and expiration for the purpose of gas exchange.

bronchiole The smallest conducting airway before alveoli appear. Bronchioles are less than 2 mm in diameter.

bronchiolitis An acute inflammation of the bronchioles

bronchitis Inflammation of the bronchi. (See Appendix F.)

bronchodilator A drug that dilates the bronchi. Bronchodilators used in asthma therapy include theophylline and beta-adrenergic agonists. (See Appendix F.)

BTPS Abbreviation for body temperature and pressure, saturated. Used to express, among other values, all lung volumes and capacities.

capacity A quantity of air made up of two or more lung volumes. For example, functional residual capacity is made up of expiratory reserve volume and residual volume.

carbon dioxide (CO_2) A by-product of metabolism. Carbon dioxide is excreted by the lungs in the process of gas exchange. In the steady state, the amount of CO_2 produced during metabolism equals the amount excreted by the lungs.

carbon monoxide (CO) A tasteless, odorless gas normally present in small amounts in the blood. Excess carbon monoxide is a poison since it prevents oxygen from combining with hemoglobin.

carbonic anhydrase The enzyme that catalyzes the hydration of CO_2 to form carbonic acid.

carboxyhemoglobin (HbCO) A combination of carbon monoxide and hemoglobin. Carbon monoxide has approximately 200 times greater affinity than oxygen for binding with hemoglobin.

carcinoma The most common form of cancer. Carcinomas arise from the epithelial cells lining various organs, e.g., the bronchi and colon. (See the section on lung cancer in Appendix F.)

carina The point at which an airway divides or branches. The main carina is the point at which the trachea divides into the right and left main bronchi.

Charles' law A law stating that at a constant pressure, the volume of a given quantity of gas is directly proportional to the absolute temperature (in degrees Kelvin):

$$\frac{V_1}{V_2} = \frac{T_1}{T_2}$$

where V_1 and V_2 are volume of the same mass of gas at corresponding absolute temperatures T_1 and T_2.

chemoreceptor Any organ or group of cells that can detect chemical change. Chemoreceptors in the brainstem are sensitive to CO_2 and normally stimulate breathing if the blood P_{CO_2} rises.

chloride (Cl^-) The principal extracellular anion. Chloride shares a reciprocal relationship with bicarbonate in the blood. Hyperchloremic states are associated with low bicarbonate.

chloride shift As carbon dioxide is taken up in the systemic capillaries, bicarbonate increases in the red cell. To preserve electrical neutrality, chloride diffuses (shifts) out of the cells into the plasma.

chylous Rich in chylomicrons; chylomicrons are fat molecules made up mainly of triglycerides.

collagen-vascular diseases A group of diseases characterized by abnormalities of connective tissue. (See Appendix F.)

compliance The quality of distensibility. Compliance is a change in volume per change in pressure; units are ml/mm Hg or l/cm H_2O. Low-compliance lungs are less distensible (i.e., stiffer) than high-compliance lungs.

conductance The reciprocal of resistance. A measure of how well air or blood flows through a tube; units are L/sec/mm Hg or L/sec/cm H_2O.

continuous positive airway pressure (CPAP) The term used in clinical practice for systems that deliver positive airway pressure without an artificial ventilator.

corticosteroids A group of hormones that are normally produced by the adrenal cortex. In doses far greater than are produced by the adrenals, corticosteroids are used to treat a variety of pulmonary disorders, especially asthma. (See the section on asthma in Appendix F.)

croup An infectious condition of childhood that involves the upper airways. Patients with croup have a high-pitched, inspiratory wheeze (stridor).

cyanosis Bluish discoloration of the skin, nailbeds, and/or mucous membranes. *Central cyanosis* occurs when at least 5 gm% of hemoglobin are desaturated in the systemic capillaries. With a normal hemoglobin content (15 gm%) this represents an Sa_{O_2} of approximately 83%. Methemoglobin is another cause of central cyanosis. *Peripheral cyanosis* may occur without oxygen desaturation, from vasoconstriction.

cystic fibrosis An inherited disease that affects exocrine secretion and often leads to severe pulmonary problems. (See Appendix F.)

cytology The technique of microscopically examining cells for malignant changes and other abnormalities.

Dalton's law The law stating that the total pressure exerted by a mixture of gases equals the sum of the separate partial pressures:

$$P_T = P_1 + P_2 + P_3 + \ldots + P_n$$

where P_T is total pressure, and $P_1 \ldots P_n$ are the pressures of individual gases. Atmospheric pressure $= P_{N_2} + P_{O_2} + P_{CO_2} + P_{H_2O}$, where P_{N_2}, P_{O_2}, P_{CO_2}, and P_{H_2O} are the partial pressure of nitrogen (plus trace amounts of other inert gases such as argon and krypton), oxygen, carbon dioxide, and water vapor, respectively. Also called the *law of partial pressures*.

dead space Any space in the lungs or upper airways that receives fresh air but that does not take part in gas exchange. *Anatomic dead space* refers to the entire airway not normally involved with gas exchange (the upper airway and much of lower airways). *Physiologic dead space* refers to the sum of anatomic dead space plus any alveolar space that is unperfused or underperfused. The ratio of physiologic dead space to tidal volume can be calculated from the P_{ECO_2} and Pa_{CO_2}. (See Bohr dead space equation.)

diffusing capacity (DL) The rate of gas transfer through a permeable membrane. *Pulmonary diffusing capacity* is measured using carbon monoxide (DL_{CO}). Units for DL are ml gas/mm Hg/min. The diffusing capacity can be decreased by a loss of alveolar surface area, thickening of the pulmonary interstitium, or anemia (decreased capillary blood volume). Diffusion impairment does not usually cause hypoxemia at rest but may lead to hypoxemia with exercise.

diffusion The passive transfer of a substance from a region of higher concentration to one of lower concentration. Diffusion is the physiologic process whereby oxygen and carbon dioxide are exchanged in the body, first between alveolar air and pulmonary capillary blood and then between the systemic capillary blood and metabolizing tissues.

dyspnea Any sensation of difficult or hard breathing. Patients who complain of shortness of breath are dyspneic. Although technically a symptom, dyspnea is also referred to as a sign; e.g., "the patient looks dyspneic."

elastic recoil The tendency of the lungs or chest wall to return to their resting state. Elastic recoil is measured as the difference between intrapleural pressure and alveolar pressure at a given lung volume; it is greatest at total lung capacity.

emphysema A chronic lung condition characterized by destruction of alveolar-capillary units. (See Appendix F.)

empyema Literally, pus in the pleural space; also used to refer to any pleural effusion infected with bacteria.

eosinophil A type of white blood cell characterized by pink-staining cytoplasmic granules. An increase in eosinophils is common in asthma and many allergic conditions.

expiratory reserve volume (ERV) The volume of air that can be exhaled from the point of functional residual capacity. ERV + residual volume = functional residual capacity.

exudate Fluid formed by inflammation or capillary leakage; generally high in protein content. (Compare transudate.)

fibrosis Scarring of tissue. Pulmonary fibrosis is a common clinical problem and a cause of restrictive lung disease.

flow Movement of gas or liquid per unit time. Units are cm/sec, L/sec, L/min, etc.

flow volume curve Plot of flow (expiratory or inspiratory) vs. volume. When expiratory and inspiratory curves are plotted on the same axes, a flow volume loop is obtained.

flow volume loop A continuous recording of air flow vs. volume during expiration and inspiration.

forced expiratory volume (FEV) A specified volume that is forced out after a full inspiration. Usually quantitated in the first second, as FEV_1.

forced vital capacity The volume of air that can be forcefully exhaled after inhalation to total lung capacity. It is measured with a spirometer and is a standard test in respiratory patients.

fraction of inspired oxygen (FIO_2) The fraction of oxygen in the inspired air. Although technically a decimal fraction (e.g., 0.21), FIO_2 is often referred to as a percentage, e.g., 21%.

functional residual capacity (FRC) The volume of air in the lungs and airways at the end of a normal tidal volume. The resting point of the lungs and thoracic cage.

gas exchange The major function of the lungs. Gas exchange involves transfer of oxygen and carbon dioxide between the atmosphere and the pulmonary capillary blood, and then between the systemic capillary blood and the metabolizing tissues.

general gas law (ideal) This law combines the laws of Charles, Boyle, and Avogadro. For an ideal gas:

$$\frac{P_1 V_1}{T_1} = \frac{P_2 V_2}{T_2}$$

where P_1, V_1, and T_1 are the initial pressure, volume, and temperature and where P_2, V_2, and T_2 are the final conditions. The general gas law is used to convert from one set of conditions to another, e.g., from BTPS to STPD.

Haldane effect The effect whereby an increase in the blood PO_2 decreases the ability of hemoglobin to combine with carbon dioxide. (Compare Bohr effect.)

helium (He) An inert gas that is lighter than air. Mixtures of helium and oxygen are used for research into mechanics of air flow.

hemodynamic monitoring The process of following the changes in cardiovascular pressures, flows, and resistances; for clinical purposes this is accomplished with the flow-directed, right heart catheter (the Swan-Ganz catheter) plus a cannula inserted into a peripheral artery.

hemoglobin (Hgb) The iron-protein complex responsible for transporting oxygen. One molecule of hemoglobin (Hgb) can combine with up to four molecules of oxygen; 1 gm Hgb can combine with up to 1.34 ml O_2. The amount of oxygen bound to hemoglobin is a function of the PaO_2; as PaO_2 increases, the oxygen saturation (SaO_2) increases. The hemoglobin-oxygen dissociation curve describes the relationship between PaO_2 and SaO_2.

Henderson-Hasselbalch equation The equation relating the three components of the bicarbonate buffer system: pH, bicarbonate, and $PaCO_2$. This equation allows calculation of one component when concentrations of the other two are known. (See equation on p. 368.)

$$pH = pK + \log \frac{HCO_3^-}{0.03\, P_{CO_2}}$$

hydrostatic pressure The pressure resulting from the weight of a liquid or from the pumping action of the heart. Hydrostatic pressure tends to force fluid out of the capillary and is opposed by oncotic pressure.

hyperbaric pressure A pressure greater than atmospheric pressure. A hyperbaric chamber allows subjects to inhale oxygen at greater than atmospheric pressure.

hypercapnia High P_{CO_2} in the blood, e.g., greater than 44 mm Hg in arterial blood.

hyperventilation A condition in which alveolar ventilation is in excess of that needed for carbon dioxide production. Hyperventilation always leads to a P_{CO_2} lower than the baseline value.

hypocapnia Low P_{CO_2} in the blood, e.g., less than 36 mm Hg in arterial blood.

hypopnea A decrease in tidal volume or respiratory rate resulting in oxygen desaturation.

hypoventilation A condition in which alveolar ventilation is less than that needed for carbon dioxide production. Hypoventilation always leads to a P_{CO_2} higher than the baseline value.

hypoxemia Low oxygen in the blood. As this term is commonly used, hypoxemia refers to either a low Pa_{O_2} or a low arterial oxygen content.

infiltrate An abnormal shadow on the chest x-ray; it is nonspecific and may refer to pneumonia, tumor, etc.

inspiratory capacity (IC) The lung capacity that can be inhaled from the point of FRC; includes tidal volume and inspiratory reserve volume.

inspiratory reserve volume (IRV) The maximal lung volume that can be inhaled after a normal inspiration. IRV + tidal volume = inspiratory capacity.

interstitium In the lungs, the area between the alveolar and capillary membranes; it includes elastic tissue and lymphatics. Many diseases predominantly affect the interstitium. (See the section on interstitial lung disease in Appendix F.)

lung capacity A named quantity of air contained within both lungs; a lung capacity comprises two or more lung volumes. The four lung capacities are inspiratory, functional residual, vital, and total lung.

lung volumes The smallest named quantities of air contained within both lungs. The four lung volumes are tidal, expiratory reserve, inspiratory reserve, and residual.

lungs The paired organs of respiration, including all airways below the trachea.

lymphoma A form of cancer. Lymphomas arise from lymphocytes in lymph nodes.

maximal midflow (MMF) The maximal midflow is customarily measured by drawing a line between points representing 25% and 75% of the forced vital capacity. When measured in this way it is called the $MMF_{25\text{-}75}$. Units are L/sec.

maximal voluntary ventilation (MVV) The maximal amount of air that can be moved during 1 min. In practice, the subject is asked to inhale and exhale as rapidly as possible for 12 or 15 sec.; the amount exhaled is then multiplied by 5 or 4, respecitvely. Maximal voluntary ventilation is a gross evaluation of the entire respiratory system, including lung and chest wall mechanics and the subject's motivation.

metabolic acidosis A primary physiologic process that results in reduced blood bicarbonate. Metabolic acidosis is compensated by hyperventilation (lowering of Pa_{CO_2}). If there is no other acid-base disorder, metabolic acidosis always results in a lower than normal blood pH. The compensatory bicarbonate excretion seen in respiratory alkalosis is not called metabolic acidosis since it is not a primary physiologic process.

metabolic alkalosis A primary physiologic process that results in excess blood bicarbonate. Compensation for metabolic alkalosis is hypoventilation, which raises the Pa_{CO_2}. If there is no other acid-base disorder, metabolic alkalosis always results in a greater than normal blood pH. The secondary bicarbonate retention seen in respiratory acidosis is not called metabolic alkalosis since it is not a primary physiologic process.

methemoglobin Hemoglobin molecule with iron in an oxidized state: Fe^{+3} instead of the normal Fe^{+2}. Methemoglobin is incapable of carrying oxygen. Methemoglobinemia causes profound cyanosis.

mixed venous blood A mixture of venous blood from all parts of the body. In practice, blood from the pulmonary artery.

nitrogen An inert gas that makes up 78% of the atmosphere and a similar amount of alveolar and arterial (dissolved) gas. Increasing the FIO_2 washes out alveolar and arterial nitrogen.

obstructive Term for any condition characterized by impediment to airflow. Airways obstruction may be present during inspiration or expiration. Obstructive airways disease includes asthma, chronic bronchitis, and emphysema.

oncotic pressure Pressure resulting from large molecular weight molecules, mainly proteins. Oncotic pressure tends to keep fluid in the capillary and is opposed by hydrostatic pressure.

Ondine's curse A condition in which the patient has lost the central breathing drive, to the point of apnea. Ondine's curse does not refer to a specific disease or cause.

orthopnea Dyspnea in the recumbent position that is relieved by sitting or standing. Orthopnea is common in patients with congestive heart failure and acute pulmonary problems such as asthma.

oxygen (O_2) Gas vital to life. Oxygen is taken up by the lungs for delivery to the tissues. Oxygen and carbon dioxide are exchanged between the blood and the atmosphere (see gas exchange).

oxygen content The amount of oxygen in the blood. Units are O_2/100 ml blood. Normal arterial oxygen content is 16 to 20 ml O_2/100 ml blood. Most oxygen is carried in the blood bound to hemoglobin.

oxygen uptake The amount of oxygen transferred by the lungs or consumed during metabolism per minute. In the steady state, the two volumes are equal. At rest, oxygen uptake is approximately 250 ml 02/min.

P_{50} The PO_2 at which hemoglobin is 50% saturated with oxygen. Normal P_{50} is approximately 27 mm Hg. A P_{50} higher than 27 mm Hg represents a rightward shift of the oxygen dissociation curve; a P_{50} lower than 27 mm Hg represents a leftward shift.

partial pressure The pressure exerted by an individual gas in a mixture of gases. Total air pressure, in the atmosphere or in the lungs, is the sum of pressures of the individual gases (See Dalton's law.)

peak flow The fastest point of flow during the forced vital capacity maneuver; it always occurs within the first second of the FVC. Peak flow is used for gauging the severity of and following the improvement from an asthma attack.

perfusion Blood flow; *pulmonary perfusion* refers to the total cardiac output as it flows through the pulmonary blood vessels. The ratio of ventilation to perfusion among the millions of alveolar-capillary units determines the efficiency of gas exchange.

pH A measure of the acidity or alkalinity of the blood. pH equals the negative log of the hydrogen ion concentration.

Pickwickian syndrome A syndrome characterized by obesity, hypoventilation, and daytime sleepiness. So named because an obese character with daytime sleepiness was first described in Dickens' *Pickwick Papers*.

plethysmograph An enclosed structure used to measure changes in volume. In pulmonary medicine, a body plethysmograph is used to measure thoracic gas volume and airway resistance.

pleura Thin membranes lining the inside of the thoracic cavity *(parietal pleura)* and the lungs *(visceral pleura)*.

pleural effusion An abnormal accumulation of fluid in the pleural space; may be an exudate or a transudate.

pleural space A potential space that exists between the parietal and visceral pleura.

pneumoconiosis A lung disease that results from inhalation of dust. (See Appendix F.)

pneumonia An infection of the alveolar spaces. Pneumonia may result from infection with viruses, bacteria, or other organisms. (See Appendix F.)

pneumothorax The collapse of a lung or of a portion of a lung, resulting from leakage of air into the intrapleural space. Air may enter the intrapleural space from the lung or from outside the chest wall.

polysomnography The continuous recording of several physiologic variables during sleep.

positive end-expiratory pressure (PEEP) PEEP is commonly employed in ventilator management of patients suffering from oxygenation respiratory failure, usually in range of 5 to 20 cm H_2O. With PEEP the airway pressure remains positive relative to atmospheric pressure at the end of exhalation.

potassium (K^+) The principal intracellular cation. Potassium is measured as part of the serum electrolytes; the normal value is 3.5 to 5 mEq/L. Elevated potassium (hyperkalemia) is often found in states of acidosis.

pressure The force exerted against a surface. Gas exerts a pressure as a result of movement of the gas molecules. At sea level, atmospheric pressure supports a column of mercury 760 mm high. In pulmonary physiology, all measured pressures are referenced to the atmospheric pressure, which is arbitrarily assigned a zero value. Thus negative pressure is less than atmospheric pressure, and positive pressure is greater than atmospheric pressure. (See also Barometric pressure, Partial pressure.)

pulmonary edema Excess fluid in the alveolar spaces that results from physiologic factors affecting the pulmonary capillary—increased hydrostatic pressure, decreased oncotic pressure, and/or increased capillary permeability.

rales Abnormal lung sounds characterized by discontinuous character. Rales signify fluid in the alveoli or terminal bronchioles or parenchymal fibrosis. Rales may be heard in a variety of conditions, including heart failure, pneumonia, and sarcoidosis.

residual volume (RV) The volume of air left in lungs after maximal exhalation.

resistance A measure of the difficulty with which air or blood flows through a tube. Resistance is pressure divided by flow; units are mm Hg/L/sec, or cm H_2O/L/sec. For a given flow, more pressure is generated in high-resistance vessels than in low-resistance vessels. The inverse of resistance is conductance.

respiratory acidosis A primary physiologic process that results in CO_2 retention. Compensation for respiratory acidosis is renal bicarbonate retention. If there is no other acid-base disorder present, respiratory acidosis always results in a blood pH that is less than normal. The secondary CO_2 retention (hypoventilation) sometimes seen in metabolic alkalosis is not called respiratory acidosis since it is not a primary physiologic process.

respiratory alkalosis A primary physiologic condition that results in CO_2 excretion. Compensation for respiratory alkalosis is bicarbonate excretion. If there is no other acid-base disorder present, respiratory alkalosis always results in a blood pH that is greater than normal. The secondary CO_2 excretion (hyperventilation) seen in metabolic acidosis is not called respiratory alkalosis since it is not a primary physiologic process.

respiratory distress syndrome Acute pulmonary edema of noncardiac origin. In infants, this is also called hyaline membrane disease. (See Adult respiratory distress syndrome.)

respiratory failure Failure of the gas exchange function of the lungs. Respiratory failure is always manifested by a lower than normal Pa_{O_2}, but it may or may not result in a high Pa_{CO_2}. The actual degree of abnormality is arbitrary when using this label.

respiratory quotient (R or RQ) The ratio of CO_2 production over oxygen uptake. In a steady state, the respiratory quotient for the lungs (the amount of CO_2 excreted over the amount of oxygen taken up by the pulmonary capillaries) equals the metabolic respiratory quotient (the amount of CO_2 produced by metabolism over the metabolic oxygen uptake).

restrictive Term for any condition characterized by inability to take in a full, deep breath. Restrictive lung diseases are manifested by a reduced total lung capacity. Examples include interstitial lung disease and chest wall weakness.

retrolental fibroplasia An eye complication seen in newborn and premature infants given high oxygen concentrations for prolonged periods. It is characterized by scarring behind the lens of the eye and may lead to blindness. It is also called retinopathy of newborns.

rhonchi Another name for wheezes. Some physicians classify as rhonchi those wheezes that are of lower pitch.

sarcoidosis A disease of unknown origin, characterized by granulomas in various organs. (See Appendix F.)

shock lung Pulmonary edema arising from severe or sudden hypotension. Shock lung is synonymous with the adult respiratory distress syndrome when shock is the precipitating event.

shunt When one thing bypasses another. In pulmonary physiology, shunts can be anatomic or physiologic. As commonly used, the term applies to blood that is either anatomically shunted past alveoli or that is inadequately oxygenated even though it courses through alveolar-capillary units (physiologic shunting).

silicosis A lung disease that results from inhalation of silica dust. (See the section on Pneumoconiosis in Appendix F.)

small airways disease Disease limited to the airways that are less than 2 mm in diameter. The diagnosis is usually made on the basis of a reduced MMF_{25-75} when the remainder of spirometry is normal.

sodium (Na^+) The principal extracellular cation. States of high and low sodium are related to extracellular water balance. High sodium (hypernatremia) and low sodium (hyponatremia) may be associated with either dehydration or overhydration.

spirometer A device used to measure the forced vital capacity and its components.

spirometry Measurement of the forced vital capacity; any test that measures forced vital capacity.

STPD Abbreviation for standard temperature and pressure, dry; used to express, among other values, oxygen uptake and CO_2 excretion.

stridor High-pitched, inspiratory wheeze resulting from upper airway obstruction (above the main carina).

tachycardia Fast heart rate. The specific rate that signifies tachycardia depends on the patient's age (newborn vs. young child vs. adult).

tachypnea Fast respiratory rate. The specific rate that signifies tachypnea depends on the patient's age (newborn vs. young child vs. adult).

tension Another word for pressure, e.g., arterial gas tension.

theophylline The basic methylxanthine bronchodilator. Theophylline is commonly used in asthma therapy. (See Appendix F.)

thoracentesis The procedure for inserting a needle into the pleural space and removing pleural fluid.

tidal volume (V$_T$) The volume of air inspired or expired during a normal breath; V$_T$ during inspiration is slightly greater than during expiration since slightly more oxygen is taken up per breath than CO_2 excreted.

torr Another name for mm Hg. Named after Evangelista Torricelli, an Italian physiologist.

total lung capacity (TLC) The volume of air within both lungs at the end of maximal inhalation. It is measured in liters or milliliters. TLC contains the four primary lung volumes: inspiratory reserve volume (IRV), tidal volume (VT), expiratory reserve volume (ERV), and residual volume (RV).

transudate Fluid formed by a decrease in oncotic pressure, an increase in hydrostatic pressure, or both. (See exudate).

tuberculosis A disease that results from infection with *Mycobacterium tuberculosis*. (See Appendix F.)

venous Pertaining to the venous system. After birth, systemic venous blood is deoxygenated, and pulmonary venous blood is oxygenated.

venous admixture The total amount of cardiac output from the right ventricle that is not fully oxygenated by the lungs. Includes blood that is shunted and that goes to areas with low ventilation-perfusion ratios.

ventilation Movement of air into and out of the lungs. Ventilation is usually qualified, as "minute," "total," "alveolar," or "dead space" ventilation.

ventilation/perfusion (V/Q) imbalance An imbalance in the normal distribution of V/Q ratios. V/Q imbalance always leads to gas exchange abnormality.

ventilation/perfusion (V/Q) ratio The ratio of alveolar ventilation to pulmonary capillary perfusion in one or more alveolar-capillary units. The ventilation/perfusion ratio of the entire lung is the alveolar ventilation divided by the cardiac output.

ventilator Any machine capable of taking over the mechanical breathing function for purposes of improving gas exchange. Also called an artificial ventilator.

vital capacity (VC) The maximal volume of gas that can be inhaled (inspiratory VC) or exhaled (expiratory VC). Forced vital capacity is a commonly employed test of lung mechanics.

volume A quantity of air contained within the lungs. There are four primary lung volumes: inspiratory reserve, tidal, expiratory reserve, and residual. Two or more lung volumes constitute a lung "capacity."

water vapor Water in the gas phase. Water vapor exerts a pressure that is a function of temperature only; at normal body temperature (37° C) water vapor pressure (PH_2O) is 47 mm Hg. PH_2O must be subtracted from any gas pressure to obtain the dry gas pressure. For example, if FIO_2 is 0.21 and if body temperature is 37° C, then at sea level PIO_2 = 0.21(760 − 47) mm Hg.

wedge pressure The measurement obtained by "wedging" a pulmonary artery (Swan-Ganz) catheter in a branch of the pulmonary artery. The wedge pressure reflects the left atrial and left ventricular end-diastolic pressures in many situations.

wheeze An abnormal breath sound of variable pitch that is continuous in character; it is generated by air going through a narrowed airway. Wheezing is usually, but not invariably, present in asthma attacks. Conversely, wheezing does not always signify asthma.

appendix F
Common clinical conditions

This appendix contains brief descriptions of the more common clinical conditions mentioned in the book. Diseases covered in the body of a chapter are listed with the chapter reference. These descriptions are necessarily brief and are included only to complement material presented in the chapters. Consult the list of general references in Appendix G for more detailed information on each diagnosis.

ADULT RESPIRATORY DISTRESS SYNDROME (See Chapter 11)

ASBESTOSIS (See Pneumoconioses)

ASTHMA

Asthma is a state of reversible airways obstruction manifested clinically by episodes of dyspnea, wheezing, and/or cough. Since many different stimuli can trigger the symptoms, asthma is sometimes referred to as a state of hyperreactive or hypersensitive airways. There are an estimated 9 million people with asthma in the United States, and approximately 2000 deaths are attributed to asthma each year.

The basic cause of asthma is unknown. The asthma response or attack occurs when one or more stimuli cause bronchial smooth muscle contraction (bronchoconstriction) and/or increased bronchial mucus production. People who do not have asthma do not manifest this airway hyperreactivity.

Common stimuli of the asthma reaction include inhaled allergens (e.g., pollen), cold air with or without exercise, some foods, medications (e.g., aspirin, penicillin), air pollution (e.g., cigarette smoke), emotional turmoil, and upper respiratory infection.

The most common trigger of an asthma attack is viral infection of the upper respiratory tract, including the common cold. Asthma is not synonymous with allergy since allergy (antigen-antibody reaction) is only one of several mechanisms that can elicit the asthma response. Most asthma attacks in the adult are not allergy-mediated. Although cigarette smoke is definitely aggravating to many asthmatics, smoking per se is not a cause of asthma (as it is of chronic bronchitis and emphysema).

Most persons with asthma have an increased number of eosinophils in their blood or sputum during an attack. The eosinophilic response is nonspecific and can occur irrespective of the stimulus.

The chest x-ray of asthmatic individuals is usually normal except for hyperinflation during attacks. An infiltrate may be present (either from pneumonia or atelectasis) but this is uncommon.

Physiologic testing (see also Chapter 3). Between asthma attacks, spirometry is usually normal or at most shows a slight decrease in MMF_{25-75}. During an asthma attack spirometry is abnormal, but it usually improves (shows reversibility) with one trial of inhaled bronchodilator. Lack of immediate reversibility is common with severe airways obstruction, particularly when caused by thick secretions and mucous plugging.

In unusual cases asthma can be manifested solely by cough, and baseline spirometry will be normal. Such patients can often be diagnosed by a bronchoprovocation test. In this test the patient inhales an agent such as methacholine, which causes bronchoconstriction (more than 15% reduction in airflow) in true asthma sufferers but not in nonasthmatic individuals.

Blood gas measurements are usually normal between asthma attacks. In the early stages of an asthma attack there is usually hyperventilation, and the PaO_2 is only slightly reduced. The more severe the attack, as gauged by peak flow rate or FEV_1, the lower is the PaO_2 and the less reduced the $PaCO_2$. When $PaCO_2$ is normal or elevated during an asthma attack, the attack must be considered severe and potentially life-threatening.

Treatment. Although almost all symptomatic persons with asthma will receive drugs, every attempt must also be made to remove the patient from possible aggravating stimuli, including cigarette smoke and pollens. Drugs from four main pharmacologic groups are used to treat the asthma attack:

Theophylline. Theophylline and its derivatives are bronchodilators and are available in a wide variety of forms (regular and slow-release capsules, elixir, and intravenous solution) and dosages. A relatively recent advance in therapy is the ability to measure serum theophylline levels, which has greatly aided accurate dosing. Therapeutic range for theophylline in most patients is 10 to 20 mg/L.

Beta-adrenergic agonists. Beta-adrenergic agonists are also classified as bronchodilators. Unlike theophylline, which cannot be given through inhalation, beta-adrenergic drugs are frequently and effectively given by the aerosol route. The time-honored drugs epinephrine and isoproterenol are now used less often than newer beta-adrenergic drugs, which last longer (when inhaled) and have fewer cardiac side effects. Among this group are metaproterenol, albuterol, and bitolterol.

Corticosteroids. Corticosteroids are probably the most potent anti-asthma drug group and are most likely to be used in persistent or severe attacks. Corticosteroids are anti-inflammatory agents, and are not considered true bronchodilators; their mechanism of action in asthma is unknown.

The more severe the asthma attack the more likely that all three drug groups will be used. For prevention of symptoms or to reverse mild bronchospasm, theophylline or a beta-adrenergic agonist alone may be sufficient.

Anticholinergics. The anticholinergics are another group of bronchodilators, of which the best known is atropine. Atropine and atropine-like drugs have been used for years in other countries but surprisingly have not yet entered the mainstream of asthma therapy in the United States. At present no anticholinergic is approved for asthma therapy in the United States, although ipratropium bromide should be released soon for inhalation use. Anticholinergics block the vagal response and provide yet another mechanism to help reverse bronchospasm.

Cromolyn sodium. A fifth drug group is represented by cromolyn sodium, which is administered only by inhalation, either in powder or liquid form. Cromolyn sodium is not a bronchodilator and is used to prevent attacks but not reverse them. The drug is used far more frequently in children than in adults.

In addition to drugs from these groups and depending on the overall clinical situation, an individual suffering from asthma may also receive antibiotics, supplemental oxygen, expectorants, and intravenous fluids. (Some of the drugs used for asthma, including bronchodilators and corticosteroids, are also used for patients with chronic obstructive pulmonary disease.)

BRONCHITIS

Bronchitis is a general term for inflammation of the bronchi. Acute bronchitis is characterized by fever, cough, and expectoration of mucus. It is usually caused by viral or bacterial infection, but it can also be the result of the inhalation of irritants (e.g., gases and fumes). Infectious bronchitis is treated with antibiotics.

Chronic bronchitis is usually caused by long-term cigarette smoking, and for this reason chronic bronchitis is often accompanied by some element of airways obstruction. (See Chronic Obstructive Pulmonary Disease.)

CARCINOMA OF THE LUNG (See Lung Cancer)

CHRONIC BRONCHITIS (See Chronic Obstructive Pulmonary Disease)

CHRONIC OBSTRUCTIVE PULMONARY DISEASE

Chronic obstructive pulmonary disease (COPD) is the term used for generalized airways obstruction that is not fully reversible with treatment. Patients with COPD often manifest one of two clinicopathologic states: chronic bronchitis or emphysema.

Chronic bronchitis is classically described by historical criteria: coughing up mucus for at least 3 months a year for 2 consecutive years. Emphysema is destruction of lung tissue that leads to abnormally large (and ineffective) airspaces. (See Chapter 11 for a further discussion of COPD.)

The patient with bronchitis may have a normal chest x-ray or one that shows only some increased bronchial wall thickening at the lung bases. Classically, severe emphysema appears with flattened diaphragms, increased retrosternal airspace (evidence of lung hyperinflation), and attenuation of pulmonary vasculature toward the lung periphery. Although there are typical radiologic patterns, COPD cannot be diagnosed by chest x-ray alone.

Clinically, both mucus production and alveolar-capillary destruction overlap in many patients. Treatment for the individual patient is based on symptoms and degree of airways obstruction, not on the specific diagnosis.

Physiologic testing. By definition, pulmonary function tests show a decrease in air flow rates, with little or no response to inhaled bronchodilators. However, as in asthma, lack of immediate bronchodilator response does not rule out clinical improvement with a long-term regimen of bronchodilators and corticosteroids.

When physiologic testing includes measurement of total lung capacity (TLC), diffusing capacity (DL_{CO}—see Chapter 5), and lung compliance, a clear distinction can often be made between emphysema and chronic bronchitis. Generally, the emphysematous patient has above normal TLC, reduced DL_{CO}, and increased compliance, all as a result of destruction of lung tissue and loss of pulmonary elastic recoil. By contrast, because lung tissue is not destroyed, these tests tend to be normal or near-normal in the stable patient with chronic bronchitis.

Blood gas measurements can vary widely in COPD. Pa_{O_2} may range from normal to very low, and Pa_{CO_2} may be normal, low, or high (see Chapter 5 for further discussion of blood gases in COPD).

Treatment. Drug treatment is practically the same as that for asthma. The main difference is in the ultimate response. The person with pure asthma should recover completely and achieve normal air flow. The patient with COPD often improves somewhat with treatment but does not achieve normal air flow.

In addition, depending on the clinical situation, patients with COPD may be treated with antibiotics, supplemental oxygen, and other medications. Breathing exercises (to increase efficiency of breathing) and aids to bronchial hygiene (such as postural drainage) are also frequently employed in cases of COPD.

COLLAGEN-VASCULAR DISEASES

Collagen-vascular diseases are a heterogeneous group of disorders characterized by inflammation in the joints, skin, and various organs, particularly the kidneys and lungs. The two most common collagen-vascular diseases are systemic lupus erythematosus (SLE) and rheumatoid arthritis (RA).

Either condition may (and commonly does) involve the lungs and pleural membranes.

Among the more common pulmonary complications (along with the disease usually implicated) are: interstitial lung disease (more common in RA—see Interstitial lung disease); noninfectious pneumonitis (SLE); pleural effusion (RA and SLE); and pulmonary nodules (RA).

Physiologic testing. See Interstitial Lung Disease; Pleural Effusions.

Treatment. In all cases treatment is of the underlying collagen-vascular process. Corticosteroids and more potent immunosuppressive drugs are commonly used in these conditions. Patients with collagen-vascular diseases may also develop classic infectious pulmonary problems, in which case appropriate antibiotics are indicated.

CYSTIC FIBROSIS

Cystic fibrosis (CF) is the most common inherited lethal disease among whites. Before the antibiotic era, virtually no patient with CF lived past puberty. Now the average life expectancy is approximately 30 years.

The inheritance of CF is autosomal recessive, meaning that both parents must be carriers (heterozygous state) for a child to inherit the disease (homozygous state). On a statistical basis one of four siblings born to CF carrier parents will have the disease. In contrast to the homozygous disease state, CF carriers are asymptomatic and healthy.

CF affects the exocrine or secreting function of many organs, especially the lungs, pancreas, and gastrointestinal tract. The major pulmonary problem is chronic mucous production, inability to clear the mucus, and recurrent bronchial infections. Infections are often from organisms that do not generally infect healthy persons (e.g., *Pseudomonas aeruginosa*). Repeated infections over a number of years can lead to pulmonary damage and respiratory failure, the major cause of death for CF patients who live past puberty.

Diagnosis of CF is first suspected on clinical grounds. For example, an infant who has failure to thrive or who suffers from repeated attacks of bronchitis should be evaluated for CF. CF is confirmed by measuring the amount of chloride in sweat collected after stimulation of the skin with a small current. In patients with CF the sweat chloride level is consistently elevated above normal.

Physiologic testing. Patients with CF usually have some degree of air flow obstruction and lung hyperinflation. The degree of abnormality is highly variable, depending on the extent and stage of the disease. Carbon dioxide retention is an end-stage finding.

Treatment. There is no therapy for the basic genetic defect. Pulmonary treatment is directed at improved bronchial hygiene (e.g., postural drainage) and any acute infection. Because of the complicated nature of this relatively uncommon condition, treatment is best given at or under the direction of a recognized CF center. (Locations are available from the National Cystic Fibrosis Foundation, 3379 Peachtree Rd., Atlanta, Georgia 30326.)

EMPHYSEMA (See Chronic Obstructive Pulmonary Disease)

GUILLAIN-BARRÉ SYNDROME (See Neuromuscular Disorders)

HEART FAILURE (See Chapter 8)

INTERSTITIAL LUNG DISEASE

Interstitial lung disease (ILD) is a general term for a heterogeneous group of conditions. These diseases usually cause an interstitial pattern on the chest x-ray, which on close inspection consists of "linear," "nodular," and/or "reticulo-nodular" infiltrates. Except for some obvious cases of sarcoidosis and pneumoconiosis, a lung biopsy is needed to make a specific diagnosis.

Patients with ILD usually complain of dyspnea. In large series, approximately 5% to 10% of patients ultimately diagnosed with ILD (from biopsy) had a negative chest x-ray initially.

There are many potential causes of ILD, including chronic pulmonary infection, dust inhalation (e.g., silicosis, asbestosis), collagen-vascular disease, and drug reactions. In addition, a large group of these diseases are of unknown cause (e.g., sarcoidosis, eosinophilic granuloma, idiopathic pulmonary fibrosis). Since there are so many different causes, the natural history and treatment vary widely, depending on the diagnosis. (See also Collagen-Vascular Diseases, Pneumoconioses, Sarcoidosis.)

Physiologic testing. Pulmonary function tests classically show restrictive impairment with reduced lung volumes and normal to increased flow rates. Some ILDs may also involve the airways (e.g., sarcoidosis), in which case there may also be some airways obstruction. Pulmonary compliance is reduced as a result of the increased elastic recoil arising from the interstitial involvement. Reduction in the diffusing capacity generally correlates with the degree of dyspnea. As a result of reduced diffusion, PaO_2 falls markedly with exercise (see Chapter 11).

Resting blood gas measurements usually show some degree of hypoxemia along with a normal $PaCO_2$ or mild hyperventilation. In advanced stages of any ILD there may also be severe hypoxemia. Only in the most severe cases—usually preterminal—does carbon dioxide retention occur.

Treatment. Treatment is directed to the basic disease and usually includes some type of drug therapy. Many patients with an ILD are treated with corticosteroids. Although corticosteroids are nonspecific therapy in any ILD, they can sometimes cause dramatic improvement. Immunosuppressive drugs, such as cyclophosphamide (Cytoxan), are also used in certain cases.

KYPHOSCOLIOSIS

Kyphosis is exaggeration of the normal posterior curve of the spine. Scoliosis is abnormal curvature of the spine laterally or sideways. Patients with kyphoscoliosis can develop pulmonary problems because of lung compression inside a distorted rib cage. Chronic pulmonary compression can lead to recurrent bronchial infections. In extreme cases respiratory failure can be the final result.

Physiologic testing. Depending on the severity of the kyphoscoliosis, patients may have normal lung function or show varying degrees of pulmonary restriction. Blood gas measurements are variable, but PaO_2 may be reduced because of basilar lung compression. $PaCO_2$ is not elevated except in the terminal stages, i.e., frank respiratory failure.

Treatment. The recurrent infections and any clinically significant hypoxemia are treated. In selected patients surgery may help to reverse the abnormal spine curvature.

LUNG CANCER

Any part of the lung can develop cancer. However, the term lung cancer usually refers to primary carcinoma—the type that arises from cells within the bronchi, bronchioles, and alveoli. Histologically, carcinoma of the lung is divided into two broad types: small cell (also called oat cell), and nonsmall cell. Nonsmall cell carcinoma is further divided into squamous (epidermoid), adenocarcinoma, and large cell carcinoma. Adenocarcinoma is the most common form of lung cancer, followed by squamous and small cell. Diagnosis must be confirmed by the presence of malignant cells found in a biopsy or sputum specimen.

Over 90% of all lung cancers are the result of cigarette smoking. Some cases are attributed to industrial pollutants (asbestos, chromium, uranium) inhaled by workers in these industries. Carcinomas can also arise in a pre-existing lung scar.

Physiologic testing. There is nothing characteristic about any pulmonary tests in lung cancer patients. Spirometry and blood gas values may range from normal to severely deranged, depending on the extent of tumor and the amount of underlying lung disease. Since most lung cancer patients are or have been heavy cigarette smokers, there is often some degree of coexisting chronic obstructive pulmonary disease.

Treatment. The three principal therapies for

lung cancer are surgical removal, radiotherapy, and anti-cancer drugs (cancer chemotherapy). However, small cell carcinoma is considered inoperable because the tumor has invariably spread (metastasized) by the time of diagnosis. For this reason small cell carcinoma is usually treated with a combination of chemotherapy and radiotherapy.

Surgical resection is the only potentially curative treatment for nonsmall cell lung cancer. Unfortunately, only a minority of patients meet the criteria for operability (no evidence of metastasis and adquate lung function) at the time of diagnosis. Patients with inoperable, nonsmall cell lung cancer are usually treated with radiotherapy, occasionally combined with chemotherapy. The results of nonsurgical therapy are dismal. In 1985 an estimated 140,000 cases of lung cancer were newly diagnosed. Based on past survival rates and considering all methods of treatment (including surgical resection), only 10% to 15% of these patients will live 5 years after diagnosis.

LUPUS ERYTHEMATOSUS (See Collagen-Vascular Disease)

MYASTHENIA GRAVIS (See Neuromuscular Disorders)

MUSCULAR DYSTROPHY (See Neuromuscular Disorders)

NEUROMUSCULAR DISORDERS

Neuromuscular disorders can affect the diaphragm and other muscles of respiration, leading to respiratory failure. Before the poliomyelitis vaccine was developed, poliomyelitis (polio) was the most common cause of neuromuscular respiratory failure. Fortunately polio is now rare in the United States. Guillain-Barré syndrome, myasthenia gravis, and muscular dystrophy are three diseases that, although relatively uncommon, can be devastating to the respiratory system.

Guillain-Barré syndrome classically begins as numbness or weakness in the lower extremities and ascends to involve the respiratory muscles and cranial nerves. The cause is presumably a viral infection of the nervous system. Guillain-Barré syndrome is usually self-limiting, and only in its most severe form does respiratory failure result. In such cases the patient must be supported by artificial ventilation until spontaneous recovery occurs. There is no effective treatment for this syndrome.

Myasthenia gravis is a generalized disorder that affects the neuromuscular junction. It is caused by a lack of acetylcholine receptors in the junction and is thought to reflect an autoimmune response (of unknown cause). Several therapies have been tried with varying success, including anticholinesterase drugs (which increase the amount of acetycholine at the neuromuscular junction), corticosteroids, immunosuppressive drugs, thymectomy (which empirically seems to help many patients), and plasmapheresis.

Muscular dystrophy is an example of a primary muscle disease that can cause respiratory failure. It is a slow, progressive wasting of the muscles and is of unknown cause. There is no specific treatment for most forms of muscular dystrophy.

Physiologic Testing. All neuromuscular diseases can cause restrictive impairment. However, if the disease affects the pharyngeal muscles, upper airways obstruction can also occur. The major airway problem is usually retained or aspirated secretions. These neuromuscular diseases do not directly affect the lung parenchyma.

PLEURAL EFFUSIONS AND PLEURAL DISEASE (See Chapter 13)

PNEUMOCONIOSES

Pneumoconiosis is lung disease that results from dust inhalation. Classically there appears an interstitial pattern on the chest x-ray (see Interstitial Lung Disease). The three most common pneumoconioses in the United States are coal worker's pneumoconiosis, silicosis, and asbestosis.

Diagnosis of any pneumoconiosis is usually based on two criteria: work history and chest x-ray. Each form of dust tends to cause a characteristic pattern on the chest x-ray which, along with a compatible work history, secures the diagnosis. Without a history of dust exposure and a chest x-ray that shows typical changes of dust inhalation, a reliable diagnosis cannot be made. A lung biopsy is not usually needed to make the diagnosis of pneumoconiosis.

Coal worker's pneumoconiosis, the most benign of the three conditions, is caused by inhalation of coal (carbon) dust. Coal dust, per se, only rarely causes serious pulmonary impairment. When there is respiratory impairment, the miner either has inhaled silica dust along with the coal or, far more commonly, has smoked cigarettes heavily.

Silicosis is caused by inhalation of silica dust and is seen in sand blasters and foundry workers (particularly moulders) and in miners exposed to underground seams of silica. Silica dust tends to be fibrogenic and can lead to massive scarring of the pulmonary parenchyma.

Asbestosis, the result of inhalation of asbestos dust, is found in asbestos miners and in people who work directly with the asbestos material, such as boiler insulators and pipe fitters. Asbestos inhalation has taken on increasing importance in recent years because of its association with lung cancer and mesothelioma (a tumor arising from pleural or peritoneal membranes). Of patients with asbestosis, 20% to 40% die from lung carcinoma. However, patients with a long history of asbestos exposure can develop lung cancer without ever manifesting classical findings of asbestosis on chest x-ray.

Physiologic testing. See Interstitial Lung Disease.

Treatment. Treatment is for symptoms only. Most patients with symptoms from respiratory impairment are cigarette smokers and tend to have coexisting obstructive lung disease; they are treated as discussed in the section on chronic obstructive pulmonary disease. Any patient still exposed to the offending dust should be removed from the work environment if at all possible.

PNEUMONIA

Broadly speaking, pneumonia is any acute inflammation of the alveolar spaces and can be caused by aspiration, inhalation of toxins, etc. When not qualified, pneumonia usually refers to airspace inflammation from infection. The infecting organisms are most commonly bacteria but may also be viruses, protozoa, fungi, etc. Among the more commonly implicated bacteria are *Streptococcus pneumoniae* (pneumococcus), *Mycoplasma pneumoniae,* and *Legionella pneumophila*. In the immunocompromised patient, so-called opportunistic organisms, which do not generally infect humans, may also cause pneumonia. The list of potential opportunistic pathogens is long and includes protozoa and fungi as well as unusual bacteria.

A good posteroanterior and lateral chest x-ray should always show the area of inflammation. However, pneumonia cannot be diagnosed by chest x-ray alone; there must be a compatible clinical picture, e.g., fever, cough, malaise, and bacteria or inflammatory cells in the sputum (in viral pneumonias there may be little or no sputum).

Physiologic testing. Patients with infectious pneumonia are often acutely ill and are not subjected to pulmonary function tests. However, when tested, patients with pneumonia usually show a restrictive pattern with decreased lung volumes.

Arterial blood gas measurements usually show some degree of hypoxemia and hyperventilation. In some patients hypoxemia can be so severe as to be life-threatening. The physiologic basis for hypoxemia is ventilation-perfusion imbalance (see Chapter 5).

Treatment. Antibiotics in some form are invariably used to treat infectious pneumonia. The specific antibiotic chosen depends on the results of the sputum examination, culture growth, and patient characteristics (e.g., age, severity of illness, and possibility of immunosuppression).

PNEUMOTHORAX (See Chapter 13)

POLIO (See Neuromuscular Disorders)

PULMONARY EDEMA (See Chapter 11)

PULMONARY EMBOLISM

In pulmonary embolism a clot or clots form in the deep veins of the legs, thighs, or pelvis or in the right heart chambers and then travel to the pulmonary arteries. Pulmonary embolism is a relatively common problem, particularly in patients with chronic heart and lung disease. An estimated 600,000 patients suffer from pulmonary embolism each year in the United States, and approximately 100,000 die directly as a result of this condition.

The principal symptoms of pulmonary emboli—chest pain and dyspnea—are nonspecific and may occur in virtually any cardiopulmonary condition. Simple mechanical blockage of the pulmonary vasculature does not explain the symptoms or the almost invariable hypoxemia seen in this condition.

Except in the most debilitated patient or in patients with severe heart disease, death from pulmonary embolism does not occur if the embolus is small and is localized to one lung segment. However, small, submassive emboli can lead to hypoxemia and substantial discomfort and may presage further emboli, making correct diagnosis imperative. Death from pulmonary emboli can occur when *massive* clots lodge in the pulmonary circulation; large clots can acutely block a major portion of the right ventricular output and cause severe, acute pulmonary hypertension.

Pulmonary embolism is one of the most difficult-to-diagnose problems in all of clinical medicine. The symptoms, chest x-ray examination, electrocardiogram, blood gas measurements, and other blood tests are all nonspecific for diagnosis. Accurate diagnosis requires at least a high-probability perfusion lung scan along with a compatible or highly suggestive clinical picture, e.g., acute onset of chest pain and pleural effusion in a postoperative patient.

The perfusion lung scan is probably the single most important test in diagnosing pulmonary embolism. The lungs are scanned after the patient has been injected with a radioactively labeled substance (e.g., albumin). The injected material is normally trapped in a homogeneous fashion throughout the pulmonary capillaries (in the aggregate only a small percentage of capillaries trap the material so there is no significant obstruction to blood flow). Absence of normal pulmonary blood flow shows up as a clear area on the lung scan—a perfusion defect. A completely normal scan rules out clinically significant pulmonary embolism with virtually 100% assurance.

When perfusion defects are present, their extent and pattern can often be interpreted as low- or high-probability for pulmonary embolism. Commonly, however, the perfusion lung scan is indeterminate, and either another test must be performed (e.g., pulmonary angiography, which requires right heart catheterization, or leg venography, in which contrast dye is injected in the leg veins), the patient must be treated on the basis of the entire clinical picture (a difficult decision), or the diagnosis must be abandoned.

Physiologic testing. Over 90% of patients with documented pulmonary embolism show some degree of hypoxemia and hyperventilation. The mechanism of hypoxemia seems to be related to release of peptides and other chemicals that alter the ventilation-perfusion ratios in the surrounding lung parenchyma (see Chapter 5). Either because of chest pain or accompanying pleural effusion or atelectasis, these patients usually manifest restrictive lung function. Again, however, the pattern of both blood gas and pulmonary function abnormality is nonspecific for diagnosis of pulmonary embolism.

Treatment. Treatment usually involves several weeks to months of anticoagulant therapy (parenteral heparin followed by oral warfarin [Coumadin]). Because anticoagulant therapy carries a risk of bleeding, the diagnosis of pulmonary embolism should be secure before embarking on therapy. Heparin therapy is aimed mainly at preventing further emboli, so there is usually no dramatic clinical response to reassure that the diagnosis is correct. On occasion, fibrinolytic therapy (e.g., Streptokinase) is used for a few days before heparin is begun to aid in dissolution of the clots.

PULMONARY HYPERTENSION (See Chapter 8)

RESPIRATORY FAILURE (See Chapter 11)

RHEUMATOID ARTHRITIS (See Collagen-Vascular Diseases)

SARCOIDOSIS

Sarcoidosis is a systemic disease of unknown cause that is characterized by multiple, noncaseating granulomas in many different organs. Caseation, another word for necrosis or dead tissue, is a common finding in the centers of granulomas caused by tuberculosis; it is almost never present in sarcoidosis. Sarcoid granulomas are found in the lungs in over 90% of sarcoidosis patients. Sarcoid granulomas are also found in the liver, spleen, skin, and eyes.

Sarcoidosis infrequently causes severe respiratory impairment. A consequence in some patients with sarcoidosis is pulmonary fibrosis; in a small percentage of all sarcoidosis patients (perhaps 5% to 10%) the fibrosis can be extensive enough to cause major respiratory disability.

Diagnosis is usually made on the basis of a compatible clinical history plus biopsy of an organ showing the noncaseating granulomas. However, for asymptomatic patients with a classic x-ray pattern of bilateral hilar adenopathy, no biopsy is necessary; for all practical purposes these patients have sarcoidosis and require no treatment.

Adjunctive tests include a gallium scan, which shows increased gallium uptake in the hilar node region, and an angiotensin converting enzyme (ACE) measurement; ACE is often elevated in sarcoidosis. Although both the ACE measurement and the gallium scan can be helpful in certain cases, the tests are nonspecific for sarcoidosis and therefore cannot be considered diagnostic.

When the patient is symptomatic or when the x-ray shows other than bilateral hilar adenopathy, a biopsy (of lung, liver, or some other organ) is usually indicated to establish the diagnosis.

Physiologic testing. The patient with sarcoidosis classically manifests restrictive pulmonary impairment. Approximately one third of these patients also have airways obstruction. The pulmonary diffusing capacity (see Chapter 5) is usually reduced as a result of the interstitial involvement. Blood gases are normal or only slightly impaired in most forms of the disease.

Treatment. The natural history of sarcoidosis is variable. There are some spontaneous remissions in milder cases (before irreversible fibrosis), and treatment is only given when there is significant organ impairment. The only effective therapy is corticosteroids, which are usually given in the form of oral prednisone. The dose and length of prednisone therapy are not standardized, but most authorities recommend a dose ranging from 15 to 40 mg per day for a period of months to a year or more.

SLEEP BREATHING DISORDERS (See Chapter 14)

TUBERCULOSIS

Tuberculosis (TB) is disease that results from infection with *Mycobacterium tuberculosis,* an acid-fast bacteria that spreads by way of the airborne route from human to human. Pathologically TB causes caseating granulomas in the involved organs (compare with Sarcoidosis).

TB has protean manifestations (tuberculous pleural effusion is discussed in Chapter 13). Since the TB organism enters the body by inhalation, the vast majority of patients manifest an abnormal chest x-ray, usually an apical infiltrate. Patients suffering from TB are usually febrile and have a history of weight loss and other symptoms such as night sweats.

The chest x-ray is essential to both diagnosis and management. Most cases are diagnosed only after a chest x-ray is obtained for nonspecific symptoms such as fever and weight loss. Diagnosis requires demonstration of the acid-fast bacilli in sputum or other tissue, and ultimately the organisms must be grown in culture. Growth of the organism takes approximately 4 to 6 weeks, but staining of the sputum for acid-fast bacilli can be done within minutes.

Physiologic testing. Pulmonary function tests are not usually obtained because of the infectious nature of TB. Except for patients with advanced disease, PaO_2 and $PaCO_2$ are not severely deranged.

Treatment. Standard antituberculous regimens include a combination of two or more drugs. The most widely employed regimens are isoniazid (INH) and rifampin daily for approximately 9 months or isoniazid and ethambutal for 2 years. The first regimen is gradually replacing the second for newly-diagnosed cases of pulmonary TB.

UPPER AIRWAY OBSTRUCTION
(See Chapter 3)

Upper airway obstruction may occur from many different causes, including aspirated foreign body, tracheal tumor, infection, and weakness of posterior pharyngeal muscles. Acute partial upper airway obstruction, which is a medical emergency, is usually characterized by stridor. Croup is a general term for infection that causes upper airway obstruction and stridor in children. Stridor is a high-pitched, inspiratory wheeze usually audible without a stethoscope. Stridor can be transmitted to the lung bases and can simulate the wheezing of asthma. (With complete upper airway obstruction, patients are unable to generate any airway sound; this condition is fatal within minutes if the airway obstruction is not relieved.) Lateral views of the neck are often helpful to demonstrate masses impinging on the lumen of the trachea or glottis. Diagnosis of upper airway obstruction during sleep usually requires polysomnography (see Chapter 14).

Chronic upper airway obstruction is usually characterized by dyspnea on exertion unless it is only during sleep, in which case daytime somnolence may be the major complaint (see Chapter 14 for a discussion of upper airway obstruction during sleep).

Physiologic testing. When in doubt about the diagnosis (upper vs. lower airway obstruction), spirometry may be useful. Upper airway obstruction shows a typical "flat-topped" pattern of flow volume loop (see Chapter 3).

Treatment. Treatment of acute upper airway obstruction always begins with securing an adequate upper airway. In extreme cases the patient may need a tracheostomy or cricothyroidotomy. Once an adequate airway is assured, treatment is directed to the specific cause, e.g., antibiotics for infection or surgery for tumor. When there is no discrete anatomic blockage, as in most patients with obstructive sleep apnea, therapy is more difficult (see Chapter 14 for discussion of therapy in this disorder).

appendix G
General references

Textbooks

The following books are considered standard reference works in the fields of pulmonary medicine or respiratory therapy. They can be consulted for further information on pulmonary physiology as it applies to clinical practice.

Baum, G.L., and Wolinsky, E., editors: Textbook of pulmonary diseases, Boston, 1983, Little, Brown & Co.

Burton, G.G., and Hodgkin, J.E., editors: Respiratory care—a guide to clinical practice, ed. 2, Philadelphia, 1984, J.B. Lippincott Co.

Crofton, J., and Douglas, A.: Respiratory diseases, ed. 3, Oxford, 1981, Blackwell Scientific Publications, Ltd.

Emerson, P.E., editor: Thoracic medicine, London, 1981, Butterworth & Co. (Publishers), Ltd.

Fishman, A.P., editor: Pulmonary diseases and disorders, New York, 1980, McGraw-Hill Book Co.

Fraser, R.G., and Pare, J.A.P.: Diagnosis of diseases of the chest, Philadelphia, 1977, W.B. Saunders Co.

George, R.B., Light, R.W., and Matthay, R.A., editors: Chest medicine, New York, 1983, Churchill Livingstone, Inc.

Guenter, C.A., and Welch, M.H.: Pulmonary medicine, Philadelphia, 1982, J.B. Lippincott Co.

Hinshaw, H.C., and Murray, J.F.: Diseases of the chest, ed. 4, Philadelphia, 1980, W.B. Saunders Co.

Scadding, J.G., Cumming, G., and Thurlbeck, W.M., editors: Scientific foundations of respiratory medicine, Philadelphia, 1981, W.B. Saunders Co.

Shapiro, B.A., Harrison, R.A., Kacmarek, R.M., et al.: Clinical application of respiratory care, ed. 3, Chicago, 1985, Year Book Medical Publishers, Inc.

Spearman, C.B., Sheldon, R.L., and Egan, D.F.: Egan's fundamentals of respiratory therapy, St. Louis, 1982, The C.V. Mosby Co.

Physiology references

The following texts concentrate on basic pulmonary physiology and/or pulmonary function testing.

Bates, D.V., Macklem, P.T., and Christie, R.V.: Respiratory function in disease, Philadelphia, 1971, W.B. Saunders Co.

Comroe, J.H., Jr.: Physiology of respiration, ed. 2, Chicago, 1974, Year Book Medical Publishers, Inc.

Cotes, J.E.: Lung function—assessment and application in medicine, ed. 3, Oxford, 1975, Blackwell Scientific Publications, Ltd.

Fishman, A.P., editor: The respiratory system. In Handbook of physiology: a critical, comprehensive presentation of physiological knowledge and concepts, sec. 3, Bethesda, Md., 1986, American Physiological Society.

Forster, R.E., DuBois, A.B., Briscoe, W.A., et al.: The lung—physiologic basis of pulmonary function tests, ed. 3, Chicago, 1986, Year Book Medical Publishers, Inc.

Gibson, G.J.: Clinical tests of respiratory function, New York, 1984, Raven Press.

Murray, J.F.: The normal lung, Philadelphia, 1976, W.B. Saunders Co.

Ruppell, G.: Manual of pulmonary function testing, ed. 3, St. Louis, 1982, The C.V. Mosby Co.

Shapiro, B.A., Harrison, R.A., and Walton, J.R.: Clinical application of blood gases, ed. 3, Chicago, 1982, Year Book Medical Publishers, Inc.

Slonim, N.B., and Hamilton, L.H.: Respiratory physiology, ed. 4, St. Louis, 1981, The C.V. Mosby Co.

Tisi, G.M.: Pulmonary physiology in clinical medicine, ed. 2, Baltimore, 1984, The Williams & Wilkins Co.

West, J.B.: Pulmonary pathophysiology—the essentials, ed. 3, Baltimore, 1985, The Williams & Wilkins Co.

West, J.B.: Respiratory physiology—the essentials, ed. 2, Baltimore, 1981, The Williams & Wilkins Co.

General references

Series

The following series carry up-to-date reviews of clinical problems.

Clinics in Chest Medicine, Philadelphia, W.B. Saunders Co. Published quarterly.

Current Pulmonology, D.H. Simmons, editor, Chicago, Year Book Medical Publishers, Inc. Published yearly.

Current Therapy of Respiratory Disease, R.M. Cherniack, editor, Philadelphia, Brian C. Decker, Publisher. Published yearly.

Lung Biology in Health and Disease, C. Lenfant, executive editor, New York, Marcel Dekker, Inc.

Pulmonary Disease Reviews, R.C. Bone, editor, New York, John Wiley & Sons, Inc. Published yearly.

Seminars in Chest Medicine, New York, Brian C. Decker, Publisher. Published quarterly.

appendix H
Microcomputer programs

In conjunction with a computer programmer, I have created several educational microcomputer programs that run on IBM PC or compatible computers. The programs are in the area of cardiopulmonary medicine and are available free to readers of this book.

Hemodynamic Profile/Blood Gas Interpretation allows the user to enter up to 30 cardiopulmonary/blood gas variables plus any cardioactive drugs the patient is receiving. After data entry, a list of entered and computer-calculated information is printed out. For example, cardiac output, if entered, will be used to calculate cardiac index and systemic vascular resistance. The hemodynamic record can be used for bedside teaching and patient care.

Respiratory Failure—Tutorial is a programmed text using the multiple-choice question format. It takes the user through the definitions, concepts, and management of respiratory failure. For each correct and incorrect response, a brief explanation is displayed on the screen. A separate glossary of terms provides textbook explanations, using appropriate figures such as the oxygen dissociation curve. The user can "skip around" among questions or alternate between the glossary and questions. The program also keeps score.

Heart-Lung Model is a computer-simulation of the oxygen cascade (Fig. 6-1). The user can change any of 10 variables and observe the effect of the change on all the other variables. This program also provides examples of the cascade in specific situations, such as pulmonary edema, shock, and high altitude.

Pleural Fluid Diagnosis is a series of interconnecting programs designed to aid in diagnosing the cause of pleural effusion. After a variety of laboratory and clinical information is entered by the user (e.g., pleural fluid protein), the program prints a list of probable causes of the pleural effusion. Numerous references and abstracts are also provided by the program, as well as a list of the algorithms used to construct the probability tables.

Author-Quiz is an authoring system for writing multiple-choice questions and entering them into a user-friendly quiz format. This program also includes "Pulmonary Trivia," a list of true-false questions on respiratory medicine.

For a copy of any program, send one blank diskette per program requested to:

Lawrence Martin, M.D.
Chief, Pulmonary Division
The Mt. Sinai Medical Center
One Mt. Sinai Drive
Cleveland, Ohio 44016

Please make sure that each diskette you send is accompanied by a *self-addressed diskette mailing envelope with sufficient return postage*. Please allow 3 weeks for delivery.

Index

A

Abbreviations and symbols, 362-363
Accessory breathing muscles, 10, 35*f*
Acid base, 364
Acid base disorders
    clinical problems, 132, 137, 140-144
    diagnosis, 132,132*p*, 140*p*-144*p*
    mixed, 143, 143*t*
    primary vs. compensatory processes, 137-138, 138*t*
    types, 135*t*
    and ventilatory weaning, 216*t*, 236*p*
Acid base map, 138-141, 139*f*
Acid base nomogram, 132-133, 134*f*
Acidemia, 134-135, 135*t*, 364
Acidosis, 134-135, 135*t*, 364
    in pleural fluid; *see* Pleural fluid acidosis and pulmonary hypertension, 149*t*, 150; *see also* Metabolic acidosis; Respiratory acidosis
Acrocyanosis, 305*p*, 309
Adult respiratory distress syndrome, 221, 225-233, 364; *see also* Infant respiratory distress syndrome
    a case, 229-233
    definition, 225
    events that may precipitate, 226*t*
    hemodynamic changes, 172*t*
    vs. infant respiratory distress syndrome, 319*t*
    management, 228
    pathology, 232*f*
    pathophysiology, 226*f*
    physiologic manifestations, 227*t*

Adult respiratory distress syndrome—cont'd
    ventilation-perfusion curve, 228*f*
    x-rays, 230-231*f*
Aerobic metabolism, 239-240, 241*t*
Air, 28-30, 29*f*
    composition of, 29*t*, 38*t*, 43
    pressure of, 28*f*; *see also* Barometric pressure
Air flow obstruction, determinants of, 60-64; *see also* Obstructive respiratory disease and impairment
Airway pressure; *see* Pressure, airway
Airway resistance, 47-49, 47*t*, 48*f*, 49*p*, 64, 360
Alkalemia, 134-135, 135*t*, 364
Alkalosis, 134-135, 135*t*, 364; *see also* Metabolic alkalosis; Respiratory alkalosis
Allergy and asthma, 372
Altitude, 21, 21*t*, 29-30, 97*pt*, 149*t*
Alveolar air equation, 92, 92*t*, 360, 364; *see also* Alveolar-arterial P_{O_2} difference
Alveolar-arterial (A-a) gradient; *see* Alveolar-arterial P_{O_2} difference
Alveolar-arterial P_{O_2} difference, 88-90, 93-95, 93*fp*, 94*fp*, 95*f*, 216*t*, 226*f*, 227*t*, 248, 360, 364
    during exercise, 248
Alveolar-capillary unit, 37*f*
Alveolar ventilation, 37, 38*p*, 74-87, 75*t*, 364
Alveoli and alveolus, 37*f*, 364
Ambient temperature and pressure
    saturated (ATPS), 31-32, 365
Aminophylline, 364
Anaerobic exercise, 364; *see also* Anaerobic threshold
Anaerobic metabolism, 239-240, 241*t*, 361
Anaerobic threshold
    clinical problems, 252-253
    definition, 240
    physiologic changes at, 240*f*, 245*f*, 246*t*, 247-249

Pages with tables and boxed material are designated by *t*. Figures are designated by *f*, and mention of the subject in a Clinical Problem is designated by *p*.

Anemia, 364
  cause of dyspnea, 21t
  cause of hypoxemia, 113t
  and diffusing capacity, 91
  vs. effect of carboxyhemoglobin, 119f
  effect on PaO_2, 107, 107t
  and oxygen saturation, 115
  and ventilator weaning, 216t
Anesthesia, 2, 5t
Angiotensin converting enzyme, 380
Anion gap, 137, 137p, 361
  causes of increased, 136t
Answers to clinical problems, 325-356
Anticholinergics, 373
Anxiety, 21
Apgar score, 304-305, 305pt
Apnea, 197p, 198t; *see also* Sleep apnea
  in newborn and infant, 308
Argon, 29t
Arterial blood gas, 3, 4, 8t, 22f, 23t; *see also* Partial pressure of carbon dioxide; Partial pressure of oxygen; Appendix F (physiologic testing in various clinical disorders)
  equipment, 19f, 119(footnote)
  measurement of, 19-20, 23
  in newborn, 303f, 314-315, 315-316f
  normal values, 20t
  in pleural effusion, 280
Arterial cannulation, 153
  measurements from, 159t
Arterial puncture, 3
Artificial blood, 190
Artificial ventilation, 3, 4, 197-218; *see also* Clinical problems (artificial ventilation)
  assist control, 202, 205p
  compliance, 209, 209p
  complications, 213-214, 214ft, 215p
  controlled, 202
  history, 4-5
  indications, 200, 200p
  intermittent mandatory, 204-205, 205fp
  intubation and, 197-200, 198ft
  mode and FIO_2, 201
  pressure patterns, 201-204, 201f, 203f, 207-208f
  settings, 206-208, 206t, 208p, 231p
  summary, 217
  weaning from, 84, 215-216, 216t, 217p
Artificial ventilator, 199f; *see also* Artificial ventilation
  development of, 4-5
Asbestos and asbestosis, 37, 256t, 262t, 364, 376-378
Asthma, 1, 12, 12p, 20-23, 67t, 68t, 69p, 71f, 98, 275t, 364, 372-374
Atelectasis, 364, 372, 379
Atmosphere, 28-30, 29f, 38t, 43

Auscultation, 11-12, 11t, 275, 312
Avogadro's law and number, 31, 365

B

Bacteria and bacterial infection, 1, 373, 378; *see also* Pneumonia
Barometric pressure, 29t, 30f, 31, 88, 92t, 365
Barometric temperature
  and pressure, saturated (BTPS), 31-32, 365
Barotrauma, 213, 214t
Base excess, 140, 365
Beta adrenergic drugs, 365, 373
Bicarbonate, 19, 23, 365
  in anion gap, 137
  arterial vs. venous, 133t
  in buffer system, 130-131, 131t
  during exercise, 245f, 246t, 248
Birth; *see* Newborn and infant
Blood count, 22f, 23t; *see also* Hemoglobin
  elevated, as cause of hypoxemia, 95-96, 96t
  in pleural effusions, 268-269
Blood gas; *see* Arterial blood gas
Blood transfusion, effect on PaO_2 and O_2 content, 190
Blood urea nitrogen (BUN), 23
Bohr dead space equation, 82-83, 83p, 360, 365
Bohr effect, 365
Boyle's Law, 31, 49
Bradycardia, 170t, 307
Bradypnea, 308
Breath sounds, 11-12, 11t
  in infant and child, 312
Breathing, 33-38, 36f, 43-46, 365
  infant, 309, 311
  normal vs. ventilator, 201
Bronchi and bronchus, 34f, 36-37, 36f, 376
Bronchiole, 37f, 365
Bronchiolitis, 365
Bronchitis, 8t, 64, 98, 373-374; *see also* Chronic bronchitis
Bronchodilator, 8t, 22, 69p, 71f, 365, 372-374
Bronchoprovocation, 24
Bronchoscope and bronchoscopy, 5t, 8t
Buffer systems, 130-131

C

Cancer, 6; *see also* Lung cancer
Capacity, 365; *see also* Lung capacity
Carbon dioxide, 365
  in air, 29t
  in bicarbonate buffer system, 131, 131f
  pressure; *see* Partial pressure carbon dioxide; Hypercapnia; Hypocapnia
  production, 75-77, 76f
    during exercise, 248

Index

Carbon dioxide—cont'd
  production—cont'd
    during sleep, 287t, 288, 288-289f
  in vivo titration curve, 139-140, 139f, 140p
Carbon dioxide dissociation curve, 107-109, 108f
Carbon dioxide pressure; see Partial pressure of carbon dioxide
Carbon monoxide, 24, 118-120, 118p, 119f, 121t, 365
  effect on PaO_2, 119
  effects of exposure, 120-121, 121t
  treatment of intoxication
    with high oxygen concentrations, 187
    with hyperbaric chamber, 187-188, 188fp
Carbon monoxide diffusing capacity; see Diffusing capacity
Carbonic anhydrase, 365
Carboxyhemoglobin, 91, 118, 120, 121p, 365; see also Carbon monoxide
Carcinoma, 365; see also Lung cancer
Cardiac catheterization, 1, 24, 153; see also Swan-Ganz
Cardiac index, 160t
Cardiac output
  during exercise, 242t, 245f, 248, 250-251
  in Fick equation, 123
  measurement, 159pt
  and oxygen delivery, 113t, 123-124, 125t
  in shunt equation, 224-225
  and ventilator weaning, 216t
Cardiac stress test, 249, 252p
Carina, 36, 365
Central nervous system, 33
  in respiratory failure, 221t
Charles' law, 31, 366
Chemoreceptor, 366
Chest bellows, 33-34
Chest cage, 35f
Chest tube drainage, 272t, 275-279, 276-279f
Chest x-ray examination, 2, 5, 12-18, 22f, 23t; see also Chest x-rays; Appendix F, 372-381 (descriptions of Common Clinical Conditions)
  pediatric, 312-313
Chest x-rays, 13-17f, 150f, 158f, 230-231f, 235f, 257-259f, 313f, 318f, 320f
Cheyne-Stokes breathing, 298-299, 299f
Chloride, 23, 365
  in anion gap, 137, 137p
  in sweat of cystic fibrosis patients, 375
Chloride shift, 365
Chronic bronchitis, 22, 60, 67t, 101, 103f, 221t, 233-237, 234f
Chronic obstructive pulmonary disease, 221t, 233-234, 374-375; see also Chronic bronchitis; Emphysema
  a case of respiratory failure, 234-237
  x-ray, 235f
Chylothorax, 262t
Chylous, 366

Chylous—cont'd
  pleural effusion, 263, 268
Cigarettes and cigarette smoking, 8t
  and asthma, 372-373
  and chronic bronchitis, 374
  CO level in smokers, 121t
  and lung cancer, 64, 376
  and pneumoconiosis, 378
  and vulnerability to dusts and pollutants, 36-37, 42
Cilia, 36
Circulation, 39-41
  fetal, 301-302, 302f
  pulmonary, 40f
  pulmonary vs. systemic, 147-148, 148t
  systemic, 40f
Cirrhosis, 223t, 256t
Clinical problems; see Answers, 325-356
  acid base disorders, 132, 137, 140-144, 230, 233, 235
  airway obstruction, 54
  airway resistance, 49
  altitude and pulmonary edema, 97
  alveolar ventilation, 79, 80, 84
  alveolar-arterial PO_2 difference, 93-94, 230, 232
  anion gap, 137
  Apgar score, 305
  arterio-venous oxygen content difference and O_2 uptake, 124
  artificial ventilation
    complications, 215
    indications, 200
    system compliance, 209
    weaning from, 217
  asthma diagnosis, 12
  arterial blood gas measurement, 39
    in COPD, 237
  carbon monoxide poisoning, 118
  chest x-ray in diagnosis, 16
  compliance
    of lung, 46, 48
    of patient and ventilator system, 209, 232
  cyanosis, 309
  dead space to tidal volume ratio (V$_D$/V$_T$), 215
  equal pressure point, 62
  exercise physiology and testing, 240-241, 248, 251-253
  fetal hemoglobin and tissue hypoxia, 303
  functional residual capacity, 51
  hemodynamic assessment
    invasive, 159, 161, 166, 168, 171-173
    noninvasive, 153
  history taking, 9
  hyperbaric oxygen therapy, 188
  hypercapnia,
    explanation of, 81
    from too much oxygen, 186, 187
  hyperventilation and hypoventilation, 79-80
  hypoventilation, explanation of, 82

Clinical problems—cont'd
  hypoxemia
    and blood gas values, 115
    and body position, 100
    and COPD, 235
    and dialysis, 98
    and hypoventilation, 98
    and pneumonia, 100, 229, 231
    and pulmonary embolism, 103
  intermittent mandatory ventilation, 205
  maximal midflow (MMF_{25-75}), 65
  minute ventilation in coma, 81
  oxygen content, 115, 119, 229, 231, 304
  oxygen delivery, 123
  oxygen partial pressure, 33
  oxygen supply in apnea, 179
  oxygen therapy, 179, 235
  oxygen uptake
    in case of ARDS, 232
    and CO_2 output, 38
    under normal conditions, 124
    under STPD conditions, 32
  Pa_{CO_2}, determinants of, 79
  partial pressure of CO_2, explanation of, 79
  partial pressure of CO_2 in liquid, 33
  partial pressure of O_2 on Mt. Everest, 30
  peak flow estimation, 54
  pleural effusion,
    blood gases, 280-281
    diagnosis, 263-264
    laboratory tests, 270
    parapneumonic, 272
    tuberculosis, 272
  pneumothorax air, 276
  positive end-expiratory pressure, 233
  respiratory failure
    oxygenation, 229-233
    ventilatory and oxygenation, in COPD, 234-237
  RV/TLC, 52
  sleep disorders, 286, 289, 295, 298
  spirometry in asthma, 69
  tachypnea, diagnosis, 12
  V_D/V_T and ventilator weaning, 83
  venous oxygen measurements, 126
  ventilator compliance, 209
  ventilator settings, 208, 236
  ventilator weaning, 215, 236
  vital capacity in infant, 315
  vital capacity measurement, 32
Coal worker's pneumoconiosis, 377-378
Collagen-vascular diseases, 366, 374-375
  and pleural effusion, 256t, 262t, 267t, 270t, 273-274, 375
Compliance, 366
  dynamic, 64, 64f

Compliance—cont'd
  frequency dependence of, 64
  left ventricular, 168, 168f, 170t
  lung, 46-48, 46p, 47ft, 48p, 73, 226f, 227t, 360, 374, 376
  ventilator, 209
Conductance, 366
Continuous positive airway pressure (CPAP), 212-213, 213f, 296t, 297, 366
Co-oximeter, 19f, 119
Cor pulmonale, 151, 152t
Corticosteroids, 5t, 8t, 229t, 366, 373-375, 377, 380
Cough
  and asthma, 372-373
  and chronic bronchitis, 374
  and pneumonia, 378
Crackles; see Rales
Cromolyn sodium, 373
Croup, 67t, 366, 381
Crying vital capacity, 313
Cuirass respirator, 5
Cyanosis, 3, 112, 121, 121p, 200, 229p, 304f, 309, 309p, 313, 366
Cystic fibrosis, 67t, 221t, 366, 375
Cytology, 266, 267t, 268, 272, 273f, 366

D

Dalton's law, 28-31, 360, 366
Dead space, 75, 82t, 366
Dead space to tidal volume ratio (V_D/V_T), 82-83, 82t, 83p, 216t, 226f, 227t
  during exercise, 245f, 248
Dead space ventilation, 75, 75f, 82
  and CO_2 retention, 81-82
  and the P_{CO_2} equation, 77, 79
Defense mechanisms, 36
Dehydration, 153p, 172t
Diaphragm, 34f, 35, 35f
  in emphysema, 374
  and neuromuscular disorders, 377
  paralysis, 67t
Diffusing capacity, 8t, 24t, 90-92, 253p, 366, 374, 376, 380
Diffusion, 38-39, 39f, 41, 366
Diffusion gradient for O_2, 89, 90f
Diffusion impairment, 39, 98
  in exercise, 251, 251p, 254f
Diphosphoglycerate, 116, 117t, 302t, 303
Dissociation curve; see Oxygen dissociation curve; Carbon dioxide dissociation curve
Drug overdose and respiratory failure, 209p, 221t
Dynamic compliance; see Compliance, dynamic
Dyspnea, 21-26, 23-24t, 25f, 367
  and ARDS, 226f
  and asthma, 372
  causes of, 5t, 21t

Dyspnea—cont'd
  and chronic airway obstruction, 381
  and CO levels, 121t
  from CO poisoning, 120
  during exercise, 239-240, 246, 249, 250t, 251
  and inadequate oxygenation, 113t
  and interstitial lung disease, 375-376
  and pleural effusion, 280, 280p
  psychogenic cause, 21, 21t
  and pulmonary embolism, 379
  routine diagnostic tests, 23t
  schema for evaluation and management, 22f, 25f
  signs and symptoms, 21t
  special diagnostic tests, 24
  summary of approach to evaluation, 26

E

Effort-dependent air flow, 63
Effort-independent air flow, 63
Elastic recoil, 50-51, 51f, 60-61, 60-62f, 67t, 367, 374, 376
Electrocardiogram (ECG), 22f, 23t, 65, 151f, 247, 249-250, 284, 286
Electroencephalogram (EEG), 284, 284t, 285f, 286, 287t, 290-291f
Electromyelogram (EMG), 284t, 285f, 290-291f
Electrolytes, 23t, 216t; see also Bicarbonate; Chloride; Sodium; Potassium
Electro-oculogram (EOG), 284t, 285f, 286, 290-291f
Emphysema, 8t, 22-23, 60-61, 64, 67t, 68t, 73, 98, 233-234, 234f, 257t, 367, 374
  equal pressure point, 62f
  and respiratory failure, 215p, 217p
  ventilation-perfusion curve, 101, 103f
Empyema, 270t, 271-272, 367
Endotracheal tube, 17, 197, 198-199f
  complications of, 214t
Eosinophil, 20, 269, 367, 372
Epiglottitis, 67t
Epinephrine, 5t
Equal pressure point, 60-62, 60-62f
Equations and formulas, 360-361; see also Individual equation or formula
Exercise physiology, 239-255; see also Anaerobic threshold; Exercise test and testing
  metabolism, 239-240, 241
  P_{CO_2} and, 240p, 241, 241fp
  summary, 255
Exercise test and testing, 23-25, 24t, 242-249; see also Clinical problems (exercise physiology and testing)
  and cardiac disease, 250-251, 250f
  clinical interpretation, 250-254, 252-253p, 255f
  clinical use, 249-250
  indications, 250t
  normal parameters, 249t

Exercise test and testing—cont'd
  poor physical fitness, 252
  respiratory disease, 251, 251pt
Expiratory positive airway pressure (EPAP), 297
Expiratory reserve volume, 49, 50f, 322f, 367
Exudate, 262-263, 367

F

Fever, 216t, 378; see also Hyperthermia; Temperature
Fibrosis, 367
  interstitial, 8t, 22, 50, 91, 275t
  pulmonary, 48p, 66, 67t, 73, 376, 378, 380
Fick equation, 123-124, 160t, 240, 361
Flail chest, 67t, 221t
Flow, 57, 367
Flow-volume curves and loops, 57-59, 57f, 58f, 59f, 63f, 66f, 367
Fluid
  balance in pleural space, 261f
  transport in lungs, 222f
Forced expiratory volume, 367
Forced expiratory volume, 1 second (FEV_1), 8t, 23, 52, 52t, 53f, 54, 54t, 55f, 68t, 69t, 70t, 70p, 71t, 71p, 72f, 373
  in calculation of MVV, 251-252
  normal values, 357-359
  over forced vital capacity (FEV_1/FVC), 8t, 52t, 54, 54t, 67, 68t, 69t, 69-71p, 73
Forced expiratory volume, 3 seconds (FEV_3), 52t, 53f, 54
  over FVC (FEV_3/FVC), 52t, 53f
Forced vital capacity (FVC), 8t, 52, 52t, 53f, 54, 54pt, 55f, 57-59f, 57-58, 65, 65f, 66f, 68t, 69-71p, 69t, 70f, 367; see also Vital capacity
  normal values, 357-359
Foreign body airway obstruction, 67t
Formulas (and equations), 360-361; see also Individual formulas
Fraction of inspired O_2 (FI_{O_2}), 88-89, 92-98, 92t, 94p, 96t, 176, 206, 206t, 216t, 367
Functional residual capacity (FRC), 49-51, 50f, 51fp, 226f, 227t, 367
  newborn, 313, 322f

G

Gallium scan, 380
Gas; see also Carbon dioxide; Oxygen; Partial pressure
  laws, 30-31, 360
  phase, 33t
  properties, 27
  in solution, 32-33
Gas exchange, 7, 8t, 27, 33-41, 88-90, 367; see also Diffusion; Ventilation-perfusion imbalance
  and correlation with lung mechanics, 71-72, 72f
  fetal, 301

General gas law; see Gas (laws)
Glucose, 23
Gravity, 29
   affect on V-Q ratios, 99-100, 100p
Gullain Barré syndrome, 67t, 221t, 377

H

Haldane effect, 367
Heart failure, 1
   congestive, 21t, 22, 67t, 143p, 256
   left, 148-149t, 151, 172t, 223t
   right, 149
   as sign of inadequate oxygenation, 113t
Heimlich valve, 277, 277f
Helium, 367
Helium-CO mixture, 91(footnote)
Helium-oxygen mixture, 176
Hemodynamic monitoring, 367
   assessment of patient, 152-153, 153p
   calculations, 160t
   in clinical practice, 171-172, 171-173p
   clinical problems, 159, 161, 166, 168, 171-173
   infant, 318-319, 318f
   interpretation of data, 171p, 172t, 172p, 173p
   measurements, 159t
   pitfalls and complications, 170, 171t
   summary, 173
Hemodynamics, 7
Hemoglobin, 367
   abnormal, 122
   chemical combination with oxygen, 32
   content, 107t, 115, 115p, 116f, 303
   deoxygenated, 121p, 309p
   fetal, 302-303, 303p, 304f
   reduced, 121p
Henderson-Hasselbalch equation, 86f, 131, 361, 367
Henry's law, 32
High-frequency ventilation, 209-211, 210t, 211f
Historical perspective, 1-6
History, from patient, 8t, 9-10, 9p, 22, 22f
   pediatric, 305-306
   with pneumoconiosis, 377-378
Home oxygen therapy, 190-194
   equipment, 191-192f, 192t
   indications, 193-194
Hydrogen ion, 129-130, 130t, 131f, 134f, 139f; see also pH
Hydrostatic pressure, 165-166, 222-223, 222f, 223t, 261-262, 261f, 361, 368
Hyperbaric pressure, 187-188, 188fpt, 368
Hypercapnia, physiologic basis for, 80, 81t; see also Hypoventilation
   in asthma, 373
   dangers of, 83
   definition, 135t, 368

Hypercapnia—cont'd
   in end-stage disease, 375-376
   and intubation, 84, 198t, 200, 200p
Hyperthermia, 96, 96t, 306
Hyperventilation, 38p, 78-79, 79p
   and asthma, 373
   as compensatory process, 135t
   criteria for intubation, 200
   during exercise, 241, 241p
   and pleural effusion, 280
   and pneumonia, 378
   and pulmonary embolism, 379
Hypocapnia, 135t, 280, 368; see also Hyperventilation
Hypopnea, 289, 292, 368
Hypoventilation, 78-79, 79p
   cause of low Pao$_2$, 98
   cause of pulmonary hypertension, 149t
   as compensatory process, 135, 221t
   criteria for intubation, 84, 198t, 200, 200p
Hypoxemia, 112-128; see also Clinical problems (hypoxemia); Oxygen content (arterial); Partial pressure of oxygen (arterial)
   causes, 113t
   clinical problems; see Clinical problems (hypoxemia)
   definition, 113, 368
   and interstitial lung disease, 91, 376
   and kyphoscoliosis, 376
   in obese patients during sleep, 283
   and oxygen content, 115, 115p
   and pleural effusion, 280
   and pneumonia, 100p, 229p, 231p, 378
   and pulmonary embolism, 103p, 379
   and pulmonary hypertension, 148-149t, 150
   and sudden infant death syndrome, 319
   after thoracentesis, 264
Hypoxia; see also Hypoxemia
   classification, 113t
   definition, 113

I

Infant; see Newborn and infant
Infant respiratory distress syndrome, 223, 319t, 320-321, 321f, 322t
Infiltrate, 368
Influenza pandemic, 4
Inspiratory capacity, 49, 50f, 322f, 368
Inspiratory plateau, 206t, 207, 208f
Inspiratory reserve volume, 49, 50f, 322f, 368
Intermittent mandatory ventilation, 204-205, 205fp
   in ventilator weaning, 216t
Interstitial fibrosis; see Fibrosis (interstitial)
Interstitial lung disease, 221t, 375-376
Interstitial space, 222f

Index

Interstitium, 368
Intubation
    and artificial ventilation, 8*t*, 197-200, 198*t*
    complications, 214*t*
    criteria for, 198*t*
    for hypercapnia, 84, 198*t*, 200, 200*p*
    in management of ARDS, 229*t*
Iron lung, 4, 5*t*, 202(footnote), 297

J

Jet ventilation, 210-211, 210*t*, 211*f*

K

Kyphoscoliosis, 221*t*, 376

L

Lactate, 241*t*, 245*f*
Lactate dehydrogenase (LDH) in pleural fluid, 263, 263-264*p*, 266, 267*t*, 268, 270-272, 272*t*
Lactic acid, 239, 251
Liquid phase, 33*t*
Lung abscess, 1
Lung biopsy, 24*t*
Lung cancer, 8*t*, 14, 20, 376-377
    and asbestosis, 378
Lung capacity, 368; *see also* Lung volumes and capacities
Lung disease and diseases, 4, 41-42; *see also* Individual lung diseases in index and Appendix F
Lung mechanics, 7, 43-73
    correlation with gas exchange, 71-73, 72*f*
    summary, 73
Lung scan
    perfusion, 24*t*, 103*p*, 379
    computerized tomographic, 17, 17*f*
Lung volumes and capacities, 24*t*, 49-50, 50*f*, 368; *see also* Individual lung volumes and capacity
    infant, 322*t*
Lungs, 34, 34*f*, 368
Lymphoma, 273, 368

M

Malignancy; *see* Lung cancer; Pleural effusion (malignancy)
Mass, 27
Maximal midflow (MMF$_{25-75}$), 52*t*, 54, 54*t*, 64-65, 65*fp*, 70*p*, 71*p*, 368, 372
Maximal voluntary ventilation (MVV), 247, 251-252, 252-253*p*, 368
Mechanics; *see* Lung mechanics
Mental status evaluation, 10-11
Mesothelial cell, 269, 269*f*, 271
Mesothelioma, 256, 274, 378
Metabolic acidosis, 135*t*, 368; *see also* Clinical problems (acid base disorders)
    acute vs. chronic, 141

Metabolic acidosis—cont'd
    clinical causes, 136*t*
    time course for compensation, 142*f*
Metabolic alkalosis, 135*t*, 221*t*, 368; *see also* Clinical problems (acid base disorders)
    acute vs. chronic, 141
    clinical causes, 136*t*
Methacholine bronchoprovocation, 373
Methemoglobin, 19, 121-122, 121*p*, 122*t*, 368
Methemoglobinemia, 121-122
    causes of, 122*t*
    and cyanosis, 121
    treatment, 122
Mitral valve disease, 152, 170*t*
Mixed venous blood, 368
Mixed venous oxygen; *see* Venous oxygen
Mt. Everest, 29-30*f*, 30*p*, 97*t*
Muscles, respiratory, 35, 35*f*
    accessory, 10, 35*f*
Muscular dystrophy, 221*t*, 377
Myasthenia gravis, 67*t*, 221*t*, 377

N

Negative pressure ventilation, 4
Neuromuscular disease and disorders, 67*t*, 377
Newborn and infant
    Apgar score; *see* Apgar score
    blood gases, 314-317, 315-316*f*
    changes at birth, 301-305
    chest x-ray, 312-313, 313*f*
    clinical problems, 303-305, 309, 315
    hemodynamic assessment, 319-320
    history-taking, 305-306
    oxygen therapy, 317-318
    physical examination, 309-312, 309-310*p*, 310-311*f*
    pulmonary function tests, 313-314, 314*f*
    respiratory distress; *see* Infant respiratory distress syndrome
    ventilation-perfusion imbalance, 317
    vital signs, 306-309, 307-308*t*
Nitrogen, 28-29, 29*t*, 38*t*, 368
Nobel prize, 5*t*, 153

O

Obesity, 67*t*
    and sleep disorders, 283, 284*t*, 286*p*, 292-295, 292*t*, 295*p*, 296*t*
Obstructive respiratory disease and impairment, 8*t*, 54, 54*pt*, 66-68, 66*f*, 67-68*t*, 369, 380
Oncotic pressure, 165-166, 222-223, 222*f*, 223*f*, 261-262, 261*f*, 361, 369
Ondine's curse, 295, 369
Orthopnea, 23, 369
Oximeter and oximetry, 20, 242, 243-244*f*, 284, 285*f*, 286*p*; *see also* Co-oximeter

Oxygen, 369; *see also* Oxygenation
   in air, 29*t*
   diffusion, 90-92, 90*f*
   discovery of, 5*t*, 175
   as a drug, 175-176, 176*t*
   liquid, 175, 191, 192*ft*
   mixed venous, 106-107, 107*t*
   partial pressure; *see* Partial pressure of O_2
   supply in apnea, 179*p*
   tent, 3
   therapy; *see* Oxygen therapy
   transfer, 88-111
   early use, 175-176, 177*f*
   wall outlets, 178*f*
Oxygen consumption; *see* Oxygen uptake
Oxygen content, 369; *see also* Clinical problems (oxygen content)
   arterial, 113-116, 114*f*, 115*p*, 360
   compensatory mechanism for reduction, 125*t*
   end-capillary, 224-225
   with fetal hemoglobin, 304*p*
   mixed venous, 106-107, 107*t*, 114*f*, 115, 224-225
   in newborn, 302*t*, 303
   and oxygen delivery, 123-124
   and venous admixture, 104-105
Oxygen delivery, 115, 123-124, 123*p*, 361
Oxygen diffusion and diffusing capacity, 90-92
Oxygen dissociation curve, 104-105, 107-109, 108*f*, 116-120, 116*f*
   effect of CO, 118, 119*f*
   effect of 2,3-DPG, 117*f*
   effect of pH, 117*f*
   effect of temperature, 117*f*
   and fetal hemoglobin, 303, 304*f*
   and P_{50}, 116-118, 116-117*f*
   shift of, in causes of reduced SaO_2, 122*t*
Oxygen extractor, 191, 191*f*, 192*t*
Oxygen pressure; *see* Partial pressure of oxygen
Oxygen-pulse, 248, 250, 250*f*, 252-253*p*
Oxygen saturation
   causes of reduced, 122-123, 122*t*
   during exercise, 245*f*, 247
   importance of direct measurement, 119
   and oxygen content, 115, 115*p*, 116*f*, 117*f*
   and pulmonary hypertension, 150, 150*f*
Oxygen therapy, 2, 175-196
   classification, 180, 180*t*
   high-flow system, 179
   history of, 2-3, 5*t*, 176(footnote), 177*f*
   home; *see* Home oxygen therapy
   low-flow system, 179
   low-supplemental, 184
   monitoring with signs and PaO_2, 188-190
   pediatric, 317

Oxygen therapy—cont'd
   positive airway pressure and, 187-188
   shunt effect and PaO_2, 189
   summary, 195
   terminology, 179, 179*p*
   toxicity from, 184-187
Oxygen toxicity, 184, 186-187, 186*fp*, 187*p*, 214*t*, 226*t*
Oxygen transport in infants, 302*t*; *see also* Oxygen delivery
Oxygen uptake, 123-127, 124*p*, 369
   during exercise, 239-240, 242*t*, 245*f*, 246-248, 246*t*, 247*f*, 249*t*
   during sleep, 288, 288*f*
   formula, 123, 160*t*, 240
   and infant body temperature, 308*f*
Oxygenation
   adequacy of, 112-127
   clinical assessment, 112-113
   failure; *see* Respiratory failure
   signs and symptoms of inadequate, 113*t*
   summary, 127
Oxygenation cycle, 114*f*
Oxyhemoglobin, 118, 121*p*; *see also* Oxygen saturation; Oxygen content

P

PAO_2; *see* Partial pressure of oxygen (alveolar)
PaO_2; *see* Partial pressure of oxygen (arterial)
Partial pressure, 28-31
Partial pressure of carbon dioxide (PCO_2)
   alveolar ($PACO_2$), 76-77, 85, 361
   and alveolar ventilation, 74-87
   arterial ($PaCO_2$), 75-87, 76*f*; *see also* Hypercapnia; Hyperventilation; Hypocapnia; Hypoventilation
      in acid-base disorders, 137-145, 138*t*
      in acid-base map/nomogram, 133, 134*f*, 139*f*, 142*f*
      in asthma, 373
      changes after birth, 303*f*
      in the clinical setting, 79-80
      in COPD, 374
      definition of respiratory failure, 219-220, 220*t*
      during exercise, 241, 241*p*, 242*f*, 245*f*, 248
      vs. FEV_1, 72*f*
      in Henderson-Hasselbalch equation, 131, 134-135
      and need for ventilatory assistance, 84
      normal range, 20*f*
      relation to oxygenation and acid-base balance, 86*f*
   capillary, 315
   end-capillary, 39*f*
   end-tidal, 85-86, 85*f*, 245*f*, 246*t*, 247
   summary, 87
   transcutaneous, 316-317, 316*f*
Partial pressure of oxygen (PO_2)
   alveolar (PAO_2), 89*f*, 88-111; *see also* Alveolar-arterial PO_2 difference

Partial pressure of oxygen (P_{O_2})—cont'd
   arterial (Pa_{O_2}), 93, 93p, 94p
     in asthma, 373
     causes of low, 95-110, 96-97t, 97-98p, 100p, 103p
     in COPD, 374
     definition of respiratory failure, 219-220, 220t
     during exercise, 245f, 248
     vs. FEV_1, 72f
     normal range, 20f, 93f
     over FI_{O_2} (Pa_{O_2}/FI_{O_2}), 95
     over PA_{O_2} (Pa_{O_2}/PA_{O_2}), 95, 95f, 364; see also Alveolar-arterial P_{O_2} difference; Clinical problems (hypoxemia)
   capillary, 315
   changes from atmosphere to blood, 89f
   changes after birth, 303f
   end-capillary, 39f, 89-90, 90f
   end-tidal, 245f, 247
   and oxygen content, 115, 115p
   transcutaneous, 316, 315f
P_{CO_2} electrode, 3
P_{CO_2} equation, 77, 79, 360
   derivation, 361
   in exercise, 241
   graph of, 83f
Peak flow, 8t, 18, 23t, 52t, 54t, 54, 54p, 55-56f, 58f, 69-71p, 369, 373
Peak flow meter, 56f
Penicillin, 5t
Perfusion, 369; see also Ventilation-perfusion
P_{50}, 24, 116-117, 116-117f, 303, 369
pH, 130, 369
   acidemia and alkalemia, 134, 135t
   acidosis and alkalosis, 134-136
   and anion gap, 137p
   changes in acid-base disorders, 137-138, 138t
   definition, 130
   during exercise, 245f, 248, 253p
   in Henderson-Hasselbalch equation, 131, 134f, 139f
   and hydrogen ion concentration, 130t
   in pleural effusion, 270-272, 270t, 274
   and pulmonary artery pressure, 150f
Physical examination, 8t, 10-12, 22f, 23, 249
   in children, 309-312, 310f, 311f
   as guide to oxygenation assessment, 112
Pickwickian syndrome, 221t, 294-295, 369
Plethysmograph, 49, 313, 369
Pleura and pleural membranes, 34, 34f, 260-261f, 261-262, 369; see also Pleural effusion
Pleural biopsy, 8t, 264, 275t
Pleural effusion, 11, 67t, 256-283, 369
   acidosis, 270-271
   cause of exudative, 266-268, 267t
   chest tube drainage, 272t, 276-279, 276-279f
   chest x-rays, 257-259f

Pleural effusion—cont'd
   chylous (chylothorax), 262t, 263, 268
   clinical problems, 263, 270, 272, 276, 280-281
   diagnostic procedures, 264-265
   diseases causing, 256t, 262t
     collagen-vascular, 273
     malignancy, 272-273, 273f
     pneumonia, 271-272, 272pt
     pulmonary embolism, 274, 377
     tuberculosis, 271, 272p
   incidence, 256t
   lung mechanics and gas exchange, 280-281, 280p, 281p
   summary, 281
   transudates vs. exudates; see also Pleural fluid dynamics; Pleural fluid laboratory tests
Pleural fluid acidosis, 270-271, 270t
Pleural fluid dynamics, 261-262
Pleural fluid laboratory tests
   amylase, 268
   CEA, 268
   cells, 268-269, 269f
   glucose, 268
   pH, 270
Pleural pressure; see Pressure (intrapleural)
Pleural space, 260-261f, 261, 369
   obliteration, 279-280
Pleuroscopy, 264
Pneumoconiosis, 37, 369, 375, 377-378
Pneumonia, 1, 3 (cases III & IV), 6, 8t, 12, 15, 21, 67t, 98, 100p, 221t, 229p, 231p, 256t, 369, 378
Pneumothorax, 2, 4, 21, 52f, 262t, 264, 274f, 275-276, 275t, 277p
P_{O_2} electrode, 3, 5t
Poliomyelitis, 221t, 377
Polycythemia, 284t
Polysomnography, 369; see also Sleep disorders
Positive end-expiratory pressure (PEEP), 206t, 207, 211-212, 212f, 227t, 228-229, 229t, 233p, 369
   and barotrauma, 213-214, 275t
   effect on cardiac output, 213, 214f
   optimal, 213-214, 214f
Positive pressure ventilation, 4-5; see also Artificial ventilation
Potassium, 23, 137, 369
P-pulmonale, 151f
Pregnancy, 21, 21t, 305
Pressure, 27, 369
   airway, 44-46, 44-45f
   alveolar, 44-45f, 48, 51f
   atmospheric, 28-30, 28-30f, 29t
   carbon dioxide; see Partial pressure of carbon dioxide
   central venous, 165, 165f
   chest wall, 44f, 311f
   in circulation
     systemic, 148t

Pressure—cont'd
  in circulation—cont'd
    pulmonary, 148t, 149-152
  dry gas, 28, 29t
  hydrostatic; see Hydrostatic pressure
  hyperbaric; see Hyperbaric pressure
  left ventricular, 167-168, 169p, 170t
  measurements; see Hemodynamic monitoring (measurements)
  mouth, 44f, 48
  oncotic; see Oncotic pressure
  oxygen; see Partial pressure of oxygen
  partial; see Partial pressure
  pleural, 44-45f, 51-52f, 60-63, 60-63f, 261-262, 261f, 275-276
  positive end-expiratory; see Positive end-expiratory pressure
  sea level, 28f, 30f
  transairway, 44f, 47t, 48
  transpulmonary, 44f, 47ft
  transthoracic, 44f
  ventilator; see Artificial ventilation (pressure patterns)
  water vapor; see Water vapor pressure
  wedge; see Pulmonary artery wedge pressure
Pressure-flow curves, 63f
Protein, in pleural fluid, 263, 263-264p, 266, 267t, 268, 270-271
Pulmonary angiogram, 24, 379
Pulmonary artery, 40f, 41
Pulmonary artery wedge pressure, 161, 161p
  during artificial ventilation, 163-165, 164f
  vs. central venous pressure, 165, 165f
  clinical problems, 161, 166, 168, 171, 172-173
  in common clinical conditions, 172
  as guide to left heart filling pressure, 166-170, 167-169f, 168p
  as guide to pulmonary capillary hydrostatic pressure, 165-166
  and left ventricular preload, 170t
  measurement, 161-164
  and PEEP, 168, 169f
Pulmonary edema, 21, 67t, 221-223, 221t, 223t, 370
  re-expansion, 264
Pulmonary emboli and embolism, 21, 98, 103p, 149t, 152, 221t, 379-380
  and pleural effusion, 256t, 262t, 263, 267t, 269, 274-275
Pulmonary fibrosis; see Fibrosis
Pulmonary function tests, 8t, 24t; see also Spirometry; Lung volumes and capacities
Pulmonary hypertension, 149-152, 172t
  causes, 148-149t
  idiopathic, 152
  and pulmonary embolism, 379

Pulmonary hypertension—cont'd
  treatment, 149t
Pursed lip breathing, 10, 62p

R

Radiology of chest; see Chest x-ray
Rale and rales, 11t, 12, 312, 370
Rapid eye movement sleep; see Sleep disorders (REM and nonREM)
Residual volume, 49, 50f, 322f, 370
Resistance
  airway; see Airway resistance
  pulmonary vascular, 160t
  systemic vascular, 160t, 172t, 360
Respiratory acidosis, 135t, 370
  acute vs. chronic, 140-141
  clinical causes, 136t
  in newborn, 302
Respiratory alkalosis, 135t, 370
  acute vs. chronic, 140-141
  clinical causes, 136t
Respiratory distress syndrome, 370; see Adult respiratory distress syndrome; Infant respiratory distress syndrome
Respiratory exchange ratio; see Respiratory quotient
Respiratory failure, 1, 8t, 41, 219-239, 370; see also Adult respiratory distress syndrome; Pulmonary edema
  acute vs. chronic, 221
  case of combined ventilatory and oxygenation failure, COPD, 234-237
  case of oxygenation failure, 229-233
  chronic obstructive pulmonary disease and, 233-237
  clinical causes, 221t
  clinical classification, 221-222
  in cystic fibrosis, 375
  definition, 219-220
  in kyphoscoliosis, 376
  in neuromuscular disorders, 376
  physiologic classification, 220, 220t
  summary, 237
Respiratory quotient, 37-38, 89, 360, 370
  in alveolar air equation, 92, 92t
  as cause of low Pa_{O_2}, 97, 98p
  during exercise, 241-242t, 245f, 246t, 248, 252-253p
  and P_{CO_2}, 77-78
Respiratory rate, 10, 12p
  and dyspnea, 21
  in newborn and children, 307-309, 307t
  and Pa_{CO_2}, 79
  ventilator, 206t, 207
Respiratory system components, 33-34, 34f
Restrictive respiratory disease and impairment, 8t, 54t, 66-67, 66f, 67, 67-68t, 73, 280, 370, 376-378

Retrolental fibroplasia, 187, 370
Rheumatoid arthritis; *see* Collagen-vascular diseases
Rhonchi and rhonchus, 11t, 370

S

Sarcoidosis, 8t, 67t, 262t, 370, 375-376, 380
Sepsis and septic shock, 172t, 223t, 226t
Shock, 1, 6, 141p, 200, 216t, 275
Shock lung, 226t, 370; *see also* Adult respiratory distress syndrome
Shunt, 103-104
   effect on PaO_2 with oxygen therapy, 189
   example of calculation, 225
   formula, 160t, 223-225, 361
   intracardiac, 96, 96t
   left-to-right, 90(footnote), 113t
   patent foramen ovale, 301, 302
   pulmonary, 96t, 98
   right-to-left, 90(footnote), 98
   in ventilator weaning, 216t
Silicosis, 37, 370, 377-378
Sleep apnea, 289-299; *see also* Pickwickian syndrome; Ondine's curse; Cheyne-Stokes breathing
   central, 291, 292f
   in infants, 319
   mixed, 291
   obstructive, 291-294, 292t, 293f
   treatment, 295-298, 295p, 296t, 297f
Sleep deprivation, 216t
Sleep disorders, 283-300
   apnea; *see* Sleep apnea
   clinical problems, 286, 289, 295, 298
   clues suggesting, 284t
   polysomnography, 284-286, 284t, 285f, 287t, 290-291f
   REM and nonREM sleep, 286, 287t, 287f
   study of, 283-284
   summary, 299
Sleep (normal), 286, 287ft, 288
   CO_2 production and ventilation, 289f
   O_2 consumption and CO_2 production, 288f
Sleep study, 24; *see also* Polysomnography
Small airways disease, 49, 54, 64-65, 370
Sodium, 23, 370
   in anion gap, 137, 137p
Spirometer, 18f, 65, 370
Spirometry, 5t, 18, 18f, 22f, 23t, 24, 371; *see also* Appendix F, 372-381 (Common clinical disorders—sections on physiologic testing)
   clinical value of, 65
   compared with ECG, 65
   criteria for assigning impairment, 69t
   interpretation of, 68-71, 69-71p

Sputum examination, 20, 24, 376, 378, 381
Standard temperature and pressure, dry (STPD), 31-32
Starling curve, 167, 167f
Starling equation, 223
Starling's law, 167
Steroids; *see* Corticosteroids
Stethoscope, 1, 5t, 11, 381; *see also* Auscultation; Breath sounds
Stridor, 12, 381
Sudden infant death syndrome, 283, 319
Sulfhemoglobinemia, 122
Surfactant, 226f, 302, 319t
Swan-Ganz catheter and catheterization, 5t, 153-158, 154-155f; *see also* Pulmonary artery wedge pressure
   calculations, 160t
   clinical problems, 159, 161, 166, 168, 171-173
   first publication, 154
   indications, 155-156
   insertion, 156-158, 157f
   in management of ARDS, 229t
   measurements, 156, 159t, 159p
   pitfalls and complications, 170, 171t
Systemic lupus; *see* Collagen vascular diseases

T

Tachycardia, 170t, 307, 371
Tachypnea, 308, 313, 371; *see also* Respiratory rate
Temperature, 27; *see also* Fever; Hyperthermia
   normal infant, 307t
   and oxygen consumption in infants, 306-307, 308f
   and PaO_2, 96
   and water vapor pressure, 92t
Tension, 371
Theophylline, 373
Thoracentesis, 8t, 24, 264, 265f, 266, 267, 275t, 280
Thoracic cage, 34
Thoracic gas volume, 313
Thoracoplasty, 2
Tidal volume, 49, 50f, 371
   in COPD, 233
   during exercise, 247
   ventilator, 202, 206, 206t
   in ventilator weaning, 216t
Torr, 33t, 371
Total lung capacity, 8t, 49, 50f, 63f, 280, 360, 371, 374
   newborn, 313, 314pf, 322f
Trachea, 34f, 36, 37f
Tracheitis, 67t
Tracheostomy, 4, 200, 283, 296t, 381
Transcutaneous PCO_2, 316-317, 316f
Transcutaneous PO_2, 19, 315f, 316
Transudate, 262-263, 371
Triglyceride, in pleural effusion, 268

Tuberculosis, 1 (Case 1), 2 (Case 3), 5t, 20, 262t, 264, 267t, 269, 270-271, 371, 380-381

U

Umbilical artery catheterization, 318, 318f
Umbilical vein catheterization, 318, 318f
Upper airway muscles, 287t, 293-295
Upper airway obstruction, 12, 67t, 312, 381
   criteria for intubation, 198t, 199-200
   flow volume curves and loops, 58, 59f
   and sleep apnea, 292-294, 293f, 297, 297f
Upper airway tract, 34f, 35, 48, 312
   infection, 372
Uvulopalatopharyngoplasty, 296t, 297

V

Vaccine (poliomyelitis), 5t
V$_D$/V$_T$; see Dead space to tidal volume ratio
Venous, 371
Venous admixture, 89f, 103-104, 371
Venous oxygen content, 106-107, 107t, 114f, 115
   aggravation of arterial hypoxemia, 98, 106-107
   use in shunt equation, 224-225
Venous oxygen pressure, 39fp, 124-126, 125t, 126p
Venous oxygen saturation, 124-127, 125t, 126p
Ventilation, 371
   alveolar; see Alveolar ventilation
   artificial; see Artificial ventilation
   dead space, 74-75, 75f
   general, 74
   high-frequency, 209-211, 210t, 211f
   minute, 74-75, 75f, 216t, 360
      during exercise, 240, 245, 245f, 247
      during sleep, 287t
Ventilation-perfusion balance, 98

Ventilation-perfusion imbalance, 40, 91, 98-110, 99-103f, 105-106f, 108-109f, 371
   in ARDS, 227, 228f
   cause of elevated PaCO_2, 104-110
   cause of reduced PaO_2, 104-110
   in chronic bronchitis, 101, 103f, 233
   in emphysema, 101, 103f, 233
   in exercise, 251
   in infants, 317, 319t, 321f
   in pleural effusion, 180
   in pulmonary embolism, 103p, 379
Ventilator, 371; see also Artificial ventilator
Ventilatory failure; see Respiratory failure
Venturi face mask, 182-184, 183-184f, 184t
Virus and viral infection, 1, 5t, 231, 226t, 372-373
Vital capacity, 32p, 40f, 49, 62-63, 63f, 216t, 314p, 322f, 371; see also Forced vital capacity; Crying vital capacity
Volume, 28, 44, 371; see also Lung volumes and capacities
V/Q ratio, 371; see also Ventilation-perfusion imbalance

W

Water vapor, 27, 371
Water vapor pressure, 27-28, 28t, 30, 36, 92t
Weaning; see Artificial ventilation (weaning)
Wedge pressure, 371; see also Pulmonary artery wedge pressure
Wheeze and wheezes, 11-12, 11t, 12p, 371-372, 381

X

X-ray, 5t; see also Chest x-ray examination; Chest x-rays

Z

Zones of lung, 162-164
   and artificial ventilation, 163
   in horizontal position, 163f
   in vertical position, 162f